The Art and Science of Physiologically-Based Pharmacokinetics Modeling

This state-of-the-art text describes the science behind the system and drug-dependent components of PBPK models, its applications in translational and regulatory science, e.g., guiding drug discovery and development, and supporting precision medicine initiatives. To incorporate state-of-the-art knowledge, each chapter is written by leaders in the field and illustrated by clear case studies. Connecting basic and applied science, this book explores the potential of PBPK modeling for improving therapeutics and is designed for a wide audience encompassing graduate students as well as biopharmaceutics scientists and clinical pharmacologists.

Features:

1. Provides a basic understanding of the physiologically-based pharmacokinetic modeling and its applications

2. Assists the reader in understanding product performance to allow for rapid product development and establish bioequivalence

3. Well-constructed content and added value of real examples

4. Illustrates how using available resources via modeling and simulation leads to a reduction in the costs related to drug development, which directly affects the costs to patients

The Art and Science of Physiologically-Based Pharmacokinetics Modeling

Edited by
Rodrigo Cristofoletti and Amin Rostami-Hodjegan

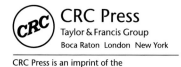

CRC Press
Taylor & Francis Group
Boca Raton London New York

CRC Press is an imprint of the
Taylor & Francis Group, an **informa** business

Designed cover image: © Shutterstock

First edition published 2025
by CRC Press
2385 Executive Center Drive, Suite 320, Boca Raton, FL 33431

and by CRC Press
4 Park Square, Milton Park, Abingdon, Oxon, OX14 4RN

© 2025 Taylor & Francis Group, LLC

CRC Press is an imprint of Taylor & Francis Group, LLC

Library of Congress Cataloging-in-Publication Data
Names: Cristofoletti, Rodrigo, editor. | Rostami-Hodjegan, Amin, editor.
Title: The art and science of physiologically-based pharmacokinetics
modeling / edited by Rodrigo Cristofoletti, Associate Director,
University of Florida, USA, Amin Rostami-Hodjegan, Chief Scientific Officer, Princeton, USA.
Description: First edition. | Boca Raton : CRC Press, 2024. |
Includes bibliographical references and index. |
Identifiers: LCCN 2023055884 (print) | LCCN 2023055885 (ebook) |
ISBN 9780367468873 (hbk) | ISBN 9781032773483 (pbk) | ISBN 9781003031802 (ebk)
Subjects: LCSH: Pharmacokinetics–Mathematical models. |
Drugs–Design–Mathematical models.
Classification: LCC RM301.5 .A78 2024 (print) | LCC RM301.5 (ebook) |
DDC 615.7–dc23/eng/20240208
LC record available at https://lccn.loc.gov/2023055884
LC ebook record available at https://lccn.loc.gov/2023055885

ISBN: 9780367468873 (hbk)
ISBN: 9781032773483 (pbk)
ISBN: 9781003031802 (ebk)

DOI: 10.1201/9781003031802

Typeset in Palatino
by codeMantra

Contents

Preface

"Everyone Only Hears What S/He Understands" (Es hört doch jeder nur, was er versteht)

Johann Wolfgang von Goethe (1749–1832)

PHYSIOLOGICALLY-BASED PHARMACOKINETICS (PBPK)
MODELING: No Longer An Academic Curiosity

In 2015, in an editorial for the *Journal of Pharmacometrics and Systems Pharmacology* (CPT:PSP) by Rowland et al (REF), the authors indicated the transition of PBPK from an *academic curiosity* to an *industrial norm* during the drug development. The latter, to a large extent, involved leading pharmaceutical companies, and not all the players in the drug development sector. It also, in many cases, concerning internal decisions rather than having any implications for drug approval and clinical applications.

What was followed played a huge role in moving the discipline from an "industrial necessity" to a "regulatory requirement', particularly in answering valid regulatory questions that could not be answered, at least easily, by conduct of clinical studies (see Chapter 11). These were waves of numerous public workshops by the drug regulatory agencies embracing the technology and encouraging its use.

The readers of this book may ask themselves 'why the need for this book?', and, 'how this is different than what is already available?'. The answer is simple: we are no longer addressing the 'academic curiosity' on what constitutes the PBPK, but providing the path for its established applications and a vision for future use. While the scientific progress in improving various corners of the PBPK modelling continues, it seems that with the availability of technology via user-friendly platforms to a wider group of scientists, beyond the relatively narrow community of traditional modelers in drug development, has broadened the applications well beyond what we knew of PBPK in the arena of toxicology quarter of century ago. Chapter 1 of this book provides the path we have taken so far and the trajectory forward quite well.

This book with all its chapters and the references therein provides many examples of practical use that lead to better decisions on drugs under development with streamlined clinical studies or even avoiding unnecessary and non-informative studies. It is a cook book to get best dishes based on ingredients and activities that are tried and tested successfully.

Although several chapters of this book look into details of how PBPK model infrastructure in terms of equations are put together (e.g. Chapters 2, 5,6), we intentionally try to focus on applications which are understood by a wider audience and are of relevance to all those concerned with drug development. Chapters 3 and 9 provide examples of such as applications to patient groups where comorbidity effect on fate of drug is not addressed as a routine practice during typical development. We also try to address many new applications that PBPK is used with the aim of drug product development (formulation) and comparative studies of various formulations (Chapters 4, 10, and 12). Although the widest application of PBPK has been related to assessing metabolism and associated drug interactions (Chapters 6 and 8), we do not put too much emphasis on that aspect as it is well established with lots of published examples in the literature regarding the methodology and case examples.

Thus, we attempt to focus on the path for applications of PBPK model for specific drugs/formulations to certain condition/population. We believe that building an infrastructure (platform) that enables to conduct PBPK modeling requires a different level of skills and understanding that concerns much narrower group of individuals who are not the target audience for this book. Nonetheless, we are grateful to all contributing authors for providing the source references, which enables the latter group to dig deeper and build their own models if they do not wish to use existing platforms as they are or by modifying them.

PHYSIOLOGICALLY-BASED PHARMACOKINETICS
(PBPK) MODELING: Prudent Use beyond Art!

Whenever people put something into the 'art' bracket in an indirect way, they admit the fact that different people have different views on the subject, and not everyone accepts and agrees on the angle that is taken by the artist! In some cases, artists intentionally leave the interpretation to the audience. Once a discipline moves from 'art' to 'science,' it defines a transition to confident usage that everyone is expected from applying certain input to a system and getting the same outcome regardless of the operator.

The name of this book suggests that we do have a spectrum in the case of PBPK, and this comes clear when we go through various applications. Some applications have been done with adequate frequency to give us the prudency in their usage (as covered in Chapter 11). De-risking the applications that are not currently used with confidence requires gathering necessary input data as well as verification to add to the credibility (see Chapters 7 and 11). Academic centers play a significant role in filling known gaps.

The transition from doubtful usage to confident application will continue and is a never-ending cycle. The existing sparse usage in certain area gets more common as we progress, and they move from 'amber' to 'green' zone; and items from the 'red' zone of no experience become the current doubtful/less prudent area of 'amber' use. However, we may not be able to exhaust moving the items from the 'red' to 'amber', and from 'amber' to 'green' for simple fact that many items that we had not even thought about are added to the list all the time! This process is captured very well by schematics that Grillo et al. of the office of clinical pharmacology (OCP) have put together and updated every now and then as shown with two versions below (also see Chapter 11):

PBPK is not a new concept, but it has shown a very rapid rise in recent years. This has been attributed to a greater connectivity to in vitro–in vivo extrapolation (IVIVE) techniques for predicting drug absorption, distribution, metabolism, and excretion (ADME) and their variability in humans. The marriage between PBPK and IVIVE under the overarching umbrella of "systems biology" has achieved a new chapter with the integration of organ-on-a-chip technology to predict the time course of drug distribution and effect (see Chapter 13).

We are grateful to all contributors who helped us with compiling this very valuable set of chapters, and we hope the readers have the opportunity in finding many practical examples that apply directly to their ongoing projects in the pharmaceutical companies. We also see benefits for the academic sector in observing the applications shown in various chapters with a view to filling the gaps identified and making improvements that are tangible.

Editors

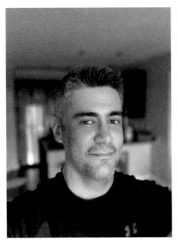

Rodrigo Cristofoletti, PhD, is an Assistant Professor of Pharmacometrics and Systems Pharmacology and Associate Director of Centre for Pharmacometrics and Systems Pharmacology, University of Florida, USA.

Dr. Cristofoletti joined the University of Florida in 2019 as a Research Assistant Professor in the Center for Pharmacometrics and Systems Pharmacology (Orlando) in the Department of Pharmaceutics. He received his B.S. in Pharmaceutical Sciences from the University of Sao Paulo, Brazil in 2004. Dr. Cristofoletti received his Ph.D. summa cum laude from the Johann Wolfgang Goethe University (Frankfurt am Main, Germany). The Clinical Pharmacology & Biopharmaceutics Office of the Brazilian Drug Regulatory Agency (ANVISA) has been Dr. Cristofoletti's place of employment for the last 15 years. While there, his research on oral drug absorption has helped in building scientific foundations for generic policies within Brazilian jurisdiction.

The work of Dr. Cristofoletti has covered wide areas of drug development over the last 30 years, ranging from pharmaceutics (e.g., drug delivery, bioavailability, and bioequivalence) to clinical pharmacology/tox (e.g., DDIs, PK/PD in special populations), translational and systems pharmacology (e.g., organotypic models and microphysiological systems for disease modeling and for *in vitro to in vivo* (IVIVE) scaling).

As a leader in the field of physiologically-based pharmacokinetics (PBPK), physiologically-based biopharmaceutics modeling (PBBM), quantitative systems pharmacology (QSP) and iPSC-derived organotypic models (e.g., intestinal, liver and brain organoids), Rodrigo is internationally recognized for his expertise in *IVIVE* to predict the behavior of drugs in the human body and understanding the associated inter-individual variabilities. He serves in the Editorial Board of many high impact journals in the field, like AAPS J, Biopharmaceutics & Drug Disposition, Frontiers in Pharmacology and Journal of Pharmacy & Pharmacology.

Dr. Cristofoletti's research is mainly funded by the federal grants (e.g., US FDA and NIH), State grants and private grants (pharma companies and not-for-profit organizations).

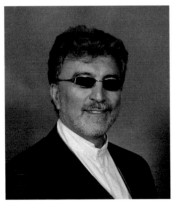

Amin Rostami-Hodjegan, PhD, FCP, FAAPS, FJSSX, FBPS, is Professor of Systems Pharmacology and Director of Centre for Applied Pharmacokinetic Research (CAPKR), University of Manchester, UK and SVP of R&D, Chief Scientific Officer (CSO), Certara, Princeton, USA.

The Institute of Scientific Information (ISI, Clativate) listed Amin as one of the world's most highly cited researchers (under 'Pharmacology & Toxicology') in 2017. Amin is also at 0.05% top rank of the Highly Cited Researchers List by Elsevier for pharmacology (2021). He has published over 300 peer-reviewed highly influential scientific articles (>22,000 citations, h-index = 80).

The work of Professor Rostami has covered wide areas of drug development over the last 30 years, ranging from pharmaceutics (e.g., bioavailability and bioequivalence) to clinical pharmacology (e.g., mixture pharmacology of drug/metabolites), translational and systems pharmacology (e.g., quantitative proteomics of enzymes and transporter for *in vitro to in vivo* (IVIVE) scaling).

Amin was co-founder of two spin-off companies from the University of Sheffield (Simcyp Limited and Diurnal PLC). As a leader in the field of physiologically-based pharmacokinetics (PBPK) and quantitative systems pharmacology (QSP), he is internationally recognized for his expertise in *IVIVE* to predict the behavior of drugs in the human body and understanding the associated inter-individual variabilities. He was one of the founding editors of *Pharmacometrics and System Pharmacology* and serves on the Editorial Boards of several other journals.

As the Senior Vice President of Research & Development (SVP) and Chief Scientific Officer at Certara, he facilitates the incorporation and integration of the latest advances in translational modeling to biosimulation platforms offered by Certara to its clients, with the aim of accelerating the development and regulatory approval of safer drug products and bringing them to the patients.

Contributors

Wen Li Kelly Chen
Pharmaceutical Sciences
China Innovation Center of Roche
Shanghai, China

Siri Kalyan Chirumamilla
Certara UK Limited
Simcyp Division
Sheffield, United Kingdom

Rodrigo Cristofoletti
Pharmaceutics Department
College of Pharmacy, University of Florida
Gainesville, Florida

Jennifer Dressman
Fraunhofer Institute of Translational Medicine
    and Pharmacology (Retired)
Frankfurt am Main, Germany

Nikoletta Fotaki
Department of Life Sciences
Centre for Therapeutic Innovation, University
    of Bath
Bath, United Kingdom

Stephen Fowler
Pharmaceutical Sciences
Roche Pharma Research and Early
    Development, Roche Innovation Center
    Basel
Basel, Switzerland

Iain Gardner
Certara UK Ltd, Simcyp Division
Sheffield, United Kingdom

Mariana Guimarães
Department of Life Sciences
Centre for Therapeutic Innovation, University
    of Bath
Bath, United Kingdom

Tycho Heimbach
Pharmaceutical Sciences and Clinical Supply
Merck & Co., Inc.
Rahway, New Jersey

Bart Hens
Drug Product Design
Pfizer
Sandwich, United Kingdom

Masoud Jamei
Certara UK Ltd, Simcyp Division
Sheffield, United Kingdom

Luis David Jiménez Franco
esqLABS GmbH
Saterland, Germany

Filippos Kesisoglou
Pharmaceutical Sciences and Clinical Supply
Merck & Co., Inc.
Rahway, New Jersey

Viera Lukacova
Simulations Plus
Lancaster, California

Haritha Mandula
Center for Drug Evaluation and Research
U.S. Food and Drug Administration
Silver Spring, Maryland

Nenad Manevski
Pharmaceutical Sciences
Roche Pharma Research and Early
    Development, Roche Innovation Center
    Basel
Basel, Switzerland

Frederico Severino Martins
esqLABS GmbH
Saterland, Germany

Mehul Mehta
Division of Neuropsychiatric Pharmacology
Office of Clinical Pharmacology, Office of
    Translational Sciences
Center for Drug Evaluation and Research
U.S. Food and Drug Administration
Silver Spring, Maryland

Maxime Le Merdy
Simulations Plus
Lancaster, California

Nicolò Milani
Pharmaceutical Sciences
Roche Pharma Research and Early
    Development, Roche Innovation
    Center Basel
Basel, Switzerland

Amitava Mitra
Clinical Pharmacology
Kura Oncology Inc.
Boston, Massachusetts

Maiara Camotti Montanha
Pfizer
Sandwich, United Kingdom

Jim Mullin
Simulations Plus
Lancaster, California

Mubtasim Murshed
Department of Life Sciences
Centre for Therapeutic Innovation, University
of Bath
Bath, United Kingdom

Helen Musther
Certara UK Ltd, Simcyp Division
Sheffield, United Kingdom

William W van Osdol
Simulations Plus
Lancaster, California

Neil Parrott
Pharmaceutical Sciences
Roche Pharma Research and Early
Development, Roche Innovation
Center Basel
Basel, Switzerland

Xavier Pepin
Regulatory Affairs
Simulations Plus
Lancaster, California

Martina Pigoni
Neuroscience and Rare Diseases
Roche Pharma Research and Early
Development, Roche Innovation
Center Basel
Basel, Switzerland

Janny Pineiro-Llanes
Pharmaceutics Department
College of Pharmacy, University of Florida
Gainesville, Florida

Stephan Schaller
esqLABS GmbH
Saterland, Germany

Armin Sepp
Certara UK Ltd, Simcyp Division
Sheffield, United Kingdom

Mohamad Shebley
Clinical Pharmacology
AbbVie Inc.
North Chicago, Illinois

Claire Simonneau
Pharmaceutical Sciences
Roche Pharma Research and Early
Development, Roche Innovation
Center Basel
Basel, Switzerland

Sreedharan Sabarinath
Division of Neuropsychiatric Pharmacology
Office of Clinical Pharmacology, Office of
Translational Sciences
Center for Drug Evaluation and Research
U.S. Food and Drug Administration
Silver Spring, Maryland

Sandra Suarez
Regulatory Affairs
Simulations Plus
Lancaster, California

Ramana Uppoor
Division of Neuropsychiatric Pharmacology
Office of Clinical Pharmacology, Office of
Translational Sciences
Center for Drug Evaluation and Research
U.S. Food and Drug Administration
Silver Spring, Maryland

Thomas Wendl
Pharmacometrics/Modeling & Simulation
Research & Development, Pharmaceuticals
Bayer AG
Leverkusen, Germany

Stefan Willmann
Pharmacometrics/Modeling & Simulation
Research & Development, Pharmaceuticals
Bayer AG
Wuppertal, Germany

Fang Wu
Center for Drug Evaluation and Research
U.S. Food and Drug Administration
Silver Spring, Maryland

Yuching Yang
Division of Pharmacometrics
Office of Clinical Pharmacology, Office of
    Translational Sciences
Center for Drug Evaluation and Research
U.S. Food and Drug Administration
Silver Spring, Maryland

Yumi Yamamoto
Pharmaceutical Sciences
Roche Pharma Research and Early
    Development, Roche Innovation
    Center Basel
Basel, Switzerland

Xinyuan Zhang
Quantitative Clinical Pharmacology
Daiichi Sankyo, Inc.
Basking Ridge, NJ

Ping Zhao
Bill & Melinda Gates Foundation
Seattle, Washington, USA

1 From a Mathematical Model to a Technology, the 100 Years' Evolution of PBPK

Xinyuan Zhang and Ping Zhao

1.1 INTRODUCTION

When we asked ChatGPT on Feb 17, 2023 to describe physiologically-based pharmacokinetic models in a layman term, it states 'Physiologically-based pharmacokinetic (PBPK) models are computer-based mathematical models that simulate how a drug or chemical moves through the body. These models take into account the properties of the drug or chemical, such as how it is absorbed, distributed, metabolized, and excreted by the body. They also incorporate information about the body itself, such as its anatomy, physiology, and blood flow'

The definition generated from ChatGPT is largely appropriate. Because we focus on medicines in this book, substances of interest are drug molecules. As illustrated in Figure 1.1, a PBPK model includes a drug-specific component and a physiology or system component. The former is composed of processes concerning permeation, active transport, metabolism, and reversible or irreversible binding of a drug; the latter is a reconstruct of virtual anatomy and physiology of a specific population (Figure 1.1a). Temporal changes of drug concentrations in the blood or a tissue of interest can be generated using simulations (Figure 1.1b).

Today, the rather complex mathematical modeling tasks to parameterize physiological and pharmacological processes and to simulate drug concentration profiles can be readily accomplished by computers. Benefited from the accumulation of biomedical knowledge over the centuries and the explosion of computational capability in the last several decades, the science and technology of PBPK evolved rapidly from academic research to routine applications by drug developers, regulators, and healthcare providers to address various questions related to the optimal use of medicines in different populations. In this chapter, we highlight the past and present of PBPK in drug development and regulation and provide our views on the future applications of the approach.

1.2 THE ORIGIN AND EARLY EVOLUTION (1937–2000)

For centuries, physicians and scientists have attempted to mathematically describe human anatomy and physiology. With the aid of mathematical equations and the laws of physics, scientists were able to describe the interconnectivity of different organs through the cardiovascular system. Such capability enables understanding of a drug's pharmacology. Nearly 90 years ago, in 1937, Torsten Teorell published two scientific papers [1,2] that mathematically described the kinetics of distribution of drug substances in the body. Drugs directly injected into the blood or transported from a depot compartment to the blood can circulate throughout the body. Tissues were connected with blood circulation in parallel. Each tissue had a certain volume. Teorell used different rate constants to describe transport of drug between tissue and the blood, and for the first time, he drew with his hands the complex scheme describing his concept of drug distribution (model) and simulated drug concentration changes from his model [1].

Teorell's hand sketches of drug movement in the body, and subsequent simulations of organ concentrations are considered by many the prototype of PBPK modeling and simulations. The model also laid the foundation of modern pharmacokinetics [3,4], a branch of pharmacology that studies what the body does to the drug.

Comparison of Figure 1.1 to Teorell's drawing [1] reveals similarities that are rooted in the same concept of describing drug behavior within the virtual physiology framework. The comparison also highlights the complexity of building PBPK models: mathematically re-constructing the interplay between a drug and human physiology requires intensive experimental data on both the drug itself and the physiological system, which demands computational power. As such, although the 1937 model represented a physician's wish to quantitatively understand the fate of the drug in the body to guide prescription, the industrialization of PBPK modeling and simulation in drug development and regulation took more than a half century.

Before 2000, PBPK remained mostly academic research and was mainly applied by toxicologists to evaluate the safety of environmental toxins starting in the 1960s. With nearly zero utility in the healthcare sector, the evolution of PBPK science over nearly six decades came along with the emergence of essential concepts and terms in pharmacokinetics and clinical pharmacology. The terms

DOI: 10.1201/9781003031802-1

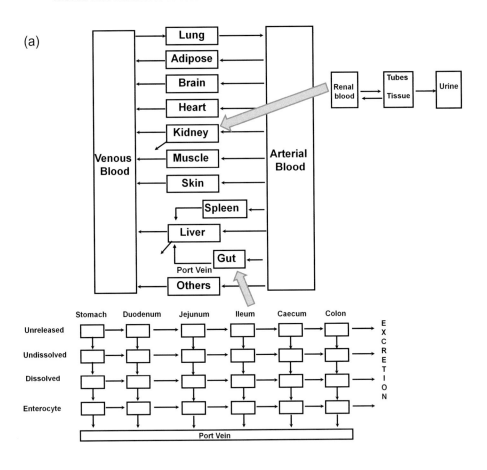

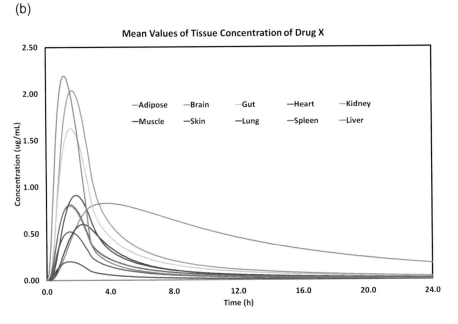

Figure 1.1 (a) Scheme of a generic PBPK model and (b) a representative simulation of drug concentrations in blood and representative tissues.

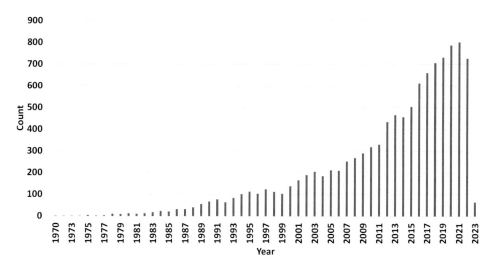

Figure 1.2 The number of publications by year (data cutoff January 2023) in PubMed by searching with key words "physiologically-based pharmacokinetic". X-axis: year; Y-axis: count.

of volume of distribution, clearance, bioavailability, and protein binding were introduced prior to the 1960s, and theoretical one- and two-compartmental models were published in the 1960s and 1970s, along with the discovery and mathematical expression of the correlation between drug effect (response) and plasma concentrations [4].

Prior to the 1980s, there were important scientific developments that further laid the foundation for future PBPK model building. These include the introduction of the concept that total body water could be divided into sub-compartments such as plasma, interstitial lymph, transcellular and intracellular components [5], the pH-partition hypothesis in the mechanism of oral absorption [6], the tissue-to-plasma partition coefficients estimation [7], and theoretical models for intestinal and hepatic clearance [8–11]. PBPK models for several drugs primarily metabolized by enzymes [12–17] were developed. The time also saw a publication on PBPK models for renally cleared drugs, highlighting the utility of PBPK models to help researchers effectively understand (learn) certain physiological processes that are commonly shared by various drugs [18]. At the same time, it had been recognized that PBPK models had the advantage to extrapolate outside the range of data if the mechanisms of transport were well understood, such as predicting the PK in humans based on the results from animal PBPK models and scaling factors [4].

Predicting oral bioavailability is of great interest as the majority of drug products on the market are oral dosage forms. Mechanistic oral absorption models consisting of drug substance properties, formulation properties, and physiological properties were developed in the 1990s. These models included quasi-equilibrium models, steady-state models, and dynamic models, depending on their dependence on spatial and temporal variables [19,20].

The turn of the millennium is a critical milestone for PBPK modeling and simulation. In their review article in 2011, Rowland et al. reported a burst in drug-related PBPK publications [21]. The change was attributed significantly to the advancement in computational technology at the same time. Since 2000, the activities in the PBPK arena have increased dramatically. Figure 1.2 represents the number of publications by year (data cutoff January 2023) in PubMed by searching with the keywords "physiologically-based pharmacokinetic".

1.3 INDUSTRIALIZATION (2000 TO PRESENT)
Nearly 90 years between Teorell's work and today's routine use of PBPK in drug development and regulation tell a tale of the industrialization of PBPK. Accumulation of biomedical knowledge, development of compartmental (non-physiological) pharmacokinetic and pharmacodynamic models, and the advancement of computer sciences together turned hand-written mathematical equations into modern-day PBPK modeling and simulation tools. The availability

of specialized software tools is arguably the main driver for the routine use of PBPK in today's drug development and clinical practice. These tools propel the dissemination of PBPK science outside of a rather small and specialized community. On the one hand, they liberated traditional modeling scientists and pharmacologists from the intensive work of model coding and literature curation; on the other hand, people outside the pharmacology modeling community tended to be reluctant to deal with mathematics and computation models. The arrival of user-friendly PBPK tools lowered the barrier for these individuals to understand and use PBPK. As such, not only did the user base of PBPK expand dramatically in the last decade, but so did the efficiency of PBPK analyses. Subsequently, PBPK science and tool innovation are accelerated, and the formulation of best practices is enabled.

As PBPK is routinely used in drug development and regulatory review, the role of quantitative models in the iterative process of product development is more comprehensively described as 'predict-learn-confirm' concept, which highlights prediction of untested scenarios. Meanwhile, industrialization is ineffective without best practice in place. The acceleration of PBPK research after 2000 was accompanied by the organization of workshops and the publication of position papers. By the end of the 2020s, regulatory agencies published guidance documents related to the use of PBPK [22,23]. A pattern of when and where PBPK can be useful has been shaping up, with consensus being reached that PBPK analyses can have high regulatory and clinical impact for certain types of intended applications. PBPK completed its first industrialization phase in supporting the development and approval of both new drugs and generic drug products [24,25].

In this section, we will review the introduction of 'predict-learn-confirm' concept, notable events in the past 20 years that have had a significant impact on advancing the applications of PBPK in drug development and regulatory assessment, and ongoing active research areas that will likely predict the trend of future applications.

1.3.1 Predict the Untested Scenarios

'Learn and confirm' is a generic concept that broadly applies to a drug development program. In a 1997 commentary, Lewis Sheiner stressed the importance of the science aspect, i.e., learning, especially through quantitative sciences, in contrast to the 'confirming' aspect in clinical drug development [26]. He illustrated how a mathematical model that described pharmacological behaviors, such as an early dose-response model, could turn 'noise' into 'signal' and support the efficacy evaluation [26]. The introduction of the 'learn and confirm' concept had significant implications. It highlighted the iterative nature of product development, in which a variety of nonclinical and clinical information is generated to test hypothesis. To this end, quantitative modeling and simulations play indispensable roles in understanding the behavior of the drug and informing subsequent development decisions.

Although well accepted, the 'learn and confirm' concept does not adequately speak to the capability of quantitative models to *predict* untested scenarios. Predictions are often needed in product development to generate hypotheses or inform decisions. Quantitative models under 'learn and confirm' generally refer to pharmacology models constructed using drug data from clinical studies. Although simulations can be performed when these models are developed, their primary utilities are to describe observed data (e.g., through model fitting techniques) and to assess potential effects of intrinsic and extrinsic factors (e.g., through covariate analyses). In contrast, a PBPK model structurally distinguishes drug-dependent components from physiology (or drug-independent) components. PBPK models, by design, are readily positioned to *predict* untested scenarios. Prediction can happen when limited drug data is available.

At any stage of drug development, questions on the effect of various patient factors, alone or in combination, are often asked. These questions dictate PBPK analyses, with modeling being a process of integrating in vitro, in silico, and in vivo data of the drug substance with prior knowledge of the anatomy and physiology of a human body to reflect the drug's pharmacological behavior. Even in the absence of clinical data, the model can be used to *predict* PK behavior when limited nonclinical data becomes available (e.g., first in human PK prediction in drug development that primarily relies on physicochemical properties and nonclinical findings on the drug's permeability, transport, and metabolism). Newly generated drug data are used to *confirm* earlier hypothesis. More importantly, the new findings can be used to optimize the model toward improved understanding of a drug's absorption, distribution, metabolism, and excretion (ADME) mechanisms. The drug-independent component (physiology) of the model enables relevant integration of drug parameters to efficiently investigate and effectively fill potential gaps in the current model. This collective *learning* rationally makes the PBPK model more predictive over time, rendering the approach greater potential to *predict* untested scenarios, guiding decisions on whether, when and how to conduct the next study(ies). Toward the later stage of the development, PBPK predictions can have a higher impact on development and regulation decisions (e.g., by replacing certain clinical studies) [30].

1.3.2 Drivers of Industrialization

In this section, we highlight notable drivers and events, in our opinion, that had made a significant impact on advancing PBPK applications, which include the development and maturation of user-friendly platforms, public workshops conducted by regulatory authorities, publication of white papers by regulators and pharma companies, and development of regulatory guidances.

1.3.2.1 A Technology, No Longer a Model

The advent of specialized PBPK software platforms has significantly lowered the entry by health-care professionals outside the rather limited modeling community to understand the concept, apply the approach, and contribute to PBPK science as important stakeholders. To this end, the authors claim that today's PBPK science should be perceived as a technology and is no longer a single mathematical model for a particular drug molecule.

A PBPK model generally involves large sets of differential equations and is expected to be computationally intensive. Both drug-dependent and drug-independent components need update when new knowledge becomes available, and parameterization of the latter in a PBPK model is particularly time- and resource-consuming. As such, a model published in a peer-reviewed journal or included in a company's study report or regulatory review only reflects a moment of the development and application of a drug's PBPK model. If one has to develop a PBPK model of the same drug molecule from scratch each time, it could be expensive (time and resource) and highly inefficient (ignorance of existing knowledgebase behind the drug-independent, physiology component). User-friendly PBPK platforms thus came into being to facilitate the PBPK applications. These platforms represent a (new) technology toward reliable and efficient prediction and description of a drug's pharmacology in humans and open new opportunities for both technological innovations and broader utilities.

In essence, a PBPK platform is a computational software that incorporates generic PBPK model structures, with anatomy and physiological parameters obtained from analyses and curation of literature or publicly available information. Within such platforms, physiological processes relevant to the ADME of drug molecules are organized through searchable/relevant databases and allow users to input drug product-related parameters. Examples of PBPK platforms include GastroPlus® (www.simulations-plus.com), PK-Sim® (www.open-systems-pharmacology.org) or Simcyp™ (www.simcyp.com).

As many PBPK analyses have been widely used and will continue to be used to support regulatory decisions [27–31], quality control and assurance of such analysis are extensively discussed. To this end, the (repeated) use of a specialized PBPK platform facilitates the assessment of consistency, model transparency, and model qualification for the intended purposes. Such qualification of a specific PBPK platform may rely on experiences across different drugs, different users, and different organizations.

1.3.2.2 Regulatory Public Workshops

Since 2010, regulatory agencies have held multiple public workshops on the PBPK topic, and here we list a few notable ones.

On March 14, 2012, the US Food and Drug Administration (FDA) called a Meeting of the Pharmaceutical Science and Clinical Pharmacology Advisory Committee to discuss the modeling and simulation in pediatric drug development. One of the voting questions was, "Should the routine use of PBPK in pediatric drug development, when possible, be recommended at the present time?". The Committee voted 7 (Yes) vs. 6 (No) on the question. The Committee members who voted 'Yes' agreed that 'the PBPK modeling approach would be beneficial in better anticipating and understanding the PK variability in the pediatric populations'. The Committee members who voted 'No' mainly concerned knowledge gaps, resource commitment, and lack of guidance on best practices. Although divergence toward the question appeared to exist, no one raised the concern that PBPK is fundamentally wrong to support pediatric drug development. Since then, many studies have been conducted to improve pediatric PBPK models.

On March 10, 2014, the FDA hosted a workshop entitled "Application of Physiologically-based Pharmacokinetic (PBPK) Modeling to Support Dose Selection". The workshop discussed the then-current status of the use and predictive performance of PBPK modeling and simulation in various clinical pharmacology applications [24]. On June 30 of the same year, the Association of the British Pharmaceutical Industry (ABPI) and Medicines and Healthcare Products Regulatory Agency (MHRA) hosted a meeting focusing on the clinical component of regulatory applications of PBPK [32]. The discussion topics included 'what are the appropriate data standards for drug input data for PBPK models' and 'verification of drug specific input parameters' [32]. Following these workshops, the number of PBPK submissions to the Office of Clinical Pharmacology (OCP) at FDA has increased dramatically [27,28].

Specifically for the use of PBPK in assessing oral drug absorption, the FDA hosted on May 19, 2016, a public workshop, entitled "Mechanistic Oral Absorption Modeling and Simulation for Formulation Development and Bioequivalence Evaluation" [25]. Questions discussed included "in which areas do we have the highest confidence in using PBPK absorption modeling, 'do we have enough experience and confidence in applying PBPK absorption models to support regulatory applications', and 'what are the gaps in the prediction and how to close them through research' [25]. Panel members expressed different opinions on the questions and agreed that the level of confidence in each area should be examined on a case-by-case basis and no general conclusions can be drawn at the moment [25].

The increased PBPK submissions call for greater attention from the regulators. On November 21, 2016, the European Medicines Agency (EMA) hosted a workshop to discuss topics to be included in its draft guideline on the qualification and reporting of PBPK analysis [33]. On March 15, 2017, the FDA held another meeting of the Pharmaceutical Science and Clinical Pharmacology Advisory Committee to discuss "what information should be included in a PBPK submission to the FDA to ensure adequacy of an analysis for its intended purpose". This Advisory Committee meeting was followed a few months later by the publication of FDA draft guidance entitled "Physiologically-Based Pharmacokinetic Analyses–Format and Content" [34].

As both EMA and FDA finalized their first PBPK guidance documents [22,34], topics on model qualification continued to be discussed at regulatory workshops. On November 18, 2019, the FDA held a public workshop entitled "Development of Best Practices in Physiologically-Based Pharmacokinetic Modeling to Support Clinical Pharmacology Regulatory Decision-Making" [35]. In this workshop, representatives from academic, industry, and regulatory provided case examples where PBPK modeling successfully helped drug development and regulatory decisions, discussed gaps, and proposed strategies to close the gaps. A credibility assessment framework was also proposed by the Agency at the workshop [36] and continuous discussion on the implementation of the credibility assessment framework was anticipated.

Meanwhile, two workshops concerning oral drug absorption and pharmaceutical quality of both new and generic drugs were held at the University of Maryland's Center of Excellence in Regulatory Science and Innovation (M-CERSI) in 2017 [37,38] and 2019 [39–41], respectively, focusing on translating in vitro product performance testing (such as the dissolution testing) to product in vivo performance. PBPK models for oral absorption, as a translational tool, were discussed intensively. These efforts later led to the publication of FDA guidance entitled "The Use of Physiologically-Based Pharmacokinetic Analyses–Biopharmaceutics Applications for Oral Drug Product Development, Manufacturing Changes, and Controls" [23].

These regulatory workshops no doubt have made PBPK broadly recognized by pharmaceutical scientists and pharmacologists.

1.3.2.3 Publication of Regulatory Guidances and Perspective Papers

As mentioned above, the increased use of PBPK in regulatory submissions accelerated the publication of several regulatory guidances by different authorities [34,42,43]. The response toward PBPK as an emerging technology was rather rapid and concerted. For example, the back-to-back publication of EMA and FDA draft guideline in 2017 was within 10 years after the two agencies began to record early PBPK submissions.

These publications further enabled harmonization among global regulators. The most prominent outcome is the draft and publication of the International Council for Harmonization (ICH) of Technical Requirements for Pharmaceuticals for Human Use M12 guideline on Drug Interaction Studies [44]. Details and comparisons of these guidances can be found in the chapter "Application of PBPK Modeling to Support Clinical Pharmacology Regulatory Decision-Making". Since 2016, FDA has begun to include greater details on PBPK in several guidances concerning specific topics. Its drug interaction guidance [45,46], especially the in vitro DDI guidance [46] has in-depth discussions on model validation and verification; FDA's guidance "The Use of Physiologically-Based Pharmacokinetic Analyses–Biopharmaceutics Applications for Oral Drug Product Development,

Manufacturing Changes, and Controls" [23] provides detailed recommendations concerning oral absorption PBPK models. Many other clinical pharmacology-related guidances also recognized PBPK modeling and simulation as a useful tool, such as guidances entitled "General Clinical Pharmacology Considerations for Pediatric Studies of Drugs, Including Biological Products" [47], "General Clinical Pharmacology Considerations for Neonatal Studies for Drugs and Biological Products" [48], "Assessing the Effects of Food on Drugs in INDs and NDAs – Clinical Pharmacology" [49], "Drug-Drug Interaction Assessment for Therapeutic Proteins Guidance for Industry" [50], and "Evaluation of Gastric pH-Dependent Drug Interactions With Acid-Reducing Agents: Study Design, Data Analysis, and Clinical Implications" [51].

1.3.3 Active Research Areas in PBPK Modeling and Simulation

Whereas this book showcases many research achievements of PBPK modeling and simulations in biomedical research and product development, we call out two related activities that are staging PBPK to make the next level impact in pharma R&D, and potentially in general medical practice in the near future: the science and the technology.

1.3.3.1 Science: Toward Qualification

As PBPK continues to play an indispensable role in the development and regulation of a particular drug of interest, the science of PBPK needs to focus on improving the PBPK model performance at the level that is beyond modeling for one drug. Learning across compounds and organizations has proven effective in the qualification of PBPK, specifically of PBPK platforms. As shown in Figure 1.3, DDI evaluation continues to dominate PBPK applications submitted by drug sponsors to the US FDA. Such dominance is attributed to extensive DDI research and the active use of PBPK by sponsors to address DDI liabilities of their drugs in the last decade. Consequently, knowledge accumulation and experience by various groups made it possible to qualify the PBPK platform for this intended use [52,53].

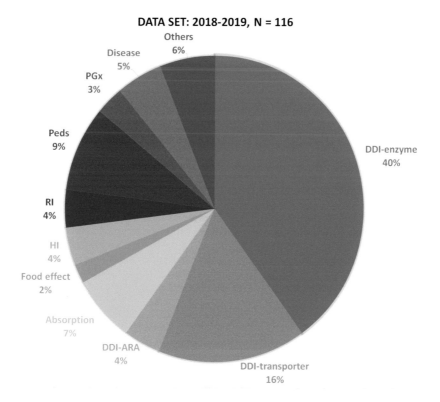

Figure 1.3   Distribution of physiologically-based pharmacokinetic submissions by application areas (2018–2019). (Reprint from Zhang et al. [27].) For special populations, percentage of submissions for pediatrics (Peds), renal impairment (RI), and hepatic impairment (HI) were each less than 10%, whereas no submissions concerned pregnant and breast-feeding women.

In other areas, especially the predictions of the effects of intrinsic factors on drug PK, PBPK has been generally considered to have low confidence [24,25]. These areas also concern special or specific populations, including subjects with renal and hepatic impairment, pediatric patients, geriatric patients, pregnant women, and breast-feeding women. Because disease (organ impairment) or specific physiological changes (age, pregnancy, and breast-feeding) can affect multiple drug ADME processes, qualification of the PBPK platform for these areas is indeed more complicated and requires extensive knowledge generation, knowledge integration, and validation using drugs whose PK in these populations are available. Our thinking in this area needs to be updated constantly, both in the awareness of scientific advancement for each intrinsic factor and in the constant refinement of our questions. In fact, progress has been made in the last decade and is heterogeneous for each intrinsic factor; and it has been increasingly recognized that within each major intrinsic factor, we need to be aware of already enhanced predictability of PBPK for certain sub-population(s) or sub-categories of intended uses. In other words, we may already be in a position to confidently predict PK in certain patients for drugs with specific ADME properties. For other scenarios, there are rooms for improvement.

Numerous publications suggest that PBPK models can effectively support pediatric development because model qualification works demonstrated robust predictability for specific scenarios [54–72]. Recently, the International Consortium for Innovation and Quality in Pharmaceutical Development (IQ Consortium) member companies published an article evaluating the PBPK model performance in renal and hepatic impairment population for 29 compounds with 106 organ impairment study arms [73]. Innovation Quality Consortium reported reasonable prediction of the effect of renal impairment on liver enzymes using the SimCYP® software platform. PBPK was an important topic in FDA's Pharmaceutical Science and Clinical Pharmacology Advisory Committee Meeting (May 7, 2019) on approaches to evaluate the effect of renal impairment on drug exposure, and workshop on "Assessing Changes in Pharmacokinetics of Drugs in Liver Disease" (2020) [74]. The increased confidence of PBPK predictability for pediatrics, renal impairment, and hepatic impairment was reflected in the US FDA's recent report (Figure 1.3). This is significant progress from FDA's 2015 report [24]. As mentioned earlier, for each intrinsic factor, there are subsets of patients for whom predictability using PBPK has not been established. For instance, not all children are equal, prediction of drug PK in pre-term babies and neonates requires more research.

In Figure 1.3, it is noticeable that no PBPK analyses have been submitted to the FDA to address drug dosing issues in pregnant and breast-feeding women. Despite efforts by the US FDA to mandate specific labeling language (The Pregnancy and Lactation Labeling Rule [PLLR]) and by the National Institute of Health, on behalf of the US Congress, to enhance pharmacotherapy in these women [Task Force on Research Specific to Pregnant Women and Lactating Women (PRGLAC)], clinical assessment continues to be delayed years, if not decades, after the approval of a new drug product. Drug companies are reluctant to conduct clinical studies in these women, and it remains difficult to design and execute an informative clinical study on pregnant and breast-feeding women. To this end, PBPK modeling is one attractive solution. Connecting (virtual) physiology between a pregnant woman and her fetus, and a lactating woman and her nursing infant, PBPK can be used to quantitatively investigate the drug exposures in relevant individuals. Mechanistic simulations can inform whether and how a medicine can be used optimally in pregnant women and breast-feeding women. It is worth noting that PBPK research concerning pregnant and breast-feeding women has been very active in recent years. There have been numerous publications [62,63,75–96], some of which demonstrate reasonable predictive performance for certain clinical scenarios, implying the readiness for PBPK to support dosing decisions for such situations. These research and workshops [97,98] of the same topic in recent years reflect the great interest by major stakeholders in applying PBPK.

1.3.3.2 Technology: Toward Reliability, Affordability and User-Friendliness

As a technology, PBPK cannot keep up if innovation stops or stagnates. Innovation transformed PBPK from a specialized pharmacological modeling technique to a technology based on highly comprehensive platforms. The advent of PBPK platforms made knowledge integration highly efficient and allowed many individuals who were not professionally trained in the field of traditional pharmacology modeling to access and to use the technology to address their clinical questions. Although a successful story of industrialization, the technology needs constant innovation by riding on the exponential growth of computer sciences and biological sciences. Today, the advancement of omics technology, such as genomics, transcriptomics, proteomics, and metabolomics can provide much richer data on genetic variation, enzyme and transporter expression, quantification of endogenous biomarkers. How can we efficiently and effectively integrate emerging research into a PBPK model or some broader virtual physiologically-based pharmacology model? As a software technology, the improvement on computational method and algorithm are expected to further enhance efficiency and accuracy of PBPK, while the models continue to integrate more complex structures and more granulated/detailed biological and biochemical processes. Machine learning and artificial intelligence will become an integral part of the next phases of PBPK industrialization.

1.4 THE VISION

We live in an information explosion age. Today, it becomes difficult to envision the future of PBPK. Ten years ago, the community worked hard to demonstrate that PBPK was "here to stay" [99], which has been evidenced by its industrialization in drug development and regulations. With the convergence of multiple disciplines in computational sciences and biomedical sciences, PBPK may evolve into something that is an integral part of a broader predictive technology for precision drug use. That said, we try to project PBPK for the next 10–20 years.

1.4.1 PBPK Modeling and Simulation in 10 Years

We envision that the development and application of PBPK modeling and simulation will continuously grow in the next 10 years in the following areas.

- **Globalization of PBPK**: The applications in low/middle confidence areas (such as evaluating the effect of intrinsic factors) will significantly increase as efforts in improving predictive performance continue, along with broader awareness and acceptance by relevant clinical communities outside clinical pharmacology. This can happen globally because of easier access of computers by low, middle income countries which in turn feedback valuable biological data contributing to efficient improvement of PBPK platforms. Recent research on changes in metabolic enzymes and transporters in liver cirrhosis suggested that there is non-uniform reduction in the abundance of enzymes and transporters, from control in cirrhosis groups with various levels of severity [96]. When simulating the effect of intrinsic factors, such as organ impairment, large variability has been observed and is a challenge in model performance evaluation. In the near future, with the commercialization of various testing for personal pharmacological parameters, PBPK models may be developed more accurately at individual level, and prediction of drug pharmacology in special populations will be improved to enhance dosing decisions both on label and off label.

- **Platform Innovation**: Innovative and collaborative PBPK platforms will emerge to facilitate the PBPK model sharing, and application. User-friendly application or a chat function on a smart device can efficiently utilize well structured, sophisticated virtual physiology and pharmacology models. This is more foreseeable today than even 5 years ago, and can further breakdown the barriers between pharmacologists and general healthcare professionals, and bridge the gaps between high income setting and low-middle income settings, enabling the next phase of PBPK industrialization.

- **Integration with Quantitative Systems Pharmacology (QSP) Models**: QSP models are mechanistic pharmacokinetic modeling. PBPK and QSP model integration provides mechanistic understanding of PK and PD interactions. The convergence may lead to a more broad predictive system to support dosing decisions.

- **Regulatory Standards and Acceptance**: Regulatory standards development and acceptance will catch up with the PBPK model development and innovation. The quality control and assurance of a PBPK platform can be a complicated topic both from a scientific and a regulatory perspective. In general, a PBPK platform is not a product regulated by health authorities, however, it generates results/evidence to support regulatory decisions. Broadly, this concern applies to any computational software that has been used for data analysis and / or modeling and simulation which supported regulatory decisions. A recent publication touched upon the topic of quality assurance of PBPK modeling platforms, in which, the authors seek consensus on the questions such as 'why', 'when', 'what', 'how' and 'by whom' to perform quality assurance for a PBPK platform [100]. We envision that this will be a topic that involves extensive discussion within and beyond the PBPK community from academic, industry, and regulatory in the coming years.

1.4.2 PBPK Modeling and Simulation in 20 Years

As technological advancements in many areas continue to converge, PBPK may disappear or become a background module of a general predictive system mentioned above. This system uses artificial intelligence and machine learning, employs a wide range of pharmacology modeling methods and integrates real-world evidence to constantly improve the backbone virtual model(s). The system then supports decisions by running real time simulations using these models. Commercialization and maturation of clinical testing and innovation in manufacturing (such as 3D printing) can be connected to this predictive system, helping developers, regulators, prescribers, and other healthcare providers to offer patients an informative dosing recommendation and a timely prescription. Continuous efforts are still warranted to make the value of PBPK being recognized by physicians, medical doctors, regulatory affairs, and other relevant disciplines.

1.5 SUMMARY

In this chapter, we briefly reflected the history of PBPK modeling and simulation, highlighted notable events, in our opinion, that have impacted the advancement of PBPK application in drug development and regulatory decisions. We discussed the active research areas that may lead PBPK to the next phase of industrialization. And finally, we envisioned that PBPK may become an indispensable background for a broader predictive system that can efficiently support prescribers and healthcare providers to make optimal dosing recommendations for the right patient.

REFERENCES

1. Teorell T. Kinetics of distribution of substances administered to the body. I. The extravascular modes of administration. *Arch Int Pharmacodyn et Ther.* 1937;57:205–25.

2. Teorell T. Kinetics of distribution of substances administered to the body. II. The intravascular modes of administration. *Arch Int Pharmacodyn et Ther.* 1937;57:226–40.

3. Paalzow LK. Torsten Teorell, the father of pharmacokinetics. *Ups J Med Sci.* 1995;100(1):41–6.

4. Wagner JG. History of pharmacokinetics. *Pharmacol Ther.* 1981;12(3):537–62.

5. Edelman IS, Leibman J. Anatomy of body water and electrolytes. *Am J Med.* 1959;27:256–77.

6. Schanker LS. On the mechanism of absorption of drugs from the gastrointestinal tract. *J Med Pharm Chem.* 1960;2:343–59.

7. Chen HS, Gross JF. Estimation of tissue-to-plasma partition coefficients used in physiological pharmacokinetic models. *J Pharmacokinet Biopharm.* 1979;7(1):117–25.

8. Pang KS, Rowland M. Hepatic clearance of drugs. I. Theoretical considerations of a "well-stirred" model and a "parallel tube" model. Influence of hepatic blood flow, plasma and blood cell binding, and the hepatocellular enzymatic activity on hepatic drug clearance. *J Pharmacokinet Biopharm.* 1977;5(6):625–53.

9. Pang KS, Rowland M. Hepatic clearance of drugs. II. Experimental evidence for acceptance of the "well-stirred" model over the "parallel tube" model using lidocaine in the perfused rat liver in situ preparation. *J Pharmacokinet Biopharm.* 1977;5(6):655–80.

10. Pang KS, Rowland M. Hepatic clearance of drugs. III. Additional experimental evidence supporting the "well-stirred" model, using metabolite (MEGX) generated from lidocaine under varying hepatic blood flow rates and linear conditions in the perfused rat liver in situ preparation. *J Pharmacokinet Biopharm.* 1977;5(6):681–99.

11. Pang KS, Gillette JR. A theoretical examination of the effects of gut wall metabolism, hepatic elimination, and enterohepatic recycling on estimates of bioavailability and of hepatic blood flow. *J Pharmacokinet Biopharm.* 1978;6(5):355–67.

12. Jacquez JA, Bellman R, Kalaba R. Some mathematical aspects of chemotherapy-II: the distribution of a drug in the body. *Bull Math Biophys*. 1960;22(3):309–22.

13. Zaharko DS, Dedrick RL, Bischoff KB, Longstreth JA, Oliverio VT. Methotrexate tissue distribution: prediction by a mathematical model. *J Natl Cancer Inst*. 1971;46(4):775–84.

14. Chen HS, Gross JF. Physiologically based pharmacokinetic models for anticancer drugs. *Cancer Chemother Pharmacol*. 1979;2(2):85–94.

15. Bischoff KB, Dedrick RL. Thiopental pharmacokinetics. *J Pharm Sci*. 1968;57(8):1346–51.

16. Bischoff KB, Dedrick RL, Zaharko DS, Longstreth JA. Methotrexate pharmacokinetics. *J Pharm Sci*. 1971;60(8):1128–33.

17. Bischoff KB, Dedrick RL, Zaharko DS. Preliminary model for methotrexate pharmacokinetics. *J Pharm Sci*. 1970;59(2):149–54.

18. Dedrick RL, Bischoff KB. Pharmacokinetics in applications of the artificial kidney. *Chem Engng Proor Syrup Ser*. 1968;64:32–44.

19. Yu LX, Lipka E, Crison JR, Amidon GL. Transport approaches to the biopharmaceutical design of oral drug delivery systems: prediction of intestinal absorption. *Adv Drug Deliv Rev*. 1996;19(3):359–76.

20. Yu LX, Amidon GL. A compartmental absorption and transit model for estimating oral drug absorption. *Int J Pharm*. 1999;186(2):119–25.

21. Rowland M, Peck C, Tucker G. Physiologically-based pharmacokinetics in drug development and regulatory science. *Annu Rev Pharmacol Toxicol*. 2011;51:45–73.

22. FDA. Physiologically Based Pharmacokinetic Analyses - Format and Content Guidance for Industry: FDA; 2018 [Available from: https://www.fda.gov/media/101469/download].

23. FDA. The Use of Physiologically Based Pharmacokinetic Analyses - Biopharmaceutics Applications for Oral Drug Product Development, Manufacturing Changes, and Controls: FDA; 2020 [Available from: https://www.fda.gov/regulatory-information/search-fda-guidance-documents/use-physiologically-based-pharmacokinetic-analyses-biopharmaceutics-applications-oral-drug-product].

24. Wagner C, Zhao P, Pan Y, Hsu V, Grillo J, Huang S, et al. Application of physiologically based pharmacokinetic (PBPK) modeling to support dose selection: report of an FDA public workshop on PBPK. *CPT: Pharmacometrics Syst Pharmacol*. 2015;4(4):226–30.

25. Zhang X, Duan J, Kesisoglou F, Novakovic J, Amidon GL, Jamei M, et al. Mechanistic oral absorption modeling and simulation for formulation development and bioequivalence evaluation: report of an FDA public workshop. *CPT Pharmacometrics Syst Pharmacol*. 2017;6(8):492–5.

26. Sheiner LB. Learning versus confirming in clinical drug development. *Clin Pharmacol Ther*. 1997;61(3):275–91.

27. Zhang X, Yang Y, Grimstein M, Fan J, Grillo JA, Huang SM, et al. Application of PBPK modeling and simulation for regulatory decision making and its impact on US prescribing information: an update on the 2018-2019 submissions to the US FDA's Office of Clinical Pharmacology. *J Clin Pharmacol*. 2020;60(Suppl 1):S160–S78.

28. Grimstein M, Yang Y, Zhang X, Grillo J, Huang SM, Zineh I, et al. Physiologically based pharmacokinetic modeling in regulatory science: an update from the U.S. Food and Drug Administration's Office of Clinical Pharmacology. *J Pharm Sci*. 2019;108(1):21–5.

29. Huang SM, Rowland M. The role of physiologically based pharmacokinetic modeling in regulatory review. *Clin Pharmacol Ther.* 2012;91(3):542–9.

30. Zhao P, Zhang L, Grillo JA, Liu Q, Bullock JM, Moon YJ, et al. Applications of physiologically based pharmacokinetic (PBPK) modeling and simulation during regulatory review. *Clin Pharmacol Ther.* 2011;89(2):259–67.

31. Zhao P, Rowland M, Huang SM. Best practice in the use of physiologically based pharmacokinetic modeling and simulation to address clinical pharmacology regulatory questions. *Clin Pharmacol Ther.* 2012;92(1):17–20.

32. Shepard T, Scott G, Cole S, Nordmark A, Bouzom F. Physiologically based models in regulatory submissions: output from the ABPI/MHRA forum on physiologically based modeling and simulation. *CPT Pharmacometrics Syst Pharmacol.* 2015;4(4):221–5.

33. Zhao P. Report from the EMA workshop on qualification and reporting of physiologically based pharmacokinetic (PBPK) modeling and simulation. *CPT Pharmacometrics Syst Pharmacol.* 2017;6(2):71–2.

34. FDA. The Use of Physiologically Based Pharmacokinetic Analyses - Biopharmaceutics Applications for Oral Drug Product Development, Manufacturing Changes, and Controls 2020 [Available from: https://www.fda.gov/media/142500/download].

35. Jean D, Naik K, Milligan L, Hall S, Mei Huang S, Isoherranen N, et al. Development of best practices in physiologically based pharmacokinetic modeling to support clinical pharmacology regulatory decision-making-A workshop summary. *CPT Pharmacometrics Syst Pharmacol.* 2021;10(11):1271–5.

36. Kuemmel C, Yang Y, Zhang X, Florian J, Zhu H, Tegenge M, et al. Consideration of a credibility assessment framework in model-informed drug development: potential application to physiologically-based pharmacokinetic modeling and simulation. *CPT Pharmacometrics Syst Pharmacol.* 2020;9(1):21–8.

37. Abend A, Heimbach T, Cohen M, Kesisoglou F, Pepin X, Suarez-Sharp S. Dissolution and translational modeling strategies enabling patient-centric drug product development: the M-CERSI workshop summary report. *AAPS J.* 2018;20(3):60.

38. Heimbach T, Suarez-Sharp S, Kakhi M, Holmstock N, Olivares-Morales A, Pepin X, et al. Dissolution and translational modeling strategies toward establishing an in vitro-in vivo link-a workshop summary report. *AAPS J.* 2019;21(2):29.

39. Pepin XJH, Parrott N, Dressman J, Delvadia P, Mitra A, Zhang X, et al. Current state and future expectations of translational modeling strategies to support drug product development, manufacturing changes and controls: a workshop summary report. *J Pharm Sci.* 2021;110(2):555–66.

40. Parrott N, Suarez-Sharp S, Kesisoglou F, Pathak SM, Good D, Wagner C, et al. Best practices in the development and validation of physiologically based biopharmaceutics modeling. A workshop summary report. *J Pharm Sci.* 2021;110(2):584–93.

41. Mitra A, Suarez-Sharp S, Pepin XJH, Flanagan T, Zhao Y, Kotzagiorgis E, et al. Applications of physiologically based biopharmaceutics modeling (PBBM) to support drug product quality: a workshop summary report. *J Pharm Sci.* 2021;110(2):594–609.

42. EMA EU. Guideline on the Reporting of Physiologically Based Pharmacokinetic (PBPK) Modelling and Simulation 2018 [Available from: https://www.ema.europa.eu/en/documents/scientific-guideline/guideline-reporting-physiologically-based-pharmacokinetic-pbpk-modelling-simulation_en.pdf].

43. PMDA. Guideline on Drug Interaction for Drug Development and Appropriate Provision of Information 2019 [Available from: https://www.pmda.go.jp/files/000228122.pdf].

44. ICH. ICH M12 Drug Interaction Studies. 2022.

45. FDA. Clinical Drug Interaction Studies - Cytochrome P450 Enzyme- and Transporter-Mediated Drug Interactions Guidance for Industry 2020 [Available from: Clinical Drug Interaction Studies - Cytochrome P450 Enzyme- and Transporter-Mediated Drug Interactions Guidance for Industry].

46. FDA. In Vitro Drug Interaction Studies - Cytochrome P450 Enzyme- and Transporter-Mediated Drug Interactions Guidance for Industry 2020 [Available from: https://www.fda.gov/media/134582/download].

47. FDA. Guidance for Industry: General Clinical Pharmacology Considerations for Pediatric Studies of Drugs, Including Biological Products 2022 [Available from: https://www.fda.gov/media/90358/download].

48. FDA. Guidance for Industry: General Clinical Pharmacology Considerations for Neonatal Studies for Drugs and Biological Products 2022 [Available from: https://www.fda.gov/media/129532/download].

49. FDA. Guidance for Industry: Assessing the Effects of Food on Drugs in INDs and NDAs - Clinical Pharmacology Considerations 2022 [Available from: https://www.fda.gov/media/121313/download].

50. FDA. Guidance for Industry: Drug-Drug Interaction Assessment for Therapeutic Proteins FDA; 2020 [Available from: https://www.fda.gov/media/140909/download].

51. FDA. Evaluation of Gastric pH-Dependent Drug Interactions with Acid-Reducing Agents: Study Design, Data Analysis, and Clinical Implications Guidance for Industry: FDA; 2020 [Available from: https://www.fda.gov/regulatory-information/search-fda-guidance-documents/evaluation-gastric-ph-dependent-drug-interactions-acid-reducing-agents-study-design-data-analysis].

52. Wagner C, Pan Y, Hsu V, Grillo JA, Zhang L, Reynolds KS, et al. Predicting the effect of cytochrome P450 inhibitors on substrate drugs: analysis of physiologically based pharmacokinetic modeling submissions to the US Food and Drug Administration. *Clin Pharmacokinet.* 2015;54(1):117–27.

53. Wagner C, Pan Y, Hsu V, Sinha V, Zhao P. Predicting the effect of CYP3A inducers on the pharmacokinetics of substrate drugs using physiologically based pharmacokinetic (PBPK) modeling: an analysis of PBPK submissions to the US FDA. *Clin Pharmacokinet.* 2016;55(4):475–83.

54. Wang K, Jiang K, Wei X, Li Y, Wang T, Song Y. Physiologically based pharmacokinetic models are effective support for pediatric drug development. *AAPS PharmSciTech.* 2021;22(6):208.

55. Small BG, Johnson TN, Rowland Yeo K. Another step toward qualification of pediatric physiologically based pharmacokinetic models to facilitate inclusivity and diversity in pediatric clinical studies. *Clin Pharmacol Ther.* 2022.

56. Emoto C, Johnson TN. Cytochrome P450 enzymes in the pediatric population: connecting knowledge on P450 expression with pediatric pharmacokinetics. *Adv Pharmacol.* 2022;95:365–91.

57. Salem F, Small BG, Johnson TN. Development and application of a pediatric mechanistic kidney model. *CPT Pharmacometrics Syst Pharmacol.* 2022;11(7):854–66.

58. Johnson TN, Small BG, Rowland Yeo K. Increasing application of pediatric physiologically based pharmacokinetic models across academic and industry organizations. *CPT Pharmacometrics Syst Pharmacol.* 2022;11(3):373–83.

59. Johnson TN, Small BG, Berglund EG, Rowland Yeo K. A best practice framework for applying physiologically-based pharmacokinetic modeling to pediatric drug development. *CPT Pharmacometrics Syst Pharmacol.* 2021;10(9):967–72.

60. Johnson TN, Ke AB. Physiologically based pharmacokinetic modeling and allometric scaling in pediatric drug development: where do we draw the line? *J Clin Pharmacol.* 2021;61(Suppl 1):S83–S93.

61. van Groen BD, Pilla Reddy V, Badee J, Olivares-Morales A, Johnson TN, Nicolai J, et al. Pediatric pharmacokinetics and dose predictions: a report of a satellite meeting to the 10th Juvenile toxicity symposium. *Clin Transl Sci.* 2021;14(1):29–35.

62. Abduljalil K, Pan X, Pansari A, Jamei M, Johnson TN. Preterm physiologically based pharmacokinetic model. Part II: applications of the model to predict drug pharmacokinetics in the preterm population. *Clin Pharmacokinet.* 2020;59(4):501–18.

63. Abduljalil K, Jamei M, Johnson TN. Fetal physiologically based pharmacokinetic models: systems information on the growth and composition of fetal organs. *Clin Pharmacokinet.* 2019;58(2):235–62.

64. Calvier EAM, Nguyen TT, Johnson TN, Rostami-Hodjegan A, Tibboel D, Krekels EHJ, et al. Can population modelling principles be used to identify key PBPK parameters for paediatric clearance predictions? An innovative application of optimal design theory. *Pharm Res.* 2018;35(11):209.

65. Emoto C, Johnson TN, Neuhoff S, Hahn D, Vinks AA, Fukuda T. PBPK model of morphine incorporating developmental changes in Hepatic OCT1 and UGT2B7 proteins to explain the variability in clearances in neonates and small infants. *CPT Pharmacometrics Syst Pharmacol.* 2018;7(7):464–73.

66. Johnson TN, Bonner JJ, Tucker GT, Turner DB, Jamei M. Development and applications of a physiologically-based model of paediatric oral drug absorption. *Eur J Pharm Sci.* 2018;115:57–67.

67. Zhou W, Johnson TN, Bui KH, Cheung SYA, Li J, Xu H, et al. Predictive performance of physiologically based pharmacokinetic (PBPK) modeling of drugs extensively metabolized by major cytochrome P450s in children. *Clin Pharmacol Ther.* 2018;104(1):188–200.

68. Johnson TN, Jamei M, Rowland-Yeo K. How does in vivo biliary elimination of drugs change with age? Evidence from in vitro and clinical data using a systems pharmacology approach. *Drug Metab Dispos.* 2016;44(7):1090–8.

69. Abduljalil K, Jamei M, Rostami-Hodjegan A, Johnson TN. Changes in individual drug-independent system parameters during virtual paediatric pharmacokinetic trials: introducing time-varying physiology into a paediatric PBPK model. *AAPS J.* 2014;16(3):568–76.

70. Salem F, Ogungbenro K, Vajjah P, Johnson TN, Aarons L, Rostami-Hodjegan A. Precision criteria to derive sample size when designing pediatric pharmacokinetic studies: which measure of variability should be used? *J Clin Pharmacol.* 2014;54(3):311–7.

71. Salem F, Johnson TN, Barter ZE, Leeder JS, Rostami-Hodjegan A. Age related changes in fractional elimination pathways for drugs: assessing the impact of variable ontogeny on metabolic drug-drug interactions. *J Clin Pharmacol.* 2013;53(8):857–65.

72. Upreti VV, Wahlstrom JL. Meta-analysis of hepatic cytochrome P450 ontogeny to underwrite the prediction of pediatric pharmacokinetics using physiologically based pharmacokinetic modeling. *J Clin Pharmacol*. 2016;56(3):266–83.

73. Heimbach T, Chen Y, Chen J, Dixit V, Parrott N, Peters SA, et al. Physiologically-based pharmacokinetic modeling in renal and hepatic impairment populations: a pharmaceutical industry perspective. *Clin Pharmacol Ther*. 2021;110(2):297–310.

74. FDA. M-CERSI Workshop: Assessing Changes in Pharmacokinetics of Drugs in Liver Disease: FDA; 2020 [Available from: https://collaboration.fda.gov/pid6pcgrjcod/?OWASP_CSRFTOKE N=50b137e978e97877b3ec12cefcbf59aa284735dfad1214683fbc9938ee1ca1f0&proto=true].

75. Zhao S, Gockenbach M, Grimstein M, Sachs HC, Mirochnick M, Struble K, et al. Characterization of plasma protein alterations in pregnant and postpartum individuals living with HIV to support physiologically-based pharmacokinetic model development. *Front Pediatr*. 2021;9:721059.

76. Mahdy WYB, Yamamoto K, Ito T, Fujiwara N, Fujioka K, Horai T, et al. Physiologically-based pharmacokinetic model to investigate the effect of pregnancy on risperidone and paliperidone pharmacokinetics: application to a pregnant woman and her neonate. *Clin Transl Sci*. 2023.

77. Chen J, You X, Wu W, Guo G, Lin R, Ke M, et al. Application of PBPK modeling in predicting maternal and fetal pharmacokinetics of levetiracetam during pregnancy. *Eur J Pharm Sci*. 2023;181:106349.

78. Liu X, Dallmann A, Brooks K, Best BM, Clarke DF, Mirochnick M, et al. Physiologically-based pharmacokinetic modeling of remdesivir and its metabolites in pregnant women with COVID-19. *CPT Pharmacometrics Syst Pharmacol*. 2023;12:148–153.

79. Alrammaal HH, Abduljalil K, Hodgetts Morton V, Morris RK, Marriott JF, Chong HP, et al. Application of a physiologically based pharmacokinetic model to predict cefazolin and cefuroxime disposition in obese pregnant women undergoing caesarean section. *Pharmaceutics*. 2022;14(6):1162.

80. Amice B, Ho H, Zhang E, Bullen C. Physiologically based pharmacokinetic modelling for nicotine and cotinine clearance in pregnant women. *Front Pharmacol*. 2021;12:688597.

81. Abduljalil K, Furness P, Johnson TN, Rostami-Hodjegan A, Soltani H. Anatomical, physiological and metabolic changes with gestational age during normal pregnancy: a database for parameters required in physiologically based pharmacokinetic modelling. *Clin Pharmacokinet*. 2012;51(6):365–96.

82. Gaohua L, Abduljalil K, Jamei M, Johnson TN, Rostami-Hodjegan A. A pregnancy physiologically based pharmacokinetic (p-PBPK) model for disposition of drugs metabolized by CYP1A2, CYP2D6 and CYP3A4. *Br J Clin Pharmacol*. 2012;74(5):873–85.

83. Lu G, Abduljalil K, Jamei M, Johnson TN, Soltani H, Rostami-Hodjegan A. Physiologically-based pharmacokinetic (PBPK) models for assessing the kinetics of xenobiotics during pregnancy: achievements and shortcomings. *Curr Drug Metab*. 2012;13(6):695–720.

84. Ke AB, Greupink R, Abduljalil K. Drug dosing in pregnant women: challenges and opportunities in using physiologically based pharmacokinetic modeling and simulations. *CPT Pharmacometrics Syst Pharmacol*. 2018;7(2):103–10.

85. Abduljalil K, Pansari A, Jamei M. Prediction of maternal pharmacokinetics using physiologically based pharmacokinetic models: assessing the impact of the longitudinal changes in the activity of CYP1A2, CYP2D6 and CYP3A4 enzymes during pregnancy. *J Pharmacokinet Pharmacodyn*. 2020;47(4):361–83.

86. Abduljalil K, Badhan RKS. Drug dosing during pregnancy-opportunities for physiologically based pharmacokinetic models. *J Pharmacokinet Pharmacodyn.* 2020;47(4):319–40.

87. Song L, Cui C, Zhou Y, Dong Z, Yu Z, Xu Y, et al. Toward greater insights on applications of modeling and simulation in pregnancy. *Curr Drug Metab.* 2020;21(9):722–41.

88. Freriksen JJM, Schalkwijk S, Colbers AP, Abduljalil K, Russel FGM, Burger DM, et al. Assessment of maternal and fetal dolutegravir exposure by integrating ex vivo placental perfusion data and physiologically-based pharmacokinetic modeling. *Clin Pharmacol Ther.* 2020;107(6):1352–61.

89. Abduljalil K, Pansari A, Ning J, Jamei M. Prediction of drug concentrations in milk during breastfeeding, integrating predictive algorithms within a physiologically-based pharmacokinetic model. *CPT Pharmacometrics Syst Pharmacol.* 2021;10(8):878–89.

90. Neeli H, Hanna N, Abduljalil K, Cusumano J, Taft DR. Application of physiologically based pharmacokinetic-pharmacodynamic modeling in preterm neonates to guide gentamicin dosing decisions and predict antibacterial effect. *J Clin Pharmacol.* 2021;61(10):1356–65.

91. Pansari A, Faisal M, Jamei M, Abduljalil K. Prediction of basic drug exposure in milk using a lactation model algorithm integrated within a physiologically based pharmacokinetic model. *Biopharm Drug Dispos.* 2022;43(5):201–12.

92. Abduljalil K, Gardner I, Jamei M. Application of a physiologically based pharmacokinetic approach to predict theophylline pharmacokinetics using virtual non-pregnant, pregnant, fetal, breast-feeding, and neonatal populations. *Front Pediatr.* 2022;10:840710.

93. Abduljalil K, Ning J, Pansari A, Pan X, Jamei M. Prediction of maternal and fetoplacental concentrations of cefazolin, cefuroxime, and amoxicillin during pregnancy using bottom-up physiologically based pharmacokinetic models. *Drug Metab Dispos.* 2022;50(4):386–400.

94. Ezuruike U, Blenkinsop A, Pansari A, Abduljalil K. Quantification of fetal renal function using fetal urine production rate and its reflection on the amniotic and fetal creatinine levels during pregnancy. *Front Pediatr.* 2022;10:841495.

95. Abduljalil K, Pansari A, Ning J, Jamei M. Prediction of maternal and fetal acyclovir, emtricitabine, lamivudine, and metformin concentrations during pregnancy using a physiologically based pharmacokinetic modeling approach. *Clin Pharmacokinet.* 2022;61(5):725–48.

96. Coppola P, Kerwash E, Cole S. Physiologically based pharmacokinetics model in pregnancy: a regulatory perspective on model evaluation. *Front Pediatr.* 2021;9:687978.

97. CERSI FUOM. FDA/M-CERSI Workshop: Pharmacokinetic Evaluation in Pregnancy 2022 [Available from: https://cersi.umd.edu/sites/cersi.umd.edu/files/Pk%20Evalutation%20in%20 Pregnancy%20Workshop%20Agenda.pdf].

98. CERSI FUOM. FDA/M-CERSI Workshop: Fetal Pharmacology & Therapeutics 2021 [Available from: https://cersi.umd.edu/sites/cersi.umd.edu/files/Agenda%20Fetal-Pharmacology.pdf].

99. Rostami-Hodjegan A Tamai I, Pang KS. Physiologically based pharmacokinetic (PBPK) modeling: it is here to stay! *Biopharm Drug Dispos.* 2012;33(2):47–50.

100. Frechen S, Rostami-Hodjegan A. Quality assurance of PBPK modeling platforms and guidance on building, evaluating, verifying and applying PBPK models prudently under the umbrella of qualification: why, when, what, how and by whom? *Pharm Res.* 2022;39(8):1733–48.

2 Basic Principles of PBPK Modeling and Simulation

Jennifer Dressman, Stefan Willmann, and Rodrigo Cristofoletti

2.1 PHARMACOKINETICS AS A MEASURE OF TEMPORAL AND SPATIAL DISTRIBUTION OF A DRUG IN THE BODY

Pharmacokinetics is often loosely defined as "what the body does to a drug". More precisely, it is a measure of temporal and spatial distribution of a drug in a system. Unless otherwise noted, the system under consideration will be the whole body. This definition of pharmacokinetics contains a spatial component, so the location of the drug in the biological system is important. From the temporal component of the definition, it follows that the amount of substance at a specific location is changing with time. Mathematically, the combination of these temporal and spatial components leads to partial differential equations (PDE). Differently from ordinary differential equations (ODE), a PDE contains an unknown function of two or more variables and its partial derivatives with respect to these variables:

$$\frac{\partial}{\partial t}, \frac{\partial}{\partial x}, \frac{\partial}{\partial y}, \frac{\partial}{\partial z}$$

where t is time, and a three-dimensional location in the system is represented by the spatial coordinates (x, y, z). In summary, ODEs are used to describe well-mixed compartments, whereas PDEs can account for drug distribution in geometrically non-uniform compartments. Although PDEs can sometimes be written for specific systems, especially to describe the delivery of an agent from a spatially restricted source to a homogeneous tissue, defining and then estimating the unknown parameters are, in most cases, impossible because of the difficulty in obtaining sufficient measurements to resolve the spatial components of the system. In pharmacokinetic applications, PDEs are used to describe distributed models. A comprehensive review on distributed models is available elsewhere [1].

Commonly, pharmacokineticists reduce the system into a finite number of components, by lumping together processes based upon time, for example, highly and poorly perfused organs. One thus moves from PDEs to ODEs, where space is not taken directly into account. This reduction in complexity results in so-called compartmental models. In this definition, compartments are kinetically homogeneous or well-mixed spaces. Reducing the system into discrete entities that contain subsets of the drug whose kinetics share a similar time frame is widely used in pharmacokinetics analysis. In compartmental analysis, lumping portions of the system together for the purpose of data analysis is based on the time frame of a particular experiment.

Another approach is to reduce the system complexity by defining compartments according to prior knowledge about organ physiology, as opposed to empirical temporal kinetic characteristics. This approach forms the basis of physiologically-based pharmacokinetic (PBPK) models. In PBPK models, a certain level of spatial realism is also preserved in the sense that different tissue compartments are connected through the arterial and venous circulation. In summary, PBPK models are multi-compartmental models consisting of a finite number of compartments (ranging from minimal to whole body models) with specified interconnections, inputs, and losses (Figure 2.1). In this context, compartmental and distributed models are actually extreme cases of PBPK models, in which compartments are assumed to be kinetically homogeneous (compartmental models) or heterogeneous (distributed models).

The basic idea behind PBPK modeling is that each mathematical compartment represents a space or region in the body that is physiologically well defined and can be parameterized based on prior physiological knowledge. In the simplest case (as depicted in Figure 2.1), one compartment represents a single organ for which, for example, the volume and blood flow rate are known *a priori*. Another very important feature in PBPK modeling is the separation between system- and drug-specific parameters. This feature distinguishes PBPK models from classical descriptive models of observed data using purely statistical/mathematical models. However, building PBPK models requires a series of drug-specific parameters that are usually, but not exclusively, measured *in vitro* or in species other than humans. On the other hand, the system parameters are derived from clinical data. So, by their nature, PBPK models are based on a "middle-out" approach, taking the advantages and strengths of both the "bottom-up" and "top-down" approaches.

Combining these top-down and bottom-up approaches is not a seamless process and is fraught with issues, as reviewed by Tsamandouras et al. [2]. If viewed purely from a mathematical point

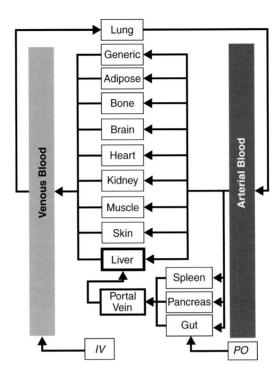

Figure 2.1 Schematic representation of a generic, whole body PBPK model.

of view, the middle-out approaches suffer from structural identifiability issues. Nevertheless, this is not the right perspective when using PBPK models. The absence of a unique correspondence between parameter values and the observed output is concerning for the researcher who wants to quantify the physiological process only based on a single observation set rather than considering a matrix of evidence from various sets. Overall, the advantage of PBPK modeling over simpler empirical compartmental models is the ability to incorporate prior knowledge of the system while verifying the model predictions beyond the clinical dataset used to optimize the input values [3].

2.2 ADDING SPATIAL REALISM TO COMPARTMENTAL PK MODELS

The assumption that every organ can be considered a well-stirred sub-compartment can often not be maintained. Permeation and diffusion within different regions of the organ can become the rate-limiting step for organ distribution instead of blood perfusion. To account for a potential permeation-limitation, the organs in a PBPK model need to be further sub-structured. A typical sub-structured PBPK model distinguishes the vascular space consisting of plasma and blood cells, the interstitial space and the intracellular space (Figure 2.2) [4]. While small molecules (e.g., molecular weight up to 500 D) can permeate quite rapidly across the vascular endothelium through transcellular pores (so-called fenestrae), passive diffusion and permeation across the cellular membrane can be hindered depending on the molecular properties of the substance (e.g., polarity/charge, lipophilicity, and shape) and the surface area that is available for intracellular uptake. The latter can largely differ between the organs and is high for an organ with dense vascularization such as the liver. In contrast, the effective surface area for intracellular uptake is low in organs with a low density of blood vessels such as, for example, the gray and white matter in the brain. A further benefit of the introduction of a permeation barrier into the PBPK model is that it facilitates the consideration of active transport processes, for example, through active influx or efflux transporters or by means of transcytosis processes.

An example for a mass-transfer equation of a typical organ for the pooled vascular (vas)/interstitial (int) volume compartment of an organ (org) is shown in Figure 2.3. The left-hand side denotes the mass-transfer per time interval from the extracellular water (consisting of plasma and interstitial fluid). The right-hand side of this equation consists of first-order terms that describe the inter-compartmental mass transfer through the plasma flow Q_{pl} of the respective organ and

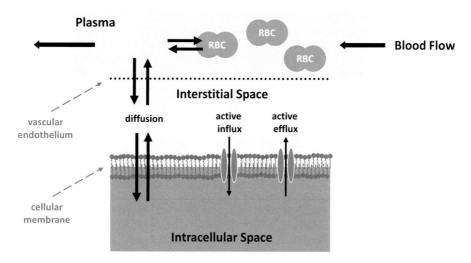

Figure 2.2 Schematic representation of an organ-substructure for a small-molecule PBPK model. (Modified from Ref. [4].)

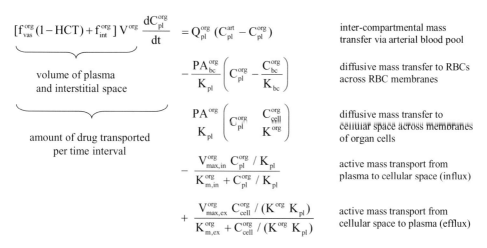

Figure 2.3 Example of a mass-transfer equation of the plasma and interstitial space considering diffusive mass transfer to red blood cells (RBC) as well as active influx and efflux processes parameterized as Michaelis–Menten processes (HCT: hematocrit).

the diffusive transport processes into the blood cells (BC) and the intracellular space (cell) that is determined by a permeability coefficient P and the effective available surface area A. If applicable, active mass transport processes through influx or efflux transporters can be added. Such saturable processes are parameterized as Michaelis–Menten kinetics with a maximum transport rate constant V_{max} and Michaelis–Menten constant K_m which denotes the drug concentration at which the transport rate is half of the maximum rate.

In addition to the permeation rate constants that determine the rate of the mass-transfer between different sub-compartments in a PBPK model, the partition coefficients (denoted as "K" in Figure 2.3) are highly relevant because they describe the concentration ratio at equilibrium between neighboring sub-compartments. The *a priori* estimation of such partition coefficients require knowledge of the fractional composition of each sub-compartment with respect to water and lipids/proteins. Various methods have been published to estimate organ/plasma partition coefficients for use in whole-body PBPK models based on physicochemical parameters such as the octanol/water coefficient (LogP) or membrane affinity (LogMA), for which standard assays that can be run with medium to high throughput are available in the pharmaceutical industry. Widely used models for organ/plasma partition coefficients have been published by Rodgers & Rowland [5–7], Poulin & Theil [8–10], and Schmitt [11]. Such models require prior physiological information about the tissue composition with respect to the fractional volume of intra- and extracellular tissue water, (phospho-)lipids, and proteins such as albumin (for details, see the original publications).

Special whole-body PBPK models have been developed that consider the specific properties and biochemical interactions of therapeutic molecules outside of the chemical space of classical small molecules. To describe the PK of antibodies, for example, specific aspects such as endosomal clearance and recycling of the antibody mediated by the neonatal FC receptor (FcRn) have been implemented in physiologically-based models [12,13]. Also, first attempts have been published to capture the unique PK properties of new modalities such as RNA interference (RNAi)-based therapeutics [14] or antisense-oligonucleotides [15] in a PBPK modeling framework.

Overall, the broad variety of existing PBPK models for the different compound classes have in common that a large number of input parameters are required to successfully execute a PBPK simulation. These parameters can be separated into systems parameters and drug parameters. Systems parameters include physiological parameters and describe either macroscopic, microscopic, or biochemical properties of the organism of interest, depending on the desired level of granularity of the PBPK model. Macroscopic physiological parameters in the PBPK context are, for example, total organ/compartment volumes and blood flow rates (that – roughly – sum up to the total body weight and cardiac output of the organism) or the glomerular filtration rate. Microscopic physiological parameters quantify, for example, the tissue composition with respect to aqueous or lipid sub-compartments, and the biochemical parameters include, for example, expression levels of metabolizing enzymes or active transporters in relevant tissues. These system parameters usually account for the majority of the required input parameters and the exact number of parameters strongly depends on the level of granularity of the PBPK model. In contrast, the number of drug-specific parameters is usually kept to a minimum in PBPK modeling. Most important drug-specific parameters are of physicochemical or biochemical nature (e.g., lipophilicity, plasma protein binding constant, solubility in water and other biorelevant media, *in vitro* metabolic or transporter rate constants, etc.).

Several whole-body PBPK modeling platforms are nowadays available either commercially (e.g., SimCYP or GastroPlus) or as open-source software (e.g., the Open Systems Biology Platform incl. PK-Sim and MoBi). In addition to easy-to-use graphical interfaces for PBPK modeling and simulation, these platforms contain large databases with validated system parameters for different animal species and humans of different age that facilitate PBPK modeling from newborns to elderly subjects.

2.3 PBPK MODELING

2.3.1 Parallel Developments in Environmental Toxicology and Drug Development

The first pharmacokinetic model to be described in the scientific literature was published by Teorell in 1937 [16]. Just a few years later, Henderson and Haggard [17] introduced the first discussion of the toxicology of inhaled gases in the context of exposure, absorption, and distribution in their book on Noxious Gases. In environmental toxicology, further work was published in 1951 by Kety [18], who proposed that the kinetics of inhaled substances is related to three tissue characteristics: tissue volume, blood flow, and partition coefficient. This concept became the basis of modern PBPK models in environmental toxicology.

In the 1950s and 1960s, the focus in the pharmaceutical world shifted to simpler models in pharmacokinetics, for which analytical solutions could be obtained. Exact mathematical solutions for drug distribution could only be obtained for simple model structures in which the body was described using a small number of compartments (usually just one or two) that did not correspond directly to the various organs. This approach resulted in the widespread application of pharmacokinetics in the pharmaceutical literature and industry, with the approach and equations represented in textbooks such as Gibaldi and Perrier [19].

However, the issues for substances with complex kinetics, or when inter-species extrapolations were required, remained, and for these substances the simple models were insufficient. As a result, research on physiological models continued. In the 1960s, the first attempts were made to solve rate equations for the concentration-time course of gases in the body using an analog computer [20]. As numerical integration algorithms became more facile with the advent of digital computing in the early 1970s, the interest in physiologically-based models was rekindled in both the pharmaceutical arena [21,22] and in environmental studies [23]. These studies included a mathematical description of non-linear processes for metabolism and excretion, which cannot be solved using the classical pharmacokinetic approaches, and paved the way to realizing PBPK models for a wide range of xenobiotics, including solvents, drugs, pesticides, and plastic monomers reaching the body from different routes of exposure (Figure 2.4).

Interest in PBPK grew in the ensuing years and by 2010, over a hundred scientific publications using PBPK models had already been published in the pharmaceutical literature, and commercial software for PBPK had become available. Since then, the field has literally exploded in terms of interest on the part of the scientific community and regulatory agencies, as documented by the growth of publications between 2000 and 2019 (Figure 2.5).

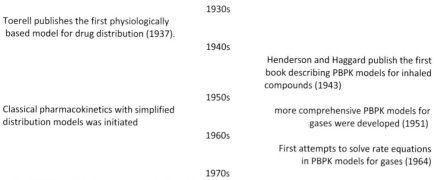

Figure 2.4 Time-Line of the early history of PBPK modeling in the pharmaceutical and environmental sciences.

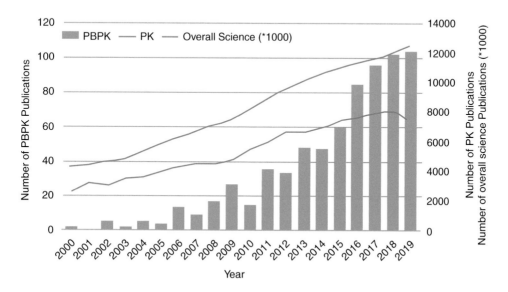

Figure 2.5 Overall original article publication trends over 20 years. Bars represent the number of PBPK modeling publications in the pharmaceutical sciences. The orange line represents the number of PK publications, and the green line represents the overall number of publications in PubMed. (From Ref. [24].)

2.3.2 From Mixing Tank to Compartment Absorption and Transit Model

The pH partition hypothesis was proposed in the 1950s as a basic guideline for predicting drug absorption trends. According to this hypothesis, weakly acidic drugs are largely unionized and lipid soluble in an acid medium and hence should be absorbed best by the stomach. In reality, the stomach does not appear to be a major site for the absorption, even of acidic drugs. In a preclinical proof-of-concept study, Hollander and co-workers perfused the stomach and small intestine of rats with acetylsalicylic acid solutions at pH 3.5 and 6.5. Even at a pH of 3.5, gastric absorption of acetylsalicylic acid was minimal, and serum levels were equivalent in all tested scenarios [25]. The surface area of the intestinal mucosa is so much greater than that of the stomach that this more than compensates for the decreased absorption rate per unit area. Furthermore, the pH partition hypothesis fails to predict the absorption of compounds that are permanently ionized. The pH partition hypothesis was expanded by Dressman and co-workers [26], leading to the quasi-equilibrium absorption potential (AP) model (Equation 2.1):

$$AP = \log\left(P * F_{non} * \frac{S_0 * V_L}{X_0} \right) \tag{2.1}$$

where P is the octanol-water partition coefficient, F_{non} is the fraction in the nonionized form at pH 6.5, S_0 is the intrinsic solubility, V_L is the volume of the intestinal fluids and X_0 is the dose administered. The validity of the AP model was demonstrated when the AP was found to increase with f_{abs} for several standard compounds with a wide variety of physicochemical properties and various degrees of extent of absorption. However, this empirical correlation is only satisfactory for drugs absorbed by passive uptake mechanisms [26].

Even though the pH partition hypothesis and AP model shed some light on the physicochemical properties affecting drug absorption, the relevance of gastrointestinal physiology was still missing. In this context, Dressman and co-workers [27,28] developed the mixing tank model, which considered the gastrointestinal tract as one or more serial mixing tanks with linear transfer kinetics. In terms of hydrodynamics, the mixing tank model assumes that both radial and axial mixing are complete, i.e., the contents are assumed to be well-stirred with instantaneous dilution of the inputted dose, which leads to uniform distribution of dissolved and solid drug. For this reason, mixing tank models are also considered compartmental models, dependent on temporal and spatial variables. For the mixing tank model, a modified Noyes–Whitney equation is used to handle drug dissolution, while the first-order absorption rate constant (k_a) accounts for the mass transport of drug across the intestinal mucosa, which can be estimated from the effective permeability (P_{eff}) and segment radius (R) ratio:

$$k_a = \frac{2P_{eff}}{R}$$

The single mixing tank model was used to predict oral absorption of digoxin and griseofulvin, successfully discriminating between dissolution rate-limited (e.g., digoxin) and dose:solubility-limited (e.g., griseofulvin) absorption [27]. Hintz and Johnson [29] extended the approach of Dressman et al. to include polydisperse drugs, in order to show the effect of particle size distribution on dissolution and absorption.

Despite the advances in modeling oral drug absorption through gastrointestinal tract, the models had not incorporated some fundamental physiological processes that can influence the rate and extent of drug absorption, namely gastric emptying and intestinal transit [30]. After an extensive review of the available human intestinal transit data, Yu and co-workers [30] concluded that the transit time throughout the human small intestine is normally distributed around 199±78 minutes and that seven compartments were optimal in describing the small intestinal transit process using a compartmental approach. This compartmental transit model was further developed into a compartment and absorption transit (CAT) model, in which the main assumptions were negligible absorption from the stomach and colon, linear absorption in the small intestine through a passive mechanism, linear transfer kinetics for each segment and instantaneous dissolution [31]. The CAT model was extended by incorporating Michaelis–Menten kinetics for active absorption across the enterocyte membrane, gastric emptying rate constants appropriate to the dosing situation, degradation rate constants where applicable and drug dissolution into the model [32,33]. Importantly, after accounting for the dissolution rate, the CAT model could be used to predict the extent and rate of absorption of poorly absorbed drugs as well as to determine the underlying mechanism (i.e. dissolution-, solubility-, or permeability-limited absorption) [32].

After further revisions and refinements, the CAT model evolved into the advanced CAT (ACAT) model, which has proven to be useful for determining the rate and extent of drug absorption as well as providing approximate gastrointestinal locations of drug release, dissolution, passive and carrier-mediated absorption, saturable metabolism, and efflux [34]. The CAT-like models can be easily linked to distribution and elimination models to predict systemic drug exposure. Combining CAT models with PBPK models has played a pivotal role in drug development and regulatory sciences [35]. In this chapter, we will discuss the current regulatory landscape and successful applications in drug development.

2.3.3 *In vitro-in vivo* Extrapolation of ADME

2.3.3.1 *z Value and Diffusion Layer Model Approaches*

A key element in *in vitro-in vivo* extrapolation of dissolution/release data is to be able to present the data in a form that is amenable to input into a PBPK model. Although in early attempts some successes in predicting the magnitude of food effects were achieved by direct comparison of dissolution profiles in biorelevant media with pharmacokinetic data [36], it was quickly identified that the prerequisite for this type of direct relationship was that the solubility of the drug would have to be the principal driver for drug absorption and that other factors like permeability and stability would only be minor considerations, as illustrated for danazol (Figure 2.6).

The next attempts centered around combining dissolution data directly with very simple models for oral absorption [38,39]. The combination resulted in reasonable predictions for a variety of poorly soluble and highly lipophilic compounds (Figure 2.7).

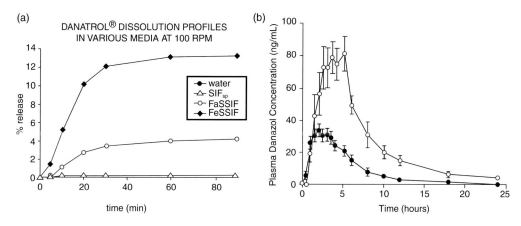

Figure 2.6 Dissolution of danazol from Danatrol® capsules in various media (a) and plasma levels after ingestion in the fasted and fed states in healthy human volunteers (b). (Data from Refs. [36,37].)

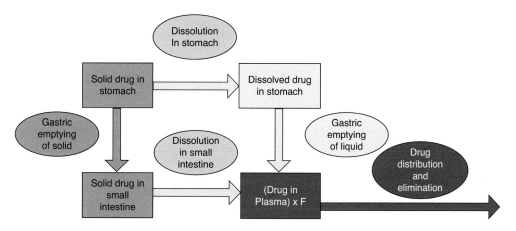

Figure 2.7 Schematic of the Nicolaides model used to obtain simulation profiles. *F* is the bioavailability constant. (Redrawn from Nicolaides et al. [40].)

Nevertheless, there was a thirst for more accurate models that could better simulate the *in vivo* pharmacokinetic profile and this led to the development of more complex *in silico* models of the gastrointestinal tract, such as the CAT, ACAT, and ADAM models. Along with the evolution of these more complex models, there was a parallel interest in building models of dissolution data that could be used to facilitate input of the data into the GI model.

Nicolaides et al. [40] addressed the modeling of dissolution data to facilitate input into the GI model by introducing the so-called z factor. To estimate *in vivo* dissolution kinetics, an *in vitro* dissolution parameter was introduced into the model by applying a modification of the Noyes–Whitney equation. This model is based on the assumption of dissolution of isometric, similarly sized particles, occurring under continuously decreasing surface area conditions with the ratio D/d, where D is the diffusion coefficient and d is the diffusion layer thickness, which is assumed to remain constant during the dissolution process. Under these conditions, the dissolution rate is given by the following equation:

$$\frac{dW_t}{dt} = \frac{D\Gamma N^{1/3}}{V\delta\rho^{2/3}} W^{2/3}(X_s - W_t) = zW^{2/3}(C_s - C)$$

where W_t is the amount dissolved at time t, W is the amount of drug remaining to be dissolved, X_s is the amount of drug which saturates the volume V of the dissolution medium, C_s is the solubility of drug, C is the concentration of the dissolved drug at time t, ρ is the particle density, Γ is the shape factor, N is the number of particles to be dissolved and z is the dissolution parameter, which is a constant equal to $D\Gamma N^{1/3}/\delta\rho^{2/3}$. Whereas sink conditions can be assumed in the small intestine if the drug is highly permeable, dissolution in the stomach is assumed to occur only until the drug concentration reaches its solubility to reflect the lack of absorption from the stomach.

An early study combining the z-value model for dissolution with a STELLA model for absorption and drug disposition was published by Shono et al. [41], who successfully simulated celecoxib pharmacokinetics in both the fasted and fed states using this approach. An important point made in that study was that the z value should be based on the initial dissolution rate rather than the entire dissolution curve, in accordance with the assumptions behind this model (Figure 2.8).

Following these and other successes, the z value was adopted by Simulations Plus for modeling dissolution behavior.

Another approach to modeling dissolution data is the Simcyp In Vitro data Analysis toolkit, or "SIVA". In a publication addressing both intraluminal and pharmacokinetic profiles of ritonavir, Fiolka et al. [42] used the SIVA® toolkit Version 3 to determine various Simcyp Simulator parameter inputs from *in vitro* experiments using the stepwise in *vitro-in vivo* extrapolation (IVIVE) approach described by Pathak et al. [43,44]. Using this approach, experimental solubility and dissolution results were analyzed mechanistically in SIVA to estimate/confirm intrinsic parameters that are essential for the simulation of *in vivo* drug absorption. In addition to input parameters for the SIVA toolkit module "Solubility" taken from the ritonavir model proposed by Arora et al. [45], the calculations of "logK$_{m:w}$ neutral" and "logK$_{m:w}$ ion" were based on in-house experimental data in FaSSIF-V1 at various physiologically relevant bile salt concentrations, while parameters defining supersaturation and precipitation behavior were extracted from two-stage and transfer experiments. The approach to setting up a mechanistic dissolution model in SIVA is shown in Figure 2.9: where $K_{m:w}$ is the partition coefficient between bile micelles and water, PRC is the precipitation rate constant calculated from transfer model experiments, CSR is the critical supersaturation ratio and the Diffusion Layer Model Scalar (DLM) is a factor used to adjust the fit of the model to the experimental data.

Using this approach, both the luminal and systemic concentration profiles of ritonavir could be simulated well (Figure 2.10).

A bonus of the mechanistic model approach for dissolution data is that it enables the modeler to explore "what if" scenarios such as what would happen if the gastric pH was higher than usual in the virtual study subject, or if the bile salt levels were lower in that individual, since without a mechanistic dissolution model, many experiments would have to be done to cover the range of potential GI physiology variations on the dissolution profile. This is particularly important for virtual bioequivalence models in which a large number of virtual subjects must be constructed – it would be, practically speaking, impossible to do this without a mechanistic model for dissolution.

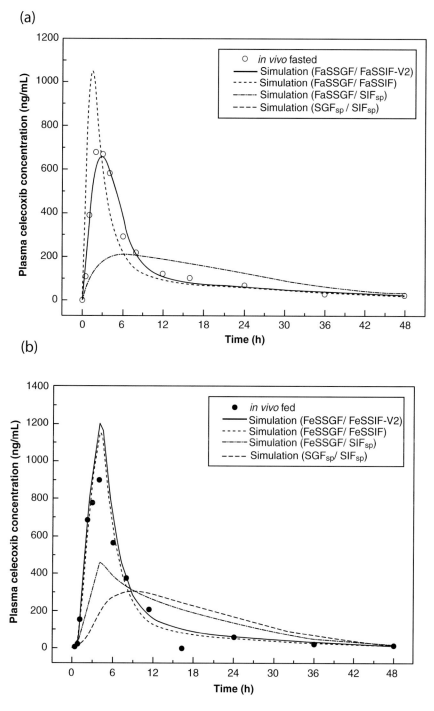

Figure 2.8 (a and b) Use of the z value in combination with STELLA to simulate fasted and fed state pharmacokinetic date for celecoxib [41].

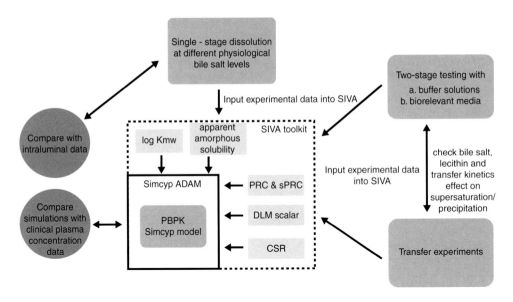

Figure 2.9 Schematic of mechanistic dissolution modeling in SIVA.

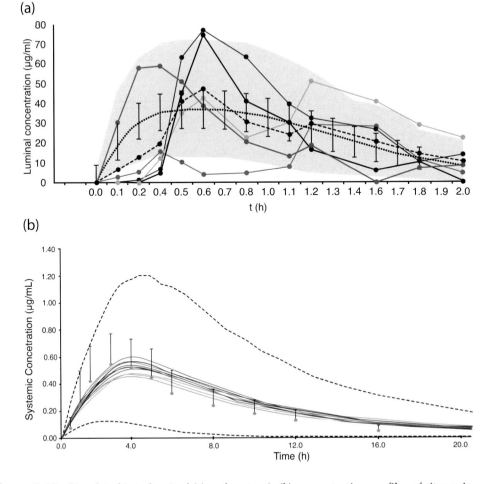

Figure 2.10 Simulated intraluminal (a) and systemic (b) concentration profiles of ritonavir, along with data from clinical studies in healthy volunteers. (Based on Ref. [42].)

2.3.3.2 P_{app}-P_{eff} Correlations

In addition to modeling the release of the drug from the dosage form as it passes through the GI tract, another crucial aspect of capturing the absorption of the drug after oral administration is to estimate the permeability of the intestinal mucosa in the human population being represented in the PBPK model to the drug in question. In most PBPK models, it is assumed that the GI mucosa is healthy, although this will obviously not be true in diseases of the GI tract such as Crohn's disease [46] and is questionable in diseases with secondary effects on the GI mucosa such as cystic fibrosis [47]. Likewise, most efforts to date to measure permeability *in vitro* or *in vivo* have focused on simulating the absorbing mucosa in healthy individuals.

Direct measurement of permeability in healthy volunteers (P_{eff}) has been limited to just a few drugs, since it requires a clinical setting with gastroenterologists familiar with the technique and is time-consuming and expensive, not to mention imposing a certain level of discomfort on the part of the subjects. The "gold standard" technique has been the Loc-i-gut perfusion, which has been described in detail in the literature [48]. However, even this method has come under some criticism in recent times, since the drug is usually perfused as a simple buffer solution and typically results in volumes in the perfusion segment which are larger than have been measured in fasted, healthy volunteers by MRI [49]. A further limitation of the method is that, thus far, almost all perfusions have been carried out in the jejunum, whereas regional absorption has been studied in very few cases, and even then using an open infusion rather than a perfusion technique. The clinical studies required to establish the regional permeability of drugs are exemplified by the publications for metoprolol from 1986 [50–52].

On the *in vitro* side, the most popular model for measuring permeability (P_{app}) is the Caco-2 cell line, immortalized from cells derived from cancer of the colon in humans, which was first introduced by Hidalgo et al. in 1989 [53]. Other immortalized cell lines such as the MDCK and LLC-PK1 have also been used to measure permeability, but these are based on kidney cells from dogs and pigs, respectively. There are also methods that do not rely on cell lines. These include the PAMPA model [54], which relies on diffusion through a synthetic membrane containing liquids representing the lipid bilayer in the cell membrane, and *in silico* methods such as QSPR based on molecular descriptors and MechPeff®, which allows for contributions to absorption from both the neutral and ionized forms of the drug [55]. A comprehensive overview of various methodologies has been published recently [56,57].

Realistically, given the experimental design of the *in vivo* perfusions, any correlation between P_{app} and P_{eff} is always going to focus on a correlation between the *in vivo* jejunal permeability and its *in vitro* estimate, and any adjustments for other regions of the GI tract will entail a knowledge of differences in uptake mechanisms as well as the structure of the mucosa and its effective surface area in those regions. Although it is accepted that most drugs are primarily taken up by passive transport across the enterocytes [58], if there is an active component to uptake, or if paracellular transport plays a role in absorption, these adjustments may be inaccurate and lead to poor estimates of absorption in the PBPK model.

Several correlations of P_{eff} to P_{app} have been published for Caco-2 cell data in the open literature. If only compounds with passive, transcellular absorption are considered, the correlation between Caco-2 cell data and fraction absorbed looks quite convincing, as demonstrated by Jarc et al. using Caco-2 cell data generated in-house and literature fraction absorbed data [59]. However, although this correlation is certainly useful for distinguishing between high and low permeability compounds, the slope of the initial part of the curve is very steep, such that compounds with similar P_{app} values between 0.7 and 0.85×10^{-6} cm/s may be absorbed to an extent of anywhere between 20% and 65%, making it difficult to extrapolate from *in vitro* to *in vivo* for PBPK modeling purposes in this range (Figure 2.11).

When data for paracellular or actively transported drugs are added to the correlation, and P_{eff} is plotted against P_{app} instead of F_{abs}, the correlation is less convincing, as shown by Tchaparian et al. [60] for 30 compounds ranging from 15% to 100% absorbed in humans (Figure 2.12).

Measurements of permeability in cell lines are usually conducted using simple buffer solutions of the drug at either pH 6.5 or 7.4. In an effort to make the measurements under more physiological conditions, Wuyts et al. [61] explored the use of FaHIF rather than simple buffer solutions as the solvent system to generate apparent permeability values (P_{app}) for a broad series of model compounds. Interestingly, P_{app} values obtained with FaSSIF as the vehicle correlated strongly to those obtained with FaHIF ($R = 0.951$). Thus, one way forward to improving correlations may be to conduct the studies with the drug dissolved in FaSSIF.

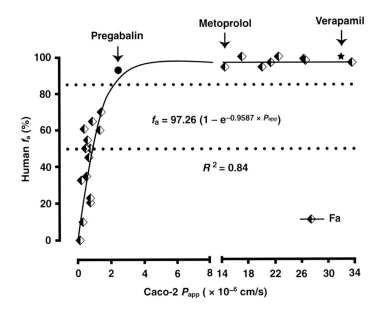

Figure 2.11 Correlation of human fraction absorbed (f_a) and apparent permeability coefficients (P_{app}) determined in Caco-2 cell models. Dotted lines represent the cutoff value for fa (fraction absorbed) 50% and 85%. (Data from Ref [60].)

Long term, a number of approaches will be necessary to improve estimates of human permeability for input into PBPK models. On the *in vivo* side, permeability from drug solutions applied using capsules that can release the drug at different sites within the gut, such as the BioPerm capsule (https://www.bioperm.se/) will aid (1) in establishing the permeability of drugs under normal physiological conditions with respect to intestinal fluid flow rates, volumes, and composition, (2) enable the regionality of permeability for drugs with various uptake mechanisms to be established and (3) provide more insight with regard to intra- and intersubject variability in permeability. On the *in vitro* side, methods based on immortalized healthy human enterocytes and 3D tissue structures are sorely needed to better simulate paracellular absorption, active transport, and exocytosis in the human gastrointestinal tract.

2.3.3.3 From in vitro Drug Metabolism Studies to Intersubject Variability in Metabolic Clearance

Overall, IVIVE of ADME properties focuses on estimating parameters in an "average individual". When estimating metabolic clearance in cryopreserved hepatocytes, researchers often average results obtained from different hepatocyte donors cultured *in vitro*. However, to efficiently design clinical studies, it is crucial to predict hepatic drug metabolism and human pharmacokinetics, not only at the level of an "average individual" but also accounting for the associated population variability. To investigate inter-individual variability *in vitro*, drug metabolism assays must be performed independently for hepatocytes obtained from different donors and with appropriate statistical analysis, like using non-linear mixed effects modeling (NLMEM), to estimate the inter-donor variability in intrinsic clearance disentangled from measurement error/uncertainty and any other types of variability (e.g., inter-well). To the best of our knowledge, NLMEM was applied in just one report focusing on describing the population variability in drug metabolism in the context of a microphysiological system [62]. Even though we applaud such an initiative, it is limited to only some covariates intrinsic to the *in vitro* setup, namely enzyme abundance. Other system parameters such as concentration of plasma proteins, liver weight, and liver blood flow are not considered in this innovative population-based IVIVE of metabolic clearance. In this context, linked PBPK-IVIVE models can incorporate different sources of variability into IVIVE approaches to simulate and predict drug metabolism in relevant populations. Rostami and Tucker integrated *in vitro* metabolism data for 15 drugs and physiological variability that is relevant to drug metabolism in both liver and gut using Simcyp Simulator and were able to estimate median

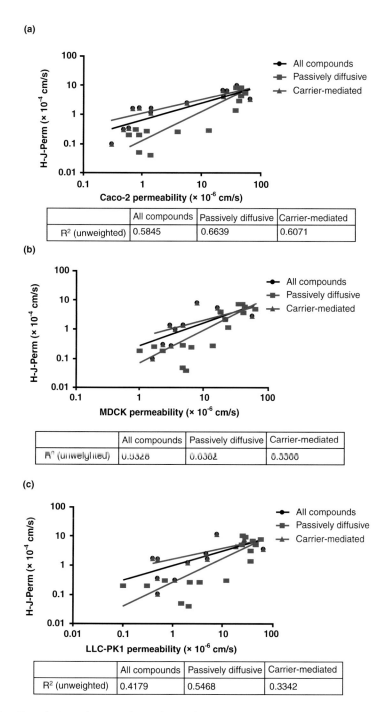

Figure 2.12 Correlation of P_{app} with P_{eff} for 30 drugs, using data from (a) Caco-2, (b) MDCK, and (c) LLC-PK1 studies [60].

clearance values that were within a twofold range criterion for 93% of the drugs given orally and 100% of the drugs given intravenously [63]. However, we still have important "unknowns". These include how to incorporate *in vitro* information on hepatic uptake and secretory transporters and phase II enzymes into predictions of drug clearance and drug–drug interactions. To do this in a fully mechanistic, but practical way, requires knowledge of the abundances of the proteins

29

and their variance within relevant organs, and a better understanding of their interplay with the cytochrome P450 system [63]. Finally, there are variables that we do not yet know exist—the as-yet-undiscovered factors that contribute to pharmacokinetic variability. The discovery and impact of these factors will be of great interest in the future.

REFERENCES

1. Morrison P. Distributed models of drug kinetics. In: Atkinson A, Lertora J, Huang S, Markey M, editors. *Principles of Clinical Pharmacology*. New York: Elsevier, 2013, pp. 117–38.

2. Tsamandouras N, Rostami-Hodjegan A, Aarons L. Combining the 'bottom up' and 'top down' approaches in pharmacokinetic modelling: fitting PBPK models to observed clinical data. *Br J Clin Pharmacol*. 2015;79(1):48–55.

3. Rostami-Hodjegan A. Reverse translation in PBPK and QSP: going backwards in order to go forward with confidence. *Clin Pharmacol Ther*. 2018;103(2):224–32.

4. Willmann S, Lippert J, Sevestre M, Solodenko J, Fois F, Schmitt W. PK-Sim®: a physiologically based pharmacokinetic 'whole-body' model. *BIOSILICO*. 2003;1(4):121–4.

5. Rodgers T, Leahy D, Rowland M. Physiologically based pharmacokinetic modeling 1: predicting the tissue distribution of moderate-to-strong bases. *J Pharm Sci*. 2005;94(6):1259–76.

6. Rodgers T, Rowland M. Physiologically based pharmacokinetic modelling 2: predicting the tissue distribution of acids, very weak bases, neutrals and zwitterions. *J Pharm Sci*. 2006;95(6):1238–57.

7. Rodgers T, Rowland M. Mechanistic approaches to volume of distribution predictions: understanding the processes. *Pharm Res*. 2007;24(5):918–33.

8. Poulin P, Nicolas JM, Bouzom F. A new version of the tissue composition-based model for improving the mechanism-based prediction of volume of distribution at steady-state for neutral drugs. *J Pharm Sci*. 2023;113(1):118–130.

9. Poulin P, Schoenlein K, Theil FP. Prediction of adipose tissue: plasma partition coefficients for structurally unrelated drugs. *J Pharm Sci*. 2001;90(4):436–47.

10. Poulin P, Theil FP. A priori prediction of tissue: plasma partition coefficients of drugs to facilitate the use of physiologically-based pharmacokinetic models in drug discovery. *J Pharm Sci*. 2000;89(1):16–35.

11. Schmitt W. General approach for the calculation of tissue to plasma partition coefficients. *Toxicol in vitro*. 2008;22(2):457–67.

12. Chetty M, Li L, Rose R, Machavaram K, Jamei M, Rostami-Hodjegan A, et al. Prediction of the pharmacokinetics, pharmacodynamics, and efficacy of a monoclonal antibody, using a physiologically based pharmacokinetic FcRn model. *Front Immunol*. 2014;5:670.

13. Niederalt C, Kuepfer L, Solodenko J, Eissing T, Siegmund HU, Block M, et al. A generic whole body physiologically based pharmacokinetic model for therapeutic proteins in PK-Sim. *J Pharmacokinet Pharmacodyn*. 2018;45(2):235–57.

14. Fairman K, Li M, Ning B, Lumen A. Physiologically based pharmacokinetic (PBPK) modeling of RNAi therapeutics: opportunities and challenges. *Biochem Pharmacol*. 2021;189:114468.

15. Monine M, Norris D, Wang Y, Nestorov I. A physiologically-based pharmacokinetic model to describe antisense oligonucleotide distribution after intrathecal administration. *J Pharmacokinet Pharmacodyn*. 2021;48(5):639–54.

16. Teorell T. Kinetics of distribution of substances administered to the body. *Archives Internationales de Pharmacodynamie et de Thérapie*. 1934;57:205–40.

17. Henderson; Y, Haggard H. *Noxious Gases and the Principles of Respiration Influencing Their Action*. New York: Rheinhold Publishing, 1943.

18. Kety SS. The theory and applications of the exchange of inert gas at the lungs and tissues. *Pharmacol Rev*. 1951;3(1):1–41.

19. Gibald M, Perrier D. *Pharmacokinetics*. New York: Marcel Dekker, 1975.

20. Mapleson WW. Mathematical aspects of the uptake, distribution and elimination of inhaled gases and vapours. *Br J Anaesth*. 1964;36:129–39.

21. Bischoff KB, Dedrick RL, Zaharko DS, Longstreth JA. Methotrexate pharmacokinetics. *J Pharm Sci*. 1971;60(8):1128–33.

22. Dedrick RL, Forrester DD, Cannon JN, el-Dareer SM, Mellett LB. Pharmacokinetics of 1-beta-D-arabinofuranosylcytosine (ARA-C) deamination in several species. *Biochem Pharmacol*. 1973;22(19):2405–17.

23. Zhoumeng L, Fisher J. A history and recent efforts of selected physiologically based pharmacokinetic modeling topics. *Physiologically Based Pharmacokinetic (PBPK) Modeling*: Academic Press, 2020, pp. 1–26.

24. El-Khateeb E, Burkhill S, Murby S, Amirat H, Rostami-Hodjegan A, Ahmad A. Physiological-based pharmacokinetic modeling trends in pharmaceutical drug development over the last 20-years; in-depth analysis of applications, organizations, and platforms. *Biopharm Drug Dispos*. 2021;42(4):107–17.

25. Hollander D, Dadufalza VD, Fairchild PA. Intestinal absorption of aspirin. Influence of pH, taurocholate, ascorbate, and ethanol. *J Lab Clin Med*. 1981;98(4):591–8.

26. Dressman JB, Amidon GL, Fleisher D. Absorption potential: estimating the fraction absorbed for orally administered compounds. *J Pharm Sci*. 1985;74(5):588–9.

27. Dressman JB, Fleisher D. Mixing-tank model for predicting dissolution rate control or oral absorption. *J Pharm Sci*. 1986;75(2):109–16.

28. Dressman JB, Fleisher D, Amidon GL. Physicochemical model for dose-dependent drug absorption. *J Pharm Sci*. 1984;73(9):1274–9.

29. Hintz R, Johnson K. The effect of particle size distribution on dissolution rate and oral absorption. *Int J Pharm*. 1989;51:9–17.

30. Yu LX, Lipka E, Crison JR, Amidon GL. Transport approaches to the biopharmaceutical design of oral drug delivery systems: prediction of intestinal absorption. *Adv Drug Deliv Rev*. 1996;19(3):359–76.

31. Yu L, Crison J, Amidon G. Compartmental transit and dispersion model analysis of small intestinal transit flow in humans. *Int J Pharm*. 1996;140(1):111–8.

32. Yu LX, Amidon GL. A compartmental absorption and transit model for estimating oral drug absorption. *Int J Pharm*. 1999;186(2):119–25.

33. Yu L, Amidon G. Characterization of small intestinal transit time distribution in humans. *Int J Pharm* 1998;171(2):157–63.

34. Agoram B, Woltosz WS, Bolger MB. Predicting the impact of physiological and biochemical processes on oral drug bioavailability. *Adv Drug Deliv Rev*. 2001;50(Suppl 1):S41–67.

35. Rowland M, Peck C, Tucker G. Physiologically-based pharmacokinetics in drug development and regulatory science. *Annu Rev Pharmacol Toxicol*. 2011;51:45–73.

36. Galia E, Nicolaides E, Horter D, Lobenberg R, Reppas C, Dressman JB. Evaluation of various dissolution media for predicting in vivo performance of class I and II drugs. *Pharm Res*. 1998;15(5):698–705.

37. Charman WN, Rogge MC, Boddy AW, Berger BM. Effect of food and a monoglyceride emulsion formulation on danazol bioavailability. *J Clin Pharmacol*. 1993;33(4):381–6.

38. Dressman JB, Reppas C. In vitro-in vivo correlations for lipophilic, poorly water-soluble drugs. *Eur J Pharm Sci*. 2000;11(Suppl 2):S73–80.

39. Nicolaides E, Galia E, Efthymiopoulos C, Dressman JB, Reppas C. Forecasting the in vivo performance of four low solubility drugs from their in vitro dissolution data. *Pharm Res*. 1999;16(12):1876–82.

40. Nicolaides E, Symillides M, Dressman JB, Reppas C. Biorelevant dissolution testing to predict the plasma profile of lipophilic drugs after oral administration. *Pharm Res*. 2001;18(3):380–8.

41. Shono Y, Jantratid E, Janssen N, Kesisoglou F, Mao Y, Vertzoni M, et al. Prediction of food effects on the absorption of celecoxib based on biorelevant dissolution testing coupled with physiologically based pharmacokinetic modeling. *Eur J Pharm Biopharm*. 2009;73(1):107–14.

42. Fiolka T, Van Den Abeele J, Augustijns P, Arora S, Dressman J. Biorelevant two-stage in vitro testing for rDCS classification and in PBPK modeling-case example ritonavir. *J Pharm Sci*. 2020;109(8):2512–26.

43. Pathak SM, Ruff A, Kostewicz ES, Patel N, Turner DB, Jamei M. Model-based analysis of biopharmaceutic experiments to improve mechanistic oral absorption modeling: an integrated in vitro in vivo extrapolation perspective using ketoconazole as a model drug. *Mol Pharm*. 2017;14(12):4305–20.

44. Pathak SM, Schaefer KJ, Jamei M, Turner DB. Biopharmaceutic IVIVE-mechanistic modeling of single- and two-phase in vitro experiments to obtain drug-specific parameters for incorporation into PBPK models. *J Pharm Sci*. 2019;108(4):1604–18.

45. Arora S, Pansari A, Kilford P, Jamei M, Gardner I, Turner DB. Biopharmaceutic in vitro in vivo extrapolation (IVIV_E) informed physiologically-based pharmacokinetic model of ritonavir norvir tablet absorption in humans under fasted and fed state conditions. *Mol Pharm*. 2020;17(7):2329–44.

46. Lechuga S, Ivanov AI. Disruption of the epithelial barrier during intestinal inflammation: quest for new molecules and mechanisms. *Biochim Biophys Acta Mol Cell Res*. 2017;1864(7):1183–94.

47. Vanuytsel T, Tack J, Farre R. The role of intestinal permeability in gastrointestinal disorders and current methods of evaluation. *Front Nutr*. 2021;8:717925.

48. Lennernas H. Human jejunal effective permeability and its correlation with preclinical drug absorption models. *J Pharm Pharmacol*. 1997;49(7):627–38.

49. Schiller C, Frohlich CP, Giessmann T, Siegmund W, Monnikes H, Hosten N, et al. Intestinal fluid volumes and transit of dosage forms as assessed by magnetic resonance imaging. *Aliment Pharmacol Ther*. 2005;22(10):971–9.

50. Godbillon J, Evard D, Vidon N, Duval M, Schoeller JP, Bernier JJ, et al. Investigation of drug absorption from the gastrointestinal tract of man. III. Metoprolol in the colon. *Br J Clin Pharmacol*. 1985;19(Suppl 2):113S–8S.

51. Jobin G, Cortot A, Godbillon J, Duval M, Schoeller JP, Hirtz J, et al. Investigation of drug absorption from the gastrointestinal tract of man. I. Metoprolol in the stomach, duodenum and jejunum. *Br J Clin Pharmacol*. 1985;19(Suppl 2):97S–105S.

52. Vidon N, Evard D, Godbillon J, Rongier M, Duval M, Schoeller JP, et al. Investigation of drug absorption from the gastrointestinal tract of man. II. Metoprolol in the jejunum and ileum. *Br J Clin Pharmacol*. 1985;19(Suppl 2):107S–12S.

53. Hidalgo IJ, Raub TJ, Borchardt RT. Characterization of the human colon carcinoma cell line (Caco-2) as a model system for intestinal epithelial permeability. *Gastroenterology*. 1989;96(3):736–49.

54. Kansy M, Senner F, Gubernator K. Physicochemical high throughput screening: parallel artificial membrane permeation assay in the description of passive absorption processes. *J Med Chem*. 1998;41(7):1007–10.

55. Pade D, Jamei M, Rostami-Hodjegan A, Turner DB. Application of the MechPeff model to predict passive effective intestinal permeability in the different regions of the rodent small intestine and colon. *Biopharm Drug Dispos*. 2017;38(2):94–114.

56. Koziolek M, Augustijns P, Berger C, Cristofoletti R, Dahlgren D, Keemink J, et al. Challenges in permeability assessment for oral drug product development. *Pharmaceutics*. 2023;15(10):2397.

57. O'Shea JP, Augustijns P, Brandl M, Brayden DJ, Brouwers J, Griffin BT, et al. Best practices in current models mimicking drug permeability in the gastrointestinal tract - An UNGAP review. *Eur J Pharm Sci*. 2022;170:106098.

58. Sugano K, Hamada H, Machida M, Ushio H, Saitoh K, Terada K. Optimized conditions of bio-mimetic artificial membrane permeation assay. *Int J Pharm*. 2001;228(1–2):181–8.

59. Jarc T, Novak M, Hevir N, Rizner TL, Kreft ME, Kristan K. Demonstrating suitability of the Caco-2 cell model for BCS-based biowaiver according to the recent FDA and ICH harmonised guidelines. *J Pharm Pharmacol*. 2019;71(8):1231–42.

60. Tchaparian E, Tang L, Xu G, Huang T, Jin L. Cell based experimental models as tools for the prediction of human intestinal absorption. *Drug Metab Rev*, 40(Suppl 3):178.

61. Wuyts B, Riethorst D, Brouwers J, Tack J, Annaert P, Augustijns P. Evaluation of fasted state human intestinal fluid as apical solvent system in the Caco-2 absorption model and comparison with FaSSIF. *Eur J Pharm Sci*. 2015;67:126–35.

62. Tsamandouras N, Kostrzewski T, Stokes CL, Griffith LG, Hughes DJ, Cirit M. Quantitative assessment of population variability in hepatic drug metabolism using a perfused three-dimensional human liver microphysiological system. *J Pharmacol Exp Ther*. 2017;360(1):95–105.

63. Rostami-Hodjegan A, Tucker GT. Simulation and prediction of in vivo drug metabolism in human populations from in vitro data. *Nat Rev Drug Discov*. 2007;6(2):140–8.

3 Oral Drug Absorption in Special Populations

In Vivo – In Vitro – In Silico Evaluation

Maiara Camotti Montanha and Bart Hens

3.1 INTRODUCTION

During the development of new drug products, the absorption of oral compounds is studied in healthy adults. However, the physiology of the gastrointestinal (GI) component can be influenced by different factors such as sex, ethnicity, age, genetics, diseases, and others.

Altered GI physiology can impact the drug absorption process, fraction absorbed, and pharmacokinetics of a drug. The main parameters that show the difference between healthy adults and patients are gastric pH and emptying time, intestinal transit time, intestinal surface area and permeability, expression of enzymes and transporters, intestinal volume and luminal fluid composition, and microbiota [1–3].

Considering that the dosage form is usually selected based on the biopharmaceutics characteristics of the drug product in healthy conditions, these altered aspects can impact the drug performance *in vivo* and result in increased variability, risk of therapeutic failure, and adverse effects. This chapter session will describe the characteristics of the targeted population and possible differences in GI tract physiology compared to healthy adults, the impact on oral drug absorption, and how to evaluate these changes *in vitro* and *in silico* from the beginning of drug and formulation development.

3.2 IMPACT OF BARIATRIC SURGERY ON ORAL DRUG ABSORPTION: In vivo, In vitro and In silico Evaluation

3.2.1 Types of Surgeries

Bariatric surgery is considered an obesity surgery treatment, leading to weight loss and metabolic disease improvement. There are several types of surgery being the most common: Sleeve Gastrectomy (SG), Roux-en-Y Gastric Bypass (RYGB), Biliopancreatic diversion with Duodenal Switch (BPD-DS), and Single Anastomosis Duodeno-Ileal bypass (SADI-S) [1].

SG and RYGB correspond to 47% and 35%, respectively, of the most common bariatric surgeries. In the SG, there is a longitudinal resection of the stomach forming a small gastric pouch without pylorus [2,3]. In the RYGB, there is a formation of a small gastric pouch and deviation of the upper part of the small intestine (the duodenum and the initial portion of the jejunum). The gastric pouch is then connected to the distal part of the small intestine in a Y configuration [2,3].

The gastrointestinal (GI) changes after the surgery can influence the disintegration, dissolution, absorption of drugs, and digestion of nutrients [4]. The complete anatomical alteration of GI physiology after bariatric surgery is still largely unknown [5].

Studies are showing the impact of these changes in the pharmacokinetics (PK) of different drugs leading to subtherapeutic or toxic effects, depending on the physicochemical and metabolic characteristics of the compound [6,7].

This chapter will focus on GI acidity changes, motility, intestinal surface area, and enzyme secretions after specific techniques of bariatric surgery and their impact on drug disintegration, dissolution, and absorption.

3.2.2 Gastrointestinal Alterations after Surgery

3.2.2.1 Gastric pH

The gastric oxyntic gland, localized in the fundus and corpus of the stomach, is responsible for the regulation of gastric acid secretion through parietal cells and maintenance of the gastric pH between 1.5 and 1.9 [4]. However, gastric acid secretion is decreased or absent after the formation of the small gastric pouch [8].

According to Smith et al. [9] and Behrns et al. [10], there is an absence of basal stimulation of gastric acid secretion and pentagastrin in patients with RYGB, resulting in an average gastric pH of 7 in the small pouch and conserved pH of 3.3 on the remaining stomach.

Patients who underwent duodenal switch and were monitored by a 24-hour pre-pyloric pH monitoring in another study [11] provided insight into the gastric pH of SG patients. The average stomach pH was 2.66, and 68.7% of the time monitored; the stomach pH was below 4.

DOI: 10.1201/9781003031802-3

The increase in the stomach pH is still not completely clear. Steenackers and colleagues showed that there is a trend for a higher median pH in patients with RYGB and with SG compared to a control group of obese participants [12]. No difference between post-surgery participants and obese patients was observed in the small intestine pH.

3.2.3 Effect on Gastric Emptying Time

The gold standard technique to investigate GI transit time is scintigraphy. Most of the published studies showed a shorter gastric emptying half-time (GET $t_{1/2}$) of semi- or solid meal compared to participants who did not undergo bariatric surgery [13–23]. For RYGB patients, the formation of a small pouch without relaxation leads to accelerated gastric emptying and transit into the jejunum. According to Goday Arno and colleagues [24], the rapid absorption and immediate maximum plasma concentration observed after the administration of paracetamol liquid suggest faster gastric transit in post-surgery patients.

Results published by another study showed an immediate gastric pouch emptying (GET $t_{1/2}$ of 1.49 ± 0.27 minutes) in participants with RYGB while obese patients showed mean GET $t_{1/2}$ of 65.8 ± 13.6 minutes. The patients with SG showed only a trend of a reduced GET $t_{1/2}$ [12].

3.2.4 Effect on Gastrointestinal Transit Time

The effect of bariatric surgery on GI transit time is controversial. Melissas and colleagues [17] demonstrated that the oral-caecal transit of a solid meal is delayed from 182 to 210 minutes after surgery; however, the small intestine transit time is decreased from 72 to 63 minutes [17]. Shah and colleagues also showed a shorter small intestine transit time in SG patients compared to healthy participants (average value of 199.0 vs. 298.1 minutes, respectively) [25].

Morínigo and colleagues used a breath test to evaluate the GI transit time before and after bariatric surgery. In their study, they showed a reduction in the transit time from 115 minutes before surgery to 75 minutes after surgery [26]. Nguyen and colleagues also observed a faster oral-caecal transit in patients who undergo RYGB surgery [27].

Contrary to the studies cited before, Carswell and colleagues did not observe any difference between obese patients and patients who had RYGB using a sulphasalazine absorption test [28].

3.2.5 Effect on Gastrointestinal Secretion

More studies are necessary to understand the effect of bariatric surgery on the gastric secretion of lipase and pepsinogen. However, Sillakivi et al. and Sundbom et al. observed a decrease in serum pepsinogen 1 in post-RYGB and SG surgery, indicating that a reduction may occur [29,30].

Because of the Y configuration and the deviation of the upper part of the intestine after the RYGB, the interaction of pancreatic enzymes and biliary secretion with food and drugs is delayed. Moreover, the undigested food presents in the distal part of the intestine inhibits secretion and motility as a trigger to potentialize nutrient absorption [31,32].

Studies showed reduced secretion rate of trypsin, amylase, and lipase [33] and reduced secretions from the pancreas [34] after gastric bypass. Published studies showed increased plasma bile acid concentration (fasted and fed conditions) in post-gastric bypass patients [35–44].

Steenackers and colleagues [12] compared the bile acid concentration in the fasted and fed state between obese, SG, and RYGB patients. In the fasted state, the bile salt concentration measured in the duodenum was higher in participants with SG (average 6.02 ± 1.05 mM) compared to obese, whereas the bile acid concentration measured in the duodenum of participants with RYGB was decreased (average 0.65 ± 1.12 mM). Both types of surgeries reflected in an increased total bile acid concentration in the jejunum, 7.5-fold higher in participants with RYGB (average 12.9 ± 2.75 mM) and 3.5-fold higher in patients with SG (average 4.82 ± 2.67 mM). The same trend was observed in the fed state.

3.2.6 Effect on Surface Area, Transporters, and Enzymes

The intestinal epithelial monolayer membrane is of extreme importance for the absorption of nutrients, solutes, electrolytes, drugs, and other species. Some preclinical and clinical studies suggest that neuroplasticity can occur after RYGB and SG because of undigested nutrients delivered into the jejunum and gastrointestinal acidity [45–54]. However, findings in humans are controversial, and more studies are necessary to conclude since mechanisms of intestinal adaptation may vary between animal species and humans.

One special note needs to be addressed, although more studies are necessary to evaluate the adaptation of the intestinal membrane, a considerable reduction in the small intestinal surface area occurs in the RYGB surgery. Since the upper part of the intestine has deviated (duodenum and initial part of the jejunum), a reduction in the extension of the absorptive site may occur.

Transporters and enzymes are important keys to absorption. The presence of P-glycoprotein (P-gp), for example, facilitates the transport of drugs back into the intestinal lumen, whereas cytochrome P450 (CYP) intermediate first-pass metabolism. P-gp is expressed in an increasing proportion from the proximal to the distal portion of the small intestine, while CYP3A4 is most abundant in the proximal portion of the small intestine decreasing the expression toward the ileum [55–57]. Considering the expression of the transporter and enzyme cited before, bypassing the CYP3A4 metabolism could increase the bioavailability of its substrates, whereas substrates of P-gp may not be affected since the main site altered by the bariatric surgery is the proximal portion of the small intestine [58].

3.2.7 Effect on Drug Bioavailability

Bariatric surgery can affect drug bioavailability in different ways, depending on the drug's physicochemical properties. Compounds that present solubility dependence on the gastric pH may be affected by the altered stomach pouch pH. The elevation of the gastric pH may contribute to the reduced solubility of basic drugs and increased solubility of acidic drugs. This was confirmed by studies that showed decreased exposure to posaconazole (a weak base) and increased plasma concentration of furosemide (weak acid) after RYGB surgery [55–57,59].

A published study evaluating immediate-release and controlled-release metoprolol formulation in postoperatively (6–8 months) compared with preoperatively bariatric patients showed that the accelerated transit did not affect the drug release rate; however, the trend toward a higher exposure in postoperative patients may be a result of the metabolism pathway bypass. Metoprolol is metabolized by CYP2D9, expressed in the proximal portion of the deviated intestine. The bypassed first-pass metabolism contributes to higher exposures [60].

The delayed secretion of enzymes and bile could reduce the dissolution and solubility of lipophilic drugs, leading to a reduction in exposure. However, a study with fenofibrate showed no effect of the RYGB on its exposure [61]. A variety of drugs have been evaluated under systematic reviews [6,7,62], highlighting that the changes in drug absorption may be drug-specific. Drugs that present poor absorption, high lipophilicity, or go through first-pass metabolism may be most affected by the changes after bariatric surgery.

3.2.8 Dissolution and PBPK Work with Bariatric Population

GI physiology is of extreme relevance for drug bioavailability. Gastric motility, for example, contributes to the disintegration of solid dosage forms; gastric pH impacts the dissolution and solubility of compounds that present pH dependency, and gastric emptying time reflects the time for the drug to be absorbed and achieve the maximum plasma concentration. The intestinal motility enables the mix of the luminal content with pancreatic and biliary secretions, improving drug solubility and dissolution and the interaction with the intestinal surface area, the main absorption site. The intestinal transit time regulates the absorption of low-solubility and low-permeability drugs and impacts the drug release of modified-release formulations. Nonetheless, the presence of transporters in the intestinal wall also contributes to the absorption of drugs [63].

To evaluate the impact of these physiological changes, modified or adapted dissolution tests, simulating conditions before and after the bariatric surgery, and/or PBPK models can be applied to estimate drug absorption by incorporating the physicochemical and metabolism characteristics of the drug.

Seaman and colleagues proposed in their work an *in vitro* drug dissolution model that reflects the GI conditions of the preoperative and post-Roux-en-Y gastric bypass (post-RYGB) [64]. They evaluated 22 common psychiatric medications. The dissolution model proposed is not based on a pharmacopeial dissolution apparatus and consists of two different media, a pH of 6.8 for post-RYGB patients and a pH of 1.2 for the control group. Electrolyte composition was identical between the models. The volume of media used was 30 mL to approximate the gastric pouch size post-RYGB. In the control group, non-crushed tablets were introduced to the gastric medium for 60 minutes, then 30 mL of the intestinal medium was added and exposed for 60 minutes. For the post-RYGB group, the tablets were crushed and exposed to the intestinal media (pH 6.8) for 2 hours. They concluded that 10 of 22 psychiatric medications had significantly decreased dissolution and two had increased dissolution in conditions post-RYGB, compared with the control group [64].

Yska et al. proposed a GI simulation system (GISS) capable of implementing variations to relevant parameters such as pH, volume, transit time, osmolality, and agitation [65]. The GISS consists of a paddle apparatus, with different media phases to represent gastrointestinal fluid. At the end of each phase, a peristaltic pump adds the next phase medium. Overall, the gastric volume is reduced, and there is no duodenum phase in the simulated post-RYGB condition. The residence time in the upper part of the intestine is shorter in the simulated post-RYGB condition (100 vs. 165 minutes in the preoperative condition). For fasted and non-fasted conditions before RYGB, the residence times in the stomach were 30 and 120 minutes, respectively. After RYGB, the residence times in the stomach pouch were 15 and 120 minutes, respectively [65].

In the previous work, they tested Metoprolol IR (100 mg) and CR (95 mg) tablets. Although in the non-fasted state in simulated conditions both before and after RYGB, a release of >85% in 25 minutes was observed for the IR formulation. In the simulated fasted state condition after RYGB, the initial dissolution was faster, achieving >85% in 15 minutes, while in the simulated fasted condition before RYGB, the same % released was achieved at 25 minutes. For CR formulation both before and after RYGB in fasted and non-fasted conditions showed a release of >90% at 22 hours, with f2 values of 81 and 84, respectively. They concluded that under the conditions applied in the GISS, Metoprolol IR, and CR did not show differences between before and after RYGB simulations, implying that no problems in the bioavailability are expected in this population [65].

Porat and colleagues [66] collected gastric content aspirated from patients before, immediately after, and the day after different bariatric technique surgeries, measured the pH and used the pH results to perform drug dissolution tests. They observed an increase of 3–4 pH units in the stomach pH one day after one-anastomosis gastric bypass (OAGB) and SG (LSG) compared to pre-surgery measurements. These values were used as a reference in the dissolution tests with dipyridamole and aspirin. Other relevant physiological parameters besides the gastric pH were implemented in the dissolution test.

In their work, they describe three different conditions: (1) before bariatric surgery; (2) after LSG, and (3) after OAGB. The dissolution settings used in each condition were: (1) 250 mL of 0.2 M maleate buffer, USP II paddle, working at 100 rpm; (2) 50 mL of 0.2 M acetate buffer; and (3) 50 mL of 0.2 M phosphate buffer, mini-paddle working at 153 rpm. The 153 rpm rotation speed was calculated based on the paddle size, reduced volume of fluid, and reduced gastric motility after bariatric surgery (fivefold decrease in contraction strength) [66].

To evaluate the impact of the post-bariatric changes on the enteric coating efficacy, they proposed a two-stage dissolution test, where the drug was initially evaluated under gastric condition (30 minutes condition 1; 15 minutes conditions 2 and 3), followed by 75 minutes of intestinal medium (pH 7). Dipyridamole (a weak base) under post-bariatric conditions (both LSG and OAGB) showed a reduced fraction dissolved (<5%) due to solubility limitation. Aspirin was not released from the enteric coat in the pre-surgery and post-LSG conditions; however, >75% was dissolved at 15 minutes in the post-OAGB condition. The type of bariatric surgery may impact enteric coating failure [66].

Some of the studies available in the literature used only *in silico* approach to investigate the impact of bariatric surgery changes on the bioavailability and PK of drugs. Darwich et al. created altered Advanced Dissolution Absorption and Metabolism (ADAM) models in Simcyp® Simulator to represent RYGB, biliopancreatic diversion with duodenal switch, SG, and jejunoileal bypass surgeries [67]. In their PBPK models, they changed the following physiological parameters post-surgery: gastric emptying (GE) of liquids, GE of solids, gastric volume, secretion rate in the stomach, initial stomach fluid volume, length of the small intestine deviation, small intestine bile secretion delay, bile concentration under fasted and fed conditions, gastrointestinal pH, the abundance of CYP3A4 and CYP3A5 enzymes, small intestine transit time, renal glomerular filtration rate, protein serum levels (albumin and α-1 Acid glycoprotein), and hepatic enzymatic function [72].

They carried out simulations with five different drugs: simvastatin, omeprazole, diclofenac, fluconazole, and ciprofloxacin. Simvastatin showed an increase in plasma exposure due to an increase in the fraction that passes the gut (F_g). This drug presents high first-pass extraction, and the deviation of the upper part of the intestine resulted in reduced gut metabolism and increased exposure. Omeprazole, a BCS Class II compound, enteric-coated formulation, showed minor F_g change and the most impacted parameter was the fraction absorbed (F_a), probably because of the reduced absorption area. Fluconazole, a BCS Class 1 compound, did not show any relevant changes in the exposure after bariatric surgery. Ciprofloxacin, a BCS class III compound, showed reduced exposure post-bariatric surgery most likely because of the reduced absorption area [67].

Chen et al. proposed an *in silico* model to understand the drug–drug interaction (DDI) potential of CYP3A4 and P-gp following RYGB surgery [68]. Initially, they simulated and verified the model with observed data from healthy volunteers, and then post-RYGB conditions were simulated by altering the population-specific parameters. The hepatic metabolism was considered to have changed in the post-RYGB population according to liver size and enzyme activity. The liver weight used in the model was based on the total body weight of the RYGB patients pre- and post-surgery (liver weight decreased from 2.67 to 2.43 kg post-RYGB). No changes were observed in the simulated F_a of midazolam, acetaminophen, digoxin, and verapamil (BCS Class I), whereas a decrease of 5%–13% in the simulated F_a was observed for posaconazole (BCS Class II). Regarding the DDI study, for midazolam-posaconazole interactions, the predicted inhibited fold-change in the maximum concentration ratio pre- and post-RYGB decreased after the surgery. For digoxin-verapamil interactions (P-gp substrates), the predicted inhibition of P-gp was comparable before and after the surgery. These results suggest that the impact of the RYGB in the DDI is dependent on the inhibitor solubility.

Montanha et al. [69] proposed a middle-out approach for parameter estimations using in vitro, in situ, and in vivo data in a non-commercial software, Berkeley Madonna, to build a PBPK model incorporating changes in the physiological parameters of the post-RYGB. Some of the physiological changes proposed in their work and incorporated into the CAT model described by Yu and Amidon [70] with a parallel physiological water model developed by Paixão et al. [71] were GE rate 2.5 times faster in the post-RYGB population, stomach pH of 6.5 due to the reduction of the number of parietal cells, decrease of the stomach secretion proportional to the decreased volume of the stomach pouch. The duodenum compartment was excluded from the model, and the upper part of the jejunum length was reduced.

Regarding the intestinal transit time, the authors explored two different scenarios: Condition A assumed that the overall peristalsis was not changed due to the surgery. Therefore, due to the 20% amount of deviated small intestine, a decrease in the intestinal transit time to 159.20 minutes was considered. Condition B assumed that the peristaltic movements could be reduced due to the surgery and an intestinal transit time of 264.67 minutes. The pH was unchanged for all intestinal compartments [69].

Their results suggested a reduction in amoxicillin exposure after RYGB surgery, and a difference in the fraction dissolved and Fa between suspension and tablet formulations. According to their results, the reduced gastrointestinal residence time may be the most likely scenario occurring following RYGB surgery. Although amoxicillin is BCS Class I, the deviation of the upper part of the intestine may impact carrier-mediated absorption.

Porat et al. proposed a well-comprehensive study integrating ex vivo, in vitro, and in silico approaches in the same work [72]. They evaluated loratadine/desloratadine pH-dependent solubility in gastric content aspirated before and after bariatric surgery. In a posterior step, they developed biorelevant dissolution methods to mimic post-SG or OAGB conditions. The variables considered in their dissolution methods were gastric volume, pH, and contractility. They studied crash tablets and syrup formulations. In a further step, they implemented the experimental data into a PBPK model.

Both drugs presented *in vitro* pH-dependent solubility decreasing at higher pH. However, the *ex vivo* solubility in the aspirated human gastric fluid after surgery showed that desloratadine solubility still allows complete dissolution, while loratadine solubility after surgery is much lower and the drug did not dissolve completely. Tablet crushing or syrup did not improve dissolution in post-OAGB conditions (stomach pH 7) but presented dissolution improvement of 40% in post-laparoscopic SG conditions (stomach pH 5). As *in vitro*, the PBPK model predicted the quick and complete dissolution of desloratadine across pre- and post-surgery conditions; however, simulations predicted a decrease of 24%–31% in the bioavailability and 28%–36% decrease in the F_a, depending on the type of the bariatric surgery.

Although the anatomy of the GI tract is substantially altered after bariatric surgery, an in-depth understanding of GI physiology is still necessary. Novel and standardized approaches are necessary to further investigate the influence on nutritional and drug therapy.

Where there is a lack of clinical studies evidence, *in vitro* dissolution studies and mechanistic PK *in silico* models would provide information about the magnitude of changes in the bioavailability of specific drugs, providing guidance on dose regimens adjustment for this population.

3.3 IMPACT OF ACHLORHYDRIC CONDITIONS ON ORAL DRUG ABSORPTION: In vivo, In vitro and In silico Evaluation

The stomach pH under normal fasted conditions presents a pH of 1.5–3.5 [73]. The pH affects the ionization of a drug, impacting the dissolution and permeation, and the release performance in the case of the modified-release formulations.

According to Feldman and Barnett [74], fasting gastric pH is higher in women than in men (2.79 ± 0.18 and 2.16 ± 0.09, respectively). This study was performed in 113 women and 252 men, and the difference can be related to reduced acid secretion in women. The basal acid output was twice as high in fasted men (4.0 ± 0.2 and 2.1 ± 0.2 mmol/h, respectively). The explanation for the increased acid secretion in men is not fully understood, but there are theories about stomach size and hormones [75].

Men and women present different physiologies and respond in different ways to medicines. However, for decades, the traditional human model used in drug development was a Caucasian Male. To overcome the disparity between sexes, the FDA and the National Institutes of Health (NIH) made mandatory the inclusion of women in clinical trials in the US in 1993 [76].

Ethnicity is considered an important aspect that contributes to significant interindividual variability in PK and pharmacodynamics (PD) of different drugs. It is known that the Japanese population, for example, presents lower gastric acidity compared to the Caucasian population.

Gastric acidity in older adults is a controversial topic. Different studies showed that there was no decrease in acid secretion with age [77,78]. Russell et al. [78] reported a median stomach pH in fasted condition of 1.3 (1.1–1.6) in the elderly compared to stomach pH of 1.7 (1.4–2.0) in young people. However, elderly people can present higher stomach pH as a consequence of atrophic gastritis and/or drug-related stomach pH increase because of the use of proton pump inhibitors.

The food intake can also impact the gastric pH and result in its elevation. In the fed state, the average pH reported in the literature is around 3.5 after 30 minutes of the ingestion of the food and 3 after 60 minutes [79–82]. Around 3 hours after the meal, the pH returns to the baseline levels [79,80]. The buffer capacity is reduced from 3.4% to 15% [82], and the intraindividual variability in pH values is lower compared to the fasted state [83].

Several studies reported contradictory results in terms of gastric secretion and stomach pH during pregnancy. Costantine [84] and Pariente and colleagues [85] demonstrated increased pH, whereas other studies showed no significant changes in gastric pH across different trimesters of pregnancy, and the same basal and peak acid secretion to non-pregnant women [86,87].

Patients with gastric cancer present higher gastric pH, around 6–7 [88], because of gastric atrophy. The reduction of the parietal cell mass causes the reduction or absence of gastric acid secretion and elevation of the pH [89].

Oral compounds and formulations with pH-dependent solubility need careful evaluation when administered to patients with *Helicobacter pylori* (*H. pylori*) infection since they can show increased or decreased stomach acidity. Infection by *H. pylori* can induce gastric alterations. The impact on gastric secretion depends on the extension of the infection and the region affected in the stomach. When the inflammation affects the antral region, the increased production of gastrin is associated, which in turn causes an increase in acid secretion in the gastric corpus. In contrast, if the inflammation is in the gastric corpus, there will be a reduced capacity to secrete acid [90].

3.3.1 Stomach pH in Patients under Co-medication with Acid-Reducing Agents (ARAs)

Proton pump inhibitors (PPIs) is a class of drug used as a single dose or short-term treatment, to treat GI diseases such as gastroesophageal reflux, peptic ulcer, or prevention of adverse effects caused by the treatment with non-steroidal anti-inflammatory drugs (NSAIDs). When used as a chronic treatment, the impact on drug absorption becomes relevant [91]

PPIs are the most potent inhibitors of gastric secretion. This effect can be extended in situations where acidic secretion is stimulated like after a meal (pH 6–7 in patients under PPIs treatment versus pH 5 without PPIs therapy) or in *H. pylori* infection [92].

According to a study published by Kirchheiner and colleagues in 2009, the overall fasted stomach pH after a single dose of PPI was 3, while this value raised to 4–6 after multiple dose administration [93]. More recent studies concluded that the average fasted stomach pH of patients in treatment with PPIs is around 5 [94,95]. A study by Miner et al. showed that esomeprazole has the longest duration effect of 14 hours, whereas rabeprazole, omeprazole, and pantoprazole presented duration of 12.1, 11.8, and 10.1 hours, respectively [96].

Most of the anticancer oral drugs approved are weak bases and present pH-dependent solubility. One example is the reduced exposure of tyrosine kinase inhibitors when co-administered with PPIs (e.g., omeprazole, lansoprazole, esomeprazole, and rabeprazole), due to the increase gastric pH [27]. Another class of drugs extensively affected is antiretrovirals, such as atazanavir [28]. The absorption of antifungal drugs is also affected by PPIs, showing reduced bioavailability when used in combination [97].

Antiacids neutralize the gastric acidic fluid and in a fasted state raise the values of pH to 3.5–5 [98]. However, the duration of the effect is short (around 30–60 minutes), after which the pH returns to its basal level [99].

Another mechanism to reduce gastric acid is by inhibition of the transmission pathway of parietal cells. Histamine type 2 receptor antagonists (H2RAs) is a class of drugs that competitively bind the histamine receptor and inhibit acid secretion. The usual mean pH values vary between 3 and 6 [100–102]. Studies reported gastric acid secretion reduction of 42%–55% with the maximum value of 94% for cimetidine [103–105], 33%–90% for ranitidine [104,106], and 60% for famotidine [103].

3.3.2 Bridging In vitro Dissolution and In vivo Exposure under Achlorhydric Conditions - In vitro Dissolution Systems

One of the parameters used to describe the in vivo solubilization of a compound in the GI tract is the dissociation constant, known as pK_a. Henderson–Hasselbalch equation illustrates the equilibrium between ionized and non-ionized species in a solution. Weak bases often show higher solubility in an acidic environment (stomach) and can precipitate upon transfer to a basic compartment (upper small intestine). Weak acids behave oppositely, showing higher solubility in the duodenum and lower solubility in the stomach.

For weak acid/basic drugs, variations in stomach pH due to the reasons listed before (differences in the physiology/diseases or co-medication with gastroprotective drugs) can impact the PK variability and bioavailability of the compound. An increase in the stomach pH will decrease the solubilization and supersaturation of a weak base drug when transferred to the intestine, impacting the absorption. Other aspects need to be considered in this process, such as permeability characteristic of the drug, dose, form of the compound (crystalline vs. amorphous), and the presence or not of precipitation inhibitors in the formulation to understand better the mechanism of supersaturation/precipitation of a weak base [83].

3.3.3 Biorelevant Medium and Dissolution Test Design to Reflect the Fasted State Gastric Fluid under Achlorhydric Conditions

The dissolution test can be applied to evaluate the impact of decreased stomach pH on the drug solubilization and the risk of precipitation upon transfer to the intestine.

Some of the aspects that need consideration when designing a dissolution test to reflect the gastric fasted state under achlorhydric conditions are the dissolution medium, the choice of the apparatus, system conditions, and the duration of the test.

3.3.4 Dissolution Medium pH

Considering the variety of the stomach pH described in the literature (ranging from pH value of 3 to 6) [93–95], one single dissolution medium pH would not describe the values *in vivo*. Segregur and colleagues proposed 2 media with pH values of 4 and 6 [91]. The pH 4 represents a patient under traditional PPI treatment, whereas the pH 6 reflects an extreme condition, under high doses and potent ARAs.

3.3.5 Buffer Capacity of the Dissolution Medium

In the dissolution medium, basic or acidic compounds can shift the dissolution pH. To counteract possible pH shifts, it is indicated the use of buffers according to their pK_a. It is recommended to use buffers whose pK_a value is less than ±1 from the pH value of the desired medium. Considering the two pHs cited above (4 and 6) to reflect the PPIs conditions, maleate buffer (pK_a 6.07) could be used for the pH 6 medium, while acetate (pK_a 4.74) for the pH 4 medium [91]. Citrate buffer could be used since the triprotic citric acid over a pH range of 2.5–7.0 presents the pK_a values of 3.13, 4.76, and 6.40, as shown in the Merck Index. McIlvaine's citrate-phosphate buffer is also an option, and it can provide buffering capacity across a very broad pH range (2–8) because of both the acid (citric acid) and the base (dibasic phosphate) groups [107].

3.3.6 Enzymes in the Dissolution Medium

The most important enzyme present in the stomach is pepsin, since it promotes the disintegration of capsule formulations, mainly when crosslink is observed. Pepsin is a protease, showing an activity that is highly dependent on pH. Gastric chief cells secrete pepsin as an inactive enzyme called pepsinogen, whereas parietal cells secrete hydrochloric acid that lowers the pH of the stomach and activates the pepsin (pepsinogen converted to pepsin) [108]. Piper and Fenton demonstrated that the peptic activity falls drastically above the pH value of 5 [109]. To reflect this loss in peptic activity under achlorhydric conditions, the content of pepsin in the FaSSGF recipe could be used for the preparation of the pH 4 medium [91], or even 70% of the pepsin content could account for the 30% decreased activity in this pH, as demonstrated by Piper and Fenton [109]. No pepsin is present in the pH 6 medium.

3.3.7 Osmolality of the Dissolution Medium

The stomach osmolality could be impacted by the PPIs' effect on gastric secretion. Considering that osmolality is relevant for the release of the drug from some tablet coating [110], this parameter should be evaluated when designing the dissolution medium. According to Litou and colleagues, the reduction of gastric acid secretion was assisted by a decrease in buffer capacity, the concentration of ion chloride, osmolality, and surface tension in the stomach [111]. As demonstrated in their results, after 35 minutes post water intake in a reduced acid secretion condition, osmolality in Phases 2 and 3 was lower than in Phase 1, but a significant difference was reached only against Phase 3. Segregur and colleagues proposed osmolality of 75 mOsmol/kg for the pH 4 medium and 50 mOsmol/kg for the pH 6 medium [91], following Litou and colleagues' results [111] (Table 3.1).

Although there is a decrease in acid secretion and volume of gastric juice under achlorhydric conditions, oral drugs are often administered with a glass of water (200–250 mL). For that reason, the recommendation is to perform the dissolution test with 250 mL of FaSSGF medium [112].

The PPIs do not affect the GE time, and then the total duration of the fasted gastric dissolution condition could be maintained as usual (30–45 minutes) [39]. However, in other cases of achlorhydric conditions where there is a change in GE time, it should be considered in the design of the dissolution test.

According to Segregur and colleagues [91], the changes observed in the surface tension under reduced gastric fluid are not significant. However, Litou et al. showed that in Phase 1 the gastric surface tension was in line with data published for healthy adults, and in Phase 2, the surface tension was lower [111].

Table 3.1: The Composition of Media Simulating Fasted Gastric Achlorhydric Conditions According to Work Proposed by Segregur and Colleagues [91]

Parameter	Medium					
	Acetate pH 4	Maleate pH 6	Citrate pH 4	Citrate pH 6	McIlvaine pH 4	McIlvaine pH 6
pH	4	6	4	6	4	6
Buffer capacity (mEq/pH/L)	7.5	1	7.5	1	7.5	1
Osmolality (mOsmol/kg)	91	50	75	50	75	50
Surface tension (mN/m)	64.49	67.21	63.32	67.86	63.20	67.58
Ingredients						
Pepsin (mg/mL)	0.1	-	0.1	-	0.1	-
Sodium taurocholate (mM)	0.08	0.08	0.08	0.08	0.08	0.08
Phosphatidylcholine (mM)	0.02	0.02	0.02	0.02	0.02	0.02
Sodium acetate (mM)	33.3	-				
Maleic acid (mM)	-	2.31				
Sodium chloride (mM)	-	22.7	7.7	22.8	17.5	21.2
Tri-Sodium citrate (mM)	-	-	11.2	1.5	-	-
Citric acid (mM)	-	-	-	-	9.00	0.86
Di-Sodium phosphate (mM)	-	-	-	-	11.29	2.94
HCl/NaOH (1 M) (mL)	qs.	qs.	qs.	qs.	qs.	qs.

Note: qs.: quantum satis (add as much of this ingredient as is needed to achieve the desired pH). Minus sign indicates the absence of component.

3.3.8 Dissolution System/Apparatus

The in vivo hydrodynamics in the fasted state stomach is complex to be represented in vitro; however, there are more than one system/apparatus that can be used to explore the PPIs effect and/or achlorhydric conditions caused by differences in the physiology/diseases.

The commonly used Pharmacopeia USP apparatus II, at 50 rpm is a good way to compare drug product dissolution under healthy and achlorhydric conditions. The use of standard pharmacopeial setups with biorelevant media reflecting the achlorhydric state is valid as suggested by Segregur and colleagues [91], although other *in vitro* models as the biorelevant GI transfer (BioGIT) system [113], mini-paddle apparatus [114], and dynamic multi-compartmental models such as TIM-1 and tiny-TIM systems.

3.3.9 Predicting In vivo Changes in Oral Absorption Using In vitro-In silico Approach

Overall, in the pharmaceutical industry, biorelevant media and in vitro tools are used in the early stages of the drug development process to predict *in vivo* performance and select formulations. Traditionally, *in vitro-in vivo* correlation (IVIVC) is established using QC dissolution data; however, there is a growing interest in using biorelevant methodologies in physiologically-based pharmacokinetic (PBPK) models to explore the *in vivo* performance [115].

In the study published by Litou and colleagues in 2017 [114], they proposed to evaluate different media under hypochlorhydria and achlorhydric conditions in the fasted state and use it in a dissolution investigation of salts of weak bases. In this work, they compared the dissolution behavior of the compound in the proposed media (Level III FaSSGFhypoc-phosphates, Level III FaSSGFhypoc-maleates, Level III FaSSGFhypoc-phosphates, and Level III FaSSGFhypoc-maleates) versus the dissolution behavior in *ex vivo* human gastric fluid from healthy adults in the fasted state without any pre-treatment, after partial inhibition of gastric acid secretion using pantoprazole and after complete inhibition of gastric acid secretion using famotidine. The dissolution work was done in the Distek® mini-paddle apparatus and the Erweka® mini-paddle apparatus. The dissolution of pioglitazone hydrochloride (doses tested at 30 and 100 mg) was estimated to be incomplete but rapid in the hypochlorhydria media achieving a plateau at a concentration less than half of that observed in normal FaSSGF. In the achlorhydric media, it also showed incomplete dissolution and a plateaued at a level slightly lower (about 8 times lower) than that observed in the dissolution performed with the human gastric fluid after administration of famotidine. These data indicate that the buffer species identity is important when trying to estimate the dissolution of pioglitazone hydrochloride in the achlorhydric stomach.

In contrast with the study cited in the previous paragraph, Fotaki and Klein integrated the dissolution results into a PBPK model to estimate the fraction absorbed of itraconazole under PPIs treatment and after intake of acidic carbonated beverages [116]. The dissolution experiments were done in a mini-paddle apparatus, and the media used were gastric fluid without pepsin (SGF) pH 1.2 and acetate buffer pH 5.0 to simulate the pH conditions of a healthy and hypochlorhydria stomach. The ADAM model implemented within the Simcyp® software was used to simulate itraconazole oral absorption. The solubility values obtained in the dissolution tests described and the dissolution profile extracted from previous works (at pH 1.2, pH 2, and pH 5) [117] were used in the model. The itraconazole solubility in different gastric media pH showed a decrease in the solubility from pH 1.2 to pH 5 of around 10 times. The simulated profiles estimated by using solubility and dissolution data of Sporanox® (itraconazole) in pH 1.2 successfully predicted the in vivo dissolution of itraconazole and the model built based on the solubility and dissolution data at pH 5 predicted 5%–8% of the administered dose absorbed. No direct comparison with *in vivo* data was done for the pH 5 condition; however, several studies reported in the literature demonstrate that itraconazole bioavailability is impaired when an acidic gastric reduction [118–120].

Another study also evaluated the dissolution of itraconazole under reduced gastric secretion but using another system, the tiny-TIM [121]. This system was designed more than 20 years ago by Minekus and colleagues to investigate food digestion [122]. TIM-1 simulates the physiological conditions of the GI tract configurated into four separate chambers, reflecting the stomach, duodenum, jejunum, and ileum. All processes are represented such as peristalsis, secretion, transfer of luminal contents, digestion, and absorption (not a proper absorption, but a filtration process). In the dissolution study using tiny-TIM with Sporanox® capsule (itraconazole), the dissolved drug concentration did not exceed 11 μg/mL in the increased gastric pH 6, contributing to higher concentrations of dispersed drug in the small intestine compartments. The decreased bioaccessibility determined in tiny-TIM correlated well with in vivo data presented in the study [121]. But some limitations need to be highlighted mainly for formulations in which the absorption aspect impacts dissolution (formation of stable micelles or nanoparticular structures), because of the inability of the plasma filter used in the system to reflect the permeation process *in vivo*.

Dissolution experiments with dipyridamole tablets were conducted using one-stage, two-stage, and transfer methods in novel biorelevant media that represent the ARA effect [123]. The results were then integrated with a PBPK model. Both two-stage and transfer experiments revealed that these in vitro setups tend to overestimate dipyridamole precipitation in the intestines in vivo. Therefore, data from one-stage dissolution testing under elevated gastric pH conditions were used for PBPK modeling of the ARA/dipyridamole interaction. The in vivo ARA effect was successfully bracketed using media representing the ARA effect in conjunction with the PBPK model.

One-stage methodology uses a single aqueous phase as a dissolution medium, whereas the two-stage method simulates the pH shift from the gastric to the small intestinal compartment through a bolus addition of an intestinal medium concentrate into the medium simulating gastric surroundings. Alternatively, a transfer model can be employed, where first-order emptying through a pump is used to empty the gastric contents into the intestinal compartment.

Dissolution test experiments were performed using a USP 2 (Paddle) apparatus with 100 mg dipyridamole (Persantin®) tablets. Dissolution in 250 mL of FaSSGF (pH 2) represented the gastric compartment, while the pH shift was induced by a bolus addition of 250 mL of FaSSIF V2 (pH 10.8) double concentrate. Two-stage dissolution methodology using ARA media as the gastric media was also developed.

A full PBPK model was created using the Simcyp Simulator software. The DLM scalar values from dissolution experiments using media representing the administration of dipyridamole after ARA pre-treatment were then substituted.

An alternative approach is to use an in vitro model like TIM-1 to reproduce luminal conditions in the GI tract. Experiments representing a lesser (pH 4) and stronger (pH 6) ARA gastric pH effect were conducted.

Dissolution in FaSSGF pH 1.6 was rapid and complete, with 100% dissolved at 10 minutes. However, dissolution experiments with dipyridamole tablets in ARA pH 4 and 6 media predicted incomplete dissolution in the stomach after ARA pre-treatment. Experiments using gastric fluid with pH 6 (TIM-1) showed a lower bioavailable fraction compared to the standard setup. The bioavailable fraction from the experiment using gastric fluid with pH 4 lies between the profiles for gastric pH 2 and pH 6.

Finally, for drugs that do not precipitate very easily or present very fast permeation across the intestinal membrane, the one-stage tests can be a useful representation of the *in vivo* drug dissolution under achlorhydric conditions.

The two-stage dissolution system is a fast tool to screen potential intestinal precipitation after co-administration of ARAs; however, the design of the experiment can cause an abrupt change of pH (not observed *in vivo*) and overestimate the precipitation of the drug.

All the dissolution tests presented here, can generate data to be used as input into a PBPK model, and predict the clinical impact on the PK of a drug product co-administrated with ARAs or reduced gastric pH caused by a disease.

It is important to highlight the differences observed between simulations based on the pH 4 and pH 6 for some drugs, as well as the difference in the dissolution profile of tests with different buffer compositions. This may suggest a high intra- and inter-variability in a population and can be further investigated *in silico*.

Moreover, the FDA published 2020 a draft guidance on "Evaluation of gastric pH-dependent drug interactions with acid-reducing agents" [124], which suggests the use of PBPK modeling simulations to investigate the PPIs effect as an alternative to clinical trials.

3.4 IMPACT OF CYSTIC FIBROSIS ON ORAL DRUG ABSORPTION:
In vivo, In vitro and In silico Evaluation

Cystic fibrosis (CF) is a genetic disorder that affects the respiratory, digestive, and reproductive systems, including the lungs, pancreas, and liver. One of the major challenges in the treatment of CF is the limited effectiveness of orally administered drugs due to the gastrointestinal (GI) complications associated with the disease [125]. The disease is characterized by the presence of a thick mucus layer that can affect the absorption of orally administered drugs. Mutations in the gene encoding the CF transmembrane conductance regulator (CFTR) protein is the responsible factor for causing the disease [126]. GI complications in CF cause thick, sticky mucus that will accumulate in the lungs, pancreas, and other organs, leading to a variety of complications. In the GI tract, CF can cause obstruction of the pancreatic ducts, resulting in reduced secretion of digestive enzymes and impaired nutrient absorption. The pancreatic enzymes are essential for the digestion of food and the absorption of nutrients. As a result, drugs (e.g., prodrugs) and drug products (e.g., lipid-based formulations) that require enzymatic digestion are poorly absorbed in CF patients [127,128]. The second mechanism is related to the thickening of the intestinal wall, which reduces the surface area available for drug absorption. The third mechanism is related to changes in the pH of the GI tract, which can alter drug solubility and ionization, affecting drug absorption. Moreover, as the secretion of bicarbonate will be hampered in CF patients, not only pH is subject of change but also the buffer capacity of the residual fluid volumes. Finally, the clinical manifestations of CF result from dysfunction of the CFTR protein/ transporter. Therefore, as in most other epithelial organs, CFTR in the intestine mediates the secretion of chloride, bicarbonate, and fluid [125]. Mutations in the CFTR gene may result in partial or total loss of function [129], resulting in secreted fluid with abnormally low volume and aberrant electrolyte composition.

Engjom and co-workers aimed to evaluate short endoscopic secretin tests for exocrine pancreatic function in CF [130]. CF patients and healthy controls underwent endoscopic collection of duodenal juice after secretin stimulation. Duodenal juice was analyzed for bicarbonate concentration and pancreatic enzyme activities, whereas stool was analyzed for fecal elastase. Based on the results, 31 CF patients and 25 healthy controls were tested, with CF patients classified as exocrine pancreatic sufficient ($n=13$) or insufficient ($n=18$). Both bicarbonate concentrations and enzyme activities in duodenal juice effectively differentiated between the two patient groups and healthy controls ($p<0.001$). A strong correlation was found between severe CF genotype in both alleles and the pancreatic insufficient phenotype ($p<0.001$). The authors concluded that the short endoscopic secretin test successfully differentiated pancreatic exocrine insufficient CF patients from exocrine sufficient patients and healthy controls. From a physiological point of view, some crucial GI changes are noted between CF patients and healthy subjects. Using a wireless motility capsule (WMC), researchers studied the intestinal pH and GI transit profiles in ten adult CF patients and ten matched healthy controls [131]. Results showed significant differences in mean pH values during the first 23 minutes of small bowel transit and a delay in reaching and sustaining pH levels necessary for pancreatic enzyme replacement therapy (PERT) dissolution in CF subjects. Small bowel transit time in CF subjects was significantly delayed, without a compensatory increase in whole gut transit time. The study demonstrated a notable delay in small intestinal transit and a deficient buffering capacity to neutralize gastric acid in the proximal small bowel of CF patients.

CF patients experience various pathological changes that can alter drug disposition [132]. Differences in the volume of drug distribution between CF patients and healthy individuals disappear when corrected for lean body mass. Hepatic dysfunction in CF patients leads to enhanced clearance for some drugs, while renal clearance is also increased despite the absence of identifiable pathological abnormalities. Optimizing antibiotic therapy in CF patients involves increasing the dose of beta-lactams and monitoring plasma concentrations of aminoglycosides, although the appropriate dosage for quinolones remains uncertain. Antibacterial drug products are crucial in managing CF patients, with adequate dosages significantly improving morbidity and mortality [133]. Optimal treatment depends on the individual patient's pharmacokinetics and the drug's effect on the relevant microorganism. Recent research suggests that the disposition of antibacterial drugs in CF patients is not as atypical as once believed, though some beta-lactam antibacterials show CF-specific increases in total body clearance. Aminoglycosides' pharmacokinetic optimization is based on measured serum drug concentrations, with the Sawchuk-Zaske method being widely used. In the future, integrating changing serum drug concentrations and killing rates of target microorganisms into a pharmacokinetic-pharmacodynamic surrogate relationship could optimize drug therapy, particularly for aminoglycoside administration, beta-lactam medication, and fluoroquinolones. Standard follow-up and symptomatic treatment have enabled most CF patients to reach young adulthood, but many still die prematurely from respiratory insufficiency. To improve therapies, researchers are exploring ways to increase airway hydration, safely reduce the inflammatory response in the lungs, and combat lung infections. Alongside, the development of modulators targeting the CF CFTR dysfunction is progressing rapidly, although current treatments are mutation-specific and can be costly. Researchers are investigating corrective treatments applicable to all patients, including gene therapy, cell-based therapies, and activation of alternative ion channels, but these are in early development stages. Efforts are also being made to advance personalized biomarkers for predicting treatment effects, especially for patients with rare mutations. Another study aimed to compare the pharmacokinetic parameters of ibuprofen administered as a suspension, chewable tablet, or tablet in children with CF and to determine optimal blood sampling times for measuring ibuprofen peak concentrations [134]. A single 20 mg/kg dose of ibuprofen was given, and blood samples were taken at various time points. The results showed that plasma T_{max} (time to peak concentration) was the only parameter with significant differences, particularly between suspension and tablet forms. The study concluded that a 20 mg/kg dose of ibuprofen suspension is recommended, with blood samples taken at 30, 45, and 60 minutes after administration. Obtaining the first blood sample 1 hour after administration could miss around 90% of peak concentrations, increasing the risk of overdosing. In addition, a randomized, double-blind, placebo-controlled study was conducted to investigate the pharmacokinetics and toxicity of ibuprofen in 19 children with CF aged 6–12 years [135]. Participants received escalating doses of ibuprofen or placebo orally twice daily for three months. Results showed that peak plasma concentration and area under the concentration-time curve (AUC) significantly increased with dose escalation. Comparing CF patients with healthy children, pharmacokinetics revealed a decreased plasma C_{max} and increased clearance and volume of distribution in CF patients. The study found no significant toxic effects, but plasma C_{max} monitoring is required for effective dosing in CF patients.

Preclinical *in vitro* models have significantly advanced CF research, a disease caused by mutations in the CFTR gene [136]. Over the last 30 years, numerous cell lines have improved the understanding of CF pathology and assisted in developing therapies targeting CFTR mutations. Recent advances in precision medicine for CF have been achieved through optimizing protocols and novel assays using human tissues and transitioning from two-dimensional monocultures to more complex three-dimensional platforms. These models help predict individual responsiveness to CFTR modulator therapies. Induced pluripotent stem cells and organ-on-a-chip systems are also being developed to more closely mimic human physiology for disease modeling and drug testing.

Researchers established conditions for long-term expansion of intestinal epithelial organoids, which mimic essential features of in vivo tissue architecture. They applied this technology to study organoids derived from CF patients, a disease caused by mutations in the CFTR gene. Forskolin, which induces rapid swelling in healthy organoids, has a reduced effect on CF organoids, and no effect on CFTR-deficient ones. This pattern is replicated by CFTR-specific inhibitors. The study's simple and robust assay will help facilitate diagnosis, functional studies, drug development, and personalized medicine approaches for CF [137]. Patient-derived intestinal organoids, *i.e.*, mini organs obtained from nasal and rectal mucosa biopsies, serve as in vitro models for CF disease, allowing for disease classification, drug development, and personalized treatment optimization [138]. However, predicting drug responses in patients remains challenging due to genetic complexity and heterogeneity. Recent advances in precision medicine for CF have been driven by patient-derived in vitro assays that can predict clinical responses to small molecule-based therapies. Primary and stem-cell-derived tissues are used to evaluate the preclinical efficacy of CFTR modulators, but they have both potential and limitations. Validation of these assays requires correlating *in vitro* responses with *in vivo* clinical biomarkers of disease outcomes. Although initial efforts have shown success, sensitive methodologies are needed to capture treatment responses in patients with mild lung disease. The development of in vitro and in vivo biomarkers will facilitate the creation of new therapeutics, especially for patients with rare mutations, ensuring access to effective targeted therapies for all CF patients [139]. Stem cells have demonstrated the ability to initiate morphogenesis *in vitro*, generating complex structures in culture that closely resemble their *in vivo* counterparts. Lgr5, a receptor for Wnt-agonistic R-spondins, marks stem cells in various adult organs in mice and humans. In R-spondin-based three-dimensional cultures, Lgr5 stem cells can grow into ever-expanding epithelial organoids that maintain their original organ identity [140]. Single Lgr5 stem cells from the intestine can form epithelial structures retaining characteristics of the *in vivo* epithelium. This technology has potential applications in stem cell research, disease modeling (such as colorectal cancer and CF), and regenerative medicine.

Pathophysiological changes affecting the GI lumen should also be considered in the framework of translational CF research. A static *in vitro* digestion model was used to study the digestion of eight foods with varying lipid contents. The enzymatic supplement dosage, intestinal pH, and bile salt concentration were manipulated as variables. Lipolysis extent was measured by analyzing free fatty acids released after digestion. The results indicated that lipolysis was influenced by intestinal pH and bile salt concentration, in addition to enzyme supplement dosage and lipid content. An evidence-based model can be developed considering these variables to better understand the digestion process [141]. In parallel, researchers investigated the therapeutic potential of an acid-resistant fungal lipase from *Aspergillus Niger* [142]. *In vitro* tests showed it had a wide pH optimum (2.5–5.5) and was resistant to pepsin and trypsin. The enzyme was given to 10 adult CF patients with pancreatic steatorrhea and showed increased acid-resistant lipase activity compared to the placebo. However, the fungal lipase had no significant effect on fecal wet weight or fat absorption compared to the placebo. In contrast, an established enteric-coated microsphere preparation (Creon) significantly improved fat absorption and reduced fecal wet weight compared to the placebo, while another microsphere preparation (Pancrex M) was also effective, but possibly less so than Creon.

From a modeling perspective, a study performed by Cicali et al. aimed to demonstrate the usefulness of quantitative modeling for extrapolating drug safety and efficacy to populations underrepresented in clinical trials, using an integrated disease/pharmacokinetics/pharmacodynamics model of ibuprofen's antipyretic efficacy in children with CF as an example [143]. The researchers developed an ibuprofen-mediated antipyresis model for febrile children with CF using published clinical trials, *in vitro* data, and drug physicochemical properties. They first created a mechanistic absorption model, followed by PBPK modeling, which was then scaled to pediatric CF patients and linked to an indirect response model of antipyresis. Results: The model simulations revealed therapeutic differences between healthy children and pediatric CF patients, with decreased plasma C_{max} and AUC in patients. Predicted pharmacodynamic time courses indicated a slower onset and faster offset of action in CF patients compared to healthy children. Exploratory simulations suggested increasing dosing frequency as a better therapeutic strategy for CF children. This work highlighted how model-informed approaches can play a crucial role in extrapolating drug efficacy and safety to underrepresented populations by leveraging knowledge obtained throughout the drug development life cycle.

3.5 IMPACT OF INFLAMMATORY BOWEL DISEASE ON ORAL DRUG ABSORPTION: In vivo, In vitro and In silico Approach

Inflammatory bowel disease (IBD), including Crohn's disease (CD) and ulcerative colitis (UC), is a global health issue with increasing incidence [144–146]. IBD results from a complex interaction between genetic, environmental, microbial factors and immune responses, with recent progress in understanding the genetic aspects of gut inflammation. A total of 163 susceptibility gene loci for IBD have been identified, with overlapping genes between childhood-onset and adult-onset IBD, suggesting similar genetic predispositions. However, the interplay between microbial, environmental factors, and genetic elements also contributes to IBD pathogenesis. Both innate and adaptive immune responses play crucial roles in inducing gut inflammation, and ongoing research is shedding light on the mechanisms underlying IBD and the interactions between various factors. The inflammatory disorders associated with the disease affect adolescents and young adults, with a rising incidence in pediatric populations [145]. IBD is caused by a dysregulated mucosal immune response to the intestinal microflora in genetically predisposed individuals. Children can present with classic symptoms like weight loss, abdominal pain, and bloody diarrhea or nonclassic symptoms like poor growth, anemia, or extraintestinal manifestations. The goals of IBD therapy are to eliminate symptoms, normalize quality of life, restore growth, prevent complications, and minimize medication side effects. Treating children and adolescents with IBD requires considering the effects of the disease on growth, development, bone health, and psychosocial functioning. Specifically related to CD, it is known that the disease state affects patients' drug metabolism due to changes in the intestine and its drug-metabolizing enzymes and transporters (DMETs) [147]. A meta-analysis was conducted to understand the system parameters affecting oral drug pharmacokinetics in CD patients. Results showed no uniform trends in reported oral bioavailability, with variations depending on the drug and formulation. Only one report was available on liver DMETs in CD, and there was limited data on protein expression in the duodenum and jejunum. Drug product performance is altered in patients with gastrointestinal (GI) diseases compared to healthy subjects due to pathophysiological alterations such as differences in GI transit time, fluid composition, and permeability [148,149]. In addition, changes in the abundance of metabolizing enzymes and transporter systems have been observed. The impact of GI diseases on each parameter may vary depending on the location and state of the disease. Drug bioavailability is influenced by the drug's physicochemical characteristics, pharmaceutical formulation, and drug metabolism. *In vitro* and *in silico* methods for predicting drug product performance in patients with GI diseases are currently limited but have the potential to improve drug therapy. Developing suitable *in vitro* dissolution and *in silico* models for patients with GI diseases relies on understanding pathophysiological alterations. Further assessment of physiological differences is essential to enhance the accuracy of these models and improve drug therapy for these patients. Current data is insufficient to enable predictive PBPK models with high confidence, and further research is needed to quantify DMETs and conduct well-defined clinical drug disposition studies. Drug product performance may be altered in CD patients due to pathophysiological changes, making it challenging to predict drug efficacy. PBPK models, integrated with *in vitro* dissolution studies, can be used to assess differences in the bioavailability of drugs between healthy and CD patients [150,151]. Using budesonide as a model drug, the performance in healthy subjects and CD patients was compared, revealing a higher exposure in CD patients due to reduced hepatic CYP3A4 enzyme abundance and lower human serum albumin concentration. PBPK modeling successfully predicted budesonide performance in healthy subjects and CD patients in both the fasted and fed state. This approach can be used to guide prescribers to adjust dosage regimens for CD patients accordingly and predict the impact of CD on the performance of other drugs.

In the case of IBD, the disease state is characterized as a result of an interplay between immune and non-immune cells, mediated by cytokines produced within the inflammatory microenvironment [152]. The role of inflammatory cytokines in IBD pathophysiology is crucial to understand and implement in *in vitro* and *in silico* framework in order to provide an overview of therapeutic options to block their function. Genome studies, *in vitro* experiments with patients' samples, and animal models of colitis have advanced understanding of cytokine modulation of mucosal inflammation in IBD. However, not all cytokines produced within the gut play a major role in IBD-associated inflammation. Anti-cytokine compounds are effective in some subgroups of IBD patients, whereas others have no benefit, making the identification of biomarkers that can predict response to therapy and facilitate a personalized therapeutic approach a major unmet need.

The introduction of biologics such as anti-TNF monoclonal antibodies and anti-integrins has transformed the therapeutic paradigm for IBD. However, many patients still fail to achieve long-term remission, highlighting the need for novel treatment targets beyond immune suppression. Recent studies have revealed the critical role of intestinal epithelial cells (IECs) in IBD pathogenesis, with barrier dysfunctions contributing to disease development. The establishment of adult stem cell-derived intestinal enteroid/organoid culture technology allows for the study of human IECs and presents a promising platform for novel drug discovery in IBD [153]. The mammalian intestine contains intestinal stem cells (ISCs), differentiated epithelial cells, and gut resident-immune cells. IBD threatens the integrity of the intestine and ISCs play a key role in the continuous renewal and repair of intestinal mucosal epithelium after injury. Inflamed mucosa healing is a new target for improving clinical symptoms, disease recurrence, and resection-free survival in IBD patients [154]. Recent advances in *in vitro* intestinal organoid culture and single-cell RNA sequencing technology have expanded knowledge of the connections between ISCs and immune cells. Transplantation of ISC to inflamed mucosa may be a new therapeutic approach to reconstruct the epithelial barrier in IBD, and the integration of biological agents and ISC transplantation may revolutionize future therapy for IBD patients. The role of epithelial cells in IBD has been extensively researched using in vitro techniques. Such studies have provided insights into the effects of microbes, immune activation, and inflammatory mediators on epithelial pathophysiology, injury, and repair in IBD. In vitro experiments have also demonstrated the ability of epithelial cells to participate in and even orchestrate immune responses in IBD [155]. Tight junction regulation and epithelial processing and presentation of antigens have also been investigated using *in vitro* studies. This information is critical in understanding the role of epithelial cells in IBD and could provide novel targets for therapeutic intervention.

3.6 IMPACT OF ALZHEIMER'S DISEASE ON ORAL DRUG ABSORPTION: In vivo, In vitro and In silico Approach

Dementia refers to a significant decrease in cognitive function that disrupts daily living. Alzheimer's disease (AD) is responsible for nearly 75% of dementia cases, while the remaining cases include vascular dementia (VaD), a combination of Alzheimer's and VaD, dementia with Lewy bodies, and frontotemporal dementia [156].

Traditionally, AD has been viewed exclusively as a neurological disorder. As a result, numerous studies have focused on identifying pathophysiological changes in the brain and blood-brain barrier of AD patients. These investigations have shed light on potential alterations in the central nervous system's drug exposure for individuals with AD. However, recent research acknowledges that AD may also impact extra-neurological systems, such as the small intestine, liver, and kidneys.

This growing area of scientific inquiry explores the potential effects of peripheral pathophysiological changes on the absorption, distribution, metabolism, and excretion (ADME) of medications for AD and related conditions. Numerous factors could potentially influence the oral absorption of medications in AD. These include alterations in GE rate, gastrointestinal microbiome, gastrointestinal system structure, intestinal permeability, and small intestinal metabolizing enzymes and transporters (Table 3.2). Both preclinical and clinical studies have reported changes in drug pharmacokinetics, which will be examined in the subsequent sections [157].

Table 3.2: A Summary of the Changes Affecting the Gastrointestinal System in AD and Their Predicted Impact on the Absorption of Orally Administered Medicines

Gastrointestinal Parameter	Parameter Increased	Parameter Decreased	Parameter Unaffected	Potential Impact on Drug Pharmacokinetics
Gastric emptying rate	No data identified	No data identified	Gastric emptying rate (APPNL-G-F mice) [34,35] (n=10–12 per genotype [34]; n=30 per genotype [35]) Gastric emptying rate (APP/PS1 mice) [34] (n=10–12 per genotype)	No effects on the rate of oral absorption anticipated
Gastrointestinal microbiome	Proteobacteria spp. (human tissues) [38] Bacteroidetes spp. in pre-onset stage of AD (human tissues) [38] (n=33 individuals with AD, 32 with MCI, and 32 with intact cognition) Actinobacteria spp. (human tissues) [39] Bacteroidetes spp. (human tissues) [39] (n=25 individuals with AD and 25 with intact cognition) Bacteroidetes spp. (APPNL-G-F mice) [35] (n=30 per genotype) Firmicutes spp. (Tg2576 mice) [40] (n=3–5 per group) Plasma LPS (human tissues) [43] (n=18 individuals with AD and 18 with intact cognition)	Firmicutes spp. (human tissues) [38,39] (n=25 individuals with AD and 25 with intact cognition [39]) Bacteroidetes spp. (human tissues) [38] (n=33 individuals with AD, 32 with MCI, and 32 with intact cognition) Firmicutes spp. (APPNL-G-F mice) [35] (n=30 per genotype) Bacteroidetes spp. (Tg2576 mice) [40] (n=3–5 mice per group)	No data identified	Oral absorption increased, as these changes in microbiota impact on intestinal permeability
Intestinal permeability	4 kDa FITC-dextran absorption (APP/PS1 mice) [34] (n=10–12 per genotype) 4 kDa FITC-dextran absorption (APP NL-G-F mice) [35] (n=30 per genotype) Serum zonulin levels (human tissues) [49] (n=110 individuals with AD, 110 with MCI, and 110 with intact cognition)	Mannitol permeation (APP/PS1 mice) [52] (n=3 per group)	4 kDa FITC-dextran absorption (APP NL-G-F mice) [34] (n=10–12 per genotype) Caffeine absorption (APP/PS1 mice) [52] Diazepam absorption (APP/PS1 mice) [52] (n=3 per group)	Oral absorption potentially reduced
Metabolizing enzymes	Ugt2b5 (APP/PS1 mice) [53] Trend toward Ugt1a1 (APP/PS1 mice) [53] (n=3 per group)	No data identified	Cyp2c29, Cyp2d22, Cyp3a11, Cyp51a1, Ugt1a9, Ugt2a3 (APP/PS1 mice) [53] (n=3 per group)	Reduced oral absorption due to increased metabolism
Transporters	Mrp2 (APP/PS1 mice) [53] (n=3 per group)	Mct1, 4F2hc, Lat2 (APP/PS1 mice) [53] (n=3 per group)	Mdr1a, Mrp3, Mrp4, Mrp6, Bcrp, Abcg5, Abcg8, Asct2, Sglt1, Sglt2, Taut, Slc22a18, Ata2, Mate1, Ostb, Oatp2b1 (APP/PS1 mice) [53] (n=3 per group)	Reduced absorption of Mrp2, Mct1, 4F2hc, and Lat2 substrates

Source: Table derived from Waller et al. [157].

Note: Conflicting results pertaining to changes to the gastrointestinal microbiome in the setting of AD are likely the result of methodological variation, including differences in sample size, study population parameters, and methods for assessing the endpoint. Please see the main text for a more in-depth discussion of these factors. Further studies are advised to resolve these inconsistencies.

Altered abundance of drug transporters at the blood-brain barrier (BBB) in AD has been widely studied, but the impact of AD on intestinal drug transporters and oral drug absorption is unknown [158]. This study examined plasma concentrations and *ex vivo* transport of four drugs in wild-type and APPswe/PSEN1dE9 transgenic mice, a mouse model of familial AD. The plasma exposure of valsartan and digoxin was significantly lower in APP/PS1 mice, while the plasma concentrations of caffeine and diazepam did not differ significantly between the two genotypes. *Ex vivo* transport studies revealed reduced permeability of 3H-digoxin and valsartan in the jejunum of APP/PS1 mice compared to WT mice. Tightened paracellular junctions were observed in the jejunal tissue of APP/PS1 mice, indicating reduced intestinal permeability. These findings suggest that modified dosing regimens may be necessary for certain drugs in people with AD to ensure effective plasma concentrations.

The pharmacological treatment of AD is crucial, and cholinesterase inhibitors like tacrine have shown cognitive and memory benefits [159]. Tacrine has nonlinear pharmacokinetics, and its plasma concentration is related to cognitive changes. Velnacrine exhibits evidence of nonlinearity in some pharmacokinetic parameters, but renal excretion is a minor route of elimination. The pharmacokinetic data of eptastigmine, a third cholinesterase inhibitor, is limited, but it can effectively inhibit acetylcholinesterase in the brain. Among the nootropic agents reviewed, oxiracetam crosses the BBB and persists longer in the CNS than in serum. Selegiline and idebenone, neuroprotective agents, are readily absorbed and can easily penetrate the CNS. Gangliosides can be administered intramuscularly or subcutaneously, and nimodipine is rapidly absorbed and does not accumulate during repeated administration. The treatment of AD with cholinesterase inhibitors, such as tacrine, can improve cognition and memory. Tacrine has nonlinear pharmacokinetics and its plasma concentration is linked to cognitive changes. Velnacrine has nonlinear pharmacokinetics and minimal renal elimination. Eptastigmine can inhibit acetylcholinesterase in the brain, but its pharmacokinetic data is limited. Among the nootropic agents, oxiracetam can cross the BBB and persist longer in the CNS. Neuroprotective agents, like selegiline and idebenone, can easily penetrate the CNS, whereas gangliosides and nimodipine are rapidly absorbed and do not accumulate during repeated administration. Gintonin is a novel lysophosphatidic acid receptor ligand derived from ginseng that exhibits anti-Alzheimer disease effects in model mice [160]. However, little is known about its intestinal absorption. This study investigated gintonin absorption using two model systems. Results showed that gintonin could permeate an artificial membrane in a dose-dependent manner and that its absorption in a mouse everted intestinal sac model increased with incubation time. Gintonin absorption was dose-dependent, and its absorption was inhibited by certain inhibitors. The study suggests that gintonin could be absorbed in the intestine through passive diffusion, paracellular diffusion, and active transport, and the lipid component of gintonin may play a crucial role in its intestinal absorption. Curcumin, a natural compound from Curcuma longa Linn, has various pharmacological activities, but its low aqueous solubility inhibits oral bioavailability, and it can be rapidly metabolized by the intestinal tract [161]. Various pharmaceutical strategies have been developed to improve the oral bioavailability of curcumin, including solid dispersions, nano/microparticles, polymeric micelles, nanosuspensions, lipid-based nanocarriers, cyclodextrins, conjugates, and polymorphs. These strategies can increase the solubility of curcumin, improve its intestinal stability, change its absorption route, and allow for co-administration with other adjuvants. *In vitro* and *in vivo* efficacy studies of curcumin nanoformulations, as well as human clinical trials, have been conducted to evaluate the effectiveness of these strategies. Tricaprilin is used as a ketogenic source for managing mild to moderate AD. It is hydrolyzed to octanoic acid and further metabolized to ketones, which act as an alternative energy substrate for the brain [162]. A physiologically-based biopharmaceutics model was developed to simulate in vivo processes following the peroral administration of tricaprilin. The model includes multiple data sources and was partially verified using data from a phase I clinical trial. A partial parameter sensitivity analysis revealed that dispersibility and lipolysis of tricaprilin, along with GE patterns, limit ketogenesis, while the conversion of octanoic acid to ketone bodies plays a minor role. The study suggests that the dispersibility and lipolysis of tricaprilin, along with GE patterns, should be considered when optimizing tricaprilin therapy for AD.

3.7 PARKINSON'S DISEASE AND ITS IMPACT ON ORAL DRUG ABSORPTION: An In vivo, In vitro, and In silico Approach

Parkinson's disease (PD) is a progressive neurodegenerative disease that can cause gastrointestinal (GI) symptoms affecting the pharmacokinetics of oral medications [163]. To develop better oral PD medications, a detailed understanding of PD-specific gastrointestinal parameters and how they affect drug release is necessary. The availability of biopredictive drug release models simulating PD-specific GI parameters would also be beneficial for this purpose. However, while there is reasonable data available on fluid volumes, motility, and passage times for some gastrointestinal segments, there is still a lack of information for others, particularly on potential disease-related changes in GI fluid composition. Delayed GE, a result of impaired motility, is evident in all stages of PD. It is underdetected in routine clinical practice but can cause upper gastrointestinal symptoms and has important implications for the absorption and action of levodopa, contributing to response fluctuations seen in people on long-term levodopa therapy [164]. The etiology of delayed GE in PD is multifactorial, at least partly related to Lewy pathology in the enteric nervous system and discrete brainstem nuclei. The neurohormonal aspects of the brain-gut axis are pertinent to discussions regarding the pathophysiology of delayed GE in PD and may contribute to the pathogenesis of PD itself. Ghrelin is a gastric-derived hormone with potential as a therapeutic agent for delayed GE and also as a novel neuroprotective agent in PD. GI disorders such as gastroparesis and *H. pylori* infection are common in PD patients, and they can adversely affect oral levodopa absorption and increase motor fluctuations [165]. Symptoms of gastroparesis include nausea, vomiting, and abdominal pain, whereas *H. pylori* infection can cause gastritis and peptic ulcers. Studies show that these conditions are associated with delayed peak levodopa plasma levels and increased incidence of motor fluctuations. Therapeutic strategies to minimize GI complications in PD patients include treatments that bypass the GI tract, such as apomorphine injection and levodopa intestinal gel delivery, as well as prokinetic agents to improve GE. The disease is associated with alpha-synucleinopathy that affects the brain-gut axis, including the central, autonomic, and enteric nervous systems [166]. The gut microbiota modulates brain-gut interactions through immunological, neuroendocrine, and neural mechanisms. Dysregulation of the brain-gut-microbiota axis in PD is linked to gastrointestinal manifestations, preceding motor symptoms, and the pathogenesis of PD, indicating that the disease's pathological process is initiated in the gut. Gut dysbiosis and bacterial overgrowth may stimulate the innate immune system, causing systemic inflammation, and may also initiate alpha-synuclein misfolding through enteric neurons and enteric glial cells. Patients often develop response fluctuations after long-term treatment with levodopa [167]. GE delays are common in these patients and are associated with fluctuations. Cisapride, a prokinetic drug, has been shown to improve these fluctuations. Levodopa ethylester injections, which bypass the stomach, have been used to reduce "delayed-on" and "no-on" phenomena in patients with severe response fluctuations. These findings highlight the stomach's contribution to PD deterioration and the potential for alternative delivery methods to improve patient outcomes. Levodopa is the most effective treatment for PD, but its oral use is complicated by erratic absorption and short plasma half-life. Long-term use leads to motor and non-motor complications. To maximize its efficacy, formulations are needed that provide consistent bioavailability and continuous dopamine formation. However, this is difficult due to levodopa's physicochemical properties and pharmacokinetic and pharmacodynamic profile [168]. Novel technologies and delivery devices are being developed to achieve more consistent and sustained delivery of levodopa to control both motor and non-motor symptoms of PD. A recent study by Wollmer and Klein aimed to establish patient-specific *in vitro* and *in silico* models to predict the *in vivo* performance of levodopa extended-release products in PD patients [169]. Current knowledge on gastrointestinal conditions in these patients was incorporated into the model development. The patient-specific *in vitro* release data were integrated into patient-specific PBPK, and levodopa plasma concentration-time profiles modeled using this approach compared far better with published average plasma profiles in PD patients than those derived from *in vitro* release data obtained from the 'average' healthy adult setup. The study highlights the importance of addressing patient-specific GI conditions when predicting drug release in such specific patient groups. Besides levodopa, the potential of quercetin, a flavonoid, as a neuroprotective agent in PD was investigated [170]. Results showed that quercetin significantly decreased catalepsy and exhibited neuroprotective effects in rotenone-induced Parkinsonism in rats by decreasing oxidative stress and apoptosis. *In silico* molecular docking studies also suggested that quercetin could be a potential drug target for aromatic L-amino acid decarboxylase and human catechol-O-methyltransferase. Quercetin possesses strong iron-chelating abilities and could be recommended as a disease-modifying therapy when administered in combination with levodopa, early on in the course of PD. These findings suggest that quercetin could be a promising agent for PD treatment, providing both symptomatic and neuroprotective benefits. Another study was conducted to develop a pulsatile oral dosage form of selegiline, a drug used in the treatment of PD [171]. The goal was to mimic the conventional tablet release from two oral administrations separated by 4 hours, to permit once-daily dosing and increase compliance. The pharmacokinetics of the pulsatile delivery system was studied in six healthy male volunteers, and it was found that the plasma concentration-time profile from the pulsatile system of selegiline and metabolites is dissimilar to that obtained from the conventional regimen. The lack of *in vivo* and *in vitro* correlation is most likely due to site-specific absorption/metabolism. The study suggests that the inequivalence of dosing regimens of the same total daily dose may ultimately be linked to the saturability of gut wall metabolism. Future studies on the role of the GI tract in the pathological progression of PD might lead to early disease detection and the development of neuroprotective approaches.

Selegiline is used in PD as an adjunct to levodopa therapy [172]. A fluorometric assay has been developed to study the pharmacokinetics of selegiline based on inhibition of rat brain monoamine oxidase-B (MAO-B) *in vitro*. The pharmacokinetics and bioavailability of selegiline were investigated in healthy volunteers after administering a 10 mg tablet or solution. Rapid absorption was observed with peak plasma concentrations between 30 and 45 minutes for the solution and 30 and 90 minutes for the tablets. There were no significant differences between the two dosage forms in terms of plasma C_{max}, T_{max}, $AUC_{0-infinity}$, and MRT. The apparent oral plasma clearance was high, indicating rapid elimination from the body, but renal clearance was negligible. Novel therapeutic options, such as modifying the gut microbiota and enhancing the intestinal epithelial barrier integrity, may influence the early stages of PD and can be promising for future drug development research in this field.

REFERENCES

1. Scopinaro N. Bariatric metabolic surgery. *Rozhl Chir*. 2014;93:404–15.

2. Nguyen NT, Varela JE. Bariatric surgery for obesity and metabolic disorders: State of the art. *Nat Rev Gastroenterol Hepatol*. 2017;14:160–9.

3. Preedy VR, Rajendram R, Martin CR. *Metabolism and Pathophysiology of Bariatric Surgery: Nutrition, Procedures, Outcomes and Adverse Effects*. Amsterdam, The Netherlands: Elsevier Science; 2016.

4. Vertzoni M, Augustijns P, Grimm M, Koziolek M, Lemmens G, Parrott N, et al. Impact of regional differences along the gastrointestinal tract of healthy adults on oral drug absorption: An UNGAP review. *Eur J Pharm Sci*. 2019;134:153–75.

5. Vella A. Enteroendocrine secretion after Roux-en-Y gastric bypass: Is it important? *Neurogastroenterol Motil*. 2013;25:1–3.

6. Yska JP, van der Linde S, Tapper VV, Apers JA, Emous M, Totté ER, et al. Influence of bariatric surgery on the use and pharmacokinetics of some major drug classes. *Obes Surg*. 2013;23:819–25.

7. Padwal R, Brocks D, Sharma AM. A systematic review of drug absorption following bariatric surgery and its theoretical implications. *Obes Rev*. 2010;11:41–50.

8. Schubert ML. Gastric acid secretion. *Curr Opin Gastroenterol*. 2016;32:452–60.

9. Smith CD, Herkes SB, Behrns KE, Fairbanks VF, Kelly KA, Sarr MG. Gastric acid secretion and vitamin B12 absorption after vertical Roux-en-Y gastric bypass for morbid obesity. *Ann Surg*. 1993;218:91–6.

10. Behrns KE, Smith CD, Sarr MG. Prospective evaluation of gastric acid secretion and cobalamin absorption following gastric bypass for clinically severe obesity. *Dig Dis Sci*. 1994;39:315–20.

11. Bekhali Z, Hedberg J, Hedenström H, Sundbom M. Large buffering effect of the duodenal bulb in duodenal switch: A wireless pH-metric study. *Obes Surg*. 2017;27:1867–71.

12. Steenackers N, Vanuytsel T, Augustijns P, Deleus E, Deckers W, Deroose CM, et al. Effect of sleeve gastrectomy and Roux-en-Y gastric bypass on gastrointestinal physiology. *Eur J Pharm Biopharm*. 2023;183:92–101.

13. Bernstine H, Tzioni-Yehoshua R, Groshar D, Beglaibter N, Shikora S, Rosenthal RJ, et al. Gastric emptying is not affected by sleeve gastrectomy--scintigraphic evaluation of gastric emptying after sleeve gastrectomy without removal of the gastric antrum. *Obes Surg.* 2009;19:293–8.

14. Kandeel AA, Sarhan MD, Hegazy T, Mahmoud MM, Ali MH. Comparative assessment of gastric emptying in obese patients before and after laparoscopic sleeve gastrectomy using radionuclide scintigraphy. *Nucl Med Commun.* 2015;36:854–62.

15. Melissas J, Daskalakis M, Koukouraki S, Askoxylakis I, Metaxari M, Dimitriadis E, et al. Sleeve gastrectomy-a "food limiting" operation. *Obes Surg.* 2008;18:1251–6.

16. Melissas J, Koukouraki S, Askoxylakis J, Stathaki M, Daskalakis M, Perisinakis K, et al. Sleeve gastrectomy: A restrictive procedure? *Obes Surg.* 2007;17:57–62.

17. Melissas J, Leventi A, Klinaki I, Perisinakis K, Koukouraki S, de Bree E, et al. Alterations of global gastrointestinal motility after sleeve gastrectomy: A prospective study. *Ann Surg.* 2013;258:976–82.

18. Michalsky D, Dvorak P, Belacek J, Kasalicky M. Radical resection of the pyloric antrum and its effect on gastric emptying after sleeve gastrectomy. *Obes Surg.* 2013;23:567–73.

19. Pilone V, Tramontano S, Di Micco R, Monda A, Hasani A, Izzo G, et al. Gastric emptying after sleeve gastrectomy: Statistical evidence of a controlled prospective study with gastric scintigraphy. *Minerva Chir.* 2013;68:385–92.

20. Sista F, Abruzzese V, Clementi M, Carandina S, Cecilia M, Amicucci G. The effect of sleeve gastrectomy on GLP-1 secretion and gastric emptying: A prospective study. *Surg Obes Relat Dis.* 2017;13:7–14.

21. Vigneshwaran B, Wahal A, Aggarwal S, Priyadarshini P, Bhattacharjee H, Khadgawat R, et al. Impact of sleeve gastrectomy on type 2 diabetes mellitus, gastric emptying time, glucagon-like peptide 1 (GLP-1), ghrelin and leptin in non-morbidly obese subjects with BMI 30–35.0 kg/m2: A prospective study. *Obes Surg.* 2016;26:2817–23.

22. Vives M, Molina A, Danús M, Rebenaque E, Blanco S, París M, et al. Analysis of gastric physiology after laparoscopic sleeve gastrectomy (LSG) with or without antral preservation in relation to metabolic response: A randomised study. *Obes Surg.* 2017;27:2836–44.

23. Keller J, Bassotti G, Clarke J, Dinning P, Fox M, Grover M, et al. Expert consensus document: Advances in the diagnosis and classification of gastric and intestinal motility disorders. *Nat Rev Gastroenterol Hepatol.* 2018;15:291–308.

24. Goday Arno A, Farré M, Rodríguez-Morató J, Ramon JM, Pérez-Mañá C, Papaseit E, et al. Pharmacokinetics in morbid obesity: Influence of two bariatric surgery techniques on paracetamol and caffeine metabolism. *Obes Surg.* 2017;27:3194–201.

25. Shah S, Shah P, Todkar J, Gagner M, Sonar S, Solav S. Prospective controlled study of effect of laparoscopic sleeve gastrectomy on small bowel transit time and gastric emptying half-time in morbidly obese patients with type 2 diabetes mellitus. *Surg Obes Relat Dis.* 2010;6:152–7.

26. Morínigo R, Moizé V, Musri M, Lacy AM, Navarro S, Marín JL, et al. Glucagon-like peptide-1, peptide YY, hunger, and satiety after gastric bypass surgery in morbidly obese subjects. *J Clin Endocrinol Metab.* 2006;91:1735–40.

27. Nguyen NQ, Debreceni TL, Burgstad CM, Wishart JM, Bellon M, Rayner CK, et al. Effects of posture and meal volume on gastric emptying, intestinal transit, oral glucose tolerance, blood pressure and gastrointestinal symptoms after Roux-en-Y gastric bypass. *Obes Surg.* 2015;25:1392–400.

28. Carswell KA, Vincent RP, Belgaumkar AP, Sherwood RA, Amiel SA, Patel AG, et al. The effect of bariatric surgery on intestinal absorption and transit time. *Obes Surg.* 2014;24:796–805.

29. Sillakivi T, Suumann J, Kirsimägi U, Peetsalu A. Plasma levels of gastric biomarkers in patients after bariatric surgery: Biomarkers after bariatric surgery. *Hepatogastroenterology.* 2013;60:2129–32.

30. Sundbom M, Mårdh E, Mårdh S, Ohrvall M, Gustavsson S. Reduction in serum pepsinogen I after Roux-en-Y gastric bypass. *J Gastrointest Surg.* 2003;7:529–35.

31. Sinclair P, Brennan DJ, le Roux CW. Gut adaptation after metabolic surgery and its influences on the brain, liver and cancer. *Nat Rev Gastroenterol Hepatol.* 2018;15:606–24.

32. Barreto SG, Soenen S, Chisholm J, Chapman I, Kow L. Does the ileal brake mechanism contribute to sustained weight loss after bariatric surgery? *ANZ J Surg.* 2018;88:20–5.

33. O'Keefe SJD, Rakitt T, Ou J, El Hajj II, Blaney E, Vipperla K, et al. Pancreatic and intestinal function post Roux-en-Y gastric bypass surgery for obesity. *Clin Transl Gastroenterol.* 2017;8:e112.

34. Ito C, Mason EE. Gastric bypass and pancreatic secretion. *Surgery.* 1971;69:526–32.

35. Pournaras DJ, Glicksman C, Vincent RP, Kuganolipava S, Alaghband-Zadeh J, Mahon D, et al. The role of bile after Roux-en-Y gastric bypass in promoting weight loss and improving glycaemic control. *Endocrinology.* 2012;153:3613–9.

36. Steinert RE, Peterli R, Keller S, Meyer-Gerspach AC, Drewe J, Peters T, et al. Bile acids and gut peptide secretion after bariatric surgery: A 1-year prospective randomized pilot trial. *Obesity (Silver Spring).* 2013;21:E660–668.

37. Albaugh VL, Flynn CR, Cai S, Xiao Y, Tamboli RA, Abumrad NN. Early increases in bile acids post Roux-en-Y gastric bypass are driven by insulin sensitizing, secondary bile acids. *J Clin Endocrinol Metab.* 2015;100:E1225–1233.

38. Patti M-E, Houten SM, Bianco AC, Bernier R, Larsen PR, Holst JJ, et al. Serum bile acids are higher in humans with prior gastric bypass: Potential contribution to improved glucose and lipid metabolism. *Obesity (Silver Spring).* 2009;17:1671–7.

39. Simonen M, Dali-Youcef N, Kaminska D, Venesmaa S, Käkelä P, Pääkkönen M, et al. Conjugated bile acids associate with altered rates of glucose and lipid oxidation after Roux-en-Y gastric bypass. *Obes Surg.* 2012;22:1473–80.

40. Kohli R, Bradley D, Setchell KD, Eagon JC, Abumrad N, Klein S. Weight loss induced by Roux-en-Y gastric bypass but not laparoscopic adjustable gastric banding increases circulating bile acids. *J Clin Endocrinol Metab.* 2013;98:E708–712.

41. De Giorgi S, Campos V, Egli L, Toepel U, Carrel G, Cariou B, et al. Long-term effects of Roux-en-Y gastric bypass on postprandial plasma lipid and bile acids kinetics in female non diabetic subjects: A cross-sectional pilot study. *Clin Nutr.* 2015;34:911–7.

42. Ahmad NN, Pfalzer A, Kaplan LM. Roux-en-Y gastric bypass normalizes the blunted postprandial bile acid excursion associated with obesity. *Int J Obes (Lond).* 2013;37:1553–9.

43. Dutia R, Embrey M, O'Brien CS, Haeusler RA, Agénor KK, Homel P, et al. Temporal changes in bile acid levels and 12α-hydroxylation after Roux-en-Y gastric bypass surgery in type 2 diabetes. *Int J Obes (Lond).* 2015;39:806–13.

44. Nemati R, Lu J, Dokpuang D, Booth M, Plank LD, Murphy R. Increased bile acids and FGF19 after sleeve gastrectomy and Roux-en-Y gastric bypass correlate with improvement in type 2 diabetes in a randomized trial. *Obes Surg.* 2018;28:2672–86.

45. Mumphrey MB, Patterson LM, Zheng H, Berthoud H-R. Roux-en-Y gastric bypass surgery increases number but not density of CCK-, GLP-1-, 5-HT-, and neurotensin-expressing entero-endocrine cells in rats. *Neurogastroenterol Motil.* 2013;25:e70–79.

46. Li L, Wang X, Bai L, Yu H, Huang Z, Huang A, et al. The effects of sleeve gastrectomy on glucose metabolism and glucagon-like peptide 1 in Goto-Kakizaki rats. *J Diabetes Res.* 2018;2018:1082561.

47. Mumphrey MB, Hao Z, Townsend RL, Patterson LM, Berthoud H-R. Sleeve gastrectomy does not cause hypertrophy and reprogramming of intestinal glucose metabolism in rats. *Obes Surg.* 2015;25:1468–73.

48. Myronovych A, Salazar-Gonzalez R-M, Ryan KK, Miles L, Zhang W, Jha P, et al. The role of small heterodimer partner in nonalcoholic fatty liver disease improvement after sleeve gastrectomy in mice. *Obesity (Silver Spring).* 2014;22:2301–11.

49. Nausheen S, Shah IH, Pezeshki A, Sigalet DL, Chelikani PK. Effects of sleeve gastrectomy and ileal transposition, alone and in combination, on food intake, body weight, gut hormones, and glucose metabolism in rats. *Am J Physiol Endocrinol Metab.* 2013;305:E507–518.

50. Bueter M, Löwenstein C, Olbers T, Wang M, Cluny NL, Bloom SR, et al. Gastric bypass increases energy expenditure in rats. *Gastroenterology.* 2010;138:1845–53.

51. Casselbrant A, Elias E, Fändriks L, Wallenius V. Expression of tight-junction proteins in human proximal small intestinal mucosa before and after Roux-en-Y gastric bypass surgery. *Surg Obes Relat Dis.* 2015;11:45–53.

52. Hansen CF, Bueter M, Theis N, Lutz T, Paulsen S, Dalbøge LS, et al. Hypertrophy dependent doubling of L-cells in Roux-en-Y gastric bypass operated rats. *PLoS One.* 2013;8:e65696.

53. Stock-Damgé C, Aprahamian M, Raul F, Marescaux J, Scopinaro N. Small-intestinal and colonic changes after biliopancreatic bypass for morbid obesity. *Scand J Gastroenterol.* 1986;21:1115–23.

54. Stearns AT, Balakrishnan A, Tavakkolizadeh A. Impact of Roux-en-Y gastric bypass surgery on rat intestinal glucose transport. *Am J Physiol Gastrointest Liver Physiol.* 2009;297:G950–957.

55. Thelen K, Dressman JB. Cytochrome P450-mediated metabolism in the human gut wall. *J Pharm Pharmacol.* 2009;61:541–58.

56. Paine MF, Khalighi M, Fisher JM, Shen DD, Kunze KL, Marsh CL, et al. Characterization of interintestinal and intraintestinal variations in human CYP3A-dependent metabolism. *J Pharmacol Exp Ther.* 1997;283:1552–62.

57. Mouly S, Paine MF. P-glycoprotein increases from proximal to distal regions of human small intestine. *Pharm Res.* 2003;20:1595–9.

58. Chan L-N, Lin YS, Tay-Sontheimer JC, Trawick D, Oelschlager BK, Flum DR, et al. Proximal Roux-en-Y gastric bypass alters drug absorption pattern but not systemic exposure of CYP3A4 and P-glycoprotein substrates. *Pharmacotherapy.* 2015;35:361–9.

59. Drozdzik M, Gröer C, Penski J, Lapczuk J, Ostrowski M, Lai Y, et al. Protein abundance of clinically relevant multidrug transporters along the entire length of the human intestine. *Mol Pharm.* 2014;11:3547–55.

60. Gesquiere I, Darwich AS, Van der Schueren B, de Hoon J, Lannoo M, Matthys C, et al. Drug disposition and modelling before and after gastric bypass: Immediate and controlled-release metoprolol formulations. *Br J Clin Pharmacol.* 2015;80:1021–30.

61. Gesquiere I, Hens B, Van der Schueren B, Mols R, de Hoon J, Lannoo M, et al. Drug disposition before and after gastric bypass: Fenofibrate and posaconazole. *Br J Clin Pharmacol.* 2016;82:1325–32.

62. Darwich AS, Henderson K, Burgin A, Ward N, Whittam J, Ammori BJ, et al. Trends in oral drug bioavailability following bariatric surgery: Examining the variable extent of impact on exposure of different drug classes. *Br J Clin Pharmacol.* 2012;74:774–87.

63. Wang G, Agenor K, Pizot J, Kotler DP, Harel Y, Van Der Schueren BJ, et al. Accelerated gastric emptying but no carbohydrate malabsorption 1 year after gastric bypass surgery (GBP). *Obes Surg.* 2012;22:1263–7.

64. Seaman JS, Bowers SP, Dixon P, Schindler L. Dissolution of common psychiatric medications in a Roux-en-Y gastric bypass model. *Psychosomatics* [Internet]. 2005 [cited 2023 Mar 29];46. Available from: https://pubmed.ncbi.nlm.nih.gov/15883146/.

65. Yska JP, Punter RJ, Woerdenbag HJ, Emous M, Frijlink HW, Wilffert B, et al. A gastrointestinal simulation system for dissolution of oral solid dosage forms before and after Roux-en-Y gastric bypass. *Eur J Hosp Pharm.* 2019;26:152–6.

66. Porat D, Vaynshtein J, Gibori R, Avramoff O, Shaked G, Dukhno O, et al. Stomach pH before vs. after different bariatric surgery procedures: Clinical implications for drug delivery. *Eur J Pharm Biopharm.* 2021;160:152–7.

67. Darwich AS, Pade D, Ammori BJ, Jamei M, Ashcroft DM, Rostami-Hodjegan A. A mechanistic pharmacokinetic model to assess modified oral drug bioavailability post bariatric surgery in morbidly obese patients: Interplay between CYP3A gut wall metabolism, permeability and dissolution. *J Pharm Pharmacol.* 2012;64:1008–24.

68. Chen K-F, Chan L-N, Lin YS. PBPK modeling of CYP3A and P-gp substrates to predict drug-drug interactions in patients undergoing Roux-en-Y gastric bypass surgery. *J Pharmacokinet Pharmacodyn.* 2020;47:493–512.

69. Montanha MC, Diniz A, Silva NMEN, Kimura E, Paixão P. Physiologically-based pharmacokinetic model on the oral drug absorption in Roux-en-Y gastric bypass bariatric patients: Amoxicillin tablet and suspension. *Mol Pharm.* 2019;16:5025–34.

70. Yu LX, Amidon GL. Saturable small intestinal drug absorption in humans: Modeling and interpretation of cefatrizine data. *Eur J Pharm Biopharm.* 1998;45:199–203.

71. Paixão P, Gouveia LF, Morais JAG. Prediction of the human oral bioavailability by using in vitro and in silico drug related parameters in a physiologically based absorption model. *Int J Pharm.* 2012;429:84–98.

72. Porat D, Dukhno O, Vainer E, Cvijić S, Dahan A. Antiallergic treatment of bariatric patients: Potentially hampered solubility/dissolution and bioavailability of loratadine, but not desloratadine, post-bariatric surgery. *Mol Pharm.* 2022;19:2922–36.

73. Koziolek M, Grimm M, Becker D, Iordanov V, Zou H, Shimizu J, et al. Investigation of pH and temperature profiles in the GI tract of fasted human subjects using the Intellicap® system. *J Pharm Sci.* 2015;104:2855–63.

74. Feldman M, Barnett C. Fasting gastric pH and its relationship to true hypochlorhydria in humans. *Dig Dis Sci.* 1991;36:866–9.

75. Freire AC, Basit AW, Choudhary R, Piong CW, Merchant HA. Does sex matter? The influence of gender on gastrointestinal physiology and drug delivery. *Int J Pharm.* 2011;415:15–28.

76. Stillhart C, Vučićević K, Augustijns P, Basit AW, Batchelor H, Flanagan TR, et al. Impact of gastrointestinal physiology on drug absorption in special populations--An UNGAP review. *Eur J Pharm Sci.* 2020;147:105280.

77. Feldman M. The mature stomach. Still pumping out acid? *JAMA.* 1997;278:681–2.

78. Russell TL, Berardi RR, Barnett JL, Dermentzoglou LC, Jarvenpaa KM, Schmaltz SP, et al. Upper gastrointestinal pH in seventy-nine healthy, elderly, North American men and women. *Pharm Res.* 1993;10:187–96.

79. Dressman JB, Berardi RR, Dermentzoglou LC, Russell TL, Schmaltz SP, Barnett JL, et al. Upper gastrointestinal (GI) pH in young, healthy men and women. *Pharm Res.* 1990;7:756–61.

80. Koziolek M, Grimm M, Garbacz G, Kühn J-P, Weitschies W. Intragastric volume changes after intake of a high-caloric, high-fat standard breakfast in healthy human subjects investigated by MRI. *Mol Pharm.* 2014;11:1632–9.

81. Koziolek M, Schneider F, Grimm M, Modeβ C, Seekamp A, Roustom T, et al. Intragastric pH and pressure profiles after intake of the high-caloric, high-fat meal as used for food effect studies. *J Control Release.* 2015;220:71–8.

82. Pentafragka C, Vertzoni M, Symillides M, Goumas K, Reppas C. Disposition of two highly permeable drugs in the upper gastrointestinal lumen of healthy adults after a standard high-calorie, high-fat meal. *Eur J Pharm Sci.* 2020;149:105351.

83. Vinarov Z, Abdallah M, Agundez JAG, Allegaert K, Basit AW, Braeckmans M, et al. Impact of gastrointestinal tract variability on oral drug absorption and pharmacokinetics: An UNGAP review. *Eur J Pharm Sci.* 2021;162:105812.

84. Costantine MM. Physiologic and pharmacokinetic changes in pregnancy. *Front Pharmacol.* 2014;5:65.

85. Pariente G, Leibson T, Carls A, Adams-Webber T, Ito S, Koren G. Pregnancy-associated changes in pharmacokinetics: A systematic review. *PLoS Med.* 2016;13:e1002160.

86. O'Sullivan GM, Bullingham RE. The assessment of gastric acidity and antacid effect in pregnant women by a non-invasive radiotelemetry technique. *Br J Obstet Gynaecol.* 1984;91:973–8.

87. Van Thiel DH, Gavaler JS, Joshi SN, Sara RK, Stremple J. Heartburn of pregnancy. *Gastroenterology.* 1977;72:666–8.

88. Lu P-J, Hsu P-I, Chen C-H, Hsiao M, Chang W-C, Tseng H-H, et al. Gastric juice acidity in upper gastrointestinal diseases. *World J Gastroenterol.* 2010;16:5496–501.

89. Ghosh T, Lewis DI, Axon ATR, Everett SM. Review article: Methods of measuring gastric acid secretion. *Aliment Pharmacol Ther.* 2011;33:768–81.

90. El-Omar EM. Mechanisms of increased acid secretion after eradication of Helicobacter pylori infection. *Gut.* 2006;55:144–6.

91. Segregur D, Flanagan T, Mann J, Moir A, Karlsson EM, Hoch M, et al. Impact of acid-reducing agents on gastrointestinal physiology and design of biorelevant dissolution tests to reflect these changes. *J Pharm Sci.* 2019;108:3461–77.

92. Williams MP, Sercombe J, Hamilton MI, Pounder RE. A placebo-controlled trial to assess the effects of 8 days of dosing with rabeprazole versus omeprazole on 24-h intragastric acidity and plasma gastrin concentrations in young healthy male subjects. *Aliment Pharmacol Ther.* 1998;12:1079–89.

93. Kirchheiner J, Glatt S, Fuhr U, Klotz U, Meineke I, Seufferlein T, et al. Relative potency of proton-pump inhibitors-comparison of effects on intragastric pH. *Eur J Clin Pharmacol.* 2009;65:19–31.

94. Foltz E, Azad S, Everett ML, Holzknecht ZE, Sanders NL, Thompson JW, et al. An assessment of human gastric fluid composition as a function of PPI usage. *Physiol Rep.* 2015;3:e12269.

95. Strand DS, Kim D, Peura DA. 25 years of proton pump inhibitors: A comprehensive review. *Gut Liver.* 2017;11:27–37.

96. Miner P, Katz PO, Chen Y, Sostek M. Gastric acid control with esomeprazole, lansoprazole, omeprazole, pantoprazole, and rabeprazole: A five-way crossover study. *Am J Gastroenterol.* 2003;98:2616–20.

97. Abuhelwa AY, Mudge S, Upton RN, Foster DJR. Mechanistic assessment of the effect of omeprazole on the in vivo pharmacokinetics of itraconazole in healthy volunteers. *Eur J Drug Metab Pharmacokinet.* 2019;44:201–15.

98. Lin MS, Sun P, Yu HY. Evaluation of buffering capacity and acid neutralizing-pH time profile of antacids. *J Formos Med Assoc.* 1998;97:704–10.

99. Sulz MC, Manz M, Grob P, Meier R, Drewe J, Beglinger C. Comparison of two antacid preparations on intragastric acidity--a two-centre open randomised cross-over placebo-controlled trial. *Digestion.* 2007;75:69–73.

100. Tripathi A, Somwanshi M, Singh B, Bajaj P. A comparison of intravenous ranitidine and omeprazole on gastric volume and pH in women undergoing emergency caesarean section. *Can J Anaesth.* 1995;42:797–800.

101. Dubin SA, Silverstein PI, Wakefield ML, Jense HG. Comparison of the effects of oral famotidine and ranitidine on gastric volume and pH. *Anesth Analg.* 1989;69:680–3.

102. Narchi P, Edouard D, Bourget P, Otz J, Cattaneo I. Gastric fluid pH and volume in gynaecologic out-patients. Influences of cimetidine and cimetidine-sodium citrate combination. *Eur J Anaesthesiol.* 1993;10:357–61.

103. Smith JL, Gamal MA, Chremos AN, Graham DY. Famotidine, a new H2-receptor antagonist. Effect on parietal, nonparietal, and pepsin secretion in man. *Dig Dis Sci.* 1985;30:308–12.

104. Longstreth GF, Go VL, Malagelada JR. Postprandial gastric, pancreatic, and biliary response to histamine H2-receptor antagonists active duodenal ulcer. *Gastroenterology.* 1977;72:9–13.

105. Richardson CT, Walsh JH, Hicks MI. The effect of cimetidine, a new histamine H2-receptor antagonist, on meal-stimulated acid secretion, serum gastrin, and gastric emptying in patients with duodenal ulcer. *Gastroenterology.* 1976;71:19–23.

106. Domschke W, Lux G, Domschke S. Furan H2-antagonist ranitidine inhibits pentagastrin-stimulated gastric secretion stronger than cimetidine. *Gastroenterology.* 1980;79:1267–71.

107. Stoll VS, Blanchard JS. Buffers: Principles and practice. *Methods Enzymol.* 2009;463:43–56.

108. Heda R, Toro F, Tombazzi CR. Physiology, Pepsin. In: *StatPearls* [Internet]. Treasure Island (FL): StatPearls Publishing; 2023 [cited 2023 Mar 29]. Available from: https://www.ncbi.nlm.nih.gov/books/NBK537005/.

109. Piper DW, Fenton BH. pH stability and activity curves of pepsin with special reference to their clinical importance. *Gut.* 1965;6:506–8.

110. Bodmeier R, Guo X, Sarabia RE, Skultety PF. The influence of buffer species and strength on diltiazem HCl release from beads coated with the aqueous cationic polymer dispersions, Eudragit RS, RL 30D. *Pharm Res.* 1996;13:52–6.

111. Litou C, Vertzoni M, Goumas C, Vasdekis V, Xu W, Kesisoglou F, et al. Characteristics of the human upper gastrointestinal contents in the fasted state under hypo- and A-chlorhydric gastric conditions under conditions of typical drug - drug interaction studies. *Pharm Res.* 2016;33:1399–412.

112. Mann J, Dressman J, Rosenblatt K, Ashworth L, Muenster U, Frank K, et al. Validation of dissolution testing with biorelevant media: An OrBiTo study. *Mol Pharm.* 2017;14:4192–201.

113. Kesisoglou F, Vertzoni M, Reppas C. Physiologically based absorption modeling of salts of weak bases based on data in hypochlorhydric and achlorhydric biorelevant media. *AAPS PharmSciTech.* 2018;19:2851–8.

114. Litou C, Vertzoni M, Xu W, Kesisoglou F, Reppas C. The impact of reduced gastric acid secretion on dissolution of salts of weak bases in the fasted upper gastrointestinal lumen: Data in biorelevant media and in human aspirates. *Eur J Pharm Biopharm.* 2017;115:94–101.

115. Butler J, Hens B, Vertzoni M, Brouwers J, Berben P, Dressman J, et al. In vitro models for the prediction of in vivo performance of oral dosage forms: Recent progress from partnership through the IMI OrBiTo collaboration. *Eur J Pharm Biopharm.* 2019;136:70–83.

116. Fotaki N, Klein S. Mechanistic understanding of the effect of PPIs and acidic carbonated beverages on the oral absorption of itraconazole based on absorption modeling with appropriate in vitro data. *Mol Pharm.* 2013;10:4016–23.

117. Buchanan CM, Buchanan NL, Edgar KJ, Klein S, Little JL, Ramsey MG, et al. Pharmacokinetics of itraconazole after intravenous and oral dosing of itraconazole-cyclodextrin formulations. *J Pharm Sci.* 2007;96:3100–16.

118. Lahner E, Annibale B, Delle Fave G. Systematic review: Impaired drug absorption related to the co-administration of antisecretory therapy. *Aliment Pharmacol Ther.* 2009;29:1219–29.

119. Jaruratanasirikul S, Sriwiriyajan S. Effect of omeprazole on the pharmacokinetics of itraconazole. *Eur J Clin Pharmacol.* 1998;54:159–61.

120. Lim SG, Sawyerr AM, Hudson M, Sercombe J, Pounder RE. Short report: The absorption of fluconazole and itraconazole under conditions of low intragastric acidity. *Aliment Pharmacol Ther.* 1993;7:317–21.

121. López Mármol Á, Fischer PL, Wahl A, Schwöbel D, Lenz V, Sauer K, et al. Application of tiny-TIM as a mechanistic tool to investigate the in vitro performance of different itraconazole formulations under physiologically relevant conditions. *Eur J Pharm Sci.* 2022;173:106165.

122. Minekus M, Marteau P, Havenaar R, Veld JHJHIT. A multicompartmental dynamic computer-controlled model simulating the stomach and small intestine. *Altern Lab Anim.* 1995;23:197–209.

123. Segregur D, Barker R, Mann J, Moir A, Karlsson EM, Turner DB, et al. Evaluating the impact of acid-reducing agents on drug absorption using biorelevant in vitro tools and PBPK modeling - case example dipyridamole. *Eur J Pharm Sci.* 2021;160:105750.

124. U.S. Food and Drug Administration. Evaluation of Gastric pH-Dependent Drug Interactions With Acid-Reducing Agents: Study Design, Data Analysis, and Clinical Implications Guidance for Industry [Internet]. U.S. Food and Drug Administration. 2023 [cited 2023 Mar

29]. Available from: https://www.fda.gov/regulatory-information/search-fda-guidance-doc-uments/evaluation-gastric-ph-dependent-drug-interactions-acid-reducing-agents-study-desi gn-data-analysis.

125. Ooi CY, Durie PR. Cystic fibrosis from the gastroenterologist's perspective. *Nat Rev Gastroenterol Hepatol.* 2016;13:175–85.

126. Castellani C, Assael BM. Cystic fibrosis: A clinical view. *Cell Mol Life Sci.* 2017;74:129–40.

127. Savant A, Lyman B, Bojanowski C, Upadia J. Cystic Fibrosis. In: Adam MP, Mirzaa GM, Pagon RA, Wallace SE, Bean LJ, Gripp KW, et al., editors. *GeneReviews®* [Internet]. Seattle (WA): University of Washington, Seattle; 1993 [cited 2023 Mar 20]. Available from: https://www.ncbi.nlm.nih.gov/books/NBK1250/.

128. Freswick PN, Reid EK, Mascarenhas MR. Pancreatic enzyme replacement therapy in cystic fibrosis. *Nutrients.* 2022;14:1341.

129. De Lisle RC, Borowitz D. The cystic fibrosis intestine. *Cold Spring Harb Perspect Med.* 2013;3:a009753.

130. Engjom T, Erchinger F, Lærum BN, Tjora E, Aksnes L, Gilja OH, et al. Diagnostic accuracy of a short endoscopic secretin test in patients with cystic fibrosis. *Pancreas.* 2015;44:1266–72.

131. Gelfond D, Ma C, Semler J, Borowitz D. Intestinal pH and gastrointestinal transit profiles in cystic fibrosis patients measured by wireless motility capsule. *Dig Dis Sci.* 2013;58:2275–81.

132. Rey E, Tréluyer JM, Pons G. Drug disposition in cystic fibrosis. *Clin Pharmacokinet.* 1998;35:313–29.

133. Touw DJ, Vinks AA, Mouton JW, Horrevorts AM. Pharmacokinetic optimisation of antibacterial treatment in patients with cystic fibrosis. Current practice and suggestions for future directions. *Clin Pharmacokinet.* 1998;35:137–59.

134. Scott CS, Retsch-Bogart GZ, Kustra RP, Graham KM, Glasscock BJ, Smith PC. The pharmacokinetics of ibuprofen suspension, chewable tablets, and tablets in children with cystic fibrosis. *J Pediatr.* 1999;134:58–63.

135. Konstan MW, Hoppel CL, Chai BL, Davis PB. Ibuprofen in children with cystic fibrosis: Pharmacokinetics and adverse effects. *J Pediatr.* 1991;118:956–64.

136. Silva IAL, Laselva O, Lopes-Pacheco M. Advances in preclinical in vitro models for the translation of precision medicine for cystic fibrosis. *J Pers Med.* 2022;12:1321.

137. Dekkers JF, Wiegerinck CL, de Jonge HR, Bronsveld I, Janssens HM, de Winter-de Groot KM, et al. A functional CFTR assay using primary cystic fibrosis intestinal organoids. *Nat Med.* 2013;19:939–45.

138. Conti J, Sorio C, Melotti P. Organoid technology and its role for theratyping applications in cystic fibrosis. *Children (Basel).* 2022;10:4.

139. Dumas M-P, Xia S, Bear CE, Ratjen F. Perspectives on the translation of in-vitro studies to precision medicine in Cystic Fibrosis. *EBioMedicine.* 2021;73:103660.

140. Sato T, Clevers H. Growing self-organizing mini-guts from a single intestinal stem cell: Mechanism and applications. *Science.* 2013;340:1190–4.

141. Calvo-Lerma J, Fornés-Ferrer V, Peinado I, Heredia A, Ribes-Koninckx C, Andrés A. A first approach for an evidence-based in vitro digestion method to adjust pancreatic enzyme replacement therapy in cystic fibrosis. *PLoS One.* 2019;14:e0212459.

142. Zentler-Munro PL, Assoufi BA, Balasubramanian K, Cornell S, Benoliel D, Northfield TC, et al. Therapeutic potential and clinical efficacy of acid-resistant fungal lipase in the treatment of pancreatic steatorrhoea due to cystic fibrosis. *Pancreas.* 1992;7:311–9.

143. Cicali B, Long T, Kim S, Cristofoletti R. Assessing the impact of cystic fibrosis on the antipyretic response of ibuprofen in children: Physiologically-based modeling as a candle in the dark. *Br J Clin Pharmacol.* 2020;86:2247–55.

144. Shapiro JM, Subedi S, LeLeiko NS. Inflammatory bowel disease. *Pediatr Rev.* 2016;37:337–47.

145. Rosen MJ, Dhawan A, Saeed SA. Inflammatory bowel disease in children and adolescents. *JAMA Pediatr.* 2015;169:1053–60.

146. Flynn S, Eisenstein S. Inflammatory bowel disease presentation and diagnosis. *Surg Clin North Am.* 2019;99:1051–62.

147. Alrubia S, Mao J, Chen Y, Barber J, Rostami-Hodjegan A. Altered bioavailability and pharmacokinetics in Crohn's disease: Capturing systems parameters for PBPK to assist with predicting the fate of orally administered drugs. *Clin Pharmacokinet.* 2022;61:1365–92.

148. Sairenji T, Collins KL, Evans DV. An update on inflammatory bowel disease. *Prim Care.* 2017;44:673–92.

149. Effinger A, O'Driscoll CM, McAllister M, Fotaki N. Impact of gastrointestinal disease states on oral drug absorption - implications for formulation design - a PEARRL review. *J Pharm Pharmacol.* 2019;71:674–98.

150. Effinger A, O'Driscoll CM, McAllister M, Fotaki N. Predicting budesonide performance in healthy subjects and patients with Crohn's disease using biorelevant in vitro dissolution testing and PBPK modeling. *Eur J Pharm Sci.* 2021;157:105617.

151. Effinger A, McAllister M, Tomaszewska I, O'Driscoll CM, Taylor M, Gomersall S, et al. Investigating the impact of Crohn's disease on the bioaccessibility of a lipid-based formulation with an in vitro dynamic gastrointestinal model. *Mol Pharm.* 2021;18:1530–43.

152. Marafini I, Sedda S, Dinallo V, Monteleone G. Inflammatory cytokines: From discoveries to therapies in IBD. *Expert Opin Biol Ther.* 2019;19:1207–17.

153. Yoo J-H, Donowitz M. Intestinal enteroids/organoids: A novel platform for drug discovery in inflammatory bowel diseases. *World J Gastroenterol.* 2019;25:4125–47.

154. Hou Q, Huang J, Ayansola H, Masatoshi H, Zhang B. Intestinal stem cells and immune cell relationships: Potential therapeutic targets for inflammatory bowel diseases. *Front Immunol.* 2020;11:623691.

155. McKay DM, Philpott DJ, Perdue MH. Review article: In vitro models in inflammatory bowel disease research--a critical review. *Aliment Pharmacol Ther.* 1997;11(Suppl 3):70–80.

156. Briggs R, Kennelly SP, O'Neill D. Drug treatments in Alzheimer's disease. *Clin Med (Lond).* 2016;16:247–53.

157. Waller ES, Yardeny BJ, Fong WY, Gan XY, Jimenez SV, Pan Y, et al. Altered peripheral factors affecting the absorption, distribution, metabolism, and excretion of oral medicines in Alzheimer's disease. *Adv Drug Deliv Rev.* 2022;185:114282.

158. Jin L, Pan Y, Tran NLL, Polychronopoulos LN, Warrier A, Brouwer KLR, et al. Intestinal permeability and oral absorption of selected drugs are reduced in a mouse model of familial Alzheimer's disease. *Mol Pharm.* 2020;17:1527–37.

159. Parnetti L. Clinical pharmacokinetics of drugs for Alzheimer's disease. *Clin Pharmacokinet.* 1995;29:110–29.

160. Lee B-H, Choi S-H, Kim H-J, Park S-D, Rhim H, Kim H-C, et al. Gintonin absorption in intestinal model systems. *J Ginseng Res.* 2018;42:35–41.

161. Ma Z, Wang N, He H, Tang X. Pharmaceutical strategies of improving oral systemic bioavailability of curcumin for clinical application. *J Control Release.* 2019;316:359–80.

162. Li Z, Ramirez G, Tang R, Paul CKX, Nair M, Henderson S, et al. Modeling digestion, absorption, and ketogenesis after administration of tricaprilin formulations to humans. *Eur J Pharm Biopharm.* 2023;182:41–52.

163. Wollmer E, Klein S. A review of patient-specific gastrointestinal parameters as a platform for developing in vitro models for predicting the in vivo performance of oral dosage forms in patients with Parkinson's disease. *Int J Pharm.* 2017;533:298–314.

164. Leta V, Klingelhoefer L, Longardner K, Campagnolo M, Levent HÇ, Aureli F, et al. Gastrointestinal barriers to levodopa transport and absorption in Parkinson's disease. *Eur J Neurol.* 2023;30:1465–80.

165. Pfeiffer RF, Isaacson SH, Pahwa R. Clinical implications of gastric complications on levodopa treatment in Parkinson's disease. *Parkinsonism Relat Disord.* 2020;76:63–71.

166. Mukherjee A, Biswas A, Das SK. Gut dysfunction in Parkinson's disease. *World J Gastroenterol.* 2016;22:5742–52.

167. Djaldetti R, Ziv I, Melamed E. Impaired absorption of oral levodopa: A major cause for response fluctuations in Parkinson's disease. *Isr J Med Sci.* 1996;32:1224–7.

168. Urso D, Chaudhuri KR, Qamar MA, Jenner P. Improving the delivery of levodopa in Parkinson's disease: A Review of approved and emerging therapies. *CNS Drugs.* 2020;34:1149–63.

169. Wollmer E, Klein S. Patient-specific in vitro drug release testing coupled with in silico PBPK modeling to forecast the in vivo performance of oral extended-release levodopa formulations in Parkinson's disease patients. *Eur J Pharm Biopharm.* 2022;180:101–18.

170. Boyina HK, Geethakhrishnan SL, Panuganti S, Gangarapu K, Devarakonda KP, Bakshi V, et al. In silico and in vivo studies on quercetin as potential anti-Parkinson agent. *Adv Exp Med Biol.* 2020;1195:1–11.

171. Rohatagi S, Barrett JS, DeWitt KE, Lessard D, Morales RJ. Pharmacokinetic evaluation of a selegiline pulsatile oral delivery system. *Biopharm Drug Dispos.* 1997;18:665–80.

172. Mahmood I, Marinac JS, Willsie S, Mason WD. Pharmacokinetics and relative bioavailability of selegiline in healthy volunteers. *Biopharm Drug Dispos.* 1995;16:535–45.

4 Physiologically-Based Absorption Models for Complex Formulations and Dosage Forms

Maxime Le Merdy, William W van Osdol, and Viera Lukacova

4.1 INTRODUCTION

Complex dosage forms comprise a large family of drug products. They can be initially classified based on their route of administration: injectable, oral, and non-oral (Figure 4.1).

Injectable drug products can be subdivided into two subcategories: direct injection into the bloodstream (intravenous administration) and injection into another tissue (e.g., subcutaneous, intramuscular administration) (Figure 4.1). Drug products injected directly into the bloodstream can be considered complex based on the formulation characteristics. For example, Doxil®, a liposome-based formulation was the first approved nano-drug on the US market used to reduce the doxorubicin side effects and enhance its anti-tumoral effect [1]. Other active pharmaceutical ingredients (APIs), formulated in injectable drug products are defined as complex, either based on their injection sites: intramuscular, subcutaneous, intraocular, intraarticular, or due to formulation characteristics.

Complex oral and non-oral drug products can be subdivided into three subcategories based on the relative contribution of the gut absorption pathway to the total absorption of the API (Figure 4.1). Orally administered drug products with absorption occurring only from the gastrointestinal (GI) tract can be defined as complex based on the formulation characteristics. For example, lipid-based formulations are utilized to enhance the absorption of highly lipophilic APIs or target the lymphatic system [2]. In addition, orally administered drug products aiming to cure GI diseases are classified as complex due to their limited bioavailability and the lack of correlation between the systemic exposure and the exposure at the site of action in the GI tract. Non-oral drug products are designed to be used locally to treat diseases directly in a specific tissue with a minimal distribution of the API in the rest of the body. For some of those drug products (e.g., dermal formulations), there is no absorption occurring through the GI tract. However, some of the locally acting drug products still present a significant GI absorption due to anatomical and physiological constraints. This is particularly the case for pulmonary drug products where a significant portion of the administered dose can be swallowed instead of being deposited into the lung airways [3].

Therefore, it should be noted that a drug product's complexity can be multifactorial: the formulation itself, the formulation interaction with a given API, the route of administration, or any combination of these factors.

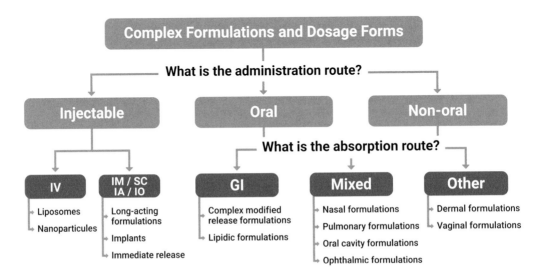

Figure 4.1 Classification diagram of complex formulations and dosage forms. Abbreviation: IV: Intravenous; IM: Intramuscular; SC: Subcutaneous; IA: Intraarticular; IO: Intraocular; GI: Gastrointestinal.

DOI: 10.1201/9781003031802-4

Regardless of the underlying cause of the complexity of a drug product, the absorption of an API into the human body is a critical first step toward clinical efficacy. A common trait of complex dosage forms is the interactions of the physicochemical properties of the API and formulation excipients with the physiology of the site of administration (e.g., gut lumen, eye tissue, skin, and subcutaneous tissue). Those interactions determine the rate and extent of API absorption and should be well understood to support the development of new and generic drug products.

To investigate these interactions, the pharmaceutical industry relies on a combination of *in vitro* (e.g., dissolution testing) and *in vivo* (e.g., preclinical pharmacokinetic studies) studies. Both present advantages and limitations. *In vitro* analyses are relatively inexpensive and permit the characterization of complex formulations systematically in a controlled, reproducible environment. Yet, *in vitro* studies cannot replicate all the nuances of API absorption *in vivo*. On the other hand, *in vivo* studies can help investigate those complex interactions. However, their costs and the lack of reproducibility limit their usage during drug product development.

To overcome those limitations, the pharmaceutical industry, supported by regulatory authorities, has identified physiologically-based pharmacokinetic (PBPK) models as a valuable tool to support the development of complex dosage forms. A PBPK core algorithm attempts to mathematically describe the interactions between the API, formulation, and physiology that govern the API's absorption and disposition. PBPK models have been employed to study numerous complex drug products administered using multiple routes of administration. He et al. reviewed how PBPK models, among other modeling tools, could support the development and regulation of liposomal drugs [4]. Le Merdy et al. developed and validated a PBPK model to study drugs administered within the knee joint [5]. Dolton et al explored the role of intestinal lymphatic transport on halofantrine GI absorption using a PBPK model [6]. Miller et al. mechanistically described the pulmonary and oral absorption pathways of inhaled nemiralisib using a PBPK model [7]. These examples showcase the vast range of PBPK applications for complex drug products.

This chapter presents, using two examples, how a PBPK model, parameterized based on *in vitro* and *in vivo* data, can predict the clinical behavior of complex ocular and dermal formulations.

4.2 OCULAR PBPK MODEL

Ophthalmic drug products are used to treat local ocular diseases in humans such as glaucoma, inflammation, or infection. The eye is divided into the anterior and posterior segments. The anterior segment includes the cornea, iris, ciliary body, and lens as well as the spaces of the anterior and posterior chambers filled with aqueous humor. The posterior segment includes the retina, choroid, and optic nerve head as well as the vitreous compartment filled with vitreous humor. Sclera is present in both segments. The globe is protected by the eyelids: mobile structures whose role is to produce and distribute tears over the eyeball and to regulate the amount of light having access to the eye. The inner layer of the eyelids and the anterior sclera are lined by a mucous membrane called conjunctiva [8].

The main challenge in ophthalmic drug development is to ensure that sufficient amount of an API can reach the site of action to obtain the desired pharmacological effect. Multiple routes of administration have been developed to treat ocular diseases.

Currently, most ophthalmic drug products are administered topically by depositing the formulation on the exposed surface of the eyeball. Following topical administration, portion of the dose (minor portion) is absorbed into the eye (productive absorption) and the majority of the dose is either lost or absorbed into the systemic circulation (non-productive absorption) [9]. Ocular bioavailability of topically administered atenolol, timolol, and betaxolol in albino rabbits was reported to be 0.07%, 1.51%, and 4.31%, respectively [10]. This results in more than 95% of the administered dose not being absorbed into the ocular tissues. Therefore, this administration route is typically employed to treat anterior segment diseases.

To overcome the limited absorption of the APIs using the topical route, multiple innovative strategies have been implemented by the pharmaceutical industry to increase APIs' exposure in the posterior segment of the eye. First, drug-eluding contact lenses or subconjunctival implants have been developed. The aim of those dosage forms is to slowly liberate an API on the surface of the eye to increase its ocular exposure. In addition, intracameral and intravitreal injections of the formulated API deliver high drug levels directly into the aqueous humor and the vitreous humor, respectively. The API can then freely diffuse into the surrounding ocular tissues. However, in addition to significant patient non-compliance [11], these injections have specific associated risks such as retinal detachment or toxic anterior segment syndrome. To limit the number of injections, ophthalmic inserts, placed between the vitreous humor and the retina have been developed [12].

Hence, significant limitations remain and must be considered in the design of all ophthalmic drug products. Therefore, to support the development and regulatory assessment of ophthalmic drug products, pharmaceutical industries, academic groups, and health authorities have developed mechanistic models to describe APIs' ocular exposure. Ocular PBPK models can provide an insight into drug partitioning in the eye tissues that are not accessible and/or are challenging to sample in humans and serve as an alternative methodology to study ophthalmic drugs PK and PD. The rabbit eyeball is anatomically and physiologically comparable to the human eyeball [13], therefore rabbits have been used as the main preclinical model to investigate ocular exposure of ophthalmic drug products. The PBPK models can be subsequently used to extrapolate preclinical data into human ocular exposure [13].

4.2.1 History of Ocular *in silico* Models

Several *in silico* PK models of ocular drug delivery have been developed to describe the absorption, distribution, and elimination of ocular drugs in the eyeball. Over time, the physiological level of complexity of the published models and the concept used for model validation improved significantly.

The early models describing ocular PK of an API following topical administration were simple one-compartment models, representing the cornea with absorption and elimination rate constants. The volume of the compartment was apparent and not linked to the eyeball physiology [13]. This basic model was extended by including a pre-corneal compartment where the formulation is administered and can be eliminated by a drainage rate. The drainage rate constant was a fitted formulation-specific first-order constant that was not correlated to an actual measured flow rate [13]. A three-compartment model including the pre-corneal space, cornea, and aqueous humor compartments had been fitted to describe the data in those biophases following topical administration of pilocarpine to albino rabbits [13]. Four- and five-compartment models have been developed to increase the model's physiological relevance by splitting the cornea into its epithelium and stroma layers. Other ocular tissues are lumped into a reservoir compartment [14,15,16]. All the models cited above assumed either unidirectional or bidirectional transfer of the API from one compartment to the adjacent one. An expanded five-compartment PK model including the pre-corneal area, cornea, aqueous humor, ICB and lens, connected in a relevant physiological pattern was developed for the intraocular disposition of pilocarpine This model also included bidirectional movement between all adjacent compartments [17]. Although this model is one of the first attempts to develop a PBPK model capable of describing ocular PK, it used a top-down approach to estimate the transfer rates between the tissue compartments. Furthermore, the volumes of distribution for each tissue were derived from *in vitro* equilibrium distribution coefficient for pilocarpine between ocular tissues and phosphate buffer [17]. Figure 4.2 presents this structural evolution of mathematical models used to describe APIs' ocular exposure.

Complexities of those models were subsequently increased by integrating additional key mechanisms involved in the ocular disposition of an API after topical administration. In 1986, Hui & Robinson published a specific model for pilocarpine and fluorometholone suspensions, incorporating drug dissolution, drug pre-cornea drainage and tear flow elimination in both solid and solution phases, and passive diffusion from cornea epithelium to the aqueous humor [18]. Tear fluid pH variation in the pre-cornea compartment was included to account for the impact of tear pH on drug solubility over time [19]. The impact of melanin binding on ocular drug delivery was modeled by Rimpelä et al [20]. A mechanistic model aimed to correlate the aqueous humor and plasma exposures. This model mechanistically describes the formulation transfer from the pre-corneal space into the nasal cavity and subsequently into the systemic circulation [21]. All these models focused on drug distribution within only a limited number of ocular tissues following topical administration and addressed only limited formulation characteristics.

Intravitreal administration of a small molecule has been described using a compartmental model. This model includes the vitreous humor, a lumped ocular tissue compartment and the systemic compartment [22]. In this model, the vitreous humor volume was fitted to a final value comparable to observed physiological values. All the other tissues' volumes and transfer rate constant were also fitted, resulting in poor physiological relevancy of this model. Multiple models focusing on the intravitreal injection of small peptides and macromolecules were recently developed [23,24,25,26,27,28,29,30]. Among those, Bussing & Shah published a full ocular PBPK model including the cornea, aqueous humor, vitreous humor, retina, choroid, sclera, and lens tissues. This model was used to predict the ocular disposition of monoclonal antibody in rabbits [30].

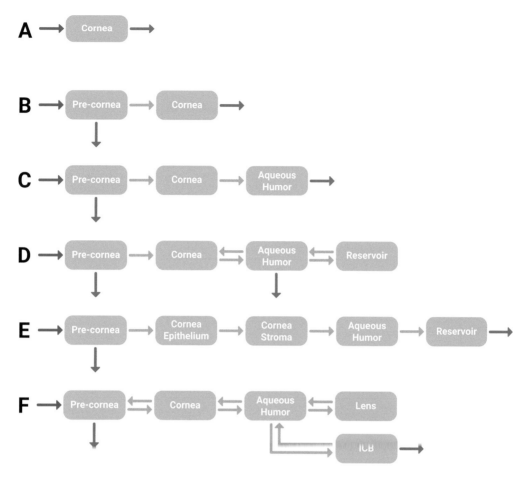

Figure 4.2 Schematic representation of the structural evolution of mathematical models used to describe APIs ocular exposure. A) single compartment model; B) two compartments model including tear drainage; C) three compartments model including tear drainage; D) four compartments model including tear drainage and a reservoir compartment; E) five compartments model including tear drainage and a reservoir compartment; F) five compartments model including tear drainage and bidirectional transfer of an API across ocular tissues. Red arrows are input functions, blue arrows are clearance parameters, and gray arrows are transfer rate parameters.

Other modeling approaches have also been used to describe the ocular PK following topical administration or injection of an API. Computational fluid dynamic (CFD) models were created to investigate the behavior of small and large molecules following their intravitreal and intracameral administrations [31,32], to discern the intravitreal drug distribution differences between the rabbit and human [33], and to simulate drug distribution in the posterior segment of the eye after intravitreal administration and ocular implantation [34]. Owing to their ability to represent the eyeball in three dimensions, these models allowed the investigation of important factors in intravitreal injection such as injection time, needle gauge or angle, and the influence of the position and the type of implant on the API concentration profile in the posterior eye segment. However, these models are computationally "expensive" and are not suitable for routine use due to computation time necessary to perform a simulation. In addition, pharmacometrics models were used to describe lampalizumab PK following intravitreal administration to patients [35]. Pharmacometrics models were also used to investigate azithromycin PK in tears following topical administration [36] or to study the ocular distribution of a tyrosine kinase inhibitor in rabbits [37]. These models used a top-down approach, and their structures have none, or minimal, physiological relevancy.

4.2.2 OCAT Model

To address the limitations of the previously published models, the Ocular Compartmental Absorption and Transit (OCAT™) model was developed and validated. The first version of the OCAT model was created in collaboration between Simulations Plus, Inc. and a large pharmaceutical company. This initial model consisted of eight ocular compartments: pre-cornea, cornea, aqueous humor, iris-ciliary body, vitreous humor, conjunctiva, sclera-choroid, and retina. The drug exchange between the ocular tissues and the systemic circulation could occur in the iris-ciliary body, conjunctiva, and retina. The model also incorporated melanin binding in relevant tissues and tear flow rate with possible clearance of drug directly into the nasolacrimal duct after topical administration. Over time, the structure of the OCAT model was expanded by separating cornea into the corneal epithelium and corneal stroma; separating conjunctiva into bulbar and palpebral sections; splitting vitreous humor and sclera compartments into anterior and posterior sections; creating a separate, vascularized, choroid compartment; adding impact of convective flows mediated by the aqueous humor dynamics on the drug distribution throughout the eye; adding protein binding in all ocular tissues; and incorporating the effect of topical formulation pH on API's productive absorption. A schematic diagram of the OCAT model (version 3) is shown in Figure 4.3.

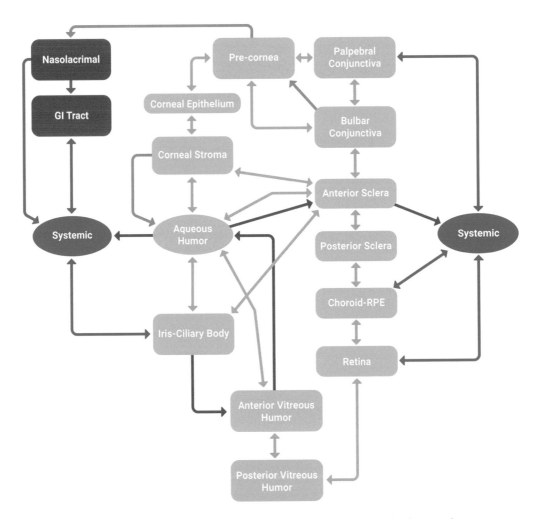

Figure 4.3   OCAT model version 3 schematic. Gray arrows represent the drug exchange between adjacent ocular compartments through passive diffusion and/or carrier-mediated transport, orange and red arrows represent the drug movement due to convective fluid flow between the compartments, blue arrows represent the drug exchange between perfused ocular tissues and systemic circulation through passive diffusion and/or carrier-mediated transport.

In this model, once the drug is dosed in a specific ocular compartment, it is subjected to a variety of mechanisms resulting in drug loss, productive and non-productive absorption, distribution, and clearance. A complete description of the OCAT model and underlying equations have been published [38]. The capacity of this model to predict local and systemic concentrations of APIs administered in rabbits as topical ophthalmic suspensions or ointments has been published [38,39]. Following this work, interspecies PK extrapolation was validated using multiple case studies [40]. Recent studies demonstrated how the OCAT model can be used to support the biopharmaceutical development of ophthalmic drug products [41,42].

4.2.3 PBPK-Based PK Preclinical to Clinical Extrapolation for Ophthalmic Drug Products

The OCAT model was employed in the development of a stepwise method for preclinical to clinical PK extrapolation [40]. First, the ocular PBPK model should be developed and validated based on the observed data obtained in albino New Zealand white rabbits and subsequently extended to include melanin binding in relevant ocular tissues using observed data from pigmented Dutch Belted rabbits. The complete model can then be used to extrapolate the ocular PK in humans. For preclinical to clinical extrapolation, the API-specific parameters remain the same for all species, and the physiological parameters are adjusted to account for the anatomical and physiological differences between humans and laboratory species. Schematic representation of the ocular PBPK-based preclinical to clinical extrapolation is presented in Figure 4.4 (left panel).

To validate the ability of the OCAT model to predict ophthalmic clinical PK/PD based on PBPK models validated against preclinical data, multiple case studies were performed by Simulations Plus scientists, in collaboration with the FDA. One of the case studies was gatifloxacin ophthalmic solution. Gatifloxacin is a topically administered fluoroquinolone for the treatment of local infections on the surface of the eye.

The initial OCAT model for gatifloxacin was developed using measured corneal and aqueous humor concentrations in New Zealand white rabbits. The cornea epithelium permeability and the iris-ciliary body systemic absorption rate were fitted to acutely describe the observed concentration time course in the two tissues, whereas all other OCAT model parameters were kept at the default values. This initial model was developed and validated by describing the observed ophthalmic concentrations in the nine preclinical studies performed on New Zealand rabbits. To account for the effect of melanin binding, the percent of drug not bound to melanin within the iris-ciliary body was fitted to 1% based on observed concentrations obtained on Dutch Belted rabbits. The same value was used for the other ocular tissues containing melanin (retina, choroid, and sclera). Once the OCAT model was fully validated using observed data obtained in both rabbit strains, extrapolation of clinical PK was performed by switching the Dutch Belted rabbit physiology to the default human ocular physiology available in the GastroPlus OCAT model. All the drug-specific parameters were kept at the same values as validated against rabbit data and the dose, dose volume, and dose administration schedule were set to match the clinical studies. Simulated human ocular PK profiles were compared with observed concentration data to assess the OCAT model's ability to predict human ocular exposure based on preclinical data. The OCAT model accurately described the observed aqueous humor clinical data obtained in healthy subjects and patients undergoing cataract, keratoplasty, or vitrectomy surgery. Representative aqueous humor predictions in both rabbit strains and humans are presented in Figure 4.4 (right panel). This case study showcased how an ocular PBPK model can be used to predict clinical ocular exposure, once validated based on preclinical data. Additional details about the gatifloxacin case study (simulations results and model parameters) as well as other case studies have been published [40].

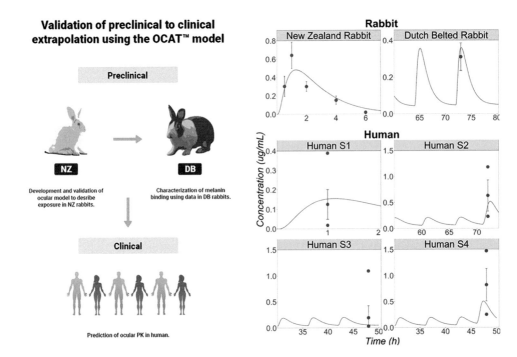

Figure 4.4 Preclinical to clinical extrapolation. Left panel: schematic representation of the extrapolation strategy using the OCAT model. Right panel: representative results obtained as part of the gatifloxacin case study: Top, observed (circles) and simulated (lines) aqueous humor concentrations in New Zealand [43] and Dutch Belted rabbits [44]; Bottom, observed (circles) and simulated (lines) aqueous humor concentrations in humans [45,46,47]. For humans, the observed mean±standard deviation, minimum and maximum concentrations are presented. (Image from [40].)

4.3 DERMAL PBPK MODEL

4.3.1 Introduction

The skin is the human body's largest organ. It is the interface between the body and the surrounding environment and provides the first biological line of defense against infection, radiation, and environmental toxins [48,49]. The skin is composed of three layers. The first and outermost layer of skin is the epidermis: a multilayer stratified squamous epithelium. The epidermis can be divided into the viable epidermis (VE) and the stratum corneum (SC). The VE comprises several anatomically distinct cell layers (stratum basale, stratum spinosam, and stratum granulosum) that undergo progressive differentiation to give rise to the SC, which is composed of a lipid matrix in which stacks of flattened cells packed with keratin bundles are embedded. The dermis is a thick layer of connective tissue lying under the epidermis. The hypodermis, or subcutaneous (SQ) tissue, is the deepest skin layer and is composed primarily of adipose tissue [50,51]. The properties and condition of the skin vary with the body site and can be influenced by various physiological factors such as age, ethnicity, sex, disease states, and nutritional status [52].

Topical and transdermal formulations, used throughout human history to manage skin and systemic conditions, have evolved to comprise a variety of delivery systems that include powders, patches, foams, gels, creams, ointments, and pastes [53]. Their development has been facilitated by advances in our understanding of the thermodynamics and rheology of complex fluids [54,55], quality by design [56,57,58], and design of experiments [59].

Topical drug delivery involves drug transport from a formulation applied to the skin surface to local target sites in one or more anatomically distinct layers of the skin, with subsequent clearance by diffusion into subcutaneous tissue and muscle, metabolism, and uptake into the systemic circulation through dermal blood flow. Advances in dermato-PK have been fostered by decades of research into the barrier function of the skin [60]. Mathematical analysis and computational simulation of permeation have been an integral part of these efforts to understand the structure [61,62,63,64] and transport [65,66,67,68] properties of the SC, VE, dermis [69,70,71,72] and hair follicles [73,74,75], and material exchange with the systemic circulation through skin blood flow [76,77,78,79].

Mathematical modeling of dermal topical formulations that are more complex than solutions or suspensions of a permeant in a single solvent date from at least the 1970s [80,81], with increasing attention paid to the fine structural details of emulsions [82,83,84] and polymeric gels [85,86,87] as their pharmaceutical application became more widespread. Moreover, the behavior of emulsion- and gel- based formulations, particularly as they evolve due to evaporative loss of volatile APIs and excipients, has become a focus of experimental study [88,89,90], mathematical modeling [91,92,93], and regulatory interest.

Great regulatory interest in fostering the development of generic equivalents to reference-listed dermal topical products has led to a need to understand topical product delivery behavior under 'in use' conditions and predicting *in vivo* response to population variations in skin barrier function and response using *in silico* and *in vitro* findings [94]. In the last decade, dermal PBPK models have been developed and validated in collaboration with the FDA [95,96,97,98,99]. Based on those collaborations, in 2020, the FDA approved the first generic topical drug product for which a PBPK model supported the BE assessment (diclofenac sodium 1% topical gel). The PBPK model integrated all available information concerning diclofenac skin permeation and systemic disposition. After model validation, the knowledge repository was leveraged to demonstrate BE between the generic and reference products at the presumed site of action in lieu of conducting a costly and lengthy in vivo comparative clinical endpoint trial in patients [100].

4.3.2 The TCAT Model

Upon the application of a topical or transdermal formulation to the skin, the API and excipients undergo a variety of processes that result in absorption, distribution, and clearance. The Transdermal Compartmental Absorption and Transit (TCAT™) model is a physiologically-based mathematical model within GastroPlus® that simulates the dermal and systemic PK of topically applied compounds. Computationally, the TCAT model is a system of ordinary differential equations that is integrated numerically with respect to time.

The structure of the TCAT model with respect to material exchange pathways is shown schematically in Figure 4.5. The skin and pilosebaceous unit are treated as a set of compartments comprising the SC, VE, dermis, subcutaneous tissue, sebum, hair lipid, and hair core. Dosage forms applied to the skin surface are represented by the vehicle compartment.

At present, the TCAT model treats the following:

- Partitioning and diffusion of a permeant among the compartments that represent the formulation, the layers of the skin, and the pilosebaceous unit

- Evaporation of a volatile permeant and excipient from the formulation through user-supplied data or equations to estimate evaporation rates

- Linear binding (as % bound) to keratin in the SC; linear and saturable binding to melanin in the VE and hair core; and linear binding to other tissue components in the VE, dermis, and SQ tissue (e.g., to albumin, and cellular lipid)

- Linear clearance (equivalently, degradation) at fixed rates (L/h) in the VE, dermis, and SQ tissue

- Saturable clearance by metabolic enzymes and saturable uptake and efflux by transporters expressed in the VE, dermis, and SQ tissue

- Permeant exchange with the systemic circulation through blood flow to the dermis and subcutaneous tissue, and lymph flow in subcutaneous tissue (primarily relevant for compounds with molecular weight greater than about 20 kilodaltons)

Physiologies for skin and pilosebaceous compartments of several sites of the human body (arm, leg, back, abdomen, face, and scalp) and minipig body (ear, snout, neck, back, flank, and abdomen) are built into the TCAT model. Whole body skin models are also available for mouse, rat, and minipig. The physiologies specify skin layer thickness, volume, pH, fractional surface area covered, blood flow rates (dermis and subcutaneous tissue), and lymph flow rate (subcutaneous tissue). The model provides default values for these parameters, which the user can change as appropriate.

The TCAT model treats the permeation of one molecular species in a single spatial dimension through mass transfer boundary conditions between compartments that approximate diffusive flux due to concentration gradients. To handle concentration gradients that may develop within

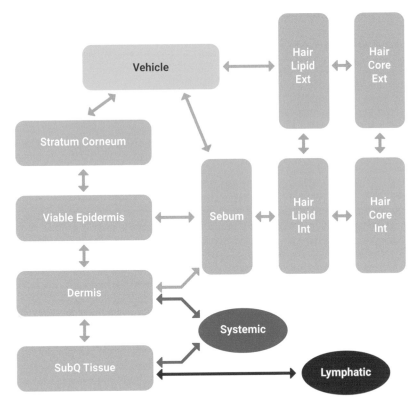

Figure 4.5 Schematic representation of the TCAT model compartments, diffusive material exchange pathways in the skin and pilosebaceous unit (gray arrows), material exchange through systemic blood (blue arrows) and lymph flows (red arrow)

a given skin layer, each model compartment, with the exception of subcutaneous tissue, can be divided into as many as 20 sub-layers.

Among the formulations that can be simulated are liquid solutions and suspensions, ointments and pastes, emulsion-based lotions, creams and gels, and patches. Below, we illustrate how one goes about using the TCAT model, by simulating the performance of a formulation that comprises an oil-in-water emulsion, dissolved API, and undissolved API particles. Because of the paramount importance of partitioning and diffusion in TCAT simulations, we present in some detail the equations for material exchange between compartments. The equation for material exchange between the continuous phase of an emulsion and the SC runs as follows:

$$\frac{dm_1^{SC}}{dt} = \frac{2 \cdot \left(SA_{skin} - SA_{ads,skin}\right)}{\dfrac{h_n^{fmln}}{D^{eff} K^{cont/w}} + \dfrac{h_1^{SC}}{D^{SC} K^{SC/w}}} \cdot \left(\frac{C_n^{cont}}{K^{cont/w}} - \frac{C_{u,1}^{SC}}{K^{SC/w}}\right) \tag{4.1}$$

in which h_n^{fmln} and h_1^{SC} are the thicknesses of the formulation and SC interfacial sub-layers, D^{eff} and D^{SC} are the effective API diffusivities in the continuous phase and SC, and $K^{cont/\tilde{w}}$ and $K^{SC/w}$ are the continuous phase and SC-water API partition coefficients with respect to a suitably chosen water reference phase. SA_{skin} and $SA_{ads,skin}$ are the skin areas to which formulation is applied and dispersed phase droplets adhere, respectively, and C_n^{cont} and $C_{u,1}^{SC}$ are the concentrations of API in the continuous phase and SC interfacial sub-layers.

Similar equations describe the material exchange between dispersed phase droplets and SC (often negligible because $SA_{ads,skin} \ll SA_{skin}$), between the sebum (if present) and VE and dermis, between dispersed and continuous phases of an emulsion, and between sub-layers of a given skin compartment. In the last instance, the mass transfer equation approximates $dm/dt = SA \cdot D \cdot \partial C/\partial z$, in which z is length along the inward pointing normal to the skin surface (assumed to be planar).

Noting that (i) $K^{\text{cont}/w}$ and $K^{\text{SC}/w}$ are approximately API solubility in the continuous phase and in SC, normalized by API solubility in the water reference phase $\left(C_{\text{sat},w}\right)$, and (ii) that KD/h defines membrane permeability in general, Equation 4.1 can be rewritten as

$$\frac{dm_1^{\text{SC}}}{dt} = \frac{2\left(\text{SA}_{\text{skin}} - \text{SA}_{\text{ads,skin}}\right)C_{\text{sat},w}}{1/P_n^{\text{cont}} + 1/P_1^{\text{SC}}} \cdot \left(F_{\text{sat},n}^{\text{cont}} - F_{\text{sat},1}^{\text{SC}}\right) \tag{4.2}$$

where $F_{\text{sat},n}^{\text{cont}}$ is API fractional saturation in the emulsion's continuous phase, and $F_{\text{sat},1}^{\text{SC}}$ is API fractional saturation in SC. As an aside, $2/\left(1/P_n^{\text{cont}} + 1/P_1^{\text{SC}}\right)$ is the harmonic mean of the two permeabilities. If, as is often the case, API permeability in the continuous phase greatly exceeds that in the SC, the rate of mass transfer is approximately:

$$\frac{dm_1^{\text{SC}}}{dt} \sim 2P_1^{\text{SC}}\left(1 - \delta\right)\left(\text{SA}_{\text{skin}} - \text{SA}_{\text{ads,skin}}\right)C_{\text{sat},w} \cdot \left(F_{\text{sat},n}^{\text{cont}} - F_{\text{sat},1}^{\text{SC}}\right) \tag{4.3}$$

where $\delta = P_1^{\text{SC}}/P_n^{\text{cont}} \ll 1$.

TCAT model simulations usually proceed under the assumption that application to the skin does not affect a formulation's characteristics despite the shearing involved in this process. There is likely large inter-individual variability in application shear rates and duration, but it may be possible to define a common scenario and begin to model its effects (e.g., see [54]), § 9.2.2).

4.3.3 Zovirax® Cream - Acyclovir

To illustrate the application of the TCAT model, we simulated the delivery of the anti-viral compound, acyclovir, from Zovirax cream [101]. The model was developed using information presented by Professors SN Murthy of the University of Mississippi [102] and MS Roberts of the Universities of Queensland and South Australia [103], articles from the peer-reviewed literature, and US patents. Zovirax creams are marketed in many countries, with, for example, the US, UK, and Austrian formulations differing in their hydrophobic components. Thus, they are not Q1 or Q2 equivalent (i.e., do not have the same composition quantitatively), but may have similar arrangements of matter, broadly speaking (Q3 similar) [104].

Acyclovir (PubChem compound 135398513) is a hydrophilic guanosine analogue. Acyclovir can be described as a low molecular weight compound of moderate aqueous solubility that is essentially uncharged between pH 4 and pH 8. This range encompasses the values of cream pH reported by Murthy [102] and Roberts [103], 7.74 and 6.4, respectively (Table 4.1).

For the simulations presented here, we have used ADMET Predictor® (Simulations Plus, Inc.)

Table 4.1: Physicochemical Properties of Acyclovir

Parameters	Values	Units	Sources
Mol Wt	225.2	g/mol	PubChem CID 135398513
Log $K_{o,w}$	−1.37		ADMET Predictor® 10.3
Water solubility	1.1	mg/mL	Diez-Sales et al. [105]
	1.45	mg/mL	ADMET Predictor 10.3
Basic pKa	2.35		ADMET Predictor 10.3
Acidic pKa	9.58		ADMET Predictor 10.3
Diffusivity in water	9.70E-06	cm²/s	ADMET Predictor 10.3

estimates for most of the parameters, retaining them from a PBPK model developed previously for oral delivery of acyclovir and valacyclovir. The sole exception is acyclovir's water solubility, for which we used the experimental value of Diez-Sales et al. [105] because they also measured acyclovir solubility in a series of water - propylene glycol (PG) mixtures, information that is relevant for simulating the Zovirax formulation.

The composition of the Zovirax cream (Table 4.2) marketed in the US was drawn from international patent application WO2000001390A1 [106] and US patent 4,963,555 [107]. The patents for the cream describe it as having a dispersed oil phase and continuous aqueous phase, although dispersed phase droplets may not always be observed [103]. Thus, initially, we simulated the cream as

Table 4.2: Weight Percent Composition of Zovirax Cream (US Patent 4963555)

Zovirax Cream US

Hydrophilic (% w/w)	Lipo- / Amphiphilic (% w/w)
Water (29%)	Mineral oil (5%)
Propylene Glycol (40%)	White Petrolatum (12.5%)
Acyclovir (5%)	Cetostearyl OH (6.75%)
	Na·Dodecyl Sulfate (0.75%)
	PEG-PPG-PEG (1%)

a suspension of undissolved acyclovir particles in an oil-in-water emulsion and subsequently as a suspension in a single-phase liquid.

PEG-PPG-PEG is Poloxamer 407, a triblock copolymer non-ionic surfactant consisting of a central hydrophobic block of polypropylene glycol (PPG) flanked by two hydrophilic blocks of polyethylene glycol (PEG). The length of each PEG chain is ~101 monomers, with ~56 monomers for the PPG chain. The molecular weight is nominally 12.6 kDa [87] and the critical micelle concentration (CMC) is 2.8 µM [108] so that polymer concentration in Zovirax greatly exceeds its CMC. In water at $T > 18°C$, the polymer forms elastic gels as a function of concentration above 12% w/v [87]. This is several-fold greater than the concentrations in Zovirax even after complete loss of water to evaporation (~ 2.5%).

Sodium dodecyl sulfate (SDS) is an anionic surfactant with a CMC of 0.2% w/w (8 mM) in water. Depending on its concentration in aqueous media, PG appears to have opposing effects on SDS micelle formation, reducing CMC at relatively low concentrations, but destabilizing micelles at higher concentrations [109,110]. Nonetheless, it would appear that Poloxamer 407 and SDS combined have great capacity to solubilize the purely hydrophobic components of the formulation: white petrolatum and mineral oil.

Simulating an emulsion through the TCAT model involves setting values for parameters that describe the thermodynamic and transport properties of a biphasic formulation. These are the solubility and diffusivity of API in the continuous major phase ($K^{cont,w}$ and D^{eff}, respectively) and in the dispersed minor phase ($K^{disp,w}$ and D^{disp}, respectively), the dispersed phase volume fraction (φ^{disp}) and droplet size (r^{disp}). API solubilities are defined as partition coefficients relative to a reference phase, and continuous phase diffusivity is denoted "effective" because it depends not only on the viscosity of the solvents used (water and PG in Zovirax) but also on φ^{disp}, and whether a gelling polymer is present. That is, emulsion formulations are complex fluids in which API diffusivity is not related simply to the macroscopic rheological properties [111,112,113].

Model input parameter values for Zovirax and acyclovir are given in Table 4.3, along with their sources or derivations. Where multiple values are given for a parameter, the value listed first was that used for simulation results presented below, and the sensitivity of model predictions to a given parameter or combination of parameters can be explored by sensitivity analysis.

It should be noted that almost 96% of the acyclovir in Zovirax cream exists as undissolved particles. Thus, acyclovir is at unit thermodynamic activity in Zovirax prior to application on the skin and, having a solubility of ~4.2 mg/mL in pure PG, remains so upon evaporative loss of water and skin permeation, assuming rapid dissolution.

Zovirax cream is applied without occlusion, allowing water to evaporate. The TCAT model can simulate linear evaporation, with the evaporation rate constant estimated by several methods [126,127] or provided by the user. Experimental evaporation data can be used as such or as fitted to a combination of up to three Weibull functions. We have used SN Murthy's Zovirax evaporation data [102] fitted to a single Weibull function as input into the simulations reported here (see Table 4.3).

The TCAT model incorporates equations to predict API permeability in the SC (Wang-Kasting-Nitsche [65,66], Potts-Guy [128,129] and Robinson [120]), VE and dermis (Kretsos [70], Bunge-Cleek [130] and Robinson [120], and sebum (Valiveti and Lu [119,131], and Yang & Lian [118,121]). In addition, the ADMET Predictor provides an estimate of overall skin permeability. We have used the Robinson model estimate (5.37e-9 cm/s), the highest among the built-in methods, as the baseline value of acyclovir SC permeability. We used the Kretsos model estimates for VE and dermis permeability.

A two-compartment pharmacokinetic model derived from human intravenous infusion data [125] and the model of Ibrahim, Nitsche and Kasting [77,78] for exchange between the dermis and skin blood flow was used to simulate the systemic distribution and clearance of acyclovir *in vivo*. Exchange between subcutaneous tissue and the systemic circulation was treated using the standard GastroPlus PBPK model equations for tissue-blood exchange. Values of the compartmental PK parameters are listed in Table 4.3.

Table 4.3: Values of TCAT Model and Compartmental PK Parameters for Acyclovir and Zovirax Cream

Parameter	Value	Units	Source/Derivation
Acyclovir content	50	mg/g cream	US prescribing information [101]
φ^{disp}	0.282		Calculated from the composition [107]
Continuous phase solubility	2.91	mg/mL	Diez-Sales et al. [105]
$K^{cont,w}$	2.64		Ratio of continuous phase and water solubilities
$K^{disp,w}$	3.98E-02		Calculated from ADMET Predictor 10.3 Log $K_{o,w}$[a]
	1.33E-03		Calculated from Log $K_{veg\,oil,w}$[a]$=1.115\cdot$Log $K_{o,w}-1.35$ [114]
D^{eff}	3.41E-08	cm^2/s	Higuchi analysis of SN Murthy's *in vitro* release data [115]
	2.21E-07	cm^2/s	Higuchi analysis of Nallagundla S et al *in vitro* release data [115,116]
D^{disp}	1.11E-08	cm^2/s	Extrapolated from ferrocene cyclic voltammetry data [117]
	2.43E-07	cm^2/s	$D_{veg\,oil}$ via Stokes-Einstein, using D_w and $\eta_{veg\,oil}$ (~ 42 cP at 32°C)
	1.83e-07	cm^2/s	Estimated as D^{Sebum}, from Yang S, Lian G et al. [118]
	2.38E-08	cm^2/s	Estimated as D^{Sebum}, using Valiveti S & Lu GW [119]
Dispersed phase droplet radius, r^{disp}	1	μm	A nominal value for emulsions
Acyclovir particle radius	1.88	μm	One half d_{50} from SN Murthy's particle size data ($d_{10}=2.07$ μm, $d_{90}=19$ μm) [102]
Evaporation time scale, τ	6.85	hours	Defined by fitting a Weibull function to SN Murthy's evaporative mass loss data:
β	0.52		$M(t)=\alpha\bullet(1-\exp[-(t/\tau)^{\beta}])$
Continuous phase volume fraction lost, α	0.341		
SC permeability, P^{SC}	5.37E-09	cm/s	Wilschut et al. [120]
VE permeability, P^{VE}	2.48E-04	cm/s	Kretsos et al. [70]
Dermis permeability, P^{De}	2.85E-05	cm/s	
Sebum / hair permeability, P^{Sebum}	8.865e-10	cm/s	$D^{Sebum}=D^{disp}$, $K^{Sebum,w}=1.04e-2$ [121] with P^{Sebum} calculated via GastroPlus 9.8.3
Fraction bound in SC	0.215		Equilibrium keratin binding model [122,123,124] in GastroPlus 9.8.3
Fraction bound to protein and lipid in VE & dermis	0.145		Bound fraction in skin (1 - $f_{u,skin}$), Lukačova Method, GastroPlus 9.8.3
CL	0.308	L/h/kg	Data from SA Spector et al. [125],
V_c	0.041	L/kg	analyzed via the PKPlus Module in
CL_2	0.735	L/h/kg	GastroPlus 9.8.3
V_2	0.671	L/kg	
K_{10}	7.507	L/h	
K_{12}	17.92	L/h	
K_{21}	1.095	L/h	

[a] The octanol-water and vegetable oil-water partition coefficients.

73

4.3.4 Simulation of Skin Permeation *In Vitro*

We used the TCAT model to simulate acyclovir transdermal permeation rates *in vitro* (IVPT), as reported by SN Murthy [102] and MS Roberts [103], and acyclovir concentrations *in vivo* in SC, as measured by tape stripping following application of the cream to the volar forearms of healthy volunteers [132]. A nominal dose of 15 mg of Zovirax cream per cm² skin was applied in each experiment. The simulations were set up to match the acyclovir dose per area of skin, skin preparation (dermatomed human skin *in vitro*), and duration of application.

Results from the simulation of the Murthy experimental data are plotted in Figure 4.6a. The initial rise of flux *in vitro* was similar in two independent experiments, but in the first an apparent maximum flux (J_{max}) was reached at 12 hours, followed by monotonic decline out to 48 hours.

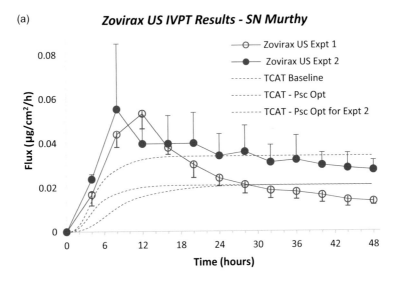

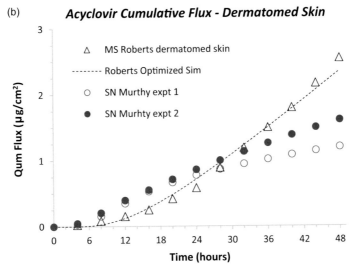

Figure 4.6 (a) Transdermal acyclovir flux reported by SN Murthy [102] for two experiments (O, ●, digitized from plots in the presentation) and flux calculated through the TCAT model (dotted lines) for the baseline values of $K^{SC,w}$ and D^{SC} that comprise baseline stratum corneum permeability (---), and the values of these parameters adjusted manually for better agreement with the initial rise in flux (---) and for better agreement with the initial rise in flux and the quasi-steady-state flux observed in Experiment 2 (---) (b) Transdermal cumulative acyclovir flux reported by MS Roberts [103] (Δ) and SN Murthy [102] (O, ●) through dermatomed human skin. Output from a TCAT simulation using $K^{SC,w}$ and D^{SC} optimized for the Roberts data is also plotted (---).

Results from the second experiment conformed more closely to expectations, with poorly defined peak flux at 8 hours and quasi-steady flux thereafter.

Using the baseline values of the parameters from Table 4.3, the initial simulation (---) reached a steady-state flux of ~ 2.1e-2 $\mu g/cm^2/h$ which was essentially the average of the experimental data at late times. Because about 24 hours were required to reach steady state, the initial rise in experimental flux at early times was underpredicted, as was J_{max}. We then manually optimized the values of acyclovir's SC-water partition coefficient ($K^{SC,w}$, reduced 1.8 fold, from 0.658 to 0.366) and SC diffusivity (D^{SC}, increased 1.8 fold, from 1.01e-11 to 1.82e-11 cm^2/s), keeping P^{SC} constant ($P^{SC} = K^{SC,w} \cdot D^{SC}/h^{SC}$, where the denominator is SC thickness), in order to better simulate the initial rise in flux, without changing steady-state flux (–··–··). Finally, by returning $K^{SC,w}$ to 90% of its baseline value (0.585) and leaving D^{SC} at its elevated value (an overall increase in P^{SC} of about 1.6-fold), we were able to simulate the initial rise in flux and the quasi-steady flux observed in the second experiment (–·–·–).

As shown in Figure 4.6b, the cumulative *in vitro* permeation data reported by Roberts [103] for dermatomed human skin stand in contrast to Murthy's data also plotted in the figure as cumulative flux. Cumulative flux was greater over 48 hours but required 24 hours to reach a quasi-steady state that showed no roll off at longer times, whereas 6–12 hours were required to reach peak flux or quasi-steady state with roll off occurring after 12–18 hours. Accurate simulation of the Roberts data thus required adjustment of the baseline model parameters. In fact, optimizing P^{SC} by increasing the baseline value of $K^{SC,w}$ from 0.658 to 3.81 and reducing the baseline value of D^{SC} from 1.01e-11 to 6.07e-12 cm^2/s allows accurate simulation of the Roberts cumulative flux data (dashed line in Figure 4.6b, $r^2 \sim 0.98$).

4.3.5 Simulation of Skin Permeation *In Vivo*

In addition to IVPT measurements, acyclovir SC concentrations from a well-designed study have been reported by Pensado et al. [132]. Simulating these results allowed us to study model performance in a way complementary to simulating IVPT. The experimental work tested three acyclovir formulations, Zovirax-US, Zovirax-UK, and Aciclovir (marketed in Austria), in pairwise fashion for bioequivalence. Two studies were conducted in which one cream (Zovirax-US or Aciclovir, respectively) served as the reference and as a positive control, with another formulation (Zovirax-UK or Zovirax-US, respectively) serving as the test. Fifteen milligram of cream/cm^2 skin was applied to six sites on each arm of healthy male and female subjects for 6 hours, at which time the formulation was removed from the skin and a set of application sites was tape-stripped. After a 17 hours clearance period, the remaining application sites were tape-stripped. The number of tape strips taken was guided by measurements of trans-epidermal water loss (TEWL), an indicator of the loss of permeability barrier function.

We first simulated the performance of Zovirax US in these experiments using the baseline parameter values listed in Table 4.3, and the human arm skin physiology provided in the TCAT model. Subsequently, while maintaining the same value of P^{SC}, we increased $K^{SC,w}$ and reduced D^{SC} 1.8-fold (denoted below as "Psc adj"); the former change increasing uptake at early times, and the latter change slowing clearance from the SC at later times. These changes to $K^{SC,w}$ and D^{SC} were the opposite of those made in these parameters for the simulation of transdermal flux *in vitro*. Thus, although the two sets of values for $K^{SC,w}$ and D^{SC} would predict the same steady-state transdermal flux *in vitro* or input rate into the systemic circulation *in vivo* (VE and dermis permeabilities were the same throughout), the approaches to steady state would differ substantially.

In Figure 4.7, simulation results are compared to the amounts of acyclovir in SC observed experimentally in Studies 1 and 2. In Study 1, the geometric mean of all measured uptake (6 hours) values was ~ 0.65 $\mu g/cm^2$, and of the clearance (23 hours) values ~ 0.42 $\mu g/cm^2$ (black). The simulations of acyclovir SC content per applied area fell within the observed distributions at uptake and clearance for both baseline (blue) and adjusted P^{SC} (red). In Study 2, the qualitative relationship between observed and predicted amounts of acyclovir in the SC was similar to that in Study 1, but the distribution of observed values differed. The geometric means of uptake and clearance values were ~ 0.89 and ~ 0.74 $\mu g/cm^2$, respectively. In both studies and for both uptake and clearance, using the adjusted P^{SC} provided a more accurate estimation of the geometric mean SC content.

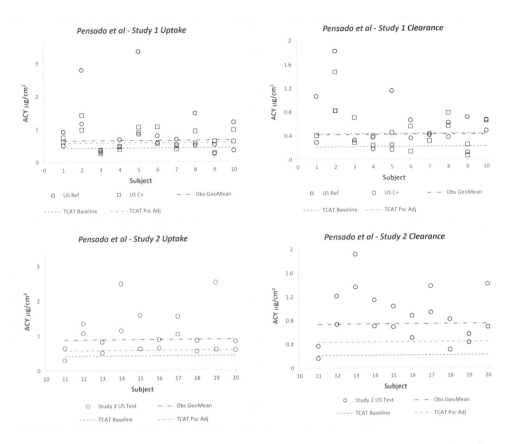

Figure 4.7 Total acyclovir concentrations (µg/cm²) in stratum corneum recovered through tape stripping on the uptake at 6 hours (left) and clearance at 23 hours (right) of Study 1 (top, US Reference and US Comparator) and Study 2 (bottom, US Test) after application of Zovirax US to the volar forearms of healthy subjects (open symbols, and geometric mean in black), with predictions for two sets of values for $K^{SC,w}$ and D^{eff}: the baseline values from the Robinson model (blue) and with $K^{SC,w}$ increased and D^{SC} reduced 1.8-fold (red). Experimental values were drawn from Pensado, Guy et al. [132]. Note the different ordinate scales for uptake and clearance.

4.3.6 Analysis of Formulation Attributes

Having shown that the baseline model with optimization of SC permeability can reproduce some important features of acyclovir skin permeation *in vitro* and *in vivo*, we investigated the sensitivity of model predictions to changes in certain formulation attributes.

Because Zovirax cream contains a reservoir of undissolved acyclovir and the compound partitions preferentially into the continuous aqueous phase ($K^{cont,disp} \sim 66$), the transport properties of that phase can contribute significantly to the rates of skin permeation achieved by the formulation. We explored this by assessing the sensitivity of acyclovir skin permeation *in vivo* to D^{eff}. This was carried out by running the TCAT model in parameter sensitivity analysis (PSA) mode: values of D^{eff} were varied systematically, while all other model inputs were held at their baseline values. Results are shown in Figure 4.8.

Cumulative mass of acyclovir input into the systemic circulation at 48 hours was almost wholly insensitive to changes in D^{eff} between 1e-10 and 1e-7 cm²/s. Only as the value of D^{eff} fell below 1e-10 cm²/s was a detectable reduction of systemic input observed (~ 20% for D^{eff}=1e-11 cm²/s). Similar behavior was observed in acyclovir concentration-time profiles in the SC and dermis compartments. Practically speaking, a reduction of greater than 300-fold in D^{eff} is perhaps unrealizable, but smaller reductions would control the transdermal flux of more highly permeable APIs. Thus, being able to estimate sensitivity to D^{eff} may generally support formulation development.

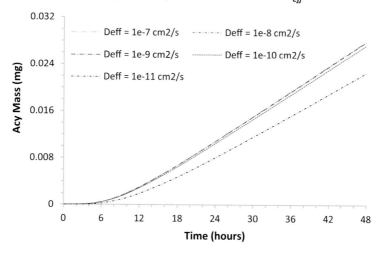

Figure 4.8 Cumulative input of acyclovir into the systemic circulation as a function of D^{eff}, the effective diffusivity of acyclovir in the continuous phase of the formulation. The curves overlap for the highest three values of D^{eff}.

We also investigated the sensitivity of transdermal flux, both *in vitro* and *in vivo*, to acyclovir crystalline particle size, through its effect on dissolution rate [133,134]. Particle radius was varied from 0.2 to 20 µm with all other model input parameters held at their baseline values. We found transdermal flux *in vitro* and mass input into the systemic circulation to be completely insensitive to particle radius over this range.

4.3.7 Discussion

We have developed and explored TCAT models for the skin permeation of the anti-viral compound acyclovir, as delivered from Zovirax cream. The cream was treated as an emulsion in which a large fraction of acyclovir existed as suspended crystalline particles. Input parameter values for the cream were derived from publicly available presentations, patents, and peer-reviewed literature.

Baseline simulations of the Murthy IVPT transdermal flux data were within three-fold of experimentally observed flux over 8–48 hours, showing a slower initial rise in flux and a steady-state flux that was not observed consistently in the experimental data. SC diffusivity and partition coefficient (D^{SC} and $K^{SC,w}$) could be optimized manually to provide accurate simulations of more of the time course acyclovir flux reported by both Murthy and Roberts.

The simulations suggest that the differences between the Roberts and Murthy IVPT results were due to differences in both acyclovir solubility and diffusivity in the SC samples. How these differences arose in the experimental setting is unknown, but high inter-sample variability in the skin permeability of compounds that span a broad range of physical properties has been reported in the literature.

Simulating the results of tape-stripping experiments, both baseline and adjusted values of D^{SC} and $K^{SC,w}$ predicted SC concentrations on uptake and clearance that were within the distribution of measured values, with the adjusted values providing the more accurate estimate of the geometric mean acyclovir concentrations during both uptake and clearance phases.

The model for Zovirax cream did not include treatment of the following processes:

- Changes in acyclovir solubility as water evaporates/PG permeates skin

- Changes in acyclovir D^{eff} as water evaporates/PG permeates

- Changes in Zovirax phase structure as water evaporates, and PG permeates the skin

- PG partitioning into the dispersed oily phase and its effect on $K^{disp,cont}$

- Effect of PG on acyclovir P^{SC} (permeation enhancement)

Extrapolating a linear fit of the Diez-Sales solubility data [105], one estimates acyclovir solubility in pure PG to be 4.3 mg/mL; 4-fold higher than in water, but only 1.5-fold higher than in the continuous phase of the cream as formulated. Thus, as water evaporates, $K^{cont/w}$ increases 1.5-fold, reducing slightly the tendency of acyclovir to partition into the SC. Moreover, despite this increase in acyclovir solubility in the residual continuous phase, the great majority of acyclovir in the formulation would remain undissolved and the formulation saturated in dissolved acyclovir throughout transdermal delivery at the rates *in vitro* and *in vivo* that we simulated.

We have also estimated the effect of evaporative water loss on D^{eff} by considering (i) the increase in viscosity of the residual continuous phase as its PG content rises (at 30°C, the viscosity of pure PG ~ 27 cP, that of water ~ 0.94 cP, and that of their relevant binary mixture ~ 5 cP); (ii) the increased volume fraction of polymer in the continuous phase[111,135]; (iii) increased crowding by the semi-permeable dispersed phase droplets (φ^{disp} rises from ~ 0.28 to ~ 0.38) [136,137]; and (iv) increased crowding by the impermeable particles of solid acyclovir [138]. The multiplicatively combined effects reduce D^{eff} ~ 4-fold (from 3.41e-8 to 9.0e-9 cm^2/s).

Given the complex composition of the hydrophobic phase, it is difficult to predict how, if at all, the formulation's phase structure changes as water evaporates and the aqueous phase becomes enriched in PG. To the best of our knowledge, this has not been examined in detail experimentally.

The Zovirax model assumed that PG does not partition into the hydrophobic phase. The $K_{o,w}$ of PG ~ 0.12 [114], suggesting some degree of partitioning, but, if the hydrophobic phase is more akin to vegetable oil or sebum than octanol, the more relevant partition coefficients might be $K_{veg\ oil,w}$ ~ 4.2e-3 [114] or $K^{Sebum,w}$ ~ 3.7e-2 [121]. Thus, our assumption may be justified. Again, this point does not seem to have been explored experimentally.

Experimental evidence has been published that PG partitions from Zovirax into the SC and enhances acyclovir permeation [103,105,139,140]. In this case, one might expect the values of $K^{SC,w}$ and D^{SC} to be time- and depth-dependent. However, we achieved good accuracy in simulating acyclovir permeation in vitro with constant values of $K^{SC,w}$ and D^{SC} (although predicted transdermal flux did not reproduce the apparent peak flux in Murthy's results [102]), and a detailed treatment of permeation enhancement by PG was beyond the scope of this chapter.

Results of the D^{eff} PSA (Figure 4.8) can be understood qualitatively by reference to Equations (4.1) and (4.2). As the value of D^{eff} declined, the value of P_n^{cont} fell and approached that of P_1^{SC}, leading to the decline of their harmonic mean, thereby reducing the rate of mass transfer from the continuous phase to the SC. But one should also note that mass transfer from Zovirax dispersed phase and through the pilosebaceous pathways was quite limited and could not compensate r reduced mass transfer from the continuous phase.

Finally, we note that Kamal et al. [139] investigated the critical quality attributes of a series of Zovirax-like formulations and observed a significant dependence of acyclovir release rate *in vitro* on acyclovir particle radius in the range of 2.5–20 μm. The measured release rates from their formulations were, however, substantially higher than our simulated delivery rates across skin: 1%–6% of dose released over 6 hours vs 0.2%–0.8% of dose delivered over 48 hours, and the authors observed no effect of particle size on the mass of acyclovir retained in human cadaver skin samples during permeation testing.

4.3.8 Conclusion

PBPK simulation through the TCAT model is a promising approach to study the absorption and transport of small molecules in the skin to changes in the thermodynamic and transport properties of topical formulations, particularly in relation to rate-limiting steps in API skin permeation. The sensitivity of API permeation to formulation attributes can be assessed for single parameters, and the combined effects of multiple parameters can be quantified through coupled PSA, bearing in mind dependencies that may exist among parameters. This in silico QbD approach may inform the design of both novel and generic formulations; in the latter case with the goal of achieving bioequivalence to a reference product.

REFERENCES

1. Barenholz, Yechezkel. 2012. "Doxil(r)--the First FDA-Approved Nano-Drug: Lessons Learned." *Journal of Controlled Release: Official Journal of the Controlled Release Society* 160 (2): 117–34. https://doi.org/10.1016/j.jconrel.2012.03.020.

2. Trevaskis, Natalie L., William N. Charman, and Christopher J. H. Porter. 2008. "Lipid-Based Delivery Systems and Intestinal Lymphatic Drug Transport: A Mechanistic Update." *Advanced Drug Delivery Reviews* 60 (6): 702–16. https://doi.org/10.1016/j.addr.2007.09.007.

3. Bäckman, Per, and Bo Olsson. 2020. "Pulmonary Drug Dissolution, Regional Retention and Systemic Absorption: Understanding Their Interactions through Mechanistic Modeling." *Respiratory Drug Delivery* 1: 113–22.

4. He, Hua, Dongfen Yuan, Yun Wu, and Yanguang Cao. 2019. "Pharmacokinetics and Pharmacodynamics Modeling and Simulation Systems to Support the Development and Regulation of Liposomal Drugs." *Pharmaceutics* 11 (3): 110. https://doi.org/10.3390/pharmaceutics11030110.

5. Le Merdy, Maxime, Jim Mullin, and Viera Lukacova. 2021. "Development of PBPK Model for Intra-Articular Injection in Human: Methotrexate Solution and Rheumatoid Arthritis Case Study." *Journal of Pharmacokinetics and Pharmacodynamics* 48 (6): 909–22. https://doi.org/10.1007/s10928-021-09781-w.

6. Dolton, Michael J., Po-Chang Chiang, and Yuan Chen. 2021. "Mechanistic Oral Absorption Modeling of Halofantrine: Exploring the Role of Intestinal Lymphatic Transport." *Journal of Pharmaceutical Sciences* 110 (3): 1427–30. https://doi.org/10.1016/j.xphs.2020.12.023.

7. Miller, Neil A., Rebecca H. Graves, Chris D. Edwards, Augustin Amour, Ed Taylor, Olivia Robb, Brett O'Brien, Aarti Patel, Andrew W. Harrell, and Edith M. Hessel. 2022. "Physiologically Based Pharmacokinetic Modelling of Inhaled Nemiralisib: Mechanistic Components for Pulmonary Absorption, Systemic Distribution, and Oral Absorption." *Clinical Pharmacokinetics* 61 (2): 281–93. https://doi.org/10.1007/s40262-021-01066-2.

8. Kels, Barry D., Andrzej Grzybowski, and Jane M. Grant-Kels. 2015. "Human Ocular Anatomy." *Clinics in Dermatology* 33 (2): 140–46. https://doi.org/10.1016/j.clindermatol.2014.10.006.

9. Farkouh, Andre, Peter Frigo, and Martin Czejka. 2016. "Systemic Side Effects of Eye Drops: A Pharmacokinetic Perspective." *Clinical Ophthalmology (Auckland, N.Z.)* 10: 2433–41. https://doi.org/10.2147/OPTH.S118409.

10. Fayyaz, Anam, Veli-Pekka Ranta, Elisa Toropainen, Kati-Sisko Vellonen, Annika Valtari, Jooseppi Puranen, Marika Ruponen, et al. 2020. "Topical Ocular Pharmacokinetics and Bioavailability for a Cocktail of Atenolol, Timolol and Betaxolol in Rabbits." *European Journal of Pharmaceutical Sciences* 155 (December): 105553. https://doi.org/10.1016/j.ejps.2020.105553.

11. Gaudana, Ripal, Hari Krishna Ananthula, Ashwin Parenky, and Ashim K. Mitra. 2010. "Ocular Drug Delivery." *The AAPS Journal* 12 (3): 348–60. https://doi.org/10.1208/s12248-010-9183-3.

12. U.S. FDA. n.d. "Orange Book: Approved Drug Products with Therapeutic Equivalence Evaluations." Accessed February 5, 2020. https://www.accessdata.fda.gov/scripts/cder/ob/index.cfm?resetfields=1.

13. Worakul, Nimit, and Joseph R. Robinson. 1997. "Ocular Pharmacokinetics/Pharmacodynamics." *European Journal of Pharmaceutics and Biopharmaceutics* 44 (1): 71–83. https://doi.org/10.1016/S0939-6411(97)00064-7.

14. Lee, Vincent Hon-Leung, and Joseph R. Robinson. 1979. "Mechanistic and Quantitative Evaluation of Precorneal Pilocarpine Disposition in Albino Rabbits." *Journal of Pharmaceutical Sciences* 68 (6): 673–84. https://doi.org/10.1002/jps.2600680606.

15. Sieg, J. W., and J. R. Robinson. 1981. "Mechanistic Studies on Transcorneal Permeation of Fluorometholone." *Journal of Pharmaceutical Sciences* 70 (9): 1026–29. https://doi.org/10.1002/jps.2600700915.

16. Makoid, M. C., and J. R. Robinson. 1979. "Pharmacokinetics of Topically Applied Pilocarpine in the Albino Rabbit Eye." *Journal of Pharmaceutical Sciences* 68 (4): 435–43.

17. Miller, Susan C., Kenneth J. Himmelstein, and Thomas F. Patton. 1981. "A Physiologically Based Pharmacokinetic Model for the Intraocular Distribution of Pilocarpine in Rabbits." *Journal of Pharmacokinetics and Biopharmaceutics* 9 (6): 653–77. https://doi.org/10.1007/BF01070899.

18. Hui, Hoa-Wah, and Joseph R. Robinson. 1986. "Effect of Particle Dissolution Rate on Ocular Drug Bioavailability." *Journal of Pharmaceutical Sciences* 75 (3): 280–87.

19. Deng, Feng, Veli-Pekka Ranta, Heidi Kidron, and Arto Urtti. 2016. "General Pharmacokinetic Model for Topically Administered Ocular Drug Dosage Forms." *Pharmaceutical Research* 33 (11): 2680–90. https://doi.org/10.1007/s11095-016-1993-2.

20. Rimpelä, Anna-Kaisa, Mika Reinisalo, Laura Hellinen, Evgeni Grazhdankin, Heidi Kidron, Arto Urtti, and Eva M. Del Amo. 2018. "Implications of Melanin Binding in Ocular Drug Delivery." *Advanced Drug Delivery Reviews* 126 (February): 23–43. https://doi.org/10.1016/j.addr.2017.12.008.

21. Grass, George M., and V. H. Lee. 1993. "A Model to Predict Aqueous Humor and Plasma Pharmacokinetics of Ocularly Applied Drugs." *Investigative Ophthalmology & Visual Science* 34 (7): 2251–59.

22. Vanhove, Marc, Jean-Marc Wagner, Bernard Noppen, Bart Jonckx, Elke Vermassen, and Alan W. Stitt. 2021. "Systemic Exposure Following Intravitreal Administration of Therapeutic Agents: An Integrated Pharmacokinetic Approach. 2. THR-687." *Journal of Pharmacokinetics and Pharmacodynamics* 48 (6): 837–49. https://doi.org/10.1007/s10928-021-09774-9.

23. Gadkar, Kapil, Cinthia V. Pastuskovas, Jennifer E. Le Couter, J. Michael Elliott, Jianhuan Zhang, Chingwei V. Lee, Sarah Sanowar, et al. 2015. "Design and Pharmacokinetic Characterization of Novel Antibody Formats for Ocular Therapeutics." *Investigative Ophthalmology & Visual Science* 56 (9): 5390–5400. https://doi.org/10.1167/iovs.15-17108.

24. Sukumaran, Siddharth, Crystal Zhang, Douglas D. Leipold, Ola M. Saad, Keyang Xu, Kapil Gadkar, Divya Samineni, et al. 2017. "Development and Translational Application of an Integrated, Mechanistic Model of Antibody-Drug Conjugate Pharmacokinetics." *The AAPS Journal* 19 (1): 130–40. https://doi.org/10.1208/s12248-016-9993-z.

25. Hutton-Smith, Laurence A., Eamonn A. Gaffney, Helen M. Byrne, Philip K. Maini, Kapil Gadkar, and Norman A. Mazer. 2017. "Ocular Pharmacokinetics of Therapeutic Antibodies Given by Intravitreal Injection: Estimation of Retinal Permeabilities Using a 3-Compartment Semi-Mechanistic Model." *Molecular Pharmaceutics* 14 (8): 2690–96. https://doi.org/10.1021/acs.molpharmaceut.7b00164.

26. Amo, Eva M. del, Kati-Sisko Vellonen, Heidi Kidron, and Arto Urtti. 2015. "Intravitreal Clearance and Volume of Distribution of Compounds in Rabbits: In Silico Prediction and Pharmacokinetic Simulations for Drug Development." *European Journal of Pharmaceutics and Biopharmaceutics: Official Journal of Arbeitsgemeinschaft Fur Pharmazeutische Verfahrenstechnik e.V* 95 (Pt B): 215–26. https://doi.org/10.1016/j.ejpb.2015.01.003.

27. Sadeghi, Amir, Jooseppi Puranen, Marika Ruponen, Annika Valtari, Astrid Subrizi, Veli-Pekka Ranta, Elisa Toropainen, and Arto Urtti. 2021. "Pharmacokinetics of Intravitreal Macromolecules: Scaling between Rats and Rabbits." *European Journal of Pharmaceutical Sciences* 159 (April): 105720. https://doi.org/10.1016/j.ejps.2021.105720.

28. Vanhove, Marc, Bernard Noppen, Jean-Marc Wagner, Tine Van Bergen, Philippe Barbeaux, and Alan W. Stitt. 2021. "Systemic Exposure Following Intravitreal Administration of Therapeutic Agents: An Integrated Pharmacokinetic Approach. 1. THR-149." *Journal of Pharmacokinetics and Pharmacodynamics* 48 (6): 825–36. https://doi.org/10.1007/s10928-021-09773-w.

29. Rimpelä, Anna-Kaisa, Iiro Kiiski, Feng Deng, Heidi Kidron, and Arto Urtti. 2019. "Pharmacokinetic Simulations of Intravitreal Biologicals: Aspects of Drug Delivery to the Posterior and Anterior Segments." *Pharmaceutics* 11 (1): 9. https://doi.org/10.3390/pharmaceutics11010009.

30. Bussing, David, and Dhaval K. Shah. 2020. "Development of a Physiologically-Based Pharmacokinetic Model for Ocular Disposition of Monoclonal Antibodies in Rabbits." *Journal of Pharmacokinetics and Pharmacodynamics.* https://doi.org/10.1007/s10928-020-09713-0.

31. Lamminsalo, Marko, Ella Taskinen, Timo Karvinen, Astrid Subrizi, Lasse Murtomäki, Arto Urtti, and Veli-Pekka Ranta. 2018. "Extended Pharmacokinetic Model of the Rabbit Eye for Intravitreal and Intracameral Injections of Macromolecules: Quantitative Analysis of Anterior and Posterior Elimination Pathways." *Pharmaceutical Research* 35 (8): 153. https://doi.org/10.1007/s11095-018-2435-0.

32. Missel, Paul J., and Ramesh Sarangapani. 2019. "Physiologically Based Ocular Pharmacokinetic Modeling Using Computational Methods." *Drug Discovery Today* 24 (8): 1551–63. https://doi.org/10.1016/j.drudis.2019.05.039.

33. Whitcomb, Julie E., Susan S. Lee, Marc Horner, Mohammad R. Kazemi, Michael R. Robinson, and Jie Shen. 2012. "3D Computational Fluid Dynamic Model Comparing Rabbit and Human Intravitreal Pharmacokinetics Using Fluorescein Dyes." *Investigative Ophthalmology & Visual Science* 53 (14): 469.

34. Jooybar, Elaheh, Mohammad J. Abdekhodaie, Fatolla Farhadi, and Yu Ling Cheng. 2014. "Computational Modeling of Drug Distribution in the Posterior Segment of the Eye: Effects of Device Variables and Positions." *Mathematical Biosciences* 255 (September): 11–20. https://doi.org/10.1016/j.mbs.2014.06.008.

35. Le, K.N., L. Gibiansky, M. van Lookeren Campagne, J. Good, T. Davancaze, K.M. Loyet, A. Morimoto, E.C. Strauss, and J.Y. Jin. 2015. "Population Pharmacokinetics and Pharmacodynamics of Lampalizumab Administered Intravitreally to Patients with Geographic Atrophy." *CPT: Pharmacometrics & Systems Pharmacology* 4 (10): 595–604. https://doi.org/10.1002/psp4.12031.

36. Wu, Feng, Xiuli Zhao, Xingang Li, and Yimin Cui. 2019. "Population Pharmacokinetic Modeling of Azithromycin Eyedrops in Tears Following Single-Dose Topical Administration in Healthy Volunteers." *European Journal of Drug Metabolism and Pharmacokinetics* 44 (3): 371–78. https://doi.org/10.1007/s13318-018-0522-6.

37. Djebli, Nassim, Sonia Khier, Florence Griguer, Anne-Laure Coutant, Alexandra Tavernier, Gerard Fabre, Caroline Leriche, and David Fabre. 2017. "Ocular Drug Distribution after Topical Administration: Population Pharmacokinetic Model in Rabbits." *European Journal of Drug Metabolism and Pharmacokinetics* 42 (1): 59–68. https://doi.org/10.1007/s13318-016-0319-4.

38. Le Merdy, Maxime, Jianghong Fan, Michael B. Bolger, Viera Lukacova, Jessica Spires, Eleftheria Tsakalozou, Vikram Patel, et al. 2019. "Application of Mechanistic Ocular Absorption Modeling and Simulation to Understand the Impact of Formulation Properties on Ophthalmic Bioavailability in Rabbits: A Case Study Using Dexamethasone Suspension." *The AAPS Journal* 21 (4): 65. https://doi.org/10.1208/s12248-019-0334-x.

39. Le Merdy, Maxime, Jessica Spires, Viera Lukacova, Ming-Liang Tan, Andrew Babiskin, Xiaoming Xu, Liang Zhao, and Michael B. Bolger. 2020. "Ocular Physiologically Based Pharmacokinetic Modeling for Ointment Formulations." *Pharmaceutical Research* 37 (12): 245. https://doi.org/10.1007/s11095-020-02965-y.

40. Le Merdy, Maxime, Farah AlQaraghuli, Ming-Liang Tan, Ross Walenga, Andrew Babiskin, Liang Zhao, and Viera Lukacova. 2022. "Clinical Ocular Exposure Extrapolation for Ophthalmic Solutions Using PBPK Modeling and Simulation." *Pharmaceutical Research*. https://doi.org/10.1007/s11095-022-03390-z.

41. Le Merdy, Maxime, Ming-Liang Tan, Andrew Babiskin, and Liang Zhao. 2020. "Physiologically Based Pharmacokinetic Model to Support Ophthalmic Suspension Product Development." *The AAPS Journal* 22 (2): 26. https://doi.org/10.1208/s12248-019-0408-9.

42. Gukasyan, Hovhannes J., Shumet Hailu, Thomas K. Karami, and Richard Graham. 2019. "Ocular Biopharmaceutics: Impact of Modeling and Simulation on Topical Ophthalmic Formulation Development." *Drug Discovery Today* 24 (8): 1587–97. https://doi.org/10.1016/j.drudis.2019.04.002.

43. Chung, Jae Lim, Eun Hye Lim, Sang Wroul Song, Byung Yeop Kim, Joon H. Lee, Francis S. Mah, and Kyoung Yul Seo. 2013. "Comparative Intraocular Penetration of 4 Fluoroquinolones after Topical Instillation." *Cornea* 32 (7): 1046–51. https://doi.org/10.1097/ICO.0b013e31828d6d9e.

44. Robertson, Stella M., Michael A. Curtis, Barry A. Schlech, Andrew Rusinko, Geoffrey R. Owen, Olga Dembinska, John Liao, and David C. Dahlin. 2005. "Ocular Pharmacokinetics of Moxifloxacin after Topical Treatment of Animals and Humans." *Survey of Ophthalmology* 50 Suppl 1 (November): S32–45. https://doi.org/10.1016/j.survophthal.2005.07.001.

45. Donnenfeld, Eric D., Timothy L. Comstock, and Joel W. Proksch. 2011. "Human Aqueous Humor Concentrations of Besifloxacin, Moxifloxacin, and Gatifloxacin after Topical Ocular Application." *Journal of Cataract and Refractive Surgery* 37 (6): 1082–89. https://doi.org/10.1016/j.jcrs.2010.12.046.

46. Solomon, Renée, Eric D. Donnenfeld, Henry D. Perry, Robert W. Snyder, Chad Nedrud, Jonathan Stein, and Adam Bloom. 2005. "Penetration of Topically Applied Gatifloxacin 0.3%, Moxifloxacin 0.5%, and Ciprofloxacin 0.3% into the Aqueous Humor." *Ophthalmology* 112 (3): 466–69. https://doi.org/10.1016/j.ophtha.2004.09.029.

47. Ong-Tone, Lindsay. 2007. "Aqueous Humor Penetration of Gatifloxacin and Moxifloxacin Eyedrops given by Different Methods before Cataract Surgery." *Journal of Cataract and Refractive Surgery* 33 (1): 59–62. https://doi.org/10.1016/j.jcrs.2006.09.015.

48. Woodby, Brittany, Kayla Penta, Alessandra Pecorelli, Mary Ann Lila, and Giuseppe Valacchi. 2020. "Skin Health from the Inside Out." *Annual Review of Food Science and Technology* 11 (March): 235–54. https://doi.org/10.1146/annurev-food-032519-051722.

49. Gravitz, Lauren. 2018. "Skin." *Nature* 563 (7732): S83. https://doi.org/10.1038/d41586-018-07428-4.

50. Yousef, Hani, Mandy Alhajj, and Sandeep Sharma. 2023. "Anatomy, Skin (Integument), Epidermis". In *StatPearls*. Treasure Island (FL): StatPearls Publishing. https://www.ncbi.nlm.nih.gov/books/NBK470464/.

51. Agarwal, Sanjay, and Karthik Krishnamurthy. 2023. "Histology, Skin." In *StatPearls*. Treasure Island (FL): StatPearls Publishing. https://www.ncbi.nlm.nih.gov/books/NBK537325/.

52. Dąbrowska, A. K., Fabrizio Spano, Siegfried Derler, Christian Adlhart, Nicholas D. Spencer, and René M. Rossi. 2018. "The Relationship between Skin Function, Barrier Properties, and Body-Dependent Factors." *Skin Research and Technology: Official Journal of International Society for Bioengineering and the Skin (ISBS) [and] International Society for Digital Imaging of Skin (ISDIS) [and] International Society for Skin Imaging (ISSI)* 24 (2): 165–74. https://doi.org/10.1111/srt.12424.

53. Pastore, Michael N., Yogeshvar N. Kalia, Michael Horstmann, and Michael S. Roberts. 2015. "Transdermal Patches: History, Development and Pharmacology." *British Journal of Pharmacology* 172 (9): 2179–2209. https://doi.org/10.1111/bph.13059.

54. Larson, Ronald G. 1999. "The Structure and Rheology of Complex Fluids". In *Topics in Chemical Engineering*. New York: Oxford University Press.

55. Prausnitz, John, Edmundo Gomes de Azevedo, and Rudiger Lichtenthaler. 1998. *Molecular Thermodynamics of Fluid-Phase Equilibria*. 3rd edition. Upper Saddle River, NJ: Pearson.

56. Simões, Ana, Francisco Veiga, Ana Figueiras, and Carla Vitorino. 2018. "A Practical Framework for Implementing Quality by Design to the Development of Topical Drug Products: Nanosystem-Based Dosage Forms." *International Journal of Pharmaceutics* 548 (1): 385–99. https://doi.org/10.1016/j.ijpharm.2018.06.052.

57. Simões, Ana, Francisco Veiga, Carla Vitorino, and Ana Figueiras. 2018. "A Tutorial for Developing a Topical Cream Formulation Based on the Quality by Design Approach." *Journal of Pharmaceutical Sciences* 107 (10): 2653–62. https://doi.org/10.1016/j.xphs.2018.06.010.

58. Miranda, Margarida, Catarina Cardoso, and Carla Vitorino. 2020. "Quality and Equivalence of Topical Products: A Critical Appraisal." *European Journal of Pharmaceutical Sciences: Official Journal of the European Federation for Pharmaceutical Sciences* 148 (May): 105082. https://doi.org/10.1016/j.ejps.2019.105082.

59. Simonoska Crcarevska, Maja, Aneta Dimitrovska, Nadica Sibinovska, Kristina Mladenovska, Renata Slavevska Raicki, and Marija Glavas Dodov. 2015. "Implementation of Quality by Design Principles in the Development of Microsponges as Drug Delivery Carriers: Identification and Optimization of Critical Factors Using Multivariate Statistical Analyses and Design of Experiments Studies." *International Journal of Pharmaceutics* 489 (1–2): 58–72. https://doi.org/10.1016/j.ijpharm.2015.04.038.

60. Gorzelanny, Christian, Christian Mess, Stefan W. Schneider, Volker Huck, and Johanna M. Brandner. 2020. "Skin Barriers in Dermal Drug Delivery: Which Barriers Have to Be Overcome and How Can We Measure Them?" *Pharmaceutics* 12 (7): 684. https://doi.org/10.3390/pharmaceutics12070684.

61. Candi, Eleonora, Rainer Schmidt, and Gerry Melino. 2005. "The Cornified Envelope: A Model of Cell Death in the Skin." *Nature Reviews. Molecular Cell Biology* 6 (4): 328–40. https://doi.org/10.1038/nrm1619.

62. Ishida-Yamamoto, Akemi, Satomi Igawa, and Mari Kishibe. 2018. "Molecular Basis of the Skin Barrier Structures Revealed by Electron Microscopy." *Experimental Dermatology* 27 (8): 841–46. https://doi.org/10.1111/exd.13674.

63. Smeden, Jeroen van, and Joke A. Bouwstra. 2016. "Stratum Corneum Lipids: Their Role for the Skin Barrier Function in Healthy Subjects and Atopic Dermatitis Patients." *Current Problems in Dermatology* 49: 8–26. https://doi.org/10.1159/000441540.

64. Bouwstra, Joke A., Richard W. J. Helder, and Abdoelwaheb El Ghalbzouri. 2021. "Human Skin Equivalents: Impaired Barrier Function in Relation to the Lipid and Protein Properties of the Stratum Corneum." *Advanced Drug Delivery Reviews* 175 (August): 113802. https://doi.org/10.1016/j.addr.2021.05.012.

65. Wang, Tsuo-Feng, Gerald B. Kasting, and Johannes M. Nitsche. 2007. "A Multiphase Microscopic Diffusion Model for Stratum Corneum Permeability. II. Estimation of Physicochemical Parameters, and Application to a Large Permeability Database." *Journal of Pharmaceutical Sciences* 96 (11): 3024–51. https://doi.org/10.1002/jps.20883.

66. Wang, Tsuo-Feng, Gerald B. Kasting, and Johannes M. Nitsche. 2006. "A Multiphase Microscopic Diffusion Model for Stratum Corneum Permeability. I. Formulation, Solution, and Illustrative Results for Representative Compounds." *Journal of Pharmaceutical Sciences* 95 (3): 620–48. https://doi.org/10.1002/jps.20509.

67. Rim, Jee E., Peter M. Pinsky, and William W. van Osdol. 2009. "Multiscale Modeling Framework of Transdermal Drug Delivery." *Annals of Biomedical Engineering* 37 (6): 1217–29. https://doi.org/10.1007/s10439-009-9678-1.

68. Naegel, Arne, Michael Heisig, and Gabriel Wittum. 2013. "Detailed Modeling of Skin Penetration--an Overview." *Advanced Drug Delivery Reviews* 65 (2): 191–207. https://doi.org/10.1016/j.addr.2012.10.009.

69. Nitsche, Johannes M., and Gerald B. Kasting. 2013. "A Microscopic Multiphase Diffusion Model of Viable Epidermis Permeability." *Biophysical Journal* 104 (10): 2307–20. https://doi.org/10.1016/j.bpj.2013.03.056.

70. Kretsos, Kosmas, Matthew A. Miller, Grettel Zamora-Estrada, and Gerald B. Kasting. 2008. "Partitioning, Diffusivity and Clearance of Skin Permeants in Mammalian Dermis." *International Journal of Pharmaceutics* 346 (1–2): 64–79. https://doi.org/10.1016/j.ijpharm.2007.06.020.

71. Calcutt, Joshua J., and Yuri G. Anissimov. 2019. "Physiologically Based Mathematical Modelling of Solute Transport within the Epidermis and Dermis." *International Journal of Pharmaceutics* 569 (October): 118547. https://doi.org/10.1016/j.ijpharm.2019.118547.

72. Wittum, Rebecca, Arne Naegel, Michael Heisig, and Gabriel Wittum. 2020. "Mathematical Modelling of the Viable Epidermis: Impact of Cell Shape and Vertical Arrangement." *Mathematics and Mechanics of Solids* 25 (5): 1046–59. https://doi.org/10.1177/1081286517743297.

73. Kattou, Panayiotis, Guoping Lian, Stephen Glavin, Ian Sorrell, and Tao Chen. 2017. "Development of a Two-Dimensional Model for Predicting Transdermal Permeation with the Follicular Pathway: Demonstration with a Caffeine Study." *Pharmaceutical Research* 34 (10): 2036–48. https://doi.org/10.1007/s11095-017-2209-0.

74. Barbero, Ana M., and H. Frederick Frasch. 2017. "Effect of Stratum Corneum Heterogeneity, Anisotropy, Asymmetry and Follicular Pathway on Transdermal Penetration." *Journal of Controlled Release: Official Journal of the Controlled Release Society* 260 (August): 234–46. https://doi.org/10.1016/j.jconrel.2017.05.034.

75. Yu, Fang, Kevin Tonnis, Gerald B. Kasting, and Joanna Jaworska. 2021. "Computer Simulation of Skin Permeability of Hydrophobic and Hydrophilic Chemicals - Influence of Follicular Pathway." *Journal of Pharmaceutical Sciences* 110 (5): 2149–56. https://doi.org/10.1016/j.xphs.2020.12.020.

76. Cevc, Gregor, and Ulrich Vierl. 2007. "Spatial Distribution of Cutaneous Microvasculature and Local Drug Clearance after Drug Application on the Skin." *Journal of Controlled Release: Official Journal of the Controlled Release Society* 118 (1): 18–26. https://doi.org/10.1016/j.jconrel.2006.10.022.

77. Ibrahim, Rania, Johannes M. Nitsche, and Gerald B. Kasting. 2012. "Dermal Clearance Model for Epidermal Bioavailability Calculations." *Journal of Pharmaceutical Sciences* 101 (6): 2094–2108. https://doi.org/10.1002/jps.23106.

78. Kapoor, Yash, Mikolaj Milewski, Amitava Mitra, and Gerald B. Kasting. 2016. "Clarifications: Dermal Clearance Model for Epidermal Bioavailability Calculations." *Journal of Pharmaceutical Sciences* 105 (3): 1341–44. https://doi.org/10.1016/j.xphs.2015.12.004.

79. Calcutt, Joshua J., Michael S. Roberts, and Yuri G. Anissimov. 2022. "Predicting Viable Skin Concentration: Modelling the Subpapillary Plexus." *Pharmaceutical Research* 39 (4): 783–93. https://doi.org/10.1007/s11095-022-03215-z.

80. Yotsuyanagi, Toshihisa, William I. Higuchi, and Abdel Halim Ghanem. 1973. "Theoretical Treatment of Diffusional Transport into and through an Oil-Water Emulsion with an Interfacial Barrier at the Oil-Water Interface." *Journal of Pharmaceutical Sciences* 62 (1): 40–43. https://doi.org/10.1002/jps.2600620106.

81. Boddé, Harry E., and Jacques G. H. Joosten. 1985. "A Mathematical Model for Drug Release from a Two-Phase System to a Perfect Sink." *International Journal of Pharmaceutics* 26 (1): 57–76. https://doi.org/10.1016/0378-5173(85)90200-5.

82. Grassi, Mario, Nicoletta Coceani, and Lorenzo Magarotto. 2000. "Mathematical Modeling of Drug Release from Microemulsions: Theory in Comparison with Experiments." *Journal of Colloid and Interface Science* 228 (1): 141–50. https://doi.org/10.1006/jcis.2000.6945.

83. Sirotti, C., N. Coceani, I. Colombo, R. Lapasin, and M. Grassi. 2002. "Modeling of Drug Release from Microemulsions: A Peculiar Case." *Journal of Membrane Science* 204 (1): 401–12. https://doi.org/10.1016/S0376-7388(02)00069-8.

84. Bernardo, Fernando P., and Pedro M. Saraiva. 2008. "A Theoretical Model for Transdermal Drug Delivery from Emulsions and Its Dependence upon Formulation." *Journal of Pharmaceutical Sciences* 97 (9): 3781–3809. https://doi.org/10.1002/jps.21268.

85. Kim, Jong-Yun, Jun-Yeob Song, Eun-Joo Lee, and Seung-Kyu Park. 2003. "Rheological Properties and Microstructures of Carbopol Gel Network System." *Colloid & Polymer Science* 281 (7): 614–23. https://doi.org/10.1007/s00396-002-0808-7.

86. R. Varges, Priscilla, Camila M. Costa, Bruno S. Fonseca, Mônica F. Naccache, and Paulo R. De Souza Mendes. 2019. "Rheological Characterization of Carbopol® Dispersions in Water and in Water/Glycerol Solutions." *Fluids* 4 (1): 3. https://doi.org/10.3390/fluids4010003.

87. Fakhari, Amir, Marta Corcoran, and Alexander Schwarz. 2017. "Thermogelling Properties of Purified Poloxamer 407." *Heliyon* 3 (8). https://doi.org/10.1016/j.heliyon.2017.e00390.

88. Bunge, Annette L., John M. Persichetti, and Jean Paul Payan. 2012. "Explaining Skin Permeation of 2-Butoxyethanol from Neat and Aqueous Solutions." *International Journal of Pharmaceutics* 435 (1): 50–62. https://doi.org/10.1016/j.ijpharm.2012.01.058.

89. Frasch, H. Frederick, Ana M. Barbero, G. Scott Dotson, and Annette L. Bunge. 2014. "Dermal Permeation of 2-Hydroxypropyl Acrylate, a Model Water-Miscible Compound: Effects of Concentration, Thermodynamic Activity and Skin Hydration." *International Journal of Pharmaceutics* 460 (1–2): 240–47. https://doi.org/10.1016/j.ijpharm.2013.11.007.

90. Ventura, Stephanie A., and Gerald B. Kasting. 2017. "Dynamics of Glycerine and Water Transport across Human Skin from Binary Mixtures." *International Journal of Cosmetic Science* 39 (2): 165–78. https://doi.org/10.1111/ics.12362.

91. Miller, Matthew A., and Gerald B. Kasting. 2015. "A Spreadsheet-Based Method for Simultaneously Estimating the Disposition of Multiple Ingredients Applied to Skin." *Journal of Pharmaceutical Sciences* 104 (6): 2047–55. https://doi.org/10.1002/jps.24450.

92. Tonnis, Kevin, Johannes M. Nitsche, Lijing Xu, Alison Haley, Joanna Jaworska, and Gerald B. Kasting. 2022. "Impact of Solvent Dry down, Vehicle PH and Slowly Reversible Keratin Binding on Skin Penetration of Cosmetic Relevant Compounds: I. Liquids." *International Journal of Pharmaceutics* 624 (August): 122030. https://doi.org/10.1016/j.ijpharm.2022.122030.

93. Yu, Fang, Kevin Tonnis, Lijing Xu, Joanna Jaworska, and Gerald B. Kasting. 2022. "Modeling the Percutaneous Absorption of Solvent-Deposited Solids over a Wide Dose Range." *Journal of Pharmaceutical Sciences* 111 (3): 769–79. https://doi.org/10.1016/j.xphs.2021.10.001.

94. Tsakalozou, Eleftheria, Khondoker Alam, Andrew Babiskin, and Liang Zhao. 2022. "Physiologically-Based Pharmacokinetic Modeling to Support Determination of Bioequivalence for Dermatological Drug Products: Scientific and Regulatory Considerations." *Clinical Pharmacology & Therapeutics* 111: 1036–49. https://doi.org/10.1002/cpt.2356.

95. Polak, Sebastian, Cyrus Ghobadi, Himanshu Mishra, Malidi Ahamadi, Nikunjkumar Patel, Masoud Jamei, and Amin Rostami-Hodjegan. 2012. "Prediction of Concentration-Time Profile and Its Inter-Individual Variability Following the Dermal Drug Absorption." *Journal of Pharmaceutical Sciences* 101 (7): 2584–95. https://doi.org/10.1002/jps.23155.

96. Patel, Nikunjkumar, James F. Clarke, Farzaneh Salem, Tariq Abdulla, Frederico Martins, Sumit Arora, Eleftheria Tsakalozou, et al. 2022. "Multi-Phase Multi-Layer Mechanistic Dermal Absorption (MPML MechDermA) Model to Predict Local and Systemic Exposure of Drug Products Applied on Skin." *CPT: Pharmacometrics & Systems Pharmacology* 11 (8): 1060–84. https://doi.org/10.1002/psp4.12814.

97. Clarke, J. F., K. Thakur, and Sebastian Polak. 2022. "A Mechanistic Physiologically Based Model to Assess the Effect of Study Design and Modified Physiology on Formulation Safe Space for Virtual Bioequivalence of Dermatological Drug Products." *Frontiers in Pharmacology* 13: 1007496. https://doi.org/10.3389/fphar.2022.1007496.

98. Mittapelly, Naresh, and Sebastian Polak. 2022. "Modelling and Simulation Approaches to Support Formulation Optimization, Clinical Development and Regulatory Assessment of the Topically Applied Formulations - Nimesulide Solution Gel Case Study." *European Journal of Pharmaceutics and Biopharmaceutics: Official Journal of Arbeitsgemeinschaft Fur Pharmazeutische Verfahrenstechnik e.V* 178 (September): 140–49. https://doi.org/10.1016/j.ejpb.2022.08.005.

99. Wiśniowska, Barbara, Susanne Linke, Sebastian Polak, Zofia Bielecka, Andreas Luch, and Ralph Pirow. 2023. "Physiologically Based Modelling of Dermal Absorption and Kinetics of Consumer-Relevant Chemicals: A Case Study with Exposure to Bisphenol A from Thermal Paper." *Toxicology and Applied Pharmacology* 459 (January): 116357. https://doi.org/10.1016/j.taap.2022.116357.

100. Tsakalozou, Eleftheria, Andrew Babiskin, and Liang Zhao. 2021. "Physiologically-Based Pharmacokinetic Modeling to Support Bioequivalence and Approval of Generic Products: A Case for Diclofenac Sodium Topical Gel, 1." *CPT: Pharmacometrics & Systems Pharmacology* 10 (5): 399–411. https://doi.org/10.1002/psp4.12600.

101. "Zovirax US Prescriping Information." 2014. US Food & Drug Administration. https://www.accessdata.fda.gov/drugsatfda_docs/label/2014/021478s007lbl.pdf.

102. Murthy, S. Narasimha. 2017. "Characterizing the Critical Quality Attributes and in Vitro Bioavailability of Acyclovir and Metronidazole Topical Products." October 20. https://www.fda.gov/media/110262/download.

103. Roberts Michael S. 2017. "Correlation of Physicochemical Characteristics and in Vitro Permeation Test (IVPT) Results for Acyclovir and Metronidazole Topical Products."

104. Chang, Rong-Kun, Andre Raw, Robert Lionberger, and Lawrence Yu. 2013. "Generic Development of Topical Dermatologic Products: Formulation Development, Process Development, and Testing of Topical Dermatologic Products." *The AAPS Journal* 15 (1): 41–52. https://doi.org/10.1208/s12248-012-9411-0.

105. Díez-Sales, O., T.M. Garrigues, J.V. Herráez, R. Belda, A. Martín-Villodre, and M. Herráez. 2005. "In Vitro Percutaneous Penetration of Acyclovir from Solvent Systems and Carbopol 971-P Hydrogels: Influence of Propylene Glycol." *Journal of Pharmaceutical Sciences* 94 (5): 1039–47. https://doi.org/10.1002/jps.20317.

106. Santus, Giancarlo, Luciano Marcelloni, and Roberto Golzi. 2000. Topical aciclovir formulations. World Intellectual Property Organization WO2000001390A1, filed July 2, 1999, and issued January 13, 2000. https://patents.google.com/patent/WO2000001390A1/en.

107. Jones, Trevor M. and Alan R. White. 1990. Formulations of Heterocyclic Compounds. 4963555, filed March 1, 1989, and issued October 16, 1990. https://image-ppubs.uspto.gov/dirsearch-public/print/downloadPdf/4963555.

108. Kabanov, Alexander V., Elena V. Batrakova, and Valery Yu Alakhov. 2002. "Pluronic(r) Block Copolymers as Novel Polymer Therapeutics for Drug and Gene Delivery." *Journal of Controlled Release* 82 (2-3): 189–212. https://doi.org/10.1016/S0168-3659(02)00009-3.

109. Gudelj, Martina, Paola Šurina, Lucija Jurko, Ante Prkić, and Perica Bošković. 2021. "The Additive Influence of Propane-1,2-Diol on SDS Micellar Structure and Properties." *Molecules (Basel, Switzerland)* 26 (12): 3773. https://doi.org/10.3390/molecules26123773.

110. Kékicheff, P., C. Grabielle-Madelmont, and M. Ollivon. 1989. "Phase Diagram of Sodium Dodecyl Sulfate-Water System: 1. A Calorimetric Study." *Journal of Colloid and Interface Science* 131 (1): 112–32. https://doi.org/10.1016/0021-9797(89)90151-3.

111. Amsden, Brian. 1998. "Solute Diffusion within Hydrogels. Mechanisms and Models." *Macromolecules* 31 (22): 8382–95. https://doi.org/10.1021/ma980765f.

112. Kalwarczyk, Tomasz, Krzysztof Sozanski, Anna Ochab-Marcinek, Jedrzej Szymanski, Marcin Tabaka, Sen Hou, and Robert Holyst. 2015. "Motion of Nanoprobes in Complex Liquids within the Framework of the Length-Scale Dependent Viscosity Model." *Advances in Colloid and Interface Science* 223 (September): 55–63. https://doi.org/10.1016/j.cis.2015.06.007.

113. Szymański, Jedrzej, Adam Patkowski, Agnieszka Wilk, Piotr Garstecki, and Robert Holyst. 2006. "Diffusion and Viscosity in a Crowded Environment: From Nano- to Macroscale." *The Journal of Physical Chemistry. B* 110 (51): 25593–97. https://doi.org/10.1021/jp0666784.

114. Leo, Albert, Corwin Hansch, and David Elkins. 1971. "Partition Coefficients and Their Uses." *Chemical Reviews* 71 (6): 525–616. https://doi.org/10.1021/cr60274a001.

115. Siepmann, Juergen, and Nicholas A. Peppas. 2011. "Higuchi Equation: Derivation, Applications, Use and Misuse." *International Journal of Pharmaceutics* 418 (1): 6–12. https://doi.org/10.1016/j.ijpharm.2011.03.051.

116. Nallagundla, Sumalatha, Srinivas Patnala, and Isadore Kanfer. 2014. "Comparison of in Vitro Release Rates of Acyclovir from Cream Formulations Using Vertical Diffusion Cells." *AAPS PharmSciTech* 15 (4): 994–99. https://doi.org/10.1208/s12249-014-0130-y.

117. Zhang, Ji, and Bozena Michniak-Kohn. 2011. "Investigation of Microemulsion Microstructures and Their Relationship to Transdermal Permeation of Model Drugs: Ketoprofen, Lidocaine, and Caffeine." *International Journal of Pharmaceutics* 421 (1): 34–44. https://doi.org/10.1016/j.ijpharm.2011.09.014.

118. Yang, Senpei, Lingyi Li, Minsheng Lu, Tao Chen, Lujia Han, and Guoping Lian. 2019. "Determination of Solute Diffusion Properties in Artificial Sebum." *Journal of Pharmaceutical Sciences* 108 (9): 3003–10. https://doi.org/10.1016/j.xphs.2019.04.027.

119. Valiveti, Satyanarayana, and Guang Wei Lu. 2007. "Diffusion Properties of Model Compounds in Artificial Sebum." *International Journal of Pharmaceutics* 345 (1–2): 88–94. https://doi.org/10.1016/j.ijpharm.2007.05.043.

120. Wilschut, Annette, Wil F. ten Berge, Peter J. Robinson, and Thomas E. McKone. 1995. "Estimating Skin Permeation. The Validation of Five Mathematical Skin Permeation Models." *Chemosphere* 30 (7): 1275–96. https://doi.org/10.1016/0045-6535(95)00023-2.

121. Yang, Senpei, Lingyi Li, Tao Chen, Lujia Han, and Guoping Lian. 2018. "Determining the Effect of PH on the Partitioning of Neutral, Cationic and Anionic Chemicals to Artificial Sebum: New Physicochemical Insight and QSPR Model." *Pharmaceutical Research* 35 (7): 141. https://doi.org/10.1007/s11095-018-2411-8.

122. Hansen, Steffi, Arne Naegel, Michael Heisig, Gabriel Wittum, Dirk Neumann, Karl-Heinz Kostka, Peter Meiers, Claus-Michael Lehr, and Ulrich F. Schaefer. 2009. "The Role of Corneocytes in Skin Transport Revised--a Combined Computational and Experimental Approach." *Pharmaceutical Research* 26 (6): 1379–97. https://doi.org/10.1007/s11095-009-9849-7.

123. Hansen, Steffi, Dominik Selzer, Ulrich F. Schaefer, and Gerald B. Kasting. 2011. "An Extended Database of Keratin Binding." *Journal of Pharmaceutical Sciences* 100 (5): 1712–26. https://doi.org/10.1002/jps.22396.

124. Wagner, Heike, Karl Heinz Kostka, Claus Michael Lehr, and Ulrich F. Schaefer. 2003. "PH Profiles in Human Skin: Influence of Two in Vitro Test Systems for Drug Delivery Testing." *European Journal of Pharmaceutics and Biopharmaceutics: Official Journal of Arbeitsgemeinschaft Fur Pharmazeutische Verfahrenstechnik e.V* 55 (1): 57–65. https://doi.org/10.1016/s0939-6411(02)00125-x.

125. Spector, S. A., J. D. Connor, M. Hintz, R. P. Quinn, M. R. Blum, and R. E. Keeney. 1981. "Single-Dose Pharmacokinetics of Acyclovir." *Antimicrobial Agents and Chemotherapy* 19 (4): 608–12. https://doi.org/10.1128/AAC.19.4.608.

126. Peress Jimmy. 2003. "Estimate Evaporative Losses from Spills." *Chemical Engineering Progress* 99 (4): 32–34.

127. Nielsen, Frands, Erik Olsen, and Aage Fredenslund. 1994. "Henry's Law Constants and Infinite Dilution Activity Coefficients for Volatile Organic Compounds in Water by a Validated Batch Air Stripping Method." *Environmental Science & Technology* 28 (12): 2133–38. https://doi.org/10.1021/es00061a022.

128. Potts, R. O., and R. H. Guy. 1992. "Predicting Skin Permeability." *Pharmaceutical Research* 9 (5): 663–69. https://doi.org/10.1023/a:1015810312465.

129. Guy, Richard H., and Russell O. Potts. 1992. "Structure-Permeability Relationships in Percutaneous Penetration." *Journal of Pharmaceutical Sciences* 81 (6): 603–4. https://doi.org/10.1002/jps.2600810629.

130. Cleek, Robert L., and Annette L. Bunge. 1993. "A New Method for Estimating Dermal Absorption from Chemical Exposure. 1. General Approach." *Pharmaceutical Research* 10 (4): 497–506. https://doi.org/10.1023/a:1018981515480.

131. Valiveti, Satyanarayana, James Wesley, and Guang Wei Lu. 2008. "Investigation of Drug Partition Property in Artificial Sebum." *International Journal of Pharmaceutics* 346 (1–2): 10–16. https://doi.org/10.1016/j.ijpharm.2007.06.001.

132. Pensado, A., Wing Sin Chiu, S. F. Cordery, Elena Rantou, A. L. Bunge, M. B. Delgado-Charro, and R. H. Guy. 2019. "Stratum Corneum Sampling to Assess Bioequivalence between Topical Acyclovir Products." *Pharmaceutical Research* 36 (12): 180. https://doi.org/10.1007/s11095-019-2707-3.

133. Wang, Jianzhuo, and Douglas R. Flanagan. 2002. "General Solution for Diffusion-Controlled Dissolution of Spherical Particles. 2. Evaluation of Experimental Data." *Journal of Pharmaceutical Sciences* 91 (2): 534–42. https://doi.org/10.1002/jps.10039.

134. Wang, Jianzhuo, and Douglas R. Flanagan. 1999. "General Solution for Diffusion-Controlled Dissolution of Spherical Particles. 1. Theory." *Journal of Pharmaceutical Sciences* 88 (7): 731–38. https://doi.org/10.1021/js980236p.

135. Cukier, R. 1984. "Diffusion of Brownian Spheres in Semidilute Polymer Solutions." https://doi.org/10.1021/MA00132A023.

136. Cheng, S. C., and R. I. Vachon. 1969. "The Prediction of the Thermal Conductivity of Two and Three Phase Solid Heterogeneous Mixtures." *International Journal of Heat and Mass Transfer* 12 (3): 249–64. https://doi.org/10.1016/0017-9310(69)90009-X.

137. Crank, John. 1975. *The Mathematics of Diffusion*. 2nd edition. Oxford, [Eng]: Clarendon Press.

138. Starov, V. M., and V. G. Zhdanov. 2008. "Effective Properties of Suspensions/Emulsions, Porous and Composite Materials." *Advances in Colloid and Interface Science* 137 (1): 2–19. https://doi.org/10.1016/j.cis.2006.11.025.

139. Kamal, Nahid S., Yellela S. R. Krishnaiah, Xiaoming Xu, Ahmed S. Zidan, Sameersingh Raney, Celia N. Cruz, and Muhammad Ashraf. 2020. "Identification of Critical Formulation Parameters Affecting the in Vitro Release, Permeation, and Rheological Properties of the Acyclovir Topical Cream." *International Journal of Pharmaceutics* 590 (November): 119914. https://doi.org/10.1016/j.ijpharm.2020.119914.

140. Trottet, L., H. Owen, P. Holme, J. Heylings, I. P. Collin, A. P. Breen, M. N. Siyad, R. S. Nandra, and A. F. Davis. 2005. "Are All Aciclovir Cream Formulations Bioequivalent?" *International Journal of Pharmaceutics* 304 (1–2): 63–71. https://doi.org/10.1016/j.ijpharm.2005.07.020.

5 Perfusion and Permeability-Limited Distribution Models

Helen Musther, Masoud Jamei, Iain Gardner, and Armin Sepp

5.1 INTRODUCTION

Regardless of the route of administration, elimination, or site of action, the movements of a drug around the body, then into and out of tissues, are critical processes that must be accounted for in understanding the pharmacokinetics of a drug. As such, these processes must also be included in physiologically-based pharmacokinetic (PBPK) models. While the movement of drug to the different tissues through the blood is described using differential equations, each required tissue is represented in the models as a compartment of a defined volume. The transfer, or distribution, of the drug across cell membranes into these tissues must then be incorporated to fully describe the time course of the drug. Once the distribution of a drug is adequately included, detailed PBPK models allow not only the capture and prediction of the systemic concentration-time profiles but also time-based distribution and accumulation of drug into specific tissues of interest.

This chapter discusses the factors affecting drug distribution into the tissues, the different mechanisms by which distribution can occur, mathematical descriptors for those processes and the incorporation of these into full-body PBPK models. The differences between perfusion-limited and permeability-limited models are described, as are the parameters needed to describe the passive and active transfer of drug into tissues. Examples of the utility of predicted concentration-time profiles are provided.

5.2 PROPERTIES AFFECTING DRUG TISSUE DISTRIBUTION

Differences in physiological factors can occur due to age, sex, genetics, ethnicity and pathology, contributing to differences in the overall observed tissue distribution of a particular drug administered to different populations or individuals. These factors can be incorporated into PBPK models by collation of the requisite data, often available in the published literature. Since this is generally completed as part of the wider PBPK model development, these will not be discussed in detail in this chapter. For example, in patients with cirrhosis observed changes (c.f. healthy volunteers) include cardiac output, reduction of liver size, reduced protein binding by both albumin and α1-acid glycoprotein, and a change in the blood flow to the liver [1]. Transporter abundances are also affected [2]. All of these parameters can affect the distribution of a drug within the body and should be accounted for within a PBPK model for a cirrhotic population. For any population, it is essential to incorporate the most relevant data for blood flows and tissue volumes while also considering whether differences will be observed in other areas such as protein binding or active transport.

The distribution of any drug into a tissue is dependent on not only these physiological parameters but also the physicochemical properties of the drug and the interaction of the drug with the constituent membrane and tissue components. These interactions form the basis of our understanding and also form the foundations on which many of the predictive and translational distribution models have been built. Drug can transfer into tissues either through passive processes or active transport, with the size of the molecule, ionisation, lipophilicity and affinity of drug to bind to blood, plasma and tissue components all impacting on the resultant drug distribution. In general, it is expected that small, neutral, lipophilic drugs will distribute into tissues through passive processes, and larger, ionised, hydrophilic drugs require active processes to permeate into the tissue [3]. This makes logical sense, as membranes are a combination of tightly packed lipid bilayers and proteins. In addition, it is widely accepted that only freely available drug, i.e., unbound drug, is available to cross from the blood to the tissues and vice-versa [4].

Assessments of size (molecular weight), lipophilicity (octanol:water partitioning, $\text{Log}P_{o:w}/\text{Log}D_{o:w}$) and ionisation (compound type, pKa) are generally available from either measurement or predictions in early drug discovery. Fraction unbound in plasma (fu_p) is commonly measured and *in silico* prediction methods have also been described. Blood-to-plasma ratio (B/P), describing the partitioning of drug into blood cells from plasma water, is another parameter of interest although this is less frequently reported for some compound types, and assumptions are sometimes made due to the lack of measured data [5,6,7]. These parameters are heavily used in the predictions and descriptions of distribution used in PBPK models. For known drugs, much of these data are published in the form of pharmacokinetic reports and can be used in model construction. Similarly, predictive *in silico* models are available for e.g., pKa and $\text{log}P_{o:w}$ if experimental data are not available, though generally experimental results are preferred.

DOI: 10.1201/9781003031802-5

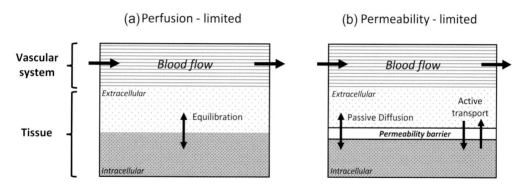

Figure 5.1 (a and b) Perfusion and permeability-limited schematic.

5.3 PERFUSION-LIMITED VERSUS PERMEABILITY-LIMITED DISTRIBUTION

Two methods are commonly used in PBPK models to describe drug distribution into tissues: perfusion-limited and permeability-limited, relating to the processes that are rate-determining for the tissue distribution of a drug [4,8]. In general, perfusion-limited models are the simplest required model for any tissue of interest, whereas permeability-limited models are more complex and can be applied to specific tissues when required. Although not discussed in this chapter, additional key processes such as metabolic clearance can be added to either perfusion or permeability-limited tissue models.

Perfusion-limited distribution, illustrated in Figure 5.1a, refers to a scenario where the distribution of the drug into the intracellular space of a tissue is not limited by any barrier and the drug can freely diffuse into and out of the tissue. In this case, the distribution of a drug is limited by the flow of blood to the tissue or perfusion of the tissue. The incorporation of perfusion-limited models in PBPK models is described in Section 5.4.

Permeability-limited distribution, illustrated in Figure 5.1b, describes a situation where there is a barrier preventing the passive movement of drug into the tissue. Therefore, in this case, the distribution is limited by the ability of the drug to cross the barrier. The permeability of the drug across the barrier rather than the delivery of the drug to the tissue by blood becomes the rate-determining step in tissue distribution [4]. This permeation of drug can take place through active transport or by some limited passive diffusion across the cell membrane, either of which can be incorporated into the PBPK model. In contrast to perfusion-limited methods, permeability-limited models are mathematically more complex, but can be applied either to individual tissues within a PBPK model, while other tissues can remain perfusion-limited, or to all of the tissues if needed. The inclusion of permeability-limited models in PBPK is described in Section 5.8.

5.4 PERFUSION-LIMITED MODELS IN PBPK

Within a perfusion-limited model each tissue, or compartment, is assumed to be well-stirred, with equilibrium across the membrane reached instantaneously [9]. Assuming that measures of tissue/blood volumes and blood flows are already known, what is still required is a mathematical description of this equilibrium, or the affinity of drug for the tissue. The relevant parameter is termed the "equilibrium distribution ratio" between the tissue and plasma, frequently referred to as a "Kp" or "$P_{t:p}$" value, and is used within perfusion-limited distribution PBPK models to describe the movement of drug into the tissue.

In vivo, when dosing to steady state for permeable compounds, passive diffusion is assumed to allow the free drug to reach an equilibrium between the plasma and the tissue. Since the components, and their concentrations, to which drugs bind (e.g., lipids and proteins) differ between plasma and tissue, the binding of drug differs between the two regions. As a result, the total relative drug concentration in plasma and each tissue are not equal and an equilibrium concentration ratio (Kp) can be calculated (Equation 5.1)

$$Kp = \frac{C_T}{C_P} \qquad (5.1)$$

where C_T is the total drug concentration in the tissue and C_P is the total drug concentration in the plasma.

These values are tissue-specific; therefore, a value is required for each tissue described within the PBPK model, termed Kp_T, where T is the tissue of interest. These values are then combined with the blood flow, tissue volume and concentration in the blood to obtain the concentration time profile for the tissue. Equation 5.2 illustrates the application for a non-eliminating tissue [9,10]:

$$\frac{dC_T}{dt} = \frac{Q_T}{V_T}\left(C_{ab} - \frac{C_T}{\dfrac{Kp_T}{B:P}}\right) \tag{5.2}$$

where C_T is the drug concentration in the tissue, Q_T is the tissue blood flow, V_T is the tissue volume, C_{ab} is the drug concentration in the arterial blood, Kp_T is the tissue-to-plasma partition coefficient, and $B:P$ is the blood-to-plasma concentration ratio of the drug.

The measurement of Kp values requires dosing a drug to steady state, followed by the determination of the concentrations in both the plasma and the tissues of interest. While sometimes determined in preclinical species, the obvious ethical and operational considerations prevent these from being routine measurements, particularly in humans. Historically, this meant that PBPK models required a significant amount of experimental work to derive appropriate input values, and this requirement hampered their widespread application. However, the development of methods to predict Kp values (Section 5.5) has allowed the wider use and further advancement of PBPK models.

5.5 PREDICTION OF TISSUE-PLASMA PARTITION COEFFICIENTS

Several types of predictive models have been utilised in the prediction of Kp values. All Kp prediction methods have their limitations, and it is up to the user to select the most appropriate model depending on the data that are available and the assessment of the applicability domain of the different models. If measured data, whether preclinical, *in vivo*, or *in vitro*, are available, these can also be incorporated into the PBPK model. Fraction unbound in tissue (fu_t) determined from *in vitro* studies can be used to calculate Kp [11]. Measured Kp values for muscle and adipose can be used in a correlation approach where Kp is predicted for other tissues using previously defined linear regressions [12]. However, these are not routine measurements. Where structural information is available, quantitative structure property/activity relationships (QSPR/QSAR), have been developed and can be used in combination with neural networks and machine-learning methods [13]. These approaches can be limited to certain compound classes used in the construction of the QSPR/QSAR model, or difficult to replicate independently.

More commonly, experimental data are available for the drug under investigation in the form of routinely measured physicochemical and blood-binding parameters. These are utilised in the most widely used Kp prediction strategy, the tissue composition models [14,15,16,17,18,19, 20,21,22,23]. These models can be incorporated into PBPK models to allowing the prediction of concentration-time profiles in both blood and tissues. The tissue composition methodology builds on the understanding of the interactions of the drug with membrane and tissue components, driven by the properties of the drug and tissue. Assumptions are made in these methods, namely that the drug distributes immediately into the tissue, that both the tissue and plasma are made up of lipids, water and proteins, and no active transport is occurring. No prior *in vivo* data are required and there is an expectation that these are applicable for "bottom-up" predictions of distribution for a wide, chemically diverse range of drugs [24]. Since this type of model is based on mechanistic principles, once a tissue composition model is established, it is assumed that it can be expanded to other drugs simply by the inclusion of the required physicochemical and blood-binding data for the new compound of interest. Predictions can also be made for other species if the relevant tissue composition data can be identified and included, with previously collated datasets available in the literature for humans [14], rats [14,16,18], dogs [25] and minipigs [26].

The model developed by Poulin and Thiel [14,15] is still widely used in PBPK modelling with some minor modifications having been proposed [27]. The Poulin and Theil method comprises two equations, one describing distribution into the adipose (Equation 5.3) and another relating to all other tissues (Equation 5.4). Here it is assumed that the global pH of both plasma and tissue is 7.4, with differential ionisation in plasma and tissue not being considered, and lipophilicity ($P_{o:w}$ and $D_{vo:w}$) is used as a measure of neutral lipid and phospholipid affinity.

$$Kp_{adipose} = \frac{\left[D_{vo:w}\cdot\left(f_{NL_T}+0.3f_{PL_T}\right)\right]+\left(f_{W_T}+0.7f_{PL_T}\right)}{\left[P_{o:w}\cdot\left(f_{NL_P}+0.3f_{PL_P}\right)\right]+\left(f_{W_P}/fu_p+0.7f_{PL_P}\right)} \tag{5.3}$$

$$Kp_{non-adipose} = \frac{\left[P_{o:w}\cdot\left(f_{NL_T}+0.3f_{PL_T}\right)\right]+\left(f_{W_T}/fu_t+0.7f_{PL_T}\right)}{\left[P_{o:w}\cdot\left(f_{NL_P}+0.3f_{PL_P}\right)\right]+\left(f_{W_P}/fu_p+0.7f_{PL_P}\right)} \tag{5.4}$$

where f_{NL_T}, f_{PL_T} and f_{W_T} refer to the fractional tissue volume of neutral lipids, phospholipids and water, respectively, and f_{NL_P}, f_{PL_P} and f_{W_P} refer to the fractional plasma volume of these same components. fu_t and fu_p are the fraction unbound in tissue and plasma, respectively. $D_{vo:w}$ refers to the antilog of the log (vegetable oil:water) partition coefficient at pH 7.4 and $P_{o:w}$ is the antilog of the log (octanol:water) partition coefficient.

Note that for the adipose tissue the alternative log$D_{vo:w}$ measure is used as a description of neutral lipid affinity in this tissue. This refers to the partitioning into vegetable oil at pH 7.4, rather than the more routine measurement in octanol, as this is considered a more representative measure for the interaction in adipose. However, this value is not routinely measured and can be calculated using Hendersen-Hasslebach principles, as generally while log$D$ refers to a partitioning measurement at a specified pH, log$P$ indicates the partitioning of the neutral species. Equation 5.5 shows the relationship for a monoprotic base:

$$\log D_{vo:w} = \log P_{vo:w} - \log\left(1+10^{pKa-pH}\right) \tag{5.5}$$

where log$P_{vo:w}$ is the vegetable oil:water partitioning of the neutral drug.

As log$P_{vo:w}$ is also not routinely measured, regression approaches have been used to develop models linking log$P_{vo:w}$ to the more commonly determined log$P_{o:w}$ as described in Equation 5.6 [15,28]. For highly lipophilic compounds (e.g., log$P_{o:w}$>4), this linear relationship overestimates the partitioning, and so the use of Equation 5.7 is presented as an alternative [29].

$$\log P_{vo:w} = 1.115\cdot\log P_{o:w} - 1.35 \tag{5.6}$$

$$\log P_{vo:w} = -4.635 + \left(\frac{7.972}{1+10^{(0.1175-0.2849\cdot\log P_{o:w})}}\right) \tag{5.7}$$

where log$P_{o:w}$ refers to the commonly measured log (octanol:water) partitioning coefficient.

One last parameter in the model not routinely measured, fu_t, refers to a global tissue binding value. If unavailable, this is calculated from the fraction unbound in plasma as shown in Equation 5.8:

$$fu_t = \frac{1}{1+\dfrac{1-fu_p}{2\cdot fu_p}} \tag{5.8}$$

where fu_p is the fraction unbound in plasma.

While appropriate for some types of drugs, e.g., neutral lipophilic compounds, this model is missing fundamental interactions for ionised drugs, particularly strongly ionised basic drugs. The models developed by Rodgers et al. address these limitations by including ionisation terms, defined using the Henderson-Hasselbalch relationship for each compound type [16,18,19]. Here it is assumed that only unionised drug can be distributed into tissue. Further, the tissue composition is subdivided to incorporate extracellular water, intracellular water, acidic phospholipid content and partitioning of albumin and lipoprotein. The generic fraction unbound in tissue is not used here, with binding to acidic phospholipids or extracellular protein being incorporated instead. As the interaction with acidic phospholipids is key for drugs with an ionised basic centre, but not for other compound types, the Rodgers and Rowland model is divided into one equation for strong bases, defined as a compound with at least one basic pKa equal to or greater than 7 (Equation 5.9), and another for other compound types (Equation 5.10):

$$\text{Kpu} = \left[\left(\frac{1+X \cdot f_{\text{IW}}}{1+Y}\right) + f_{\text{EW}} + \left(\frac{\text{Ka}_{\text{AP}} \cdot [\text{AP}] \cdot X}{1+Y}\right) + \left(\frac{P_{o:w} \cdot f_{\text{NL}} + (0.3P_{o:w} + 0.7) \cdot f_{\text{NP}}}{1+Y}\right)\right] \quad (5.9)$$

$$\text{Kpu} = \left[\left(\frac{1+X \cdot f_{\text{IW}}}{1+Y}\right) + f_{\text{EW}} + \left(\text{Ka}_{\text{PR}} \cdot [\text{PR}]_T\right) + \left(\frac{P_{o:w} \cdot f_{\text{NL}} + (0.3P_{o:w} + 0.7) \cdot f_{\text{NP}}}{1+Y}\right)\right] \quad (5.10)$$

where X and Y are terms describing ionisation of the compound (see Table 5.1), calculated using the Henderson-Hasselbalch relationship with the drug pKa and pH of the intracellular water and plasma, respectively. $P_{o:w}$ is the antilog of $\log P_{o:w}$. $f_{\text{IW}}, f_{\text{EW}}, f_{\text{NL}}$ and f_{NP} are the fractions of intracellular water, extracellular water, neutral lipids and neutral phospholipids present in the tissue, and [AP] is the concentration of acidic phospholipids in the tissue. Ka_{AP} is the binding affinity of the ionised compound to acidic phospholipids, $[\text{PR}]_T$ is the concentration of extracellular protein, and Ka_{PR} is the binding affinity of the compound of interest to these proteins.

Ka_{AP} and Ka_{PR} are not routinely measured but can be calculated as follows. Ka_{AP} using measured blood-binding data (B/P) as per Equation 5.11, and Ka_{PR} from plasma binding as shown in Equation 5.12, and the relevant lipid composition data. Where calculation leads to a negative value, these affinity values are set to 0.

$$\text{Ka}_{\text{AP}} = \left[\text{Kpu}_{\text{BC}} - \left(\frac{1+Z}{1+Y} \cdot f_{\text{IW}}\right) - \left(\frac{P_{o:w} \cdot f_{\text{NL}} + (0.3P_{o:w} + 0.7) \cdot f_{\text{NP}}}{1+Y}\right)\right] \cdot \left(\frac{1+Y}{[\text{AP}] \cdot Z}\right) \quad (5.11)$$

$$\text{Ka}_{\text{PR}} = \left[\frac{1}{\text{fu}_p} - 1 - \left(\frac{P_{o:w} \cdot f_{\text{NL}} + (0.3P_{o:w} + 0.7) \cdot f_{\text{NP}}}{1+Y}\right)\right] \cdot \left(\frac{1}{[\text{PR}]}\right) \quad (5.12)$$

where K_{puBC}, the unbound partition coefficient between plasma and blood cells, is calculated from fu_p, B/P and the haematocrit, $P_{o:w}$ is the antilog of $\log P_{o:w}$. $f_{\text{IW}}, f_{\text{NL}}$ and f_{NP} are the fractions of intracellular water, neutral lipids and neutral phospholipids present in the blood cells or plasma, [AP] is the concentration of acidic phospholipids in blood cells and [PR] is the concentration of extracellular protein in plasma. Z and Y are terms describing the ionisation of the compound using the intracellular blood cell or plasma pH as appropriate (see Table 5.1).

Table 5.1: Ionisation Terms for Kpu Predictions

Compound Type	X	Y	Z
Neutral	0	0	n/a
Monoprotic acid	$10^{\text{pHIW} - \text{pKa}}$	$10^{\text{pHP} - \text{pKa}}$	n/a
Monoprotic base	$10^{\text{pKa} - \text{pHIW}}$	$10^{\text{pKa} - \text{pHP}}$	$10^{\text{pKa} - \text{pHIW,rbc}}$
Diprotic acid	$10^{\text{pHIW} - \text{pKa1}} + 10^{\text{pHIW} - \text{pKa2}}$ $+ 10^{2\text{pHIW} - (\text{pKa1} + \text{pKa2})}$	$10^{\text{pHP} - \text{pKa1}} + 10^{\text{pHP} - \text{pKa2}}$ $+ 10^{2\text{pHP} - (\text{pKa1} + \text{pKa2})}$	n/a
Diprotic base	$10^{\text{pKa1} - \text{pHIW}} + 10^{\text{pKa2} - \text{pHIW}}$ $+ 10^{(\text{pKa1} + \text{pKa2}) - 2\text{pHIW}}$	$10^{\text{pKa1} - \text{pHP}} + 10^{\text{pKa2} - \text{pHP}}$ $+ 10^{(\text{pKa1} + \text{pKa2}) - 2\text{pHP}}$	$10^{\text{pKa1} - \text{pHIW,rbc}} + 10^{\text{pKa2} - \text{pHIW,rbc}}$ $+ 10^{(\text{pKa1} + \text{pKa2}) - 2\text{pHIW,rbc}}$
Ampholyte	$10^{\text{pHIW} - \text{pKa1}} + 10^{\text{pKa2} - \text{pHIW}}$ $+ 10^{\text{pKa2} - \text{pKa1}}$	$10^{\text{pHP} - \text{pKa1}} + 10^{\text{pKa2} - \text{pHP}}$ $+ 10^{\text{pKa2} - \text{pKa1}}$	$10^{\text{pKa2} - \text{pHIW,rbc}}$

Note: For ampholytes pKa1 is the acidic pKa and pKa2 is the basic pKa.
P, plasma; IW, intracellular; rbc, red blood cells.

Equations 5.9 and 5.10 calculate Kpu rather than Kp, and are easily converted using fraction unbound in plasma using Equation 5.13:

$$Kp = Kpu \cdot fu_p \tag{5.13}$$

While the overall structure of the models remains the same, variations on these tissue composition models can be explored to address specific concerns, for example incorporating measured phospholipid partitioning [20,21] or fraction unbound in microsomes in place of $\log P_{o:w}$ as a phospholipid binding descriptor [22,30,31].

5.6 EXTENSIONS TO Kp PREDICTION MODELS

For basic drugs, a phenomenon where drug is sequestered in acidic subcellular organelles, lysosomes, is suggested to contribute to tissue distribution through passive processes. Lysosomes can comprise a significant proportion of some tissues (e.g. lung), and the difference in the pH between the organelle and the cytosol leads to the distribution of cations into the subcellular space, resulting in increased overall equilibrium distribution to those tissues. Partitioning into the subcellular compartment, considering this pH differential, in line with the previously described model, has been incorporated into Kp prediction models to account for this increased distribution [32,33].

In the models discussed previously, it has generally been assumed that ionised, or polar, drug does not permeate passively across a membrane, however, this is not strictly true. Ionised drug can be distributed passively, but the rate is significantly slower than for unionised drug and is generally expected to be of relevance only for highly ionised drugs. This distribution can be incorporated by determining the flux of both neutral and ionised forms of the drug across a membrane, and incorporating it into cell or tissue distribution models [34,35]. Existing Kp prediction models have been extended to incorporate this ion permeation, utilising local tissue intracellular pH and membrane potential in a Fick-Nernst Plank framework [34,36] to describe transfer of the ionised species as well as the neutral species across the membrane.

5.7 USE OF THE STEADY-STATE VOLUME OF DISTRIBUTION IN PBPK MODELLING

The volume of distribution at steady-state (V_{ss}) is a routinely obtained parameter in *in vivo* clinical pharmacokinetic investigations, describing the overall amount of drug in the tissues versus the plasma at a steady-state or equilibrium condition. It is determined using non-compartmental analysis of intravenous concentration-time profiles [37]. A dataset of collated V_{ss} information for 1,300 drugs in humans has been published [38]. In a full-body PBPK model, where the tissue volumes and Kp values are specified individually, V_{ss} is not used as an input parameter but can be predicted to provide useful information for model verification purposes. This is achieved by summing the combination of Kp value and tissue volume across all the tissues in the body or model (Equation 5.14):

$$V_{ss} = V_p + \left(V_{rbc} \cdot \frac{E}{P} \right) + \sum V_t \cdot Kp \tag{5.14}$$

where V_p is the volume of plasma, V_{rbc} is the volume of red blood cells, E/P is the erythrocyte-to-plasma partition coefficient, V_t is the volume of tissues, and Kp is the tissue-to-plasma partition coefficient.

This predicted V_{ss} can then be compared to in *in vivo* data, if available, to allow assessment of whether Kp values are adequately predicted and whether adjustments need to be made to the model. If human V_{ss} data are not available e.g., if a PBPK model is developed to predict the pharmacokinetics in a first time in human (FIH) study, the assumptions of the different Kp prediction methods can be assessed by comparing the PBPK model in preclinical species to observed *in vivo* distribution data to verify the validity of different Kp prediction methods. The distribution model may then be adjusted to better fit the preclinical data before making prospective predictions in human, which may be achieved by adjusting Kp values manually, applying a global "Kp scalar" across all predicted values (e.g. [39]), or fitting other values to give the desired outcome (e.g. [40]).

Prediction of V_{ss}, using predicted Kp values, assumes that only passive processes contribute to tissue distribution and if active transport processes occur for a particular drug in one or several tissues, this would influence the V_{ss} value determined *in vivo* and can lead to mismatches between predictions and observations. Active transport processes can be incorporated into the PBPK model using permeability-limited models (Section 5.8).

5.8 PERMEABILITY-LIMITED MODELS IN PBPK

Active, or carrier-mediated, transport is important for several key tissues in the body, in particular the liver, kidney, gut and brain. It is relevant for a large, rapidly increasing, number of drugs as the chemical space utilised in drug discovery and development projects expands. It occurs through transporter proteins that are part of the cell membrane structure, which vary according to tissue type and are also subject to inter-individual variability in terms of abundance and function. While specific transporters will not be discussed here, numerous publications are available in the literature describing the location and function of drug transporters, (e.g. [41,42]).

Active transport is incorporated into PBPK models using permeability-limited models. In contrast to the perfusion-limited scenario, where Kp and blood flow drive the transfer of drug across the membrane, permeability-limited models require estimates of the uptake, efflux and passive transport processes for the drug in the tissue(s) of interest. This section discusses the structure of permeability-limited tissue models, while Section 5.9 describes the *in vitro* assessments, systems data and calculations required to include transport processes in the PBPK models.

At the simplest level, a permeability-limited model may only represent a permeability barrier between the blood/extracellular water and the intracellular space of the tissue without consideration of active transport. The level of complexity that is needed for a particular PBPK model needs to be defined by the modeller according to the processes that need to be included. This is true whether drug is transported only into the intracellular water of the tissue, then subject to metabolism, or is subject to further transport processes either back into the blood or to another compartment (e.g. bile or urine).

Considering the liver as an example, drugs can be transported by both passive and active processes, with transport occurring both on the sinusoidal (blood flow) membrane and on the canalicular side, which leads to the bile (Figure 5.2). Known liver transporters indicate uptake occurs on the sinusoidal membrane only, with efflux occurring on both sinusoidal and canalicular membranes.

This knowledge is translated into a mathematical description of the processes involved, in the form of differential equations. These equations can become quite complex; therefore, readers are referred to Jamei et al. [9] as an example for a detailed set of equations for a permeability-limited liver model.

In general, the tissue is defined as several compartments, with an equation required for each compartment in the model. This requires definitions of volumes, initial concentrations and blood flows. Multiple uptake and efflux processes can be incorporated, including passive and active uptake in and out of the compartments. Mass balance should be maintained, i.e., drug transported from one compartment should appear in the other. Metabolism can also be incorporated to account for clearance of the drug. As per perfusion-limited models, there is an assumption that only unbound drug is available for passive diffusion or active transport, with either unbound or unbound+unionised concentration at the site of action driving the transport/diffusion processes.

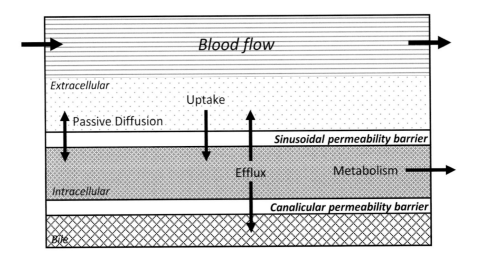

Figure 5.2 Generic liver transport processes.

This liver example represents a relatively simple permeability-limited model. However, permeability-limited models can increase significantly in complexity by the definition of multiple compartments within the tissue, with further rate-limiting steps incorporated between those compartments or additional binding components within a compartment being considered (e.g. [43]). While permeability-limited PBPK models increase the computational resources required, the applications allow the exploration of the different components of drug disposition in the specified tissue [41]. Therefore, highly mechanistically defined models have been developed and published for some tissues (e.g. kidney [41,44,45], brain [46,47], lung [48] and liver [45,49,50].

5.9 IN VITRO – IN VIVO EXTRAPOLATION OF TRANSPORTER-MEDIATED KINETICS

In vitro data relating to the transport of the drug is required to incorporate transport processes within the permeability-limited tissue model(s). The systems used depend on the tissue of interest and include, to name a few: hepatocytes [49,51, 52], Human Embryonic Kidney (HEK) cells transfected with specific transporters [53], kidney slices [41] and brain slices [47]. Passive diffusion processes (CL_{PD}) are assessed by the use of transport inhibitors or cells with knocked out transporters or null transfected cells. For many of these *in vitro* systems, the results require modelling of the *in vitro* system in order to obtain the required transporter data for inclusion in PBPK models [54]. It is commonly assumed that simple Michaelis-Menten kinetics are appropriate to describe these transporter data, with rates represented by K_m and J_{max} determined from fitting, and intrinsic transporter clearance, $CL_{int,T}$, calculated as shown in Equation 5.15:

$$CL_{int} = \frac{J_{max}}{K_m + Cu} \tag{5.15}$$

where J_{max} is the *in vivo* maximum rate of transport, K_m is the Michaelis constant, and Cu is the relevant unbound concentration for the transporter.

However, it is acknowledged that this assumption is not appropriate for all transporters and drugs, and expansions of fitting to two-site, or models incorporating additional binding or dependencies may be required [44,54]. When performing modelling of transporter data care is therefore advised in selecting the most appropriate model.

Suitable *in vitro* data are required to be scaled from the *in vitro* system-specific parameters to physiologically relevant values *in vivo* for inclusion in the model. There are at least two general approaches that are commonly used, relative expression or activity scaling and absolute abundance scaling.

Relative scaling approaches use a comparative activity or amount of transporter in the *in vitro* system vs. a system representative of *in vivo* transport, which could be a native tissue cell (e.g. hepatocytes) or potentially a whole body. Often this will require using scaling factors in combination with physiological data (Figure 5.3) to bring an *in vitro* observed value to a whole organ *in vivo* transporter clearance. There are two types of relative scaling approach: relative activity factor (RAF) and relative expression factor (REF).

RAF refers to the relative transporter clearance between the two systems. This approach requires a transporter-selective probe substrate to be identified and administered in both *in vitro* and representative *in vivo* systems, and clearance of the probe is compared [52] (Equation 5.16).

$$RAF = \frac{In\ vitro\ \text{transporter activity}\,(Unit)}{In\ vivo\ \text{transporter activity}\,(Unit)} \tag{5.16}$$

where the units must be the same.

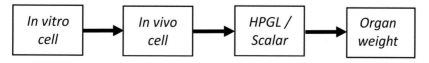

Figure 5.3 Example of generic scaling approach where transporter activity or expression has been measured in the *in vitro* system and a native tissue cell. HPGL refers to hepatocytes per gram of liver, different scalars are used here dependent on the tissue of interest.

REF refers to the relative amount of transporter, e.g., per million cells or per pmol/mg protein, in different systems and is determined by the quantification of the relative abundance [55] of the transporter in the expression system and in native tissue cells (Equation 5.17). An experimental technique that can be used to achieve this is western blotting, although data from high-powered liquid chromatography with tandem mass spectrometry (LC-MS/MS) proteomics can also be used. Care needs to be taken with these measurements to ensure that the same thing is measured in both cases, and consideration needs also to be made to the recovery of protein and the site of expression, e.g., membrane expression versus total cell/tissue concentration [56].

$$\text{REF} = \frac{\textit{In vivo } \text{transporter abundance(Unit)}}{\textit{In vitro } \text{transporter abundance(Unit)}} \tag{5.17}$$

where the units must be the same.

Application of either of these values, when scaling through a native tissue cell, rather than directly to whole body, requires the use of physiological scalars to calculate a whole organ value. For example, in the liver, a measured value in transfected HEK cells expressing the transporter of interest uses the REF or RAF to convert to a value representative of the transport in human hepatocytes, which can then be scaled to a whole liver value using hepatocytes per gram of liver (HPGL) and the liver weight (Equation 5.18), with the physiological scaling data obtained from the literature.

$$\text{CLu}_{\text{int,T}} \text{ per Liver} = \text{CLu}_{\text{int,T}} \textit{ in vitro} \cdot \text{REF or RAF} \cdot \text{HPGL} \cdot \text{Liver weight} \tag{5.18}$$

where $\text{CLu}_{\text{int,T}}$ refers to the unbound intrinsic transporter clearance.

Care should be taken to ensure that units of clearance are converted in an appropriate manner for consistency with the wider PBPK model. This same approach can be applied to any other tissues/transporters provided the appropriate scalars are applied. Note that if the *in vivo* system used in the determination of a RAF is the whole body (i.e., probe substrate is administered to a subject) then additional physiological scalars such as HPGL and liver weight are not required [57], the *in vitro* obtained clearance is simply multiplied by the RAF value to give an *in vivo* intrinsic clearance for this specific transporter.

REF and RAF approaches can also be combined to account for both the differences in activity and expression between the systems [55]. It should not be assumed that, for example, scaling for transporter expression alone will fully account for the differences.

Absolute abundance scaling approaches take the *in vitro* measured transporter clearance per unit of transporter and scale it by measured transporter abundance data in the tissues. Owing to the development and use of the LC-MS/MS proteomics methods, the availability of these data is rapidly expanding, and best practices have been suggested [58]. The overall strategy for the absolute abundance scaling follows a similar structure as the relative scaling process, where the *in vitro* data are scaled to an *in vivo* relevant value using system-specific and physiological scalars. However, for absolute abundance scaling, the clearance from the *in vitro* system must be expressed relative to the abundance of transporter protein and is then scaled by an intersystem extrapolation factor for transport (ISEF,T) [54]. This ISEF,T is not a direct comparison of transporter abundance in the systems, but rather the relative intrinsic clearance per functional abundance of transporter (Equation 5.19), incorporating differences in activity between the two systems:

$$\text{ISEF,T} = \frac{\text{CL}_{\text{int,T}} \textit{ in vitro} / \text{Transporter abundance } \textit{in vitro}}{\text{CL}_{\text{int,T}} \textit{ in vivo} / \text{Transporter abundance } \textit{in vivo}} \tag{5.19}$$

This ISEF,T will differ for each transporter studied and is currently not widely determined as the abundance both in the *in vitro* system and *in vivo* is required. An analogous ISEF approach is used in scaling metabolism [59].

Depending on the tissue of interest, the *in vivo* value may be expressed as either abundance in whole tissue (e.g. in jejunum for intestinal data) or a value relevant to the number of cells (e.g. hepatocytes for liver).

Returning to the liver example, the scaling approach can be illustrated as follows, with units in brackets for clarity.

1. HEK cell determined J_{max} (pmol/min/pmol transporter)/K_m (μM) or CLu_{int} (μL/min/pmol transporter) data, is scaled through an appropriate ISEF,T (no units) from HEK cells to an equivalent clearance in hepatocytes (μL/min/pmol transporter).

2. This then uses the absolute abundance (pmol transporter/10^6 hepatocytes) to convert to a clearance per million hepatocytes (μL/min/10^6 hepatocytes).

3. This is then scaled through HPGL (10^6 hepatocytes/g) to a CLu_{int} per gram of liver (μL/min/g Liver), which is then scaled by the liver weight (g) to give an overall liver CLu_{int} in μL/min. It is important to note that this value may need conversion to different units for use in the wider PBPK model.

This process is reflected in Equation 5.20:

$$CLu_{int} = \left[\sum_{j=1}^{n} \left[\frac{\text{ISEF,T}_j \cdot J_{max,j} \cdot \text{Transporter abundance } in \ vivo}{K_{m,j}} \right] \right] \cdot \text{HPGL} \cdot \text{Liver Weight} \tag{5.20}$$

where the summation is performed across the different contributing transporter isoforms, and transporter abundance *in vivo* in the described example refers to pmol transporter/10^6 hepatocytes. Where the ISEF,T is determined using whole tissue, step 3, scaling using physiological scalars is not required; however, for tissues such as the intestine, care should be taken in accounting for any regional differences in the organ.

5.10 ENDOCYTOSIS FOR SMALL MOLECULES

While perfusion and permeability-limited models are the most commonly used in PBPK, these do not cover all potential modes of distribution. In recent years, nanoparticle delivery systems have been employed to improve the pharmacokinetics of small molecule drugs, and these systems exploit endocytosis to distribute into cells or tissues. While a number of endocytic mechanisms exist [60], this process broadly involves the formation of an envelope of membrane lipid bilayer around the drug, referred to as an endosome, which then carries the drug into the intracellular space. Receptor-mediated endocytosis is one such mechanism, and, as the name suggests, requires interactions with a specific receptor.

To include this or any other endocytosis process in PBPK models, a combination of perfusion-limited or permeability-limited approaches can be used [61]. A simple approach to include uptake into the tissue would be to use a perfusion-limited model and update the total tissue-plasma partition coefficients to values including the contribution of the endocytic pathway [62]. It is important to note that existing Kp prediction models cannot be used here since nanoparticles behave differently from normally dosed small molecule drugs [63].

A more mechanistic approach is to incorporate an additional endosome compartment. The positioning of this compartment could be within the tissue, suitable where endocytosis relates to the uptake of drug already within the tissue, e.g., for phagocytes [63,64]. Alternatively, it could be situated between the blood and tissue if uptake into the tissue is to be modelled. In adding an endocytic compartment, volume or capacity of the endocytic space/process is required. Similarly, uptake and release must be defined, either in a perfusion-limited manner defining an endocytic partition coefficient, or in permeability-limited models [64], with uptake and release defined separately. Owing to the complexity of endocytosis processes, one approach is to use empirical fitting of data to determine the relevant parameters [61], although attempts to adjust model parameters to allow the use of a general model structure for different species have been made [63]. The incorporation of endocytosis into small molecule PBPK models is currently not widespread, unlike the models previously discussed, and further developments may well be made in the forthcoming years.

5.11 APPLICATIONS OF TISSUE CONCENTRATIONS
DETERMINED IN FULL-BODY PBPK MODELS

PBPK models, even with the standard reported result, or output, of a blood or plasma concentration-time profile, give the user wide ranging options to explore "what if" scenarios that can be difficult to study *in vivo*, including the impact of dosing regimen changes or administration to special populations. However, the structure of the complex PBPK models, with an equation describing each compartment, allows not only these standard concentration-time profiles to be visualised and reported, but an equivalent profile can be plotted for any tissue or compartment of interest. These individual tissue concentrations extend the utility of PBPK modelling, allowing the user to, for example, explore the potential for accumulation of drug in specific tissues over time, use a particular simulated concentration to drive a process or interaction, or link a tissue concentration-time profile to an observed effect.

Traditionally, attempts to link the predicted pharmacokinetics to observed pharmacodynamics (PBPK-PD modelling) have used the predicted plasma concentration-time profile to drive the effect model, although this could be seen as a mismatch when the site of action is expected to be intracellular. An example using a tissue-specific intracellular concentration to drive a PD model was published by Rose et al. [65], where a PBPK model was developed to assess the impact of OATP1B1 genotype differences on rosuvastatin action. In this instance, all compartments were perfusion-limited, with the exception of the liver where a permeability-limited model was incorporated to allow for the inclusion of active transport. Comparisons were made between the use of the predicted plasma concentration and unbound intracellular liver concentration to drive the PD response model, use of the liver concentration resulted in more representative capture of the *in vivo* observed PD profile. Similar approaches have used predicted concentrations for: free heart [66], mid myocardium [67], lumen (small intestine) and proximal tubule [68], and brain [69], to drive PD response models.

Tissue-specific concentration profiles can also be manipulated to provide further useful information. One example of this is the determination of a profile at an alternative sampling site. While the plasma or blood concentration-time profile output from a PBPK model is normally equivalent to the central venous compartment, sampling *in vivo* usually occurs at a peripheral site, such as the lower arm. By using a combination of the concentration-time profiles of the tissues most relevant to the sampling site (e.g., fat, muscle, and skin), a more relevant profile could be obtained [70].

5.12 LARGE MOLECULE (BIOLOGICS) PBPK MODELS

Large molecule PBPK models share many fundamental features with small molecule PBPK, like the physiological layout of the body, blood flow connections between the organs, their overall and capillary volume values. There are notable differences too, reflecting the diverging properties between small and large molecules. First and foremost, while most small molecule drugs are entirely synthetic entities that do not exist in nature and their physicochemical properties are (often) designed to conform to Lipinski's rules of five [71], the opposite holds for biologics, which are mostly proteins containing same naturally occurring monomer units (amino acids) as the endogenous ones and, as such, they generally flout each and every one of Lipinski's rules. Proteins are highly charged and polar macromolecules, with molecular weights reaching from tens to hundreds kDa. Any notion of logP, calculated or experimental, is irrelevant as they don't dissolve in organic solvents, even if they happen to contain plasma membrane-embedded hydrophobic domains.

As a result, while small molecule PBPK can be successfully handled in frameworks outlined in Figures 5.1 and 5.2 where intra- and extravascular spaces often exist in equilibrium, supplemented with passive and active transport across the plasma membranes, and extravascular space forming a well-stirred continuum, this is insufficient for biologics. Proteins, endogenous or dosed, do not diffuse across the plasma membrane; their extravasation involves transcytosis or paracellular diffusion-filtration, plasma circulation is supplemented with lymphatic circulation and cellular uptake involves pinocytosis [72,73].

The characteristic structural and physicochemical features of small and large molecule drugs also have consequences for their respective therapeutic uses. While small molecule drugs can reach intracellular targets, those of the large molecule drugs, e.g. monoclonal antibodies (mAbs), are all extracellular. While small molecule drugs often function as inhibitors, agonists and antagonists, fitting well into the limited confines of their targets' active sites, large molecule drugs like mAbs mostly engage in competitive inhibition of protein-protein interactions between receptors and their respective soluble or membrane-bound protein ligands that small molecule drugs are less effective at disrupting at clinically relevant doses.

The distinct physicochemical features of large molecule drugs thus mean that the organ frameworks shown in Figures 5.1 and 5.2 for small molecule drugs need to be adapted, as shown in Figure 5.4.

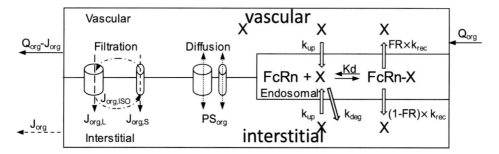

Figure 5.4 Generic organ layout for biologics showing fluid transfer and protein X transport from the vascular space to the interstitial space through small and large pores according to the two-pore hypothesis, pinocytosis, catabolism and FcRn-mediated recycling in the endosomal space, where active. Q_{org} denotes plasma flow into to organ, while J_{org} denotes organ-specific lymph flow. $J_{org,L/S}$ denotes linear plasma flow leaving the capillary plasma compartment through large or small paracellular pores respectively, further modified by isogravimetric flow $J_{org,ISO}$. $PS_{org,L/S}$ denotes permeability-surface area product values for large and small pores respectively for the diffusional flux. Macropinocytosis K_{up} accounts for the endocytosis of protein X, followed by endosomal recycling/transcytosis of the FcRn-bound protein. FR accounts for the FcRn-bound fraction that is recycled to the vascular side of the endothelium. (Figure reproduced from [74] with permission from Springer (License Number 5481501449430).)

In addition to drug transport and distribution, those of the target/s and any interaction/s with the drug can also be included in any interaction scheme.

The main structural and transport features of biologics PBPK models are therefore defined as follows;

1. Extravascular space is separated from the vascular space by endothelial cell layer and is further divided into intracellular and interstitial spaces by plasma membrane of parenchymal cells. Interstitial space contains interstitial fluid (ISF) [75] which constitutes around ¾ of the total of 12 L of extracellular fluid in humans [76], the rest being plasma.

2. Vascular plasma and ISF are connected through paracellular pores of approximately 5–50 nm in diameter [77] through which a small fraction of plasma is understood to be flowing continuously into interstitial space, where it becomes ISF. Any plasma proteins are subject to filtration and diffusion en route, with major proteins undergoing around two-fold dilution on average [78]. Protein extravasation is relatively slow compared with vascular circulation and experimentally manifests as about half of the intravenously dosed mAb or albumin leaving the plasma compartment during the 3–5 day long distribution phase but not the body [79]. ISF, in turn, leaves the interstitial space through lymphatic vessels and lymph nodes, of which there are approximately 500 in humans [80], before emptying into venous plasma. Lymphatic circulation is an integral part of large molecule PBPK, as shown in Figure 5.5. In humans, the total lymph flow rate measured in the thoracic duct is relatively slow at about 2–8 L/day, compared with 3.1 L/min plasma cardiac output [81].

3. All eukaryotic cells are involved in macropinocytosis where they continuously take up fluid (alongside with anything that it contains) from their surrounding environment [72]. In biologics PBPK models, this is denoted in the model as K_{up}, though typically assigned only to endothelial cells. The pinocytosed fluid ends up in endosomal space where its content undergoes sorting and processing. A fraction of those protein molecules which bind the neonatal Fc receptor (FcRn), e.g. mAbs of IgG1, IgG2 and IgG4 isotypes, as well as albumin, are then recycled back to the cell surface where they dissociate from the receptor and re-enter the circulation [82], while the rest end up being degraded into constituent amino acids in lysosomes. The recycling process is accomplished through pH-dependent binding of these proteins to FcRn in the acidic pH of endosomes and forms a central feature of biologics PBPK models and is often the focus of antibody engineering efforts. In the endothelium, FcRn-mAb complex can also be released to either side of the cell layer, giving rise to FcRn-mediated transcytosis. The net result of

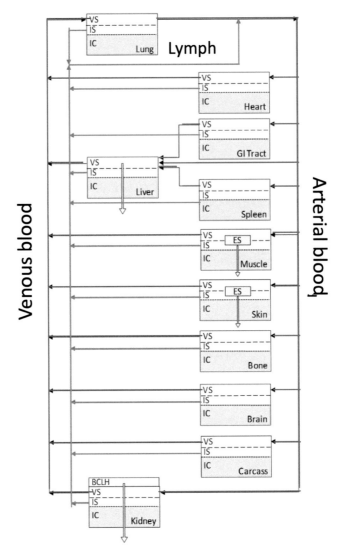

Figure 5.5 The overall tissue layout and plasma flows of large molecule PBPK are the same as in small molecule PBPK but, in addition, it also contains lymphatic circulation and distinct vascular, interstitial, endosomal and, optionally, intracellular (cytoplasm + nucleus etc.) compartments. (Figure reproduced from [74] with permission from Springer (License Number 5481501449430).)

FcRn-mediated recycling is diminished non-specific degradation of macropinocytosed mAbs (as well as endogenous albumin and relevant endogenous IgG isotypes) which leads to longer half-lives, especially if combined with pH-dependent binding of target antigens (pH-switch, as described by Igawa et al. [83]). For the proteins which don't bind FcRn (or receptor of similar function, e.g. transferrin receptor for transferrin) the combination of pinocytosis, degradation and recycling sets the upper limit of plasma half-life at around 100 hours in humans [84]. This is the terminal half-life value for endogenous IgG observed in humans both in the absence of functionally active FcRn [85] or the limit value as the receptor becomes saturated at very high levels of circulating IgG [86].

The mathematical framework that quantitatively relates plasma fluid paracellular flow with protein transport was formulated in the form of two-pore hypothesis (2PH) by Rippe and Haraldsson [87], on the basis of Patlak formalism [88]. According to 2PH, the plasma proteins move across the vascular endothelial cell layer through paracellular waterfilled channels by means of convection and diffusion. Convection is driven by hydrostatic blood pressure and aligns with flow from vascular to interstitial space, while diffusion is driven by any concentration gradients and can proceed in either direction.

A number of alternative implementations of 2PH to biologics PBPK have been developed by Baxter, Ferl and others [89, 90, 91,92] but they follow the general schematic of Figure 5.4, e.g. [74]

$$V_{org,VS} \frac{dC_{org,VS}}{dt} = Q_{org,X} \cdot C_A - \left(Q_{org} - J_{org}\right) \cdot C_{org,VS} - CL_{org} \cdot C_{org,VS} - Kup_{org} \cdot C_{org,VS} + k_{rec} \cdot FR \cdot V_{org,EN} \cdot C_{org,EN}^{bound}$$

(5.21)

$$V_{org,IS} \frac{dC_{org,IS}}{dt} = -J_{org} \cdot C_{org,IS} + CL_{org} \cdot C_{org,VS} - Kup_{org} \cdot C_{org,IS} + k_{rec} \cdot (1 - FR) \cdot V_{org,EN} \cdot C_{org,EN}^{bound}$$

(5.22)

$$V_{org,EN} \frac{C_{org,EN}^{free}}{dt} = Kup_{org} \cdot \left(C_{org,IS} + C_{org,VA}\right) - k_{deg} \cdot V_{org,EN} \cdot C_{org,EN}^{free}$$

$$- k_{on,FcRn} \cdot V_{org,EN} \cdot C_{org,EN}^{free} \cdot C_{org,EN}^{FcRn,free} + k_{off,FcRn} \cdot V_{org,EN} \cdot C_{org,EN}^{FcRn,bound}$$

(5.23)

$$V_{org,EN} \frac{C_{org,EN}^{bound}}{dt} = V_{org,EN} \cdot k_{on,FcRn} \cdot C_{org,EN}^{free} \cdot C_{org,EN}^{FcRn,free} - V_{org,EN} \cdot k_{off,FcRn} \cdot C_{org,EN}^{FcRn,bound} - V_{org,EN} \cdot k_{rec} \cdot C_{org,EN}^{bound}$$

(5.24)

In Equations 5.21–5.24, $V_{org,VS}$, $V_{org,IS}$ and $V_{org,EN}$ correspond to organ vascular, interstitial and endosomal volumes. Q_{org} is organ plasma flow entering the organ and J_{org} the lymph flow leaving the organ. C_A, $C_{org,VS}$ and $C_{org,IS}$ correspond to drug concentrations in plasma entering the organ, vascular and interstitial compartments, respectively. $C_{org,EN}^{free}$ and $C_{org,EN}^{bound}$ correspond free and FcRn-bound drug in endosomal compartment, where $C_{org,EN}^{FcRn,free}$ and $C_{org,EN}^{FcRn,bound}$ denote free and drug-bound FcRn fractions respectively. Kup_{org} corresponds to organ-specific macropinocytosis uptake, k_{rec} to endosomal recycling rate constant and k_{deg} to non-specific endosomal degradation. FR denotes the fraction of FcRn-drug complex recycled to the vascular compartment. $k_{on,FcRn}$ and $k_{off,FcRn}$ denote the association and dissociation rate constants of drug interaction with endosomal FcRn.

Organ-specific two-pore clearance CL_{org} is the sum of contributions from transport through large and small pores respectively:

$$CL_{org} = CL_{org,L} + CL_{org,S}$$

(5.25)

Organ- and pore type-specific clearance $CL_{org,X}$ where X denotes large or small pores, respectively, is based on the Patlak equation for filtration-diffusion across the microporous membrane:

$$CL_{org,X} = J_{org,X} \cdot \left(1 - \sigma_{org,X}\right) + PS_{org,X} \cdot \left(1 - \frac{C_{org,IS}}{C_{org,VS}}\right) \cdot \frac{Pe_{org,X}}{e^{Pe_{org,X}} - 1}$$

(5.26)

$J_{org,X}$ denotes the respective organ-specific small or large pore lymph flow rate, $s_{org,x}$ is the reflection coefficient, $PS_{org,X}$ is permeability-surface area product and $Pe_{org,X}$ the Peclet coefficient.

$J_{org,X}$ is determined by total tissue lymph flow rate J_{org}, hydraulic conductance a_X and isogravimetric flow $J_{org,X}$

$$J_{org,L} = J_{iso,org} + \alpha_L \cdot J_{org}$$

(5.27)

$$J_{org,S} = -J_{iso,org} + \alpha_S \cdot J_{org}$$

(5.28)

Given that both diffusion and filtration proceed through the same pores, it can be shown that in the case of biologics PBPK the permeability-surface area product $PS_{org,X}$ and organ-specific isogravimetric flow rates $J_{iso,org}$ are linear functions from organ-specific lymph flow rate J_{org}

$$PS_{org,X} = X_{P,org} \cdot \left(\frac{A_X}{A_{oX}}\right)_{org} \cdot \frac{\alpha_{org,X}}{r_{X,org}^2} \cdot J_{org}$$

(5.29)

$$J_{iso,org} = X_{J,org} \cdot J_{org}$$

(5.30)

In Equations 5.29 and 5.30, $X_{P,\text{org}}$, $X_{J,\text{org}}$ and other parameters can be calculated from first principles according to 2PH

$$X_{P,\text{org}} = \frac{8 \cdot R \cdot T}{6\pi \cdot N \cdot a_e \cdot \left(\Delta P - \bar{\sigma}_{\text{org,alb}} \cdot \Delta\pi\right)} \tag{5.31}$$

$$X_{J,\text{org}} = \frac{\alpha_{L,\text{org}} \cdot \alpha_{S,\text{org}} \cdot \left(\sigma_{S,\text{org,alb}} - \sigma_{L,\text{org,alb}}\right) \cdot \Delta\pi}{6\pi \cdot N \cdot a_e \cdot \left(\Delta P - \bar{\sigma}_{\text{org,alb}} \cdot \Delta\pi\right)} \tag{5.32}$$

In these conditions, the Peclet coefficients are organ-specific constants characteristic to the protein of interest where higher value aligns with higher contribution from the convection component:

$$\text{Pe}_{\text{org},X} = \frac{J_{\text{org},X} \cdot \left(1 - \sigma_{\text{org},X}\right)}{\text{PS}_{\text{org},X}} = \frac{\left(X_{J,\text{org}} + \alpha_{X,\text{org}}\right) \cdot \left(1 - \sigma_{X,\text{org}}\right) \cdot r_{X,\text{org}}^2}{X_{P,\text{org}} \cdot \left(\dfrac{A_X}{A_{oX}}\right)_{\text{org}} \cdot \alpha_{\text{org},X}} \tag{5.33}$$

The ratios of $\left(\dfrac{A_X}{A_{oX}}\right)_{\text{org}}$ account for the fraction of total pore area available for diffusion as a function of the ratio $\gamma_{X,\text{org}}$ of protein hydrodynamic radius a_e to that of the pore $r_{X,\text{org}}$, while R is universal gas constant, T is absolute temperature and N is Avogadro number.

$$\left(\frac{A_X}{A_{oX}}\right)_{\text{org}} = (1 - \gamma_{X,\text{org}})^2 \cdot \frac{1 - 2.105\gamma_{X,\text{org}} + 2.087\gamma_{X,\text{org}}^3 - 1.707\gamma_{X,\text{org}}^5 + 0.726\gamma_{X,\text{org}}^6}{1 - 0.7586\gamma_{X,\text{org}}^5} \tag{5.34}$$

$$\gamma_{X,\text{org}} = \frac{a_e}{r_{X,\text{org}}} \tag{5.35}$$

ΔP stands for hydrostatic pressure gradient across the vasculature, while $\Delta\pi$ denotes oncotic pressure gradient. $\sigma_{X,\text{org,alb}}$ denotes albumin reflection coefficient at the large or small pores of a given organ, with $\bar{\sigma}_{\text{org,alb}}$ denotes its weighed average for an organ.

$$\bar{\sigma}_{\text{org,alb}} = \alpha_{L,\text{org}} \cdot \sigma_{L,\text{org,alb}} + \alpha_{S,\text{org}} \cdot \sigma_{S,\text{org,alb}} \tag{5.36}$$

Equations 5.25–5.36 define the correlations between organ physiological parameters and the respective two-pore flux rates (5.25), the most important of which are 5.29 and 5.30 which define the correlation between organ net lymph flow rate J_{org} on one hand and PS_{org} and $J_{\text{iso,org}}$ one other hand. This means the diffusion and filtration processes are cross-correlated as expected, given that both take place at the same time through the same pores. The rest of the parameters encountered in Equations 5.31–5.36 are familiar from school days or collected from literature as independently measured values [74,92].

Two approaches have been taken to implementing Equations 5.25–5.36. Gill et al. [91] used estimated human organ-specific lymph flow rate values to fit the sizes and ratios of organ-specific small and large pores to capture the observed dependencies of lymph/plasma protein concentration ratios measured in different species. Sepp et al. [74] and Sepp et al. [92] used published organ-specific pore size and ratio values to estimate respective lymph flow values the tissue distribution and elimination time course data measured in mice and rats for a number of inert proteins of different sizes, followed by validation in monkeys [93] and humans [94] using positron emission tomography of mAbs and an albumin-binding antibody fragment, respectively.

The relative contributions of diffusion and convection to the overall rate of extravasation depend on the size of the protein [95]. For mAb-sized (and larger) proteins, the two-pore filtration-diffusion model approximates to filtration pathway only, as exemplified by Shah and Betts in their platform PBPK model [96], for small proteins, e.g. insulin and cytokines, diffusion dominates and the latter is important in the case of subcutaneous and intramuscular dosing of such biologics.

Organ-specific adjustments to the default generic layout shown in Figure 5.4 need to be implemented to incorporate essential physiological features of select organs.

Kidneys: The kidney model is supplemented by a lumped compartment corresponding to the combined volumes of, glomerulus, Bowman's capsule and loops of Henle. This compartment is supplied by way of glomerular filtration from kidney alveolar compartment at the glomerular filtration rate and empties into bladder at urine formation rate. The latter is about 200-fold lower than the former, thus capturing the process of 99.5% reabsorption of water from raw glomerular filtrate, with corresponding accumulation of filtered proteins in the kidney cortical region. The glomerular filtration coefficient is treated as a function of protein hydrodynamic radius (i.e. molecular weight) [74], empirically fitted to experimental data by Venturoli and Rippe [97].

Lung model in PBPK contains an alveolar compartment which is in passive protein-size-dependent diffusional exchange with lung interstitium and is characterised by rapid local non-specific degradation of proteins [74,98]. The alveolar compartment allows to evaluate pulmonary delivery of biologics both from the local and systemic exposure perspectives as well as pulmonary exposure after systemic delivery.

Brain: brain interstitial space has been supplemented with cerebrospinal fluid (CSF) flow which draws its intake through aquaporins [99,100], that only allow the passage of water [77]. In effect, the brain represents a three-pore system where the two-pore pathway provides negligible CNS access to the proteins while aquaporin-enabled water flow dominates brain ISF turnover and discharge into the central circulation [74]. More mechanistic models have been developed by Shah et al. which treat the central nervous system as a cascade of fluid flowing from the brain towards the spinal cord [99,100,101]. In practice, plasma protein concentration in the brain ISF/CSF is around 300-fold lower than in circulation and, within the margin of experimental error in the case of imaging or tissue homogenate studies, the average brain concentration is entirely accounted for by the vascular component. More invasive in situ sampling enables reliable insight into protein extravasation in CNS [99,100].

Solid tumour is a frequent feature of PBPK models given the importance of oncological targets and is mostly treated as a typical organ except that the lymph flow rate is assigned as zero [102,103]. This follows from the observation that tumours often lack functioning lymphatics [75], which renders the convection pathway of mAb extravasation inoperative. The diffusional flux is driven by the drug concentration gradient across tumour vasculature and this has two consequences. First, solid tumour penetration of antibody-sized molecules is slow, even if the tumour vascular porosity is higher than that of normal tissues [104]. Second, slow tumour penetration can become rate-limiting in the case of cancer cell surface antigens with strong TMDD as a result of high copy number, rapid internalisation or both. In this case, most of the extravasated mAb are internalised in tumour cell layers close to the capillary and the interstitial space of solid tumour cannot be treated as a well-stirred environment anyore, leaving the interior of tumour underexposed. This phenomenon is known as the affinity barrier [105]. Mathematical description of the latter can be expressed in terms of partial differential equations [106,107,108].

Subcutaneous (SC) and intramuscular (IM) dosing sites: While intravenous (IV) dosing is the most effective in terms of 100% bioavailability of the drug and instant (plasma) exposure, given that cardiac output per minute equals to the entire peripheral vascular volume, it requires medical assistance with its associated costs and patient inconvenience. For that reason, both SC and IM dosing options are used where possible since they can be performed by the patient, both reducing the costs and improving compliance and convenience. The maximum dose level of about 3 mg/kg largely arises from the volume, which is limited to around 1.5 mL and the maximum 150 mg/mL concentration of the mAb [109]. For modelling purposes, the SC and IV dosing sites are being separated from total skin and skeletal muscle, respectively, as the dosed drug will not become well-mixed in the entire organ volume and will be absorbed locally [110], where the lymphatic pathway subject the dose to first-pass local catabolism in haematopoietic cells in the draining lymph nodes [111]. The values of plasma C_{max}, T_{max} and bioavailability $F\%$ depend on the size of the protein, dose and FcRn-binding activity [110, 112, 113, 114].

Most large molecule models have been and are being constructed by traditional means where differential equations corresponding to transport and reactions, including any supporting calculations for each molecular species in each organ compartment (hundreds of them in total) are manually encoded in graphical or text editor environments [90,91,92,96]. Given that the models can easily contain more than a dozen compartments, each divided into at least three sub-compartments involving transport and any chemical reactions, the effort required for building and debugging soon becomes rate-limiting and confines the frameworks to one or two molecular species at most. This limitation has been overcome with the introduction of computer-assisted biologics PBPK model construction where MATLAB SimBiology-compliant bug-free models containing large number reactants requiring thousands of ordinary differential and algebraic equations can be rapidly created without human intervention, yielding models fit for simulation and curve-fitting purposes [74,98].

In summary, while even the most complex PBPK models do not capture the full physiological complexity due to lack of scientific insight or computational limitations, they can be useful for analysing the results, drawing conclusions and making predictions, occasionally even from first principles. In this context, it is important to appreciate the assumptions that the biologics PBPK framework and the underlying 2PH rely on: all compartments are well-stirred, the hydrostatic and oncotic pressure differences across the endothelial barrier are the same in all organs and macropinocytosis is limited to the FcRn-expressing cells only, usually identified as endothelium. Patlak equation, which underpins 2PH, meanwhile describes a steady-state system where infinitely diluted spherical uncharged particles move in perfectly shaped cylindrical channels. In practice, the paracellular pores are tortuous, plasma crowded with albumin and endogenous IgG, while hardly any protein is spherical at all, differing in shape, charge and hydrophobicity.

Nevertheless, several important conclusions can be drawn from biologics PBPK. First, biologics' tissue distribution, concentration gradients and extravasation do not represent equilibrium but reflect the steady state that is maintained by unceasing cardiac output which drives central circulation and paracellular fluid flows. Equilibrium only arrives after death. Second, well-conserved antibody biodistribution coefficients (ABC) by Shah and Betts [115] suggest that the respective tissue properties are well-conserved across species. This, combined with the limited variation of biophysical properties of mAb is the underlying reason why the intrinsic PK properties of different antibodies vary little between species, as shown by Betts et al. after stripping out the target-mediated effects [116]. While some variation in antibody PK is observed and can reflect the marginal impact of Fab regions on Fc complex with FcRn [117], it's contribution is relatively small [118] and can be screened out experimentally or in silico [119] before progressing, so that only leads with likely typical baseline 18–22 day terminal half-life in humans will be taken to the clinic. Finally, given that the two-pore framework only uses the size of the protein and its affinity for FcRn to quantitatively describe its extravasation kinetics, it can be proposed with high confidence that biologics PBPK also applies to endogenous soluble proteins, which should come as no surprise either as these were used throughout the two-pore model development [87].

5.13 DRUG-TARGET INTERACTIONS FOR LARGE MOLECULE PBPK

As mentioned in Section 5.12, most of the intrinsic PK, tissue distribution and elimination properties of soluble proteins are described in terms of their size and FcRn-binding activity, once the target-mediated effects are taken into account. This is unsurprising given that differences between mAbs are confined to the antigen-binding paratope region of the variable domain is coded by around 5% of the total sequence, i.e. 95% of the mAb sequence is invariant from one drug to another. The surface area of typical paratope of $\approx 100 \text{ Å}^2$ is sufficient for mAbs with pM-range affinities to be developed, which leaves ample room for target engagement and protein-protein interaction inhibition even at very low concentrations, given that typical mAb plasma concentration after 10 mg/kg IV dose starts from approximately 1 mM value.

The overall pharmacokinetic formalism for target-mediated effects has been described before [120,121] where it revolves around the formation of drug-target complex and the rate of its elimination vs. that of the free drug and the free target. The critical parameters are the concentrations of the drug and the target, the turnover of free target, affinity of the interaction and elimination of the drug-target complex.

The soluble target case is more straightforward. The two binding sites of mAbs engage such targets independently from each other with little to now impact on FcRn-binding affinity-at least for small ligands, where affinity values from surface plasmon resonance with antibody on the surface (or its Fab in solution) usually provide reliable guidance. Likewise, while the molecular weights and hydrodynamic radii of such complexes will be higher than that of the free mAb, from the two-pore PBPK perspective the impact is negligible with largely unchanged clearance/terminal half-life of the mAb complex relative to the free molecule. While this has minimal impact on the behaviour of the antibody, the consequences for the target can be dramatic, if its free state is in fast turnover, where half-life values for typical cytokine (or other small protein) targets can often be in the region of 1–2 hours, or even less [122,123]. Given the ≈450 hour half-life of the mAb, the end result is 200- to 4,400-fold accumulation of soluble target in complex with the mAb [124,125,126], as the target secretion rate remains often largely unaffected. While it is sometimes argued to be irrelevant given the neutralising nature of most mAbs, this is not necessarily so, as accumulating target even in bound form undoes much of the reduction in free target concentration that's still in circulation and exercises its physiological role according to mass action equilibrium equation, as shown in Equations 5.37 and 5.38

$$K_d = \frac{\text{Target}_{\text{free}} \cdot \text{mAb}_{\text{free}}}{\text{Complex}} \qquad (5.37)$$

In the conditions $\text{mAb}_{\text{total}} \gg K_d$ and $\text{mAb}_{\text{total}} \gg \text{Complex}$, typically met for cytokine-like ligands, Equation 5.37 transforms to

$$\text{Target}_{\text{free}} \approx K_d \cdot \frac{\text{Target}_{\text{total}}}{\text{mAb}_{\text{total}}} \qquad (5.38)$$

where

$$\text{mAb}_{\text{free}} \approx \text{mAb}_{\text{total}} \text{ and } \text{Target}_{\text{total}} \approx \text{Complex} \qquad (5.39)$$

For example, at $K_d = 100$ pM mAb present at 100 nM to inhibit 1 pM (pre-dosing steady state) concentration target with 2.25 hour half-life, the concentration of free circulating target, which still exercises its physiological effect, is reduced only five-fold, hardly a ground-breaking achievement despite ≈100,000-fold molar excess of the circulating high-affinity drug over the pre-dosing level of the target. With dosing limit in practice being at around 10 mg/kg, the only way to further decrease the level of free target fraction is by affinity maturation of the drug affinity (K_d) into low single-digit pM range (or involve protein advanced protein engineering methods, pH-switch or pH-sweep [127]). The second insight from Equation 5.38 should come in the form of realisation that *in vitro* cellular potency assays performed at physiological target levels underestimate the drug concentrations required *in vivo* for reaching a similar kind of effect. More informative insight would be obtained *in vitro* at target concentrations applied at levels equal to that of total target at its highest plasma concentration value (which is largely predictable from first principles) [84].

Antibody interaction with membrane targets is more complex and typically non-linear, with terminal half-life being a function of time and depending on the mAb concentration [128]. First of all, due to its bivalent nature, a mAb will typically cross-link two cell surface molecules, the copy number of which can range from low hundreds to over a million per cell, while internalisation half-life can vary from minutes to hours [129]. Target cross-linking on cell membrane enhances the binding efficiency of the mAb, termed avidity effect, which typically ranges from 100- to 1,000-fold and has theoretical limit around 10,000 [130] but is also epitope-dependent and hence only partly predictable. Non-linearity of the cell membrane protein-targeting antibody PK manifests itself when the elimination through target-mediated clearance (which is saturable) becomes comparable with non-specific macropinocytosis-mediated clearance and can become dominating, e.g. anti-CD4 mAb ibalizumab which has around two-day terminal half-life at low nanomolar concentrations.

From the practical perspective, it's not always easy to distinguish membrane TMDD from the impact of anti-drug immune response, which also results in accelerated drug clearance. Mouse anti-human immune response typically develops by the end of the first week following the dosing event and will get more dominant upon repeat dosing. In primates, the immune response humanised antibodies can be weaker but remains target-dependent. Multiple dose levels can be helpful in identifying the situation.

In summary, the underlying PK properties of different mAbs can be very similar, unless distorted by suboptimal biophysical properties [131,132,133] or, as discussed above, by TMDD. While the former belongs to the realm of protein engineering, the latter reflects the pharmacology of the target/s, as each will have different tissue distribution properties and engage in physiological interactions in their own right. The latter can be incorporated into biologics PBPK for mechanistic pharmacodynamic purposes according to the three pillars concept of drug discovery [134].

Biologics PBPK has come a long way and can by now also incorporate endogenous proteins, if desired, including cellular entities [135,136,137]. As such, time may well be right to shift the emphasis from purely reflective analysis to that which also provides predictive modelling in the form of target druggability analysis. An example of how this could have been used for developing complement C5-neutralising biweekly dosed eculizumab into bimonthly dosed ravulizumab by combining pH-switch and half-life extension technologies into a single molecule has been provided [94].

5.14 SUMMARY/CONCLUDING REMARKS

This chapter has discussed perfusion and permeability-limited distribution models utilised in PBPK, including the practicalities that should be taken into consideration when building or using such models to simulate pharmacokinetics for either a small or large molecule.

Distribution models can provide valuable information about the free and bound drug concentrations in various tissues assisting with understanding where the drug goes around the body and what are the concentrations driving desired or side effects. Similar overall model structures are applied for small and large molecules, with key differences being incorporated into the descriptions of vascular and plasma membrane permeability due to the mechanisms of tissue distribution (diffusion/transport across lipid membranes vs convection/diffusion through paracellular pores). For small molecules, this prediction and description of distribution is well established after many years of investment in PBPK modelling, with perfusion and permeability models utilised for predictions and understanding beyond simple PK profiles. Some challenges still remain – particularly when making de novo predictions for highly lipophilic compounds ($\log P_{o:w} > 5$) or compounds outside the applicability domain of the mechanistic, tissue composition methods. From the biologics perspective, where PBPK is less established but moving swiftly, quantitative early-stage translational modelling can encourage mechanistic analysis to support target druggability evaluation and reduce attrition en route to the clinic. As a bonus, the more flexible cross-modality/cross-species versions of biologics PBPK can be expected to be applicable also to endogenous soluble proteins of any size. This opens up the possibility of incorporating into the model also the target molecule/s to capture their dynamics before, during and after drug administration, including any interactions with their own cognate soluble or membrane-linked interaction partners at system-level integration for advanced pharmacodynamic analysis.

In a broader sense, the similarities between small and large molecule models may even run deeper than similar overall model structure given that both describe the physiology of the same organism, albeit from slightly different angles. Both small and large molecules can be subject to degradation by the respective enzymatic processes and carrier-mediated transport, both in circulation and in cells. The models also need to describe situations where both small and large molecules need to be modelled simultaneously within the same framework, e.g. in the case of antibody-drug conjugates (ADC). In this case, the intact drug (ADC) behaves like a large molecule while the small molecule payload molecules, once released from the mAb in target cells or non-specifically in solution, will follow the small molecule formalism.

REFERENCES

1. Johnson, T. N., Boussery, K., Rowland-Yeo, K., Tucker, G. T. and Rostami-Hodjegan, A. (2010). A semi-mechanistic model to predict the effects of liver cirrhosis on drug clearance. *Clin Pharmacokinet* **49**(3): 189–206.

2. El-Khateeb, E., Achour, B., Al-Majdoub, Z. M., Barber, J. and Rostami-Hodjegan, A. (2021). Non-uniformity of changes in drug-metabolizing enzymes and transporters in liver cirrhosis: Implications for drug dosage adjustment. *Mol Pharm* **18**(9): 3563–3577.

3. Jones, H. M., Gardner, I. B. and Watson, K. J. (2009). Modelling and PBPK simulation in drug discovery. *AAPS J* **11**(1): 155–166.

4. Tozer, T. N. and Rowland, M. (2006). *Introduction to Pharmacokinetics and Pharmacodynamics: The Quantitative Basis of Drug Therapy.* Lippincott Williams & Wilkins. Philadelphia, PA.

5. Riley, R. J., McGinnity, D. F. and Austin, R. P. (2005). A unified model for predicting human hepatic, metabolic clearance from in vitro intrinsic clearance data in hepatocytes and microsomes. *Drug Metab Dispos* **33**(9): 1304–1311.

6. Soars, M. G., Grime, K., Sproston, J. L., Webborn, P. J. and Riley, R. J. (2007). Use of hepatocytes to assess the contribution of hepatic uptake to clearance in vivo. *Drug Metab Dispos* **35**(6): 859–865.

7. Grime, K., Ferguson, D. D. and Riley, R. J. (2010). The use of HepaRG and human hepatocyte data in predicting CYP induction drug-drug interactions via static equation and dynamic mechanistic modelling approaches. *Curr Drug Metab* **11**(10): 870–885.

8. Rowland, M. and Tozer, T. N. (1995). *Clinical Pharmacokinetics: Concepts and Applications.* Lippincott Williams & Wilkins. Philadelphia, PA.

9. Jamei, M., Bajot, F., Neuhoff, S., Barter, Z., Yang, J., Rostami-Hodjegan, A. and Rowland-Yeo, K. (2014). A mechanistic framework for in vitro-in vivo extrapolation of liver membrane transporters: Prediction of drug-drug interaction between rosuvastatin and cyclosporine. *Clin Pharmacokinet* **53**(1): 73–87.

10. Musther, H., Harwood, M. D., Yang, J., Turner, D. B., Rostami-Hodjegan, A., & Jamei, M. (2017). The constraints, construction, and verification of a strain-specific physiologically based pharmacokinetic rat model. *J Pharm Sci* **106**(9): 2826–2838.

11. Berry, L. M., Roberts, J., Be, X., Zhao, Z. and Lin, M. H. (2010). Prediction of V(ss) from in vitro tissue-binding studies. *Drug Metab Dispos* **38**(1): 115–121.

12. Bjorkman, S. (2002). Prediction of the volume of distribution of a drug: Which tissue-plasma partition coefficients are needed? *J Pharm Pharmacol* **54**(9): 1237–1245.

13. Freitas, A. A., Limbu, K. and Ghafourian, T. (2015). Predicting volume of distribution with decision tree-based regression methods using predicted tissue:plasma partition coefficients. *J Cheminform* **7**: 6.

14. Poulin, P. and Theil, F. P. (2002). Prediction of pharmacokinetics prior to in vivo studies. 1. Mechanism-based prediction of volume of distribution. *J Pharm Sci* **91**(1): 129–156.

15. Poulin, P. and Theil, F. P. (2002). Prediction of pharmacokinetics prior to in vivo studies. II. Generic physiologically based pharmacokinetic models of drug disposition. *J Pharm Sci* **91**(5): 1358–1370.

16. Rodgers, T., Leahy, D. and Rowland, M. (2005). Physiologically based pharmacokinetic modeling 1: Predicting the tissue distribution of moderate-to-strong bases. *J Pharm Sci* **94**(6): 1259–1276.

17. Rodgers, T., Leahy, D. and Rowland, M. (2005). Tissue distribution of basic drugs: Accounting for enantiomeric, compound and regional differences amongst beta-blocking drugs in rat. *J Pharm Sci* **94**(6): 1237–1248.

18. Rodgers, T. and Rowland, M. (2006). Physiologically based pharmacokinetic modelling 2: Predicting the tissue distribution of acids, very weak bases, neutrals and zwitterions. *J Pharm Sci* **95**(6): 1238–1257.

19. Rodgers, T. and Rowland, M. (2007). Mechanistic approaches to volume of distribution predictions: Understanding the processes. *Pharm Res* **24**(5): 918–933.

20. Schmitt, W. (2008). General approach for the calculation of tissue to plasma partition coefficients. *Toxicol in Vitro* **22**(2): 457–467.

21. Ruark, C. D., Hack, C. E., Robinson, P. J., Mahle, D. A. and Gearhart, J. M. (2014). Predicting passive and active tissue:plasma partition coefficients: Interindividual and interspecies variability. *J Pharm Sci* **103**(7): 2189–2198.

22. Holt, K., Ye, M., Nagar, S. and Korzekwa, K. R. (2019). Prediction of tissue - plasma partition coefficients using microsomal partitioning: Incorporation into physiologically-based pharmacokinetic models and steady state volume of distribution predictions. *Drug Metab Dispos* **40**(10):1050–1060.

23. Utsey, K., Gastonguay, M. S., Russell, S., Freling, R., Riggs, M. M. and Elmokadem, A. (2020). Quantification of the impact of partition coefficient prediction methods on physiologically based pharmacokinetic model output using a standardized tissue composition. *Drug Metab Dispos* **48**(10): 903–916.

24. Zou, P., Zheng, N., Yang, Y., Yu, L. X. and Sun, D. (2012). Prediction of volume of distribution at steady state in humans: Comparison of different approaches. *Expert Opin Drug Metab Toxicol* **8**(7): 855–872.

25. Rodgers, T., Jones, H. M. and Rowland, M. (2012). Tissue lipids and drug distribution: Dog versus rat. *J Pharm Sci* **101**(12): 4615–4626.

26. Poulin, P., Collet, S. H., Atrux-Tallau, N., Linget, J. M., Hennequin, L. and Wilson, C. E. (2019). Application of the tissue composition-based model to minipig for predicting the volume of distribution at steady state and dermis-to-plasma partition coefficients of drugs used in the physiologically based pharmacokinetics model in dermatology. *J Pharm Sci* **108**(1): 603–619.

27. Berezhkovskiy, L. M. (2004). Volume of distribution at steady state for a linear pharmacokinetic system with peripheral elimination. *J Pharm Sci* **93**(6): 1628–1640.

28. Leo, A., Hansch, C. and Elkins, D. (1971). Partition coefficients and their uses. *Chem. Rev.* **71**(6): 525–616.

29. Bartels, M., Rick, D., Lowe, E., Loizou, G., Price, P., Spendiff, M., Arnold, S., Cocker, J. and Ball, N. (2012). Development of PK- and PBPK-based modeling tools for derivation of biomonitoring guidance values. *Comput Methods Programs Biomed* **108**(2): 773–788.

30. Korzekwa, K. and Nagar, S. (2017). Drug distribution part 2. Predicting volume of distribution from plasma protein binding and membrane partitioning. *Pharm Res* **34**(3): 544–551.

31. Nagar, S. and Korzekwa, K. (2017). Drug distribution. Part 1. Models to predict membrane partitioning. *Pharm Res* **34**(3): 535–543.

32. Assmus, F., Houston, J. B. and Galetin, A. (2017). Incorporation of lysosomal sequestration in the mechanistic model for prediction of tissue distribution of basic drugs. *Eur J Pharm Sci* **109**: 419–430.

33. Schmitt, M. V., Reichel, A., Liu, X., Fricker, G. and Lienau, P. (2021). Extension of the mechanistic tissue distribution model of Rodgers and Rowland by systematic incorporation of lysosomal trapping: Impact on unbound partition coefficient and volume of distribution predictions in the rat. *Drug Metabo Dispos* **49**(1): 53–61.

34. Trapp, S., Rosania, G. R., Horobin, R. W. and Kornhuber, J. (2008). Quantitative modeling of selective lysosomal targeting for drug design. *Eur Biophys J* **37**(8): 1317–1328.

35. Reynolds, D. P., Lanevskij, K., Japertas, P., Didziapetris, R. and Petrauskas, A. (2009). Ionization-specific analysis of human intestinal absorption. *J Pharm Sci* **98**(11): 4039–4054.

36. Fisher, C., Siméon, S., Jamei, M., Gardner, I. and Bois, Y. F. (2019). VIVD: Virtual in vitro distribution model for the mechanistic prediction of intracellular concentrations of chemicals in in vitro toxicity assays. *Toxicol in Vitro* **58**: 42–50.

37. Obach, R. S., Lombardo, F. and Waters, N. J. (2008). Trend analysis of a database of intravenous pharmacokinetic parameters in humans for 670 drug compounds. *Drug Metab Dispos* **36**(7): 1385–1405.

38. Lombardo, F., Berellini, G. and Obach, R. S. (2018). Trend analysis of a database of intravenous pharmacokinetic parameters in humans for 1352 drug compounds. *Drug Metab Dispos* **46**(11): 1466–1477.

39. Mathew, S., Tess, D., Burchett, W., Chang, G., Woody, N., Keefer, C., Orozco, C., Lin, J., Jordan, S., Yamazaki, S., Jones, R. and Di, L. (2021). Evaluation of prediction accuracy for volume of distribution in rat and human using In Vitro, In Vivo, PBPK and QSAR methods. *J Pharm Sci* **110**(4): 1799–1823.

40. Shimizu, H., Yoshida, K., Nakada, T., Kojima, K., Ogasawara, A., Nakamaru, Y. and Yamazaki, H. (2019). Prediction of human distribution volumes of compounds in various elimination phases using physiologically based pharmacokinetic modeling and experimental pharmacokinetics in animals. *Drug Metab Dispos* **47**(2): 114–123.

41. Neuhoff, S., Gaohua, L., Burt, H., Jamei, M., Li, L., Tucker, G. T. and Rostami-Hodjegan, A. (2013). Accounting for transporters in renal clearance: Towards a Mechanistic Kidney Model (Mech KiM). In: *Transporters in Drug Development: Discovery, Optimization, Clinical Study and Regulation.* Y. Sugiyama and B. Steffansen, New York, Springer New York: pp. 155–177.

42. Zamek-Gliszczynski, M. J., Sangha, V., Shen, H., Feng, B., Wittwer, M. B., Varma, M. V. S., Liang, X., Sugiyama, Y., Zhang, L., Bendayan, R. and Consortium, I. T. (2022). Transporters in drug development: international transporter consortium update on emerging transporters of clinical importance. *Clin Pharmacol Therapeut* **112**(3): 485–500.

43. Kawai, R., Mathew, D., Tanaka, C. and Rowland, M. (1998). Physiologically based pharmaco-kinetics of cyclosporine A: Extension to tissue distribution kinetics in rats and scale-up to human. *J Pharmacol Exp Therapeut* **287**(2): 457–468.

44. Burt, H. J., Neuhoff, S., Almond, L., Gaohua, L., Harwood, M. D., Jamei, M., Rostami-Hodjegan, A., Tucker, G. T. and Rowland-Yeo, K. (2016). Metformin and cimeti-dine: Physiologically based pharmacokinetic modelling to investigate transporter mediated drug-drug interactions. *Eur J Pharm Sci* **88**: 70–82.

45. Asaumi, R., Nunoya, K. I., Yamaura, Y., Taskar, K. S. and Sugiyama, Y. (2022). Robust physi-ologically based pharmacokinetic model of rifampicin for predicting drug-drug interac-tions via P-glycoprotein induction and inhibition in the intestine, liver, and kidney. *CPT Pharmacometrics Syst Pharmacol* **11**(7): 919–933.

46. Gaohua, L., Neuhoff, S., Johnson, T. N., Rostami-Hodjegan, A. and Jamei, M. (2016). Development of a permeability-limited model of the human brain and cerebrospinal fluid (CSF) to integrate known physiological and biological knowledge: Estimating time varying CSF drug concentra-tions and their variability using in vitro data. *Drug Metab Pharmacokinet* **31**(3): 224–233.

47. Murata, Y., Neuhoff, S., Rostami-Hodjegan, A., Takita, H., Al-Majdoub, Z. M. and Ogungbenro, K. (2022). In vitro to in vivo extrapolation linked to physiologically based phar-macokinetic models for assessing the brain drug disposition. *AAPS J* **24**(1): 28.

48. Gaohua, L., Wedagedera, J., Small, B. G., Almond, L., Romero, K., Hermann, D., Hanna, D., Jamei, M. and Gardner, I. (2015). Development of a multicompartment permeability-limited lung PBPK model and its application in predicting pulmonary pharmacokinetics of antitu-berculosis drugs. *CPT Pharmacometrics Syst Pharmacol* **4**(10): 605–613.

49. Sato, M., Toshimoto, K., Tomaru, A., Yoshikado, T., Tanaka, Y., Hisaka, A., Lee, W. and Sugiyama, Y. (2018). Physiologically based pharmacokinetic modeling of bosentan identifies the saturable hepatic uptake as a major contributor to its nonlinear pharmacokinetics. *Drug Metab Dispos* **46**(5): 740–748.

50. Zhang, M., Fisher, C., Gardner, I., Pan, X., Kilford, P., Bois, F. Y. and Jamei, M. (2022). Understanding interindividual variability in the drug interaction of a highly extracted CYP1A2 substrate tizanidine: Application of a permeability-limited multicompartment liver model in a population based physiologically based pharmacokinetic framework. *Drug Metab Dispos* **50**(7): 957–967.

51. Bi, Y. A., Mathialagan, S., Tylaska, L., Fu, M., Keefer, J., Vildhede, A., Costales, C., Rodrigues, A. D. and Varma, M. V. S. (2018). Organic anion transporter 2 mediates hepatic uptake of tolbutamide, a CYP2C9 probe drug. *J Pharmacol Exp Ther* **364**(3): 390–398.

52. Izumi, S., Nozaki, Y., Kusuhara, H., Hotta, K., Mochizuki, T., Komori, T., Maeda, K. and Sugiyama, Y. (2018). Relative activity factor (RAF)-based scaling of uptake clearance mediated by organic anion transporting polypeptide (OATP) 1B1 and OATP1B3 in human hepatocytes. *Mol Pharm* **15**(6): 2277–2288.

53. Bi, Y. A., Lin, J., Mathialagan, S., Tylaska, L., Callegari, E., Rodrigues, A. D. and Varma, M. V. S. (2018). Role of hepatic organic anion transporter 2 in the pharmacokinetics of R- and S-warfarin: In vitro studies and mechanistic evaluation. *Mol Pharm* **15**(3): 1284–1295.

54. Harwood, M. D., Neuhoff, S., Carlson, G. L., Warhurst, G. and Rostami-Hodjegan, A. (2013). Absolute abundance and function of intestinal drug transporters: A prerequisite for fully mechanistic in vitro-in vivo extrapolation of oral drug absorption. *Biopharm Drug Dispos* **34**(1): 2–28.

55. Hirano, M., Maeda, K., Shitara, Y. and Sugiyama, Y. (2004). Contribution of OATP2 (OATP1B1) and OATP8 (OATP1B3) to the Hepatic Uptake of Pitavastatin in Humans. *J Pharmacol Exp Ther* **311**(1): 139–146.

56. Harwood, M. D., Russell, M. R., Neuhoff, S., Warhurst, G. and Rostami-Hodjegan, A. (2014). Lost in centrifugation: Accounting for transporter protein losses in quantitative targeted absolute proteomics. *Drug Metab Dispos* **42**(10): 1766–1772.

57. Kumar, A. R., Prasad, B., Bhatt, D. K., Mathialagan, S., Varma, M. V. S. and Unadkat, J. D. (2020). In vivo-to-in vitro extrapolation of transporter-mediated renal clearance: Relative expression factor versus relative activity factor approach. *Drug Metab Dispos* **49**(6): 470–478.

58. El-Khateeb, E., Vasilogianni, A. M., Alrubia, S., Al-Majdoub, Z. M., Couto, N., Howard, M., Barber, J., Rostami-Hodjegan, A. and Achour, B. (2019). Quantitative mass spectrometry-based proteomics in the era of model-informed drug development: Applications in translational pharmacology and recommendations for best practice. *Pharmacol Ther* **203**: 107397.

59. Proctor, N. J., Tucker, G. T. and Rostami-Hodjegan, A. (2004). Predicting drug clearance from recombinantly expressed CYPs: intersystem extrapolation factors. *Xenobiotica* **34**(2): 151–178.

60. Rennick, J. J., Johnston, A. P. R. and Parton, R. G. (2021). Key principles and methods for studying the endocytosis of biological and nanoparticle therapeutics. *Nat Nanotechnol* **16**(3): 266–276.

61. Utembe, W., Clewell, H., Sanabria, N., Doganis, P. and Gulumian, M. (2020). Current Approaches and Techniques in Physiologically Based Pharmacokinetic (PBPK) Modelling of Nanomaterials. *Nanomaterials (Basel)* **10**(7): 1267.

62. Chen, W. Y., Cheng, Y. H., Hsieh, N. H., Wu, B. C., Chou, W. C., Ho, C. C., Chen, J. K., Liao, C. M. and Lin, P. (2015). Physiologically based pharmacokinetic modeling of zinc oxide nanoparticles and zinc nitrate in mice. *Int J Nanomed* **10**: 6277–6292.

63. Deng, L., Liu, H., Ma, Y., Miao, Y., Fu, X. and Deng, Q. (2019). Endocytosis mechanism in physiologically-based pharmacokinetic modeling of nanoparticles. *Toxicol Appl Pharmacol* **384**: 114765.

64. Carlander, U., Li, D., Jolliet, O., Emond, C. and Johanson, G. (2016). Toward a general physiologically-based pharmacokinetic model for intravenously injected nanoparticles. *Int J Nanomed* **11**: 625–640.

65. Rose, R. H., Neuhoff, S., Abduljalil, K., Chetty, M., Rostami-Hodjegan, A. and Jamei, M. (2014). Application of a physiologically based pharmacokinetic model to predict OATP1B1-related variability in pharmacodynamics of rosuvastatin. *CPT: Pharmacometrics Syst Pharmacol* **3**(7): e124–e124.

66. Chetty, M., Rose, R. H., Abduljalil, K., Patel, N., Lu, G., Cain, T., Jamei, M. and Rostami-Hodjegan, A. (2014). Applications of linking PBPK and PD models to predict the impact of genotypic variability, formulation differences, differences in target binding capacity and target site drug concentrations on drug responses and variability. *Front Pharmacol* **5**: 258.

67. Lang, J., Vincent, L., Chenel, M., Ogungbenro, K. and Galetin, A. (2020). Simultaneous ivabradine parent-metabolite PBPK/PD modelling using a bayesian estimation method. *AAPS J* **22**(6): 129.

68. Mori, K., Saito, R., Nakamaru, Y., Shimizu, M. and Yamazaki, H. (2016). Physiologically based pharmacokinetic-pharmacodynamic modeling to predict concentrations and actions of sodium-dependent glucose transporter 2 inhibitor canagliflozin in human intestines and renal tubules. *Biopharm Drug Dispos* **37**(8): 491–506.

69. Yang, F., Wang, B., Liu, Z., Xia, X., Wang, W., Yin, D., Sheng, L. and Li, Y. (2017). Prediction of a therapeutic dose for buagafuran, a potent anxiolytic agent by physiologically based pharmacokinetic/pharmacodynamic modeling starting from pharmacokinetics in rats and human. *Front Pharmacol* **8**: 683.

70. Musther, H., Gill, K. L., Chetty, M., Rostami-Hodjegan, A., Rowland, M. and Jamei, M. (2015). Are physiologically based pharmacokinetic models reporting the right Cmax? Central venous versus peripheral sampling site. *AAPS J* **17**(5): 1268–1279.

71. Lipinski, C. A., Lombardo, F., Dominy, B. W. and Feeney, P. J. (2001). Experimental and computational approaches to estimate solubility and permeability in drug discovery and development settings. *Adv Drug Deliv Rev* **46**(1–3): 3–26.

72. Pavelka, M. and Roth, J. (2010). Fluid-phase endocytosis and phagocytosis. In: *Functional Ultrastructure: Atlas of Tissue Biology and Pathology*. M. Pavelka and J. Roth, Vienna, Springer Vienna: pp. 104–105.

73. Swanson, J. A. and King, J. S. (2019). The breadth of macropinocytosis research. *Philos Trans R Soc Lond B Biol Sci* **374**(1765): 20180146–20180146.

74. Sepp, A., Meno-Tetang, G., Weber, A., Sanderson, A., Schon, O. and Berges, A. (2019). Computer-assembled cross-species/cross-modalities two-pore physiologically based pharmacokinetic model for biologics in mice and rats. *J Pharmacokinet Pharmacodyn* **46**(4): 339–359.

75. Wagner, M. and Wiig, H. (2015). Tumor interstitial fluid formation, characterization, and clinical implications. *Front Oncol* **5**: 115.

76. Feher, J. (2012). Regulation of arterial pressure. In: *Quantitative Human Physiology*. Boston, MA, Academic Press: pp. 538–548.

77. Sarin, H. (2010). Physiologic upper limits of pore size of different blood capillary types and another perspective on the dual pore theory of microvascular permeability. *J Angiogenes Res* **2**(1): 1–19.

78. Wiig, H. and Swartz, M. A. (2012). Interstitial fluid and lymph formation and transport: Physiological regulation and roles in inflammation and cancer. *Physiol Rev* **92**(3): 1005–1060.

79. Rossing, N. (1978). Intra- and extravascular distribution of albumin and immunoglobulin in man. *Lymphology* **11**(4): 138–142.

80. Melody, A. S. (2001). The physiology of the lymphatic system. *Adv Drug Deliv Rev* **50**(1–2): 3–20.

81. Moore Jr., J. E. and Bertram, C. D. (2018). Lymphatic system flows. *Ann Rev Fluid Mech* **50**(1): 459–482.

82. Pyzik, M., Sand, K. M. K., Hubbard, J. J., Andersen, J. T., Sandlie, I. and Blumberg, R. S. (2019). The neonatal Fc Receptor (FcRn): A misnomer? *Front Immunol* **10**: 1540.

83. Igawa, T., Tsunoda, H., Tachibana, T., Maeda, A., Mimoto, F., Moriyama, C., Nanami, M., Sekimori, Y., Nabuchi, Y., Aso, Y. and Hattori, K. (2010). Reduced elimination of IgG antibodies by engineering the variable region. *Protein Eng Des Sel* **23**(5): 385–392.

84. Muliaditan, M. and Sepp, A. (2022). Application of quantitative protein mass spectrometric data in the early predictive analysis of target engagement by monoclonal antibodies. *Clin Transl Sci* **15**(7): 1634–1643.

85. Waldmann, T. A. and Terry, W. D. (1990). Familial hypercatabolic hypoproteinemia. A disorder of endogenous catabolism of albumin and immunoglobulin. *J Clin Invest* **86**(6): 2093–2098.

86. Brambell, F. W., Hemmings, W. A. and Morris, I. G. (1964). A theoretical model of gamma-globulin catabolism. *Nature* **203**: 1352–1354.

87. Rippe, B. and Haraldsson, B. (1994). Transport of macromolecules across microvascular walls: The two-pore theory. *Physiol Rev* **74**(1): 163–219.

88. Patlak, C. S., Goldstein, D. A. and Hoffman, J. F. (1963). The flow of solute and solvent across a two-membrane system. *J Theor Biol* **5**(3): 426–442.

89. Baxter, L. T., Zhu, H., Mackensen, D. G. and Jain, R. K. (1994). Physiologically based pharmacokinetic model for specific and nonspecific monoclonal antibodies and fragments in normal tissues and human tumor xenografts in nude mice. *Cancer Res* **54**(6): 1517–1528.

90. Ferl, G., Wu, A. and DiStefano, J. (2005). A predictive model of therapeutic monoclonal antibody dynamics and regulation by the Neonatal Fc Receptor (FcRn). *Ann Biomed Eng* **33**(11): 1640–1652.

91. Gill, K., Gardner, I., Li, L. and Jamei, M. (2016). A bottom-up whole-body physiologically based pharmacokinetic model to mechanistically predict tissue distribution and the rate of subcutaneous absorption of therapeutic proteins. *AAPS J.* 18: 156–170.

92. Sepp, A., Berges, A., Sanderson, A. and Meno-Tetang, G. (2015). Development of a physiologically based pharmacokinetic model for a domain antibody in mice using the two-pore theory. *J Pharmacokinet Pharmacodyn* **42**(2): 97–109.

93. Aweda, T. A., Cheng, S.-H., Lenhard, S. C., Sepp, A., Skedzielewski, T., Hsu, C.-Y., Marshall, S., Haag, H., Kehler, J., Jagdale, P., Peter, A., Schmid, M. A., Gehman, A., Doan, M., Mayer, A. P., Gorycki, P., Fanget, M., Colas, C., Smith, B., Maier, C. C. and Alsaid, H. (2022). In vivo biodistribution and pharmacokinetics of sotrovimab, a SARS-CoV-2 monoclonal antibody, in healthy cynomolgus monkeys. *Eur J Nucl Med Mol Imaging* 50(3):667–678.

94. Sepp, A., Bergström, M. and Davies, M. (2020). Cross-species/cross-modality physiologically based pharmacokinetics for biologics: 89Zr-labelled albumin-binding domain antibody GSK3128349 in humans. *mAbs* **12**(1): e1832861.

95. Li, Z., Yu, X., Li, Y., Verma, A., Chang, H. P. and Shah, D. K. (2021). A two-pore physiologically based pharmacokinetic model to predict subcutaneously administered different-size antibody/antibody fragments. *AAPS J* **23**(3): 62.

96. Shah, D. K. and Betts, A. M. (2012). Towards a platform PBPK model to characterize the plasma and tissue disposition of monoclonal antibodies in preclinical species and human. *J Pharmacokinet Pharmacodyn* **39**(1): 67–86.

97. Venturoli, D. and Rippe, B. (2005). Ficoll and dextran vs. globular proteins as probes for testing glomerular permselectivity: Effects of molecular size, shape, charge, and deformability. *Am J Physiol - Renal Physiol* **288**(4): F605–F613.

98. Jagdale, P., Sepp, A. and Shah, D. K. (2022). Physiologically-based pharmacokinetic model for pulmonary disposition of protein therapeutics in humans. *J Pharmacokinet Pharmacodyn* **49**(6): 607–624.

99. Chang, H.-Y., Wu, S., Li, Y., Guo, L., Li, Y. and Shah, D. K. (2022). Effect of the Size of Protein Therapeutics on Brain Pharmacokinetics Following Systematic Administration. *AAPS J* **24**(3): 62.

100. Wu, S., Le Prieult, F., Phipps, C. J., Mezler, M. and Shah, D. K. (2022). PBPK model for antibody disposition in mouse brain: Validation using large-pore microdialysis data. *J Pharmacokinetics Pharmacodyn* **49**(6): 579–592.

101. Chang, H.-Y., Wu, S., Meno-Tetang, G. and Shah, D. K. (2019). A translational platform PBPK model for antibody disposition in the brain. *J Pharmacokinet Pharmacodyn* **46**(4): 319–338.

102. Li, Z., Li, Y., Chang, H. P., Yu, X. and Shah, D. K. (2021). Two-pore physiologically based pharmacokinetic model validation using whole-body biodistribution of trastuzumab and different-size fragments in mice. *J Pharmacokinet Pharmacodyn* **48**(5): 743–762.

103. Chang, H.-P., Li, Z. and Shah, D. K. (2022). Development of a physiologically-based pharmacokinetic model for whole-body disposition of MMAE containing antibody-drug conjugate in mice. *Pharm Res* **39**(1): 1–24.

104. Sarin, H., Kanevsky, A. S., Wu, H., Sousa, A. A., Wilson, C. M., Aronova, M. A., Griffiths, G. L., Leapman, R. D. and Vo, H. Q. (2009). Physiologic upper limit of pore size in the blood-tumor barrier of malignant solid tumors. *J Transl Med* **7**: 51.

105. Rudnick, S. I. and Adams, G. P. (2009). Affinity and avidity in antibody-based tumor targeting. *Cancer Biother Radiopharm* **24**(2): 155–161.

106. Thurber, G. M., Schmidt, M. M. and Wittrup, K. D. (2008). Antibody tumor penetration: Transport opposed by systemic and antigen-mediated clearance. *Adv Drug Deliv Rev* **60**(12): 1421–1434.

107. Thurber, G. M. and Wittrup, K. D. (2008). Quantitative spatiotemporal analysis of antibody fragment diffusion and endocytic consumption in tumor spheroids. *Cancer Res* **68**(9): 3334–3341.

108. Wittrup, K. D., Thurber, G. M., Schmidt, M. M. and Rhoden, J. J. (2012). Practical theoretic guidance for the design of tumor-targeting agents. In: *Methods in Enzymology*. K. D. Wittrup and L. V. Gregory, Academic Press. Volume 503: pp. 255–268.

109. Viola, M., Sequeira, J., Seiça, R., Veiga, F., Serra, J., Santos, A. C. and Ribeiro, A. J. (2018). Subcutaneous delivery of monoclonal antibodies: How do we get there? *J Control Release* **286**: 301–314.

110. Richter, W. F. and Jacobsen, B. (2014). Subcutaneous absorption of biotherapeutics: Knowns and unknowns. *Drug Metabol Dispos* **42**(11): 1881–1889.

111. Richter, W. F., Christianson, G. J., Frances, N., Grimm, H. P., Proetzel, G. and Roopenian, D. C. (2018). Hematopoietic cells as site of first-pass catabolism after subcutaneous dosing and contributors to systemic clearance of a monoclonal antibody in mice. *mAbs* **10**(5): 803–813.

112. Porter, C. J. H. and Charman, S. A. (2000). Lymphatic transport of proteins after subcutaneous administration. *J Pharm Sci* **89**(3): 297–310.

113. Kagan, L. and Mager, D. E. (2013). Mechanisms of subcutaneous absorption of rituximab in rats. *Drug Metab Dispos* **41**(1): 248–255.

114. Kagan, L., Turner, M. R., Balu-Iyer, S. V. and Mager, D. E. (2012). Subcutaneous absorption of monoclonal antibodies: Role of dose, site of injection, and injection volume on rituximab pharmacokinetics in rats. *Pharm Res* **29**(2): 490–499.

115. Shah, D. K. and Betts, A. M. (2013). Antibody biodistribution coefficients: Inferring tissue concentrations of monoclonal antibodies based on the plasma concentrations in several preclinical species and human. *mAbs* **5**(2): 297–305.

116. Betts, A., Keunecke, A., van Steeg, T. J., van der Graaf, P. H., Avery, L. B., Jones, H. and Berkhout, J. (2018). Linear pharmacokinetic parameters for monoclonal antibodies are similar within a species and across different pharmacological targets: A comparison between human, cynomolgus monkey and hFcRn Tg32 transgenic mouse using a population-modeling approach. *mAbs* **10**(5): 751–764.

117. Neuber, T., Frese, K., Jaehrling, J., Jager, S., Daubert, D., Felderer, K., Linnemann, M., Hohne, A., Kaden, S., Kolln, J., Tiller, T., Brocks, B., Ostendorp, R. and Pabst, S. (2014). Characterization and screening of IgG binding to the neonatal Fc receptor. *mAbs* **6**(4): 928–942.

118. Jensen, P. F., Schoch, A., Larraillet, V., Hilger, M., Schlothauer, T., Emrich, T. and Rand, K. D. (2017). A two-pronged binding mechanism of IgG to the neonatal Fc receptor controls complex stability and IgG serum half-life. *Mol Cell Proteom* 16(3): 451–456.

119. Datta-Mannan, A. (2019). Mechanisms influencing the disposition of monoclonal antibodies and peptides. *Drug Metab Dispos* 47(10): 1100–1110.

120. Gibiansky, L., Gibiansky, E., Kakkar, T. and Ma, P. (2008). Approximations of the target-mediated drug disposition model and identifiability of model parameters. *J Pharmacokinet Pharmacodyn* 35(5): 573–591.

121. Davda, J. P. and Hansen, R. J. (2010). Properties of a general PK/PD model of antibody-ligand interactions for therapeutic antibodies that bind to soluble endogenous targets. *mAbs* **2**(5): 576–588.

122. Bocci, V. (1991). Interleukins. Clinical pharmacokinetics and practical implications. *Clin Pharmacokinet* **21**(4): 274–284.

123. Liu, C., Chu, D., Kalantar-Zadeh, K., George, J., Young, H. A. and Liu, G. (2021). Cytokines: From clinical significance to quantification. *Adv Sci* **8**(15): 2004433.

124. Berkhout Lea, C., l'Ami Merel, J., Ruwaard, J., Hart Margreet, H., Heer Pleuni, O.-d., Bloem, K., Nurmohamed Michael, T., van Vollenhoven Ronald, F., Boers, M., Alvarez Daniel, F., Smith Catherine, H., Wolbink Gerrit, J. and Rispens, T. (2019). Dynamics of circulating TNF during adalimumab treatment using a drug-tolerant TNF assay. *Sci Transl Med* **11**(477): eaat3356.

125. Staton, T. L., Peng, K., Owen, R., Choy, D. F., Cabanski, C. R., Fong, A., Brunstein, F., Alatsis, K. R. and Chen, H. (2019). A phase I, randomized, observer-blinded, single and multiple ascending-dose study to investigate the safety, pharmacokinetics, and immunogenicity of BITS7201A, a bispecific antibody targeting IL-13 and IL-17, in healthy volunteers. *BMC Pulm Med* **19**(1): 5.

126. Borski, A., Eskandary, F., Haindl, S., Doberer, K., Mühlbacher, J., Mayer, K. A., Budde, K., Halloran, P. F., Chong, E., Jilma, B., Böhmig, G. A. and Wahrmann, M. (2023). Anti-interleukin-6 antibody clazakizumab in antibody-mediated renal allograft rejection: Accumulation of antibody-neutralized interleukin-6 without signs of proinflammatory rebound phenomena. *Transplantation* 107(2): 495–503.

127. Igawa, T., Maeda, A., Haraya, K., Tachibana, T., Iwayanagi, Y., Mimoto, F., Higuchi, Y., Ishii, S., Tamba, S., Hironiwa, N., Nagano, K., Wakabayashi, T., Tsunoda, H. and Hattori, K. (2013). Engineered monoclonal antibody with novel antigen-sweeping activity in vivo. *PLoS One* **8**(5): e63236.

128. Mager, D. E. and Krzyzanski, W. (2005). Quasi-equilibrium pharmacokinetic model for drugs exhibiting target-mediated drug disposition. *Pharm Res* **22**(10): 1589–1596.

129. Stüber, J. C., Kast, F. and Plückthun, A. (2019). High-Throughput Quantification of Surface Protein Internalization and Degradation. *ACS Chem Biol* **14**(6): 1154–1163.

130. Sengers, B. G., McGinty, S., Nouri, F. Z., Argungu, M., Hawkins, E., Hadji, A., Weber, A., Taylor, A. and Sepp, A. (2016). Modeling bispecific monoclonal antibody interaction with two cell membrane targets indicates the importance of surface diffusion. *mAbs* **8**(5): 905–915.

131. Datta-Mannan, A., Lu, J., Witcher, D. R., Leung, D., Tang, Y. and Wroblewski, V. J. (2015). The interplay of non-specific binding, target-mediated clearance and FcRn interactions on the pharmacokinetics of humanized antibodies. *mAbs* **7**(6): 1084–1093.

132. Datta-Mannan, A., Croy, J. E., Schirtzinger, L., Torgerson, S., Breyer, M. and Wroblewski, V. J. (2016). Aberrant bispecific antibody pharmacokinetics linked to liver sinusoidal endothelium clearance mechanism in cynomolgus monkeys. *mAbs* **8**(5): 969–982.

133. Datta-Mannan, A., Estwick, S., Zhou, C., Choi, H., Douglass, N. E., Witcher, D. R., Lu, J., Beidler, C. and Millican, R. (2020). Influence of physiochemical properties on the subcutaneous absorption and bioavailability of monoclonal antibodies. *mAbs* **12**(1): 1770028.

134. Morgan, P., Van Der Graaf, P. H., Arrowsmith, J., Feltner, D. E., Drummond, K. S., Wegner, C. D. and Street, S. D. A. (2012). Can the flow of medicines be improved? Fundamental pharmacokinetic and pharmacological principles toward improving Phase II survival. *Drug Discov Today* 17(9–10): 419–424.

135. Zhu, H., Melder, R. J., Baxter, L. T. and Jain, R. K. (1996). Physiologically based kinetic model of effector cell biodistribution in mammals: Implications for adoptive immunotherapy. *Cancer Res* **56**(16): 3771–3781.

136. Ganusov, V. V. and Auerbach, J. (2014). Mathematical modeling reveals kinetics of lymphocyte recirculation in the whole organism. *PLoS Comput Biol* **10**(5): e1003586.

137. Brown, L. V., Coles, M. C., McConnell, M., Ratushny, A. V. and Gaffney, E. A. (2022). Analysis of cellular kinetic models suggest that physiologically based model parameters may be inherently, practically unidentifiable. *J Pharmacokinet Pharmacodyn.* 49(5): 539–556.

6 Modeling Drug Metabolism and Excretion

Frederico Severino Martins, Stephan Schaller, and Luis David Jiménez Franco

6.1 METABOLIC CLEARANCE

Clearance is the parameter that determines total systemic exposure to the drug, which is simply the sum of all processes by which drugs are removed from the body or inactivated, primarily renal excretion and metabolism [1].

Drug metabolism plays an essential role in the pharmacokinetics (PK), pharmacodynamics (PD), and safety profiles of drug candidates in drug research and development (R&D). Drug metabolism and pharmacokinetics (DMPK) studies are used throughout drug discovery. DMPK studies aim to accelerate the drug discovery cycle by determining the drug properties that yield the desired efficacy and safety to enable clinical use [2].

Determining the clearance with an appropriate experimental design is the first step in R&D to improve the PK properties of a drug candidate. Characterization of drug clearance can be challenging as it may be associated with different pathways (e.g., metabolic and renal). The total drug clearance is described by:

$$CL = CL_h + CL_r + CL_{other} \qquad (6.1)$$

where CL_h reflects hepatic clearance, CL_r renal clearance, and CL_{other} combines all other causes of clearance, such as extracorporeal elimination (e.g., dialysis) or metabolism by pH-dependent plasma esterases (e.g., CES and Est-A).

Drug metabolism comprises two phases (Figure 6.1). Though most Phase I metabolic reactions are catalyzed by cytochrome P450 enzymes (also known as CYP, P450 or CYP450 enzymes) (Table 6.1), other enzymes such as oxidoreductases, esterases, and oxidases can also play a role in Phase I drug oxidation, reduction, and hydrolysis. Phase II reactions occur when Phase I metabolites are glucuronidated, sulfonated, methylated, acetylated, and amino acids conjugated. The principal enzymes involved in Phase II metabolism are glucuronosyltransferases (UGTs), sulfotransferases (SULTs), and N-acetyltransferase (NATs) [3–5].

During Phase I metabolism, the drug or prodrug is converted into more polar, water-soluble, active metabolites by unmasking or inserting a polar functional group. The enzymes take effect to integrate an atom of oxygen into nonactivated hydrocarbons, which results in the introduction of hydroxyl groups or N-, O- and S-dealkylation of substrates. In most cases, oxidation is responsible for converting a prodrug to an active drug or non-toxic to toxic molecules. Drugs that already have –OH, –NH$_2$ or COOH groups can bypass Phase I and directly enter Phase II.

During Phase II, the parent drug is transformed into more polar inactive metabolites by conjugation of subgroups. Phase II conjugation reactions include carboxy (–COOH), hydroxy (–OH), amino (NH$_2$), and thiol (–SH) groups. As for Phase I enzymes, Phase II enzymes (Figure 6.1) are also associated with elevated interindividual variability and risk for drug–drug interactions (DDIs).

A specific concern is a high clearance mediated by a single CYP enzyme, as it would not only necessitate high and frequent dosage but also carry the risk of DDI and substantial variation in exposure. On the other hand, having multiple clearance mechanisms is advantageous in mitigating the DDI risks [4].

The characterization and mapping of metabolic pathways involve separation (i.e., isolation of the biotransformed molecules by chromatographic methods) and drug structural elucidation (i.e., compound identification by analytical methods). Failure to characterize the metabolic clearance can be an issue during drug discovery as a wrongly mapped metabolic clearance may lead to late detection of undesired drug–drug interactions, poor bioavailability or metabolite-related toxicities [6].

6.2 IMPROVING PK PROPERTIES

A drug must reach the organ of action to exert its pharmacological effect. However, suppose a drug shows poor PK properties, for example, high clearance and low bioavailability after oral dosing. In that case, exposure is likely too low to exert a substantial PD effect. If a drug candidate exhibits a high enzyme-dependent clearance, efforts should be made to stabilize its chemical structure to reduce clearance.

DOI: 10.1201/9781003031802-6

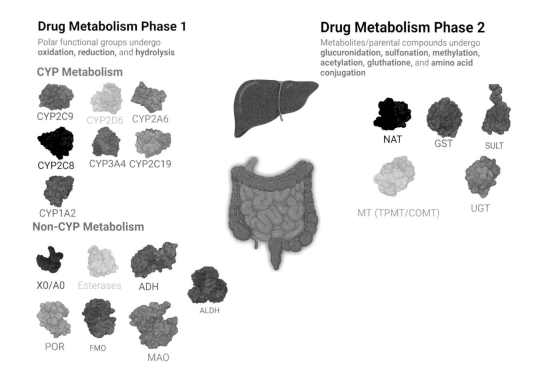

Drug Metabolism Phase 1

Polar functional groups undergo
oxidation, **reduction**, and **hydrolysis**

CYP Metabolism

CYP2C9 CYP2D6 CYP2A6

CYP2C8 CYP3A4 CYP2C19

CYP1A2

Non-CYP Metabolism

X0/A0 Esterases ADH

ALDH

POR FMO

MAO

Drug Metabolism Phase 2

Metabolites/parental compounds undergo
glucuronidation, **sulfonation**, **methylation**,
acetylation, **gluthatione**, and **amino acid**
conjugation

NAT GST SULT

MT (TPMT/COMT) UGT

Figure 6.1 Outline of drug metabolism mediated by CYP and non-CYP enzymes and transport in the liver. The metabolism is divided into Phase I and Phase II reactions.

Table 6.1: Example of Drugs Metabolized by CYP Enzymes

Enzyme	Tissue Expression	Substrate
CYP3A4	+++ Liver + Kidney ++ Gut mucosa	Midazolam Triazolam Alfentanil
CYP2C19	+++ Liver + Kidney ++ Gut mucosa	Omeprazole Lansoprazole Citalopram
CYP2C9	+++ Liver + Kidney ++ Gut mucosa	Warfarin Phenytoin Losartan
CYP2D6	+++ Liver ++ Kidney ++ Gut mucosa	Haloperidol Sertraline Paroxetine
UGT1A1	+++ Liver + Kidney ++ Gut mucosa	Raltegravir Dapagliflozin

+++ high expression; ++ moderate expression; + low expression

There are different strategies to optimize a drug's PK properties. One of the first steps is to identify the molecule's *soft spot* (i.e., the molecular group prone to be metabolized) and modify the "culprit" substructure. The *soft spot* identification method combines *in silico* prediction and ranking of *soft spots* as well as mass spectrometric confirmation (Figure 6.2), aiming to reduce drug clearance and, thus, increase drug half-life [7].

The structure-metabolism relationship is complex and not entirely known. An approach to reduce or prevent the metabolism on a specific *soft spot* of a molecule is to use a substituent (e.g., a deuterium or halogen atom) replacing the H-atom of a C-H bond to reduce or block the

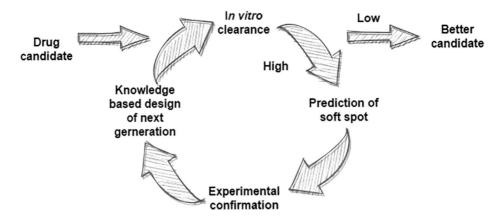

Figure 6.2 Proposed drug optimization workflow. (Adapted from Ref. [7].)

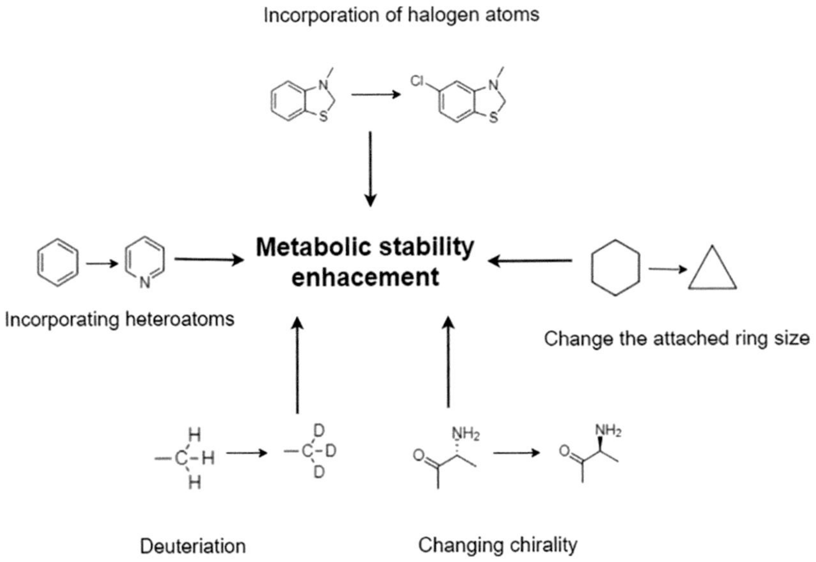

Incorporation of halogen atoms

Metabolic stability enhacement

Incorporating heteroatoms

Change the attached ring size

Deuteriation

Changing chirality

Figure 6.3 Approaches to metabolic stability enhancement.

accessibility of the iron-bound oxidizing species of the P450 enzyme and thus improving the metabolic stability [2,8]. It is commonly accepted that CYP enzymes have a large active site and frequently metabolize lipophilic substrates. Overall, increasing the drug hydrophilicity or polarity by blocking or replacing metabolic *soft spots* with more stable molecular groups enhances metabolic stability. Furthermore, reducing the drug lipophilicity decreases drug binding to CYP enzymes due to reduced hydrophobic interactions [9]. Figure 6.3 illustrates the main approaches to improving the metabolic stability of a compound [10].

Unfortunately, the approaches presented in Figure 6.3 are not always efficient. CYP enzymes have multiple metabolism sites, and modifications in a drug can cause the molecule to attach to other binding sites of the metabolizing enzyme, resulting in metabolism on a different *soft spot*. This pattern, called alternative metabolic switching, is not uncommon [9].

Another strategy used in R&D is using prodrugs or active metabolites as new drug candidates. Prodrugs are inactive compounds, enzymatically activated or chemically transformed to a pharmacologically active form *in vivo* [8]. Carbamates, phosphates, esters, amides, or carbonates are frequently functional groups in prodrugs cleaved enzymatically or chemically in the body. The use of prodrugs helps to overcome problems associated with the absorption barrier, route of administration, metabolism, excretion, and toxicity (Table 6.2) [11].

Table 6.2: Use of Prodrugs to Improve DMPK [11]

Prodrug Name and Therapeutic Area	Functional Group	Structure	Strategy
Enalapril (angiotensinconverting enzyme inhibitor)	Monoethyl ester of enalaprilat		• Bioconversion by esterases. • Oral bioavailability of enalaprilat in humans is 36%–44%. • 53%–74% of the administered dose is absorbed.
Oseltamivir (anti-influenza)	Ethyl ester of oseltamivir carboxylate		• Bioconversion by esterases. • Oral bioavailability of less than 5% in rats and marmosets for oseltamivir carboxylate is increased to 80% when using oseltamivir in humans.
Tenofovir disoproxil (antiviral)	Bis-(isopropyloxy-carbonyloxy methyl) ester of tenofovir		• Bioconversion by esterases and phosphodiesterases. • Oral bioavailability of tenofovir from tenofovir disoproxil is 39% in the fed state
Ximelagatran (anticoagulant)	Hydroxyamidine and ethyl ester of melagatran		• Bioconversion by esterases and reductive enzymes. • Oral bioavailability of 3%–7% for melagatran increased to 20% for ximelagatran.

6.3 RENAL CLEARANCE

The kidney is a vital organ for drug excretion as approximately 60% of all medicines, and their metabolites are excreted renally. Renal clearance results from four biological processes: glomerular filtration, active tubular secretion, active reabsorption, and passive reabsorption. Filtration is a passive flow-dependent process. Passive reabsorption removes useful molecules and water from the filtrate in the distal tubules and returns them to systemic circulation. Active secretion and reabsorption utilize membrane transporters to excrete or reabsorb molecules (e.g., administered drugs) and typically occur within the proximal tubule of the kidney [12,13].

Mathematically, the renal clearance is represented by the equation:

$$CL_r = (F_u \times GFR) + CL_{secretion} - CL_{reabsorption} \tag{6.2}$$

where F_u is the fraction unbound of drug that can be filtered, GFR is the glomerular filtration rate, and $CL_{secretion}$ and $CL_{reabsorption}$ are the increase and decrease in the clearance through secretion and reabsorption, respectively [14]. Not all of these processes are relevant in the renal clearance for every compound. Understanding the interaction between these processes is vital to allow accurate predictions of renal clearance.

6.3.1 Glomerular Filtration

The primary parameter clinicians consider for a drug and its metabolite when cleared by the kidney is the GFR. The GFR is a calculation that determines how well the blood is filtered by the kidneys, which is one way to measure the kidney function. Creatinine-based estimate equations are not appropriate for all populations. The kidneys receive 25% of cardiac output, with glomerular filtration driven by hydrostatic pressure within glomerular capillaries. The GFR is estimated

Table 6.3: Equations for Estimating GFR Expressed for the Specified Race, Sex, and Serum Creatinine Level [15]

Race	Sex	Serum Creatinine, S_{cr} (mg/dL)	Equation (Age in Years ≥ 18)
Black	Female	≤ 0.7	$GFR = 166 \times (S_{cr}/0.7)^{-0.329} \times (0.993)^{Age}$
Black	Female	> 0.7	$GFR = 166 \times (S_{cr}/0.7)^{-1.209} \times (0.993)^{Age}$
Black	Male	≤ 0.9	$GFR = 163 \times (S_{cr}/0.9)^{-0.411} \times (0.993)^{Age}$
Black	Male	> 0.9	$GFR = 163 \times (S_{cr}/0.9)^{-1.209} \times (0.993)^{Age}$
White or other	Female	≤ 0.7	$GFR = 144 \times (S_{cr}/0.7)^{-0.329} \times (0.993)^{Age}$
White or other	Female	> 0.7	$GFR = 144 \times (S_{cr}/0.7)^{-1.209} \times (0.993)^{Age}$
White or other	Male	≤ 0.9	$GFR = 141 \times (S_{cr}/0.9)^{-0.411} \times (0.993)^{Age}$
White or other	Male	> 0.9	$GFR = 141 \times (S_{cr}/0.9)^{-1.209} \times (0.993)^{Age}$

Table 6.4: Morphine Dosage Reductions for Reduced Glomerular Filtration Rate

GFR (mL/min)	Morphine Dosage (% of Normal Dose)
20–50	75
10–20	50
<10	25

by measuring substances or drugs that are eliminated solely by glomerular filtration, such as creatinine or inulin (Table 6.3) [12]. Creatinine is only helpful when the renal function is stable, while unstable creatinine values will not provide precise GFR estimations [15]. Glomerular filtration occurs only with unbound small molecules (molecular weight $\lesssim 30$ kDa [16]), while larger molecules such as protein or bound drugs are mostly not filtered at the glomerulus.

As a practical example, morphine is metabolized in the liver to morphine-3-glucuronide (55%), morphine-6-glucuronide (10%), and normorphine (4%). These metabolites and 10% of the parent compound are excreted renally in subjects with normal renal function. In patients with renal failure, the dose of morphine needs to be adjusted (Table 6.4) because high levels of morphine-6-glucuronide can cause respiratory depression as morphine-6-glucuronide is a depressant to the central nervous system (CNS) [17,18].

6.3.2 Tubular Secretion

In the tubular secretion, the drug requires access to the proximal tubule cells from the blood via the basolateral membrane, or the drug is removed into the luminal fluid via the apical membrane. Both can happen passively, but a transporter facilitates drug movement across membranes for most medications, making compounds with active tubular secretion have a CL_r higher than the glomerular filtration [19].

The kidney transporters are divided into two superfamilies: the solute carrier (SLC) and the ATP binding cassette (ABC) (see Transporter-mediated clearance). Drugs with similar structures compete for the same transport family. For example, probenecid and fluoroquinolones compete with penicillin for the same transport system, decreasing the CL_r for these drugs [19].

6.3.3 Renal Reabsorption

Renal reabsorption is usually a non-saturable passive back-diffusion process driven by a concentration gradient. Approximately two-thirds of the filtrate in the proximal tubule is reabsorbed isosmotically, creating a concentration gradient that favors the passive reabsorption of drug molecules. The extension of drug reabsorption depends on the molecular size, protein binding, solubility, acid dissociation (pK_a), and urine pH. The renal clearance of drugs predominantly reabsorbed by passive diffusion will generally display a linear relationship with the urine production rate. Active reabsorption occurs in the kidney's proximal tubules and is mediated by specific anion and cation transporters expressed at the apical and basolateral membranes (e.g., MCTs, SMCTs).

6.4 TRANSPORTER-MEDIATED CLEARANCE

Transporters are membrane proteins facilitating molecules and ions' permeation across biological membranes. Permeation mediated by transporters is characterized by saturability. Higher substrate concentrations increase the total transport velocity, but the transport velocity eventually reaches a steady state. The effect of saturable mechanisms on the uptake and subsequent excretion of different drug types have been demonstrated *in vivo* and *in vitro*, determining the specific tissues to which these drugs are delivered and how they are eliminated [20]. Many transporters are expressed in the liver and kidneys, two major organs associated with clearance. Compared with the SLC family, which comprises 364 proteins arranged into 48 subfamilies, the ABC family consists of only 49 proteins organized into seven subfamilies. The mechanisms of SLC-type transporters involve facilitated diffusion and secondary active transport, combined with ion symport or antiport to provide the driving force. ABC transporters act as catalysts for ATP hydrolysis and mediate active transport in unidirectional efflux [21,22].

In vitro transport studies using human cells, e.g., cryopreserved hepatocytes and membrane vesicles, indicate the importance of transporters and their clinical relevance. Polymorphisms in transporter genes have also been studied, which can cause interindividual, gender, and ethnic differences in drug disposition and response (Table 6.5) [23].

6.4.1 Hepatic Transporters

After being absorbed, the drug goes into the liver through the portal vein or the hepatic artery. Various uptake transporters are located on the liver plasma membrane driving the movement of drugs from blood to the interstitial compartment of hepatocytes. In contrast, the efflux transporters occur in two places: on the basolateral membrane, where drugs are transferred back to the systemic circulation, and on the canalicular membrane, where drugs are exported into bile. The multidrug resistance-associated proteins MRP3, MRP4, and MRP6 are basolateral membrane transporters. In comparison, the canalicular membrane transporters include the multidrug resistance protein 1 (MDR1 or P-gp), MRP2, the breast cancer resistance protein (BCRP), and the multidrug and toxin extrusion protein 1 (MATE1) (see Table 6.5). These transporters influence the free intracellular concentrations and thus impact the toxicity and efficacy of substrate drugs [22,24] (Figure 6.4).

Table 6.5: Transporters Involved in Drug Disposition

Transporter	Gene Name	Tissue	*In vivo* Function	Substrates
OATP1A2	SLCO1A2	Brain, liver	Intestinal absorption and tissue uptake	Ouabain, digoxin
OATP1B1	SLCO1B2	Liver	Intestinal absorption and liver active uptake	Pravastatin, pitavastatin, rosuvastatin, fexofenadine repaglinide, nateglinide
OATP1B3	SLCO1B3	Liver	Liver active uptake, renal active secretion	Valsartan, telmisartan, pravastatin
OATP4C1	SLCO4C1	Kidney	Renal active secretion	Digoxin
OCT1	SLC22A1	Liver	Liver uptake	Cimetidine, ranitidine, famotidine
OCT2	SLC22A26	Kidney	Renal active secretion	Cimetidine, ranitidine, famotidine
OAT1	SLC22A6	Kidney	Renal active secretion	Adefovir, tenofovir
OAT3	SLC22A8	Kidney	Renal active secretion	Cimetidine, ranitidine, famotidine
MATE1	SLC47A1	Liver, kidney, skeletal muscle	Renal active secretion, and liver uptake	Metformin, cimetidine, procainamide, fluoroquinolones
MDR1	ABCB1	Brain, liver, kidney, intestine	Renal active secretion, and liver uptake	Desloratadine, ebastine, verapamil, digoxin
BCRP	ABCG2	Liver and intestine	Liver active uptake, biliary clearance, gut absorption	Mitoxantrone, irinotecan, topotecan, imatinib, rosuvastatin

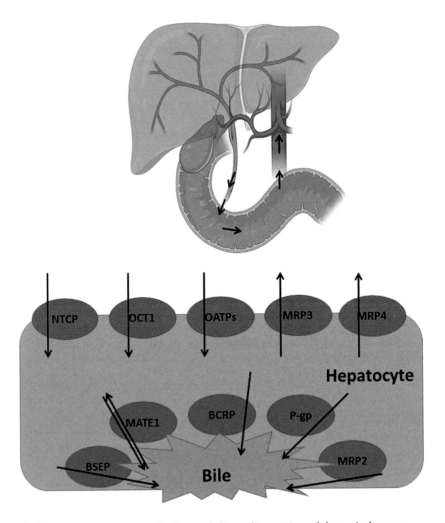

Figure 6.4 Transporters acting in the hepatobiliary disposition of drugs in humans.

Organic-anion-transporting polypeptides (OATP) transporters show a broad substrate affinity, and it has been clinically demonstrated that they considerably impact drug PK [25]. This has been supported by clinical evidence, DDI-, and pharmacogenomic studies. For example, cerivastatin shows a fourfold increase in plasma exposure when coadministered with the OATP1B1 inhibitor cyclosporine A. Also, genetic polymorphisms of OATP transporter affect drug disposition. Nishizato et al. [26] demonstrated that the OATP1B1 T521C mutation results in the formation of the OATP1B1*15 haplotype in the Japanese population, which makes the plasma concentration of pravastatin after oral administration higher when compared with healthy subjects with the *1b allele (A388G mutation). Comparable clinical conclusions have been related to the *15 and other T521C alleles for other drugs, such as ezetimibe, irinotecan, atorvastatin, pitavastatin, rosuvastatin, valsartan, and temocapril [24,26].

6.4.2 Renal Transporters

In drug discovery, renal transporter substrate studies aim to understand the mechanism of active renal secretion and to predict clearance and the risk of renal DDIs. The three major organic uptake transporters are the cation transporter 2 (OCT2), the anion transporter 1 (OAT1), and the OAT3, expressed on the basolateral side of the renal proximal tubule cells. These transporters mediate the uptake of metformin, cimetidine, and cidofovir. The major renal transporters expressed in the apical side of the renal proximal tubule cells include P-gp, BCRP, and MATEs (Table 6.5 and Figure 6.5) [12,27].

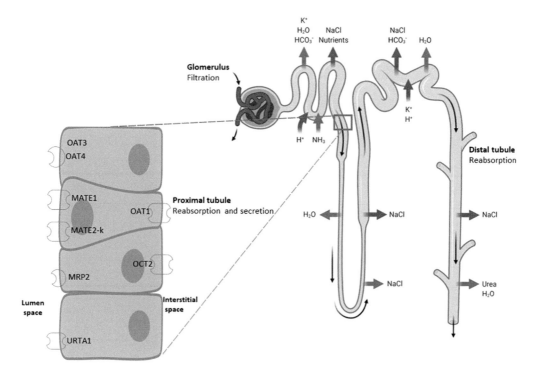

Figure 6.5 Transporters acting in the kidneys disposition of drugs in humans.

Transporter inhibitions at the basolateral and apical membranes have opposite effects, with the drug concentration in the proximal tubular cells either decreasing or increasing. Moreover, inhibition of the tubular secretion at the apical membrane has a more intense impact on intracellular drug concentrations, but it produces only small AUC alterations. Unfortunately, it is technically challenging to assess the effect of DDIs at the organ level, and, therefore, the effects of the proximal tubule transporters may be underestimated [13].

6.5 MEASURING AND MODELING DRUG METABOLISM AND EXCRETION

Metabolism and excretion generally occur in multiple tissues, such as the gut mucosa, lungs, kidneys, blood, and skin. Understanding and selecting the most appropriate *in vitro* assays, combined with *in vivo* pharmacokinetic data, are essential to elucidate the metabolic pathway of a drug. Many *in* vitro assays are used during drug discovery. Regarding the optimization of pharmacokinetic parameters, the metabolic stability of new chemical entities can be divided into four groups: organs, cells (primary cultures and cell lines), subcellular fractions (S9, cytosol, and microsomes), and isolated enzymes (purified and recombinant enzymes) (Table 6.6).

6.5.1 *In vitro* to *in vivo* Extrapolation (IVIVE) of Hepatic Metabolism

The **hepatocyte metabolic stability** is considered the "gold standard" for *in vitro* evaluation of metabolism as it allows the measurement of Phases I and II metabolism. In addition, *in vitro* clearance experiments can be used to rank molecules and to predict *in vivo* hepatic clearance. Cells from different species can be used to identify inter-species differences, which is essential when generating first-in-human predictions.

In vitro hepatocyte assays allow to investigate drug uptake, clearance, hepatotoxicity, and drug–drug interactions. It is an effective model, as most drug-metabolizing enzymes are abundantly found in this type of cell. Thus, hepatocyte assays are a convenient and cost-effective alternative to *in vivo* testing.

Optimized *in vitro* conditions have been developed to eliminate dedifferentiation, which decreases the enzymatic activity over time (especially for CYP2E1 and 3A4), thereby enabling long-term cultures of hepatocytes. These conditions include specific culture media, hormones, and

Table 6.6: In vitro Tools for Drug Metabolism Studies and Their Applications [28]

In vitro Tools	Metabolic Profiling	Metabolic Clearance	Inhibitory Potential	Phenotyping	Induction	Advantages	Disadvantages
Liver slices	+	+	na	+/−	+	Contains the whole complement of DMEs and cell-cell connections. The induction effect of an NCE can be studied.	Requires specific techniques and well-established procedures. Limited viability
Intestine slices	+	+	na	na	na		Difficult to obtain. Fresh tissue needed.
Hepatocytes	++	++	+	+/−	++	Cryopreservation possible. Non-limited source of enzymes.	Expression of most DMEs is poor. Genotype/phenotype instability.
Enterocytes	+	+	na	na	na		
S9	+	na	+/−	+/−	na	Can be used to evaluate Phase I metabolism and some conjugation in Phase II	Metabolism is often lower.
Microsomes (liver, intestine, etc.)	++	++	++	++	na	Contains most important rate-limiting enzymes. Relatively inexpensive. Easy storage.	Contains only Phase I enzymes and UGTs. Requires strictly specific substrates or antibodies for individual DMEs. Cofactor addition necessary.

++, model used in first intention; +, model used in second intention; +/−, model used only to address a specific question; na, not applicable; DME, drug-metabolizing enzyme; NCE, new chemical entity matrix composition. The poor availability of fresh human hepatocytes and their short lifespan in standard cultures have led to the development of hepatocyte cell lines. HepG2 is the most commonly used and best-characterized human hepatoma cell line. Other cell lines such as HLE, THLE, BC2, or Fa2N-4 are also frequently used.

The **microsomal metabolic assay** uses liver microsomes to determine intrinsic hepatic clearance (CL_{int}). This assay contains cytochrome P450, FMO carboxylesterases, and UGT. Hepatocytes and liver microsomes are fast and cost-effective to determine a drug candidate's CL_{int}. These assays, alongside other parameters such as protein binding and blood-to-plasma ratio, frequently allow a good prediction of *in vivo* hepatic clearance. Additionally, determining drug degradation in the stomach or intestinal lumen is essential not to overestimate the first-pass metabolism.

S9 metabolic stability is a supernatant fraction obtained from organs, usually for the liver (CYP and UGT) and kidney (CYP3A4, CYP4B UGT1A6, UGT2B7, SULT1C2, and NQO1). The S9 can be used to evaluate Phase I metabolism and some conjugation in Phase II. It can also be applied to determine sulfatation and glucuronidation. Compared to other drug metabolism systems (e.g., microsomes and hepatocytes), the metabolism in S9 is often much lower. S9 incubation is frequently used for qualitative purposes to determine the formation of metabolites by cytosolic enzymes [29].

6.5.2 Scaling Factors for Different Experimental Systems

Generally, *in vitro–in vivo* extrapolation (IVIVE) of metabolic reactions has two main objectives: predicting the intrinsic hepatic clearance (CL_{int}) and screening potential drug–drug interactions. *In vivo* parameters such as volume of distribution, protein binding, oral bioavailability, and plasma half-life need to be considered to estimate *in vivo* kinetics based on *in vitro* studies. A simple approach for IVIVE is presented in Figure 6.6. Details of the equations for the well-stirred and parallel tube hepatic models to determine first-pass metabolism are described below.

The basic assumption of the **well-stirred model** for hepatic clearance is that the efficiency of hepatic drug removal from the blood is proportional to the efficiency of blood delivery to the liver. The former is described by the hepatic extraction ratio, and the latter is simply the blood flow to the liver. Thus, the equation below (Equation 6.3) is basically "flow times extraction ratio" [30,31].

$$CL_h = Q_h \cdot \frac{fu \cdot CL_{int}}{Q_h + fu \cdot CL_{int}} \tag{6.3}$$

where CL_h is the hepatic clearance, Q_h the liver blood flow, fu the fraction unbound in plasma, and CL_{int} is the intrinsic clearance. The CL_{int} is the inherent capability of the liver to remove the drug from the body – in the absence of any flow limitation – and is related to the sum of enzymatic activities that metabolize the drug (Equation 6.4).

$$CL_{int} = \sum_{i=1}^{n} \frac{V_{max,i}}{K_{m,i} + C_u} \tag{6.4}$$

where V_{max}, K_m are the maximum velocity of the metabolic reaction and the Michaelis-Menten constant, respectively, and C_u is the unbound concentration of the drug in the liver.

The **parallel tube model** assumes that the liver is composed of many identical and parallel tubes with enzymes distributed evenly in each cross-section of the sinusoidal vascular and perisinusoidal space. At any point along the tubes, the concentration of the equilibrating drug at the hepatocyte is the same as that in the sinusoidal space. For the parallel tube model, the calculations for E_h (extraction ratio), F_h (hepatic availability), and CL_h which are based on fu_b (free fraction of the drug in the blood), CL_{int} (intrinsic clearance), and Q_h (hepatic blood flow) are given below (Equations 6.5–6.7) [31]:

$$E_h = 1 - e^{\frac{-fu_b \cdot CL_{int}}{Q_h}} = 1 - e^{\frac{-CL_{int}}{Q_h}} \tag{6.5}$$

$$F_h = 1 - E_h = e^{\frac{-fu_b \cdot CL_{int}}{Q_h}} = 1 - e^{\frac{-CL_{int}}{Q_h}} \tag{6.6}$$

$$CL_h = Q_h * E_h = Q_h \left(1 - e^{\frac{-fu_b \cdot CL_{int}}{Q_h}} \right) = Q_h \left(1 - e^{\frac{-fu_b \cdot CL_{int}}{Q_h}} \right) \tag{6.7}$$

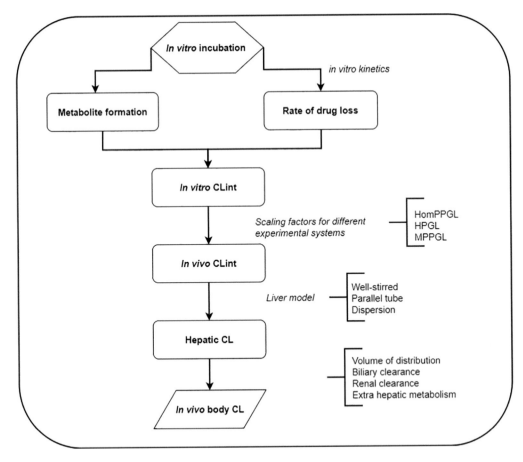

Figure 6.6 Workflow of *in vitro–in vivo* extrapolation of hepatic clearance. HomPPGL, homogenate protein per gram of liver; HPGL, hepatocellularity per gram of liver; MPPGL, microsomal protein per gram liver; CL, clearance; CL_{int}, intrinsic clearance.

Both models assume that the permeability of the drug across the interstitial space and hepatocyte membranes is much higher than the CL_{int} of the drug. Therefore, permeability is not the rate-limiting step in elimination. However, these models need to be adapted if permeability becomes an issue. In this case, the membrane permeability needs to be accounted for.

6.6 CONCLUSION

Metabolism and excretion are determinant factors in drug pharmacokinetics and pharmacody-namics. Therefore, considerable resources are spent during drug development to determine and optimize drug candidates' chemical and pharmacological properties that define the desired clearance characteristics. However, the mechanisms involved in these processes are often complex and challenging to measure *in vivo*. Thus, surrogate *in vitro* experiments and/or indirect measurements together with *in vitro*-to *in vivo* extrapolation techniques are usually performed to determine drug metabolism and excretion. Measured and/or estimated metabolic and excretion values in combination with a deep understanding of the drug's characteristics and the involved physiological processes are essential for pharmacokinetic and pharmacodynamic modeling. In addition, PK/PD models require the inclusion of potential drug–drug interactions with their corresponding mechanisms of action to be able to produce meaningful estimations that could be used to optimize drug development and preclinical and clinical trials.

REFERENCES

1. "Clearance - An Overview | ScienceDirect Topics." https://www.sciencedirect.com/topics/immunology-and-microbiology/clearance (accessed Jan. 18, 2022).

2. P. Ballard et al., "Metabolism and Pharmacokinetic Optimization Strategies in Drug Discovery," In *Drug Discovery and Development*, Elsevier, 2013, pp. 135–155. doi: 10.1016/B978-0-7020-4299-7.00010-X.

3. A. Galetin, M. Gertz, and J. B. Houston, "Potential role of intestinal first-pass metabolism in the prediction of drug-drug interactions," *Expert Opin Drug Metab Toxicol*, vol. 4, no. 7, pp. 909–922, 2008, doi: 10.1517/17425255.4.7.909.

4. S. Jana and S. Mandlekar, "Role of phase II drug metabolizing enzymes in cancer chemoprevention," *Curr Drug Metab*, vol. 10, no. 6, pp. 595–616, 2009, doi: 10.2174/138920009789375379.

5. M. Bortolato, K. Chen, and J. C. Shih, "Monoamine oxidase inactivation: From pathophysiology to therapeutics," *Adv Drug Deliv Rev*, vol. 60, no. 13–14, pp. 1527–1533, 2008, doi: 10.1016/j.addr.2008.06.002.

6. N. Zhang, S. T. Fountain, H. Bi, and D. T. Rossi, "Quantification and rapid metabolite identification in drug discovery using API time-of-flight LC/MS," *Anal Chem.*, vol. 72, no. 4, pp. 800–806, 2000, doi: 10.1021/ac9911701.

7. M. Trunzer, B. Faller, and A. Zimmerlin, "Metabolic soft spot identification and compound optimization in early discovery phases using metasite and LC-MS/MS validation," *J Med Chem*, vol. 52, no. 2, pp. 329–335, 2009, doi: 10.1021/jm8008663.

8. Z. Zhang and W. Tang, "Drug metabolism in drug discovery and development," *Acta Pharmaceutica Sinica B*, vol. 8, no. 5, pp. 721–732, 2018, doi: 10.1016/j.apsb.2018.04.003.

9. M. J. Humphrey and D. A. Smith, "Role of metabolism and pharmacokinetic studies in the discovery of new drugs--present and future perspectives," *Xenobiotica*, vol. 22, no. 7, pp. 743–755, 1992, doi: 10.3109/00498259209053137.

10. G. N. Kumar and S. Surapaneni, "Role of drug metabolism in drug discovery and development," *Med Res Rev*, vol. 21, no. 5, pp. 397–411, 2001, doi: 10.1002/med.1016.

11. J. Rautio et al., "Prodrugs: Design and clinical applications," *Nat Rev Drug Discov*, vol. 7, no. 3, pp. 255–270, 2008, doi: 10.1038/nrd2468.

12. E. F. Barreto, T. R. Larson, and E. J. Koubek, "Drug Excretion," In *Reference Module in Biomedical Sciences*, Elsevier, 2021, p. B9780128204727000000. doi: 10.1016/B978-0-12-820472-6.99999-7.

13. E. J. Cafruny, "Renal Tubular Handling of Drugs," *Am J Med*, vol 62, no. 4, pp.490–496, 1977, doi: 10.1016/0002-9343(77)90403-X.

14. T. N. Lea-Henry, J. E. Carland, S. L. Stocker, J. Sevastos, and D. M. Roberts, "Clinical pharmacokinetics in kidney disease: Fundamental principles," *CJASN*, vol. 13, no. 7, pp. 1085–1095, 2018, doi: 10.2215/CJN.00340118.

15. "Estimating Glomerular Filtration Rate | NIDDK," National Institute of Diabetes and Digestive and Kidney Diseases. https://www.niddk.nih.gov/health-information/professionals/clinical-tools-patient-management/kidney-disease/laboratory-evaluation/glomerular-filtration-rate/estimating (accessed Jan. 20, 2022).

16. A. Ruggiero et al., "Paradoxical glomerular filtration of carbon nanotubes," *Proc Natl Acad Sci*, vol. 107, no. 27, pp. 12369–12374, 2010, doi: 10.1073/pnas.0913667107.

17. F. Coluzzi et al., "Safe use of opioids in chronic kidney disease and hemodialysis patients: Tips and tricks for non-pain specialists," *TCRM*, vol. 16, pp. 821–837, 2020, doi: 10.2147/TCRM. S262843.

18. M. Dean, "Opioids in renal failure and dialysis patients," *J Pain Symptom Manage*, vol. 28, no. 5, pp. 497–504, 2004, doi: 10.1016/j.jpainsymman.2004.02.021.

19. D. M. Moss, M. Neary, and A. Owen, "The role of drug transporters in the kidney: Lessons from tenofovir," *Front Pharmacol*, vol. 5, 2014, doi: 10.3389/fphar.2014.00248.

20. H. Kusuhara and Y. Sugiyama, "In vitro-in vivo extrapolation of transporter-mediated clearance in the liver and kidney," *Drug Metab Pharmacokinet*, vol. 24, no. 1, pp. 37–52, 2009, doi: 10.2133/dmpk.24.37.

21. "Structures and General Transport Mechanisms by the Major Facilitator Superfamily (MFS) | Chemical Reviews." https://pubs.acs.org/doi/10.1021/acs.chemrev.0c00983 (accessed Jan. 20, 2022).

22. "Membrane Transporters in Drug Development | Nature Reviews Drug Discovery." https://www.nature.com/articles/nrd3028 (accessed Jan. 19, 2022).

23. T. M. Sissung, A. K. L. Goey, A. M. Ley, J. D. Strope, and W. D. Figg, "Pharmacogenetics of membrane transporters: A review of current approaches," *Methods Mol Biol*, vol. 1175, pp. 91–120, 2014, doi: 10.1007/978-1-4939-0956-8_6.

24. M. J. Zamek-Gliszczynski, K. A. Hoffmaster, D. J. Tweedie, K. M. Giacomini, and K. M. Hillgren, "Highlights from the international transporter consortium second workshop," *Clin Pharmacol Ther*, vol. 92, no. 5, pp. 553–556, 2012, doi: 10.1038/clpt.2012.126.

25. A. Kalliokoski and M. Niemi, "Impact of OATP transporters on pharmacokinetics," *Br J Pharmacol*, vol. 158, no. 3, pp. 693–705, 2009, doi: 10.1111/j.1476-5381.2009.00430.x.

26. Y. Nishizato et al., "Polymorphisms of OATP-C (SLC21A6) and OAT3 (SLC22A8) genes: Consequences for pravastatin pharmacokinetics," *Clin Pharmacol Ther*, vol. 73, no. 6, pp. 554–565, 2003, doi: 10.1016/S0009-9236(03)00060-2.

27. M. A. Felmlee, R. A. Dave, and M. E. Morris, "Mechanistic models describing active renal reabsorption and secretion: A simulation-based study," *AAPS J*, vol. 15, no. 1, pp. 278–287, 2013, doi: 10.1208/s12248-012-9437-3.

28. Y. Parmentier, M.-J. Bossant, M. Bertrand, and B. Walther, "In Vitro Studies of Drug Metabolism," In *Comprehensive Medicinal Chemistry II*, Elsevier, 2007, pp. 231–257. doi: 10.1016/B0-08-045044-X/00125-5.

29. D. C. Ackley, K. T. Rockich, and T. R. Baker, "Metabolic Stability Assessed by Liver Microsomes and Hepatocytes," In *Optimization in Drug Discovery: In Vitro Methods*, Z. Yan and G. W. Caldwell, Eds. Totowa, NJ: Humana Press, 2004, pp. 151–162. doi: 10.1385/1-59259-800-5:151.

30. K. S. Pang, Y. R. Han, K. Noh, P. I. Lee, and M. Rowland, "Hepatic clearance concepts and misconceptions: Why the well-stirred model is still used even though it is not physiologic reality?," *Biochem Pharmacol*, vol. 169, p. 113596, 2019, doi: 10.1016/j.bcp.2019.07.025.

31. K. S. Pang and M. Rowland, "Hepatic clearance of drugs. I. Theoretical considerations of a 'well-stirred' model and a 'parallel tube' model. Influence of hepatic blood flow, plasma and blood cell binding, and the hepatocellular enzymatic activity on hepatic drug clearance," *J Pharmacokinet Biopharm*, vol. 5, no. 6, pp. 625–653, 1977, doi: 10.1007/BF01059688.

7 Platform Qualification and Model Verification

Mohamad Shebley

7.1 INTRODUCTION

PBPK modeling and simulation, which integrates system- and drug-dependent parameters [1], is a well-established approach in the model-informed drug development paradigm. Applications of PBPK modeling can impact various stages of drug development, ranging from early compound selection for first in human (FIH) trials to dosing recommendations in product labeling. The rise of PBPK applications in drug development and the increasing number of submissions to regulatory agencies have recently prompted the FDA and EMA to issue PBPK guidelines for industry [2,3]. In the EMA guideline, special emphasis has been given to "qualification" of platform and reporting of PBPK modeling and simulation, while the FDA guidance focuses on the format and content of reporting PBPK analyses for regulatory submissions. In this chapter, each component that relates to the PBPK platform and model qualification and verification procedures will be discussed.

7.2 TERMINOLOGY

The terms "Qualification," "verification," and "validation" have been referred to in the PBPK literature and regulatory guidelines when PBPK platforms and models are discussed. These terms will be discussed in more detail in the following sections; however, a brief definition of each term will be useful upfront. The term qualification seems to be appropriate for discussing the PBPK platform as the first level of its ability to perform the intended task. While verification applies to the test, refine, and confirm steps during the development of a PBPK model to demonstrate its ability to predict available datasets (i.e., PK profiles and parameters of several drugs) related to the intended use (i.e.,– CYP-mediated drug–drug interaction). The term validation adds a higher level of scrutiny for the PBPK platform and is intended to test its ability to predict a different scenario outside of the datasets and scenarios that were involved in the verification procedure. For example, a PBPK platform has been qualified for simulating PK profiles and parameters of various drugs, and the PBPK model within the platform is verified for its ability to predict CYP3A-mediated inhibition by multiple drugs using available clinical datasets. The PBPK model is then used to predict an untested scenario (intended use), where the clinical data become available later demonstrating a successful prediction, such model will be considered validated.

7.3 PLATFORM QUALIFICATION

A PBPK platform is an integrated software environment that allows building and running PBPK models that may or may not provide compound or population-specific databases. From a software perspective, a platform includes various components such as graphical user interface (GUI), data structures, collections of various models, computational engine, as well as interfaces for presenting the simulation results. The PBPK models within a platform are developed to handle specific tasks based on certain assumptions. For example, a minimal PBPK model is developed to predict the drug plasma concentration-time profile and some of the derived PK parameters such as area under the curve (AUC), maximum concentration (C_{max}), time to achieve maximum concentration (T_{max}), and clearance values. If the general model structure and assumptions are valid and the correct drug and system parameters are used, the model can be used to simulate any drug regardless of how the drug is eliminated or what enzymes are involved. An example of such a model is the liver well-stirred model, which is a common element of PBPK models used for a wide range of compounds where hepatic and intestinal enzymes are the primary routes of elimination, but hepatic transporters are not involved. Regulatory agencies have also provided guidance on the level of platform qualification needed, depending on the level and impact of the intended use [3]. For example, the US FDA and EMA require demonstration of the ability of a PBPK platform to predict the clinical observations of a pre-specified independent dataset for the intended use, to consider the platform qualified [2,3]. Some remaining challenges for PBPK platform qualification remain, such as identifying "sufficient" clinical datasets for a given qualification process, according to the EMA description, may be challenging or impossible in some cases. For example, to qualify a platform for DDI predictions, the current EMA guideline proposes that a variety of substrates, covering a wide range of fm values be assessed against an inhibitor 'test' model file to qualify the said file. Conversely, a range of inhibitors of various potencies should presumably be

DOI: 10.1201/9781003031802-7

identified to assess the predictability of a given test substrate model file. The requirement for such a range of qualifying files, with the accompanying relevant PK characteristics and clinical data may not even exist for certain scenarios. Qualification of system-related information (i.e., CYPs abundance and turnover rates) along with qualification of the mechanism of interest (i.e., CYP3A reversible inhibition) should allow for the extension of the qualification to other enzymes (i.e., CYP2C9) without the need for an extensive clinical data set. In our experience, the abundance of data that would fit the EMA criteria is only available in the literature for specific scenarios, such as CYP3A interactions. Such requirements are not justifiable and could therefore limit the application of PBPK modeling approaches in drug development. To further the science and test the boundaries of what PBPK can accomplish, in the absence of such databases, it should be acceptable to qualify models using a much smaller dataset based on the viability of the mechanistic understanding. As long as the drug used for qualification, a PBPK platform is similar to the test molecule with regard to PK characteristics (i.e., is appropriate for the intended purpose), there should not be a problem using a limited clinical dataset for qualification. Once a particular version of the platform is qualified for a particular purpose (i.e., CYP3A inhibition), subsequent versions should be deemed qualified. The need to requalify every version would impose a significant overhead and is not scientifically warranted. A clear separation of drug and platform components of qualification is also needed to help the sponsor provide necessary submission package. Finally, harmonized requirements for qualification between Regulatory Agencies can help conserve resources and speed up delivering safe and efficacious drugs to patients.

Therefore, when models within a PBPK platform are developed based on generally acceptable scientific and physiological principles, reliable systems data, and reasonable assumptions, these models are considered qualified for the intended use.

7.3.1 Computational Framework

Design Qualification (DQ): DQ is the documented collection of activities that define the processes of design, implementation, functional, and operational specifications and intended purpose of an instrument or a software platform. These processes are often part of a comprehensive quality assurance (QA) framework. DQ may be performed by the instrument manufacturer [4] or the user [5]. The supplier is generally responsible for robust design and maintaining documentation describing how the platform is developed and how data in databases are analyzed and populated. Nonetheless, the user should ensure that the platform and relevant databases are suitable for their intended application and may evaluate whether the supplier has adopted a quality system that provides reliable software and databases. As an example, the QA system used to develop the Simcyp platform is described in Jamei et al. [6]

Installation Qualification: When a user receives a software package and installs it onto their computer, it may have different settings from the machine used to develop the software. Therefore, it is necessary to ensure the correct installation of the platform and confirm that results can be robustly reproduced on the users' computers. To this end, specific test simulations should be carried out to verify that the platform uses the same input file and generates similar output files as provided by the platform producer. These procedures ensure that the results are reproducible and that no unintended issues are introduced while installing the platform. For example, a specific set of workspaces and the relevant Excel output files are provided with each release of the Simcyp Simulator to test and qualify the platform installation. To test the robustness of installation of the Simcyp PBPK platform, a simulation was conducted by an individual in one location and the design of the simulation was saved as a workspace. The workspace was subsequently sent to five additional individuals each in different companies and different geographical locations. These additional individuals ran the workspace and the results from all six simulations were compared. The results from all these simulations were identical in terms of the summary parameters such as CL, CL_{po}, C_{max}, T_{max}, and AUC. In all locations, the number of differential equations in the PBPK model was the same and when examined closely the results for numerical values were identical to at least 13 decimal places. This demonstrates that if appropriately installed along with proper installation qualification documentation, a PBPK platform should give reproducible results for the same simulation regardless of the location and user.

7.3.2 System Parameters

A PBPK model is a mathematical model consisting of tissue and organ compartments, which are connected by circulating arterial and venous blood systems. Each compartment is defined by tissue-specific volume and blood flow rate. These compartments generally include, but are not restricted to, adipose tissue, bone, brain, gut, heart, kidney, liver, lung, muscle, pancreas, skin, and spleen. Basic PBPK models assume perfusion rate-limited distribution in all tissue compartments, whereas permeability rate-limited distribution with active transport processes can be incorporated for specific organs, depending on the software. In addition, the gut compartment, which typically consists of the lumen and enterocytes for unabsorbed and absorbed drugs, respectively, is more complex to incorporate drug absorption processes.

The gut compartment is generally divided further into sub-compartments serially arranged corresponding to the different regions of the gastrointestinal tract such as duodenum, jejunum, and ileum. Each sub-compartment requires specific system parameters such as tissue volume, surface area, fluid dynamics, pH, gastric emptying time, and intestinal transit time. Furthermore, some tissue/organ compartments, mainly the gut, liver, and kidney, require physiological system parameters of drug-metabolizing enzymes/transporters, such as their abundances or activities including genotypes and synthesis/degradation rates. There are also other important system parameters such as plasma protein and hematocrit concentrations, amounts of microsomal protein/hepatocytes per liver, and glomerular filtration rate of the kidney.

These system parameters depend on specific population demographics such as age, gender, genotype, and disease state and may exhibit different variability and covariance in each population. Therefore, the system parameters should be defined in specific virtual populations of interest such as healthy adult subjects of certain ethnicities, patients with impairment of organ function (e.g., liver and kidney), pediatric and geriatric patients, and cancer patients.

7.3.3 Drug Parameters

Information pertaining to specific compounds (built-in compound files in PBPK platforms) should be accompanied by documentation detailing the intended use and performance verification for the compound files. In general, the verification process of a compound file whether provided as part of the PBPK platform or newly developed is the same and is discussed in more detail in the "Drug model verification" section of this chapter. Information on the source of the parameters used in the model should be provided (i.e., whether they are derived solely from in vitro data or from clinical studies). The mechanistic components included in a compound file will vary from compound to compound and are dependent also on the intended use of the compound file. For example, if a compound file is developed for an inhibitor of a CYP isozyme that is not involved in its own metabolism and is primarily cleared by metabolism, then it may be sufficient to have a model that accurately describes the concentration of the compound at the site of inhibition with appropriate information on its potency (K_i) as an inhibitor of the CYP isozyme in question. In contrast, when developing a compound file for a substrate of a particular CYP isozyme it is necessary to ensure that in addition to describing the plasma concentration vs. time profile of the compound accurately, the fraction of the systemic clearance occurring through the isozyme in question is also accurately described. Parameters obtained by estimation techniques should be clearly identified and the data used in the fitting procedure described. Although the ideal scenario is to have separate sets of data for model building and model verification, in many cases, there is insufficient data to achieve this. When this arises, this limitation of the model should be acknowledged. It is also helpful to list mechanisms not considered in the model. For instance, if a compound file is developed to enable the file to be used as a CYP 3A4 inhibitor and the compound is also known to inhibit other transporters or enzymes, but these are not considered in the model, this should be stated.

If the compound file is developed as a potential DDI victim, it is useful to show performance verification in both the uninhibited and inhibited states. Likewise, for a perpetrator of DDI, it is useful to show the performance of the compound model after single and multiple dosing, as well as showing the ability of the compound model to recover published or available drug interactions.

7.4 MODEL VERIFICATION

Development and Verification of Drug Models: PBPK model development is an iterative process that may involve multiple cycles of "predict, learn, confirm." Usually, a base model is first developed using experimentally determined or in silico predicted physicochemical and in vitro drug absorption, distribution, metabolism, and excretion (ADME) parameters. The predictions from the base model are then compared with the observed clinical PK data (e.g., PK from single ascending dose (SAD) or multiple ascending dose (MAD) studies) where a selection of model parameters may be adjusted to improve the drug model predictive performance based on sound physiological and scientific evidence. The predictive performance of the refined model will then be confirmed by comparing the prediction with the additional clinical PK data such as results from a DDI study that were not used in previous steps. Since the complexity of the model increases as additional mechanisms are identified from new in vitro or clinical data, at any given stage during the drug model development process, a compound model can be considered verified for a particular use or application if the predictive performance for that particular use or application is assessed to be satisfactory based on commonly accepted criteria (see below for criteria). For example, a drug may initially have been only identified as an inhibitor of CYP3A, but later found to be an inhibitor of a drug transporter as well. If the compound PBPK model is able to satisfactorily demonstrate its predictive performance of a DDI with a sensitive CYP3A substrate, the model is considered verified for its predictive performance for a DDI through CYP3A inhibition, although its predictive performance may have not yet been verified for a drug transporter inhibition. An exception would be if multiple mechanisms affect the same enzyme or transporter, or enzyme–transporter interplay. For example, if a drug inhibits and induces CYP3A4, the model needs to be verified for both mechanisms prior to declaring that the model is verified for CYP3A-related applications.

It is important to distinguish the studies used for initial model development and refinement (the training dataset), from the dataset from studies used for model verification. The design of a clinical study and the use of data to support model verification should be based on the purpose of the application. If a substrate PBPK model is to be applied for DDI predictions with moderate and/or weak inhibitors, it is preferable to evaluate the predictive performance against the observed DDI with a strong inhibitor of the same enzyme. For both model refinement and verification, C_{max}, T_{max}, CL_{po} (and CL and V if intravenous PK data are available), and AUC are some key parameters that may be used for comparison between predicted and observed values. Visual inspection of overlays of predicted and observed PK profiles is also performed. When evaluating the accuracy and acceptability of predictions, a commonly applied criterion is for values to be within twofold of the observed values. However, results from one controlled clinical study may not be representative of the larger population, especially for drugs that exhibit high variability in PK or if the sample size was small in such studies. As a result, the twofold criterion may be unreasonable for such drugs or studies. Instead, Abduljalil et al. [7] proposed to evaluate the success of model predictions considering the study sample size and the observed variance of the parameter of interest. Separately, the predictive performance of DDI simulations is usually evaluated by comparing the geometric mean ratios of C_{max} and AUC in the presence or absence of an interaction, and their respective 90% CI. Guest et al. [30] proposed that the predictive performance for DDI be based on the observed AUC ratios, instead of the twofold rule, which tends to introduce bias at lower interaction levels. We encourage PBPK modelers to consider incorporating the above approaches when evaluating the accuracy of model predictions. However, depending on the intended use, therapeutic area, safety, and efficacy factors, the acceptable performance may be adjusted accordingly.

7.5 INTERNAL AND EXTERNAL VERIFICATION

As part of the PBPK model development best practices, the predictive performance of compound models is evaluated by assessing the model's ability to recover clinically observed data. The observed data may also be used to refine and/or improve the model performance. In such cases, the model is fit to the data to estimate a few of the model parameters to improve the model's predictive performance [8]. There may be combinations of parameter values in a PBPK model that equally well fit or describe the observed data, potentially introducing identifiability issues. The problem may be reduced or avoided through rational selection of parameters to be fitted based on in-depth knowledge of the compounds' physicochemical properties and elimination pathways, as well as the intended use of the model. Generally, sensitivity analysis is recommended to be undertaken prior to selecting the model parameters for fitting, as this helps to decide which parameters should, or can, be fitted.

7.6 UNCERTAINTY AND VARIABILITY

Uncertainty in a PBPK model is introduced by two main sources: (i) the underlying biology or mechanisms, and (ii) drug-related parameters. As discussed elsewhere in this chapter, the model assumptions and their potential impact on the predictions should be justified and explained based on available scientific evidence.

Additionally, there can be significant variation and thus uncertainty in the experimentally determined values of drug parameters. Further, some parameter values may be derived entirely from in silico predictions or parameter estimations from observed data and should be evaluated using sensitivity analysis. However, the parameters and their ranges should be based on what is known about the mechanism and should not be chosen arbitrarily. The scientific rationale should be made clear.

Variability in drug exposure could lead to variability in patients' response (safety and efficacy), particularly for drugs that exhibit an exposure-response relationship. PBPK models can consider identifying physiological and molecular ADME factors that lead to between subject variability (BSV) and within subject variability (WSV) in drug exposure, to ultimately inform dosing scenarios. A useful example of demonstrating the value of PBPK modeling to identify baseline physiological factors that influence BSV is the case of dabrafenib trough exposure [9]. The impact of population characteristics on dabrafenib exposure was simulated using virtual populations, where covariates such as gender, age, body composition, ethnicity, and diseases were accounted for. The model was then used to assess potential associations between physiological and molecular characteristics and dabrafenib exposure, using univariate logistic regression analysis. Subsequently, a baseline multivariate regression model was employed for the baseline characteristics that were significant in the univariate analysis. The PBPK model results suggested that a combined consideration of baseline weight, BMI, and CYP2C8, CYP3A4, and P-gp liver abundance, are possible physiological and molecule characteristics that drive BSV in dabrafenib exposure.

To assess the impact of physiological parameters that may influence WSV, an example of posaconazole bioequivalence was described by Bego et al. [10] The PBPK framework was used to estimate the plausible WSV in GI physiology parameters that would describe more realistically the observed variation in the PK parameters. The model was then subjected to local and global sensitivity analyses to identify the GI parameters that may impact the systemic exposure, and virtual twins were simulated by varying the coefficient of variation of a given physiological parameter (i.e., luminal pH, or bile salt levels, etc.) based on known ranges. This in turn was used for virtual bioequivalence trial simulations and compared with observed WSV from repeated trials to mimics scenario where the probability of bioequivalence failure between two formulations could be evaluated using the PBPK model.

7.7 IDENTIFIABILITY ISSUES IN PBPK

A PBPK model consists of many parameters, some of which may have unknown values either due to technical difficulties in measurement techniques or because they may have never been measured before. The unknown parameters are usually estimated through fitting of the model to the observed data from well-defined study sets using a known specific dosing regimen [8,11]. A controlled input specifies data with observations from well-defined study sets, e.g., at a known specific dose in a specific population. However, estimation of model parameters through this approach can have limitations when the number of unknown parameters is large relative to the information contained in the available data. Various sets of parameter values can result in an equally good model fit to the data in a way that individual parameters cannot be uniquely identified. In this case, the model loses mechanistic meaning and applicability and is said to be "unidentifiable." As a result, extrapolation to populations outside the studied conditions is unjustified or may lead to false conclusions [8,11]. Various mathematical identifiability analysis approaches have been previously described in the literature [12,13]. Proposed approaches to deal with identifiability issues when fitting a PBPK model include measuring some of the unknown physiological parameter values, if possible (e.g., collecting additional information on absolute bioavailability using intravenous drug administration in order to distinguish between gut extraction and poor solubility), reduction in the number of parameters (i.e., by grouping several unidentifiable parameters into a single identifiable parameter), redefining parameters or reparameterization, or generating data that could be used in calibration with a different in vivo dataset [11,12,14,15]. Several statistical approaches can also be used to declare a PBPK model as identifiable [16]. Overall, structural identifiability is not an issue for PBPK models when the model structure and parameter values are justified mechanistically, and the PK properties are verified against observed data [17].

Another aspect of increasing confidence in mechanistic models, such as PBPK models, is to reduce the number of model parameters, especially when fitting the model to high-level clinical data, with the objective of generating a PBPK model that is numerically more stable [18]. This is generally referred to as PBPK model reduction or parameter lumping process, where the reduced or simplified PBPK model could be viewed as more 'identifiable' and stable relative to the original whole body PBPK model. It is important to note that reduction or lumping of PBPK model parameters, especially those of the system (i.e., blood flows, organ compartments, and clearance pathways) still needs to consider physiological plausibility and avoid pure mathematical fitting that may lead to non-physiological parameter values.

7.8 SENSITIVITY ANALYSIS

During the development of a specific compound or population model, there can be uncertainty in the true value of some of the parameters. This may be due, for example, to the absence of a specific parameter or unreliability of the in vitro data. In these cases, it is useful to assess the impact of uncertainty in those specific parameters or specific modeling assumptions may have on the simulation outcome. This is commonly done through a sensitivity analysis where the selected parameters are changed within a given reasonable range and a selected set of endpoints are investigated. Identifying whether an input parameter has a significant impact on the outcome of a simulation is highly valuable, as it assists with making decisions on which in vitro assays, or clinical study should be performed at what stage of drug development and how much resource should be invested in obtaining a particular parameter for a given compound [19,20].

In addition to verification with observed data, sensitivity analysis of drug parameters that have high impact on prediction results and/or have high uncertainty is another important step in attaining confidence in the drug model.

A global sensitivity analysis for every parameter that can influence the simulation outcome is unlikely to be informative since many parameters may impact the outcome within these complex models. For instance, changing tissue blood flow and organ sizes will change the PK profile of a drug, but it is not clear how such an analysis would be informative within the same intended population without scientific justification.

Sensitivity analysis is important and appropriate, however, only when there are uncertain parameters in the model but not on all parameters of the model. For example, if a drug K_i value was measured in vitro and the assay had a known error associated with it, a sensitivity analysis would be warranted to cover a range of values that would span the uncertainty space. In the late stages of drug development, much of a PBPK model will be based on data with higher quality and certainty. At such stages, the parameters which are uncertain may be few, and the level of uncertainty in the parameters may be minimal which allows for constraining of the sensitivity analysis space. In addition, a PBPK model may be sensitive to a certain physiological parameter such as hepatic blood flow, which is known with high certainty in the general healthy population. In this case, a sensitivity analysis exercise on this parameter is not warranted nor justified. Ultimately, deriving plausible drug or system model parameters using the PBPK model could be achieved by estimating the in vitro parameters based on clinical PK or DDI data or by estimating scaling factors such as transporter in vitro-to-in vivo extrapolation scaling factors, respectively [20,21].

7.9 CONCLUSION

The technical and strategic aspects for ensuring a successful PBPK modeling package for regulatory approval during drug development can be simplified in a framework that captures PBPK platform qualification, drug model verification, model assumptions and uncertainty, data variability, parameter identifiability solutions, and sensitivity analyses. Addressing each of these components as described in this chapter would enable a harmonized approach of best practice for conducting and applying PBPK modeling in drug development. By dissecting various components of a PBPK analysis package, the sponsor would be able to successfully address regulatory requirements based on the intended use.

REFERENCES

1. Zhao, P., Rowland, M. & Huang, S.M. Best practice in the use of physiologically based pharmacokinetic modeling and simulation to address clinical pharmacology regulatory questions. *Clin. Pharmacol. Ther.* 92(1), 17–20 (2012).

2. U.S. Food and Drug Administration. (2018). Guidance for Industry, Physiologically Based Pharmacokinetic Analyses- Format and Content, Guidance for Industry. https://www.fda.gov/media/101469/download.

3. European Medicines Agency. (2019). Guideline on the reporting of physiologically based pharmacokinetic (PBPK) modelling and simulation. https://www.ema.europa.eu/en/documents/scientific-guideline/guideline-reporting-physiologically-based-pharmacokinetic-pbpk-modelling-simulation_en.pdf.

4. Shebley, M., Sandhu, P. & Emami Riedmaier, A. et al. Physiologically based pharmacokinetic model qualification and reporting procedures for regulatory submissions: a consortium perspective. *Clin. Pharmacol. Ther.* 104(1), 88–110 (2018). doi: 10.1002/cpt.1013.

5. Frechen, S., Solodenko, J., Wendl, T., Dallmann, A., Ince, I., Lehr, T., Lippert, J. & Burghaus, R. A generic framework for the physiologically-based pharmacokinetic platform qualification of PK-Sim and its application to predicting cytochrome P450 3A4-mediated drug-drug interactions. *CPT Pharmacometrics Syst Pharmacol.* 10(6), 633–644 (2021). doi: 10.1002/psp4.12636.

6. Jamei, M. et al. The Simcyp population based simulator: architecture, implementation, and quality assurance. *In Silico Pharmacol.* 1, 9 (2013).

7. Abduljalil, K., Cain, T., Humphries, H. & Rostami-Hodjegan, A. Deciding on success criteria for predictability of pharmacokinetic parameters from in vitro studies: an analysis based on in vivo observations. *Drug Metab. Dispos.* 42, 1478–1484 (2014).

8. Tsamandouras, N., Rostami-Hodjegan, A. & Aarons, L. Combining the 'bottom up' and 'top down' approaches in pharmacokinetic modelling: fitting PBPK models to observed clinical data. *Br. J. Clin. Pharmacol.* 79, 48–55 (2015).

9. Rowland, A., van Dyk, M., Hopkins, A.M., Mounzer, R., Polasek, T.M., Rostami-Hodjegan, A. & Sorich, M.J.; Physiologically based pharmacokinetic modeling to identify physiological and molecular characteristics driving variability in drug exposure. *Clin. Pharmacol. Ther.* 104(6), 1219–1228 (2018). doi: 10.1002/cpt.1076.

10. Bego, M., Patel, N., Cristofoletti, R. & Rostami-Hodjegan, A. Proof of concept in assignment of within-subject variability during virtual bioequivalence studies: propagation of intra-subject variation in gastrointestinal physiology using physiologically based pharmacokinetic modeling. *AAPS J.* 24(1), 21 (2022). doi: 10.1208/s12248-021-00672-z.

11. Slob, W., Janssen, P.H. & van den Hof, J.M. Structural identifiability of PBPK models: practical consequences for modeling strategies and study designs. *Crit. Rev. Toxicol.* 27, 261–272 (1997).

12. Yates, J.W. Structural identifiability of physiologically based pharmacokinetic models. *J. Pharmacokinet. Pharmacodyn.* 33, 421–439 (2006).

13. Godfrey, K.R., Jones, R.P. & Brown, R.F. Identifiable pharmacokinetic models: the role of extra inputs and measurements. *J. Pharmacokinet. Biopharm.* 8, 633–648 (1980).

14. Cheung, S.Y., Majid, O., Yates, J.W. & Aarons, L. Structural identifiability analysis and reparameterisation (parameter reduction) of a cardiovascular feedback model. *Eur. J. Pharm. Sci.* 46, 259–271 (2012).

15. Cheung, S.Y., Yates, J.W. & Aarons, L. The design and analysis of parallel experiments to produce structurally identifiable models. *J. Pharmacokinet. Pharmacodyn.* 40, 93–100 (2013).

16. Garcia, R.I., Ibrahim, J.G., Wambaugh, J.F., Kenyon, E.M. & Setzer, R.W. Identifiability of PBPK models with applications to dimethylarsinic acid exposure. *J. Pharmacokinet. Pharmacodyn.* 42, 591–609 (2015).

17. Agoram, B. Evaluating systems pharmacology models is different from evaluating standard pharmacokinetic-pharmacodynamic models. *CPT Pharmacometrics Syst. Pharmacol.* 3, e101 (2014).

18. Wendling, T., Tsamandouras, N., Dumitras, S., Pigeolet, E., Ogungbenro, K., Aarons, L., Reduction of a whole-body physiologically based pharmacokinetic model to stabilise the bayesian analysis of clinical data. *AAPS J.* 18(1), 196–209 (2016). doi: 10.1208/s12248-015-9840-7.

19. Arya, V., Zhao, P., Reynolds, K.S., Mishra, P. & Younis, I.R. Utilizing PBPK modeling to evaluate the potential of a significant drug-drug interaction between clopidogrel and dasabuvir: a scientific perspective. *Clin. Pharmacol. Ther.* (2017). doi: 10.1002/cpt.1699.

20. Shebley, M., Fu, W., Badri, P., Bow, D. & Fischer, V. Physiologically based pharmacokinetic modeling suggests limited drug-drug interaction between clopidogrel and dasabuvir. *Clin. Pharmacol. Ther.* (2017). doi: 10.1002/cpt.1689.

21. Harwood, M.D., Achour, B., Neuhoff, S., Russell, M.R., Carlson, G., Warhurst, G. & Rostami-Hodjegan, A. In vitro-In vivo extrapolation scaling factors for intestinal P-glycoprotein and breast cancer resistance protein: part II. The impact of cross-laboratory variations of intestinal transporter relative expression factors on predicted drug disposition. *Drug Metab. Dispos.* 44(3), 476–80 (2016). doi: 10.1124/dmd.115.067777.

8 Applying PBPK Modelling to Predict Drug–Drug Interactions

Thomas Wendl

8.1 INTRODUCTION

8.1.1 Background

Drug–drug interactions (DDIs) are distinguished into (i) pharmacokinetic interactions in which one drug alters the drug concentration-time profile of another drug by modulating enzymes, transporters or binding partners involved in the absorption, distribution, metabolism, or elimination (ADME) of the victim drug, (ii) pharmacodynamic interactions in which the co-administered drug modulates the drug effect and (iii) physicochemical interactions in which one drug or excipient may increase or decrease the solubility of the other. This is of interest because it can alter the exposure of and/or response to a drug and may require dose adaption or warnings for involved drugs as part of their label guided use. At an earlier stage during drug development, it may also indicate potential restrictions to be accepted for further drug development or not to be accepted that may then lead to further substance optimization and/or termination of drug development. The PBPK DDI submissions to regulatory authorities as well as the regulatory DDI guidance documents related to PBPK modelling almost exclusively deal with pharmacokinetic drug interactions through CYP enzymes and transporters, they currently rarely address therapeutic proteins, gastric pH change-dependent, protein displacement-mediated, and phase 2 enzyme-mediated or pharmacodynamic DDIs [1–5]. Pharmacodynamic interactions, apart from pharmacodynamic effects related to pharmacokinetics, are usually very diverse and usually do not share common underlying mechanisms, hence, no general modelling principles as in the case of pharmacokinetic interactions have evolved. Therefore, this chapter will focus on pharmacokinetic interactions through CYP enzymes and transporters in humans.

Over the last two decades, PBPK modelling has become an integral part of drug discovery and development while concepts of ensuring the quality of specialized PBPK software platforms and credibility of PBPK model-based derived conclusion have evolved [6]. Among PBPK modelling applications, the modelling of DDIs including the prediction of DDIs for drug combinations, which have not been tested in clinical studies, has taken a leading role [7]. Recent publications underline that the vast majority of PBPK submissions to regulatory health authorities are related to DDIs, in particular, DDIs involving Cytochrome P450 (CYP) enzymes [8–10].

Important reasons for this development go back to pioneer cases of PBPK DDI modelling approaches like the ibrutinib example (see also the Case example in Section 8.3.7), which were accepted by regulatory authorities in lieu of dedicated clinical DDI trials. In addition, examples like this as well as systematic elaborations on this topic [11,12] also led to the inclusion of specific recommendations in regulatory guidance documents for the use of PBPK models for the conduct of clinical and in-vitro DDI studies. Specifically, the guidance documents of the US Food and Drug Administration (FDA) [2,3] and the European Medicines Agency (EMA) [4,5] now explicitly promote the use of PBPK models in place of clinical DDI studies. Additionally, the success of DDI predictions also lies in the ability to be able to make use of *in-vitro* data. Particularly, interaction parameters for CYP enzymes such as the inhibition constant K_i can be estimated with low to moderate uncertainty leading to moderate to high confidence in PBPK DDI predictions [13].

Moreover, many established PBPK platforms such as GastroPlus® (Simulations Plus, Inc., www.simulations-plus.com), PK-Sim® (Open Systems Pharmacology, www.open-systems-pharmacology.org) or Simcyp™ (Certara, www.certara.com) already come with compound libraries that include verified, ready-to-use interaction partner substance models to facilitate the simulation of DDIs.

8.1.2 Substrates, Inhibitors and Inducers

Pharmacokinetic DDIs involve at least two substances on the one hand, which interact through an enzyme or transporter on the other hand. The substances can be distinguished in a victim drug, in the following called **substrate**, whose exposure may be altered by another drug, and a perpetrator drug that affects the pharmacokinetics of the substrate, in the following simply called **perpetrator**. Perpetrators can be classified as **inhibitors** if they decrease the activity and/or abundance of unbound enzyme or transporter and are classified as **inducers** if they increase it.

The most prominent example of pharmacokinetic interactions are enzymatic DDIs where the activity and/or abundance of the enzyme, and, consequently, the metabolic clearance through this enzyme is altered.

DOI: 10.1201/9781003031802-8

Inhibitors and inducers are classified according to their potential to increase or decrease the area under the substrate plasma concentration-time curve (AUC, i.e., inversely proportional to the clearance of the drug) of sensitive probe substrates *in-vivo* [2]. Such sensitive probe substrates are characterized by a high fraction metabolized (f_m) through this enzyme, and, thus, the AUC is sensitive to alterations of enzyme activity/abundance. For perpetrator classification, the AUC ratio (AUCR) is calculated as

$$AUCR = \frac{AUCi}{AUC}$$

where AUCi and AUC are the AUCs in presence or absence of the inhibitor or inducer, respectively.

Table 8.1 shows the general classification of inhibitors and inducers based on the AUC changes of sensitive substrates proposed by the FDA as of 2022 [2].

Table 8.1: Classification of Inhibitors and Inducers Based on AUC Changes of a Sensitive Substrate

	Strong	Moderate	Weak
Inhibitors	≥ 5-fold increase in AUC	≥ 2- to < 5-fold increase in AUC	≥ 1.25- to < 2-fold increase in AUC
Inducers	≥ 80 % decrease in AUC	≥ 50 to < 80 % decrease in AUC	≥ 20 to < 50 % decrease in AUC

Note: FDA – Clinical Drug Interaction Studies [2].

CYP enzymes represent the most important group of enzymes in the metabolization of drugs, hence, PBPK modelling of CYP interactions plays a major role in DDI modelling [9]. To facilitate the choice of appropriate interaction partner substances for the drug of interest, regulatory guidance documents recommend the use of specific index substrates and index perpetrators in clinical DDI studies. Such **index substrates** exhibit a well-characterized exposure increase due to inhibition or decrease due to induction of a specific enzyme, whereas **index perpetrators** generate a defined degree of inhibition or induction of a given enzyme or transporter [2]. Furthermore, index drugs proposed by the FDA are selected in view of their specificity, safety profiles, and adequate number of reported clinical DDI studies with different in vivo inhibitors. A list of CYP3A4 index substrates, inhibitors and inducers proposed by the FDA [14] is given in Table 8.2.

Table 8.2: Examples of Clinical Index Substrates, Inhibitors and Inducers for P450-Mediated Metabolisms (For Use in Index Clinical DDI Studies)

	Sensitive Index Substrates	Strong Index Inhibitors	Moderate Index Inhibitors	Strong Inducers	Moderate Inducers
CYP1A2	Caffeine, Tizanidine	Fluvoxamine[d]			
CYP2B6					Rifampin[j]
CYP2C8	Repaglinide[a]	Clopidogrel[e], Gemfibrozil[f]			Rifampin[j]
CYP2C9	Tolbutamide[b], S-warfarin[b]		Fluconazole[g]		Rifampin[j]
CYP2C19	Lansoprazole[b,c], Omeprazole	Fluvoxamine[d]		Rifampin[j]	
CYP2D6	Desipramine, Dextromethorphan, Nebivolol	Fluoxetine[h], Paroxetine	Mirabegron		
CYP3A	Midazolam, Triazolam	Clarithromycin[i], Itraconazole[i]	Erythromycin, Fluconazole[g], Verapamil[i]	Phenytoin[k], Rifampin[j]	

Note: FDA: Drug Development and Drug Interactions | Table of Substrates, Inhibitors and Inducers [14].
[a] Also OATP1B1 substrate.
[b] Moderate sensitive substrates.
[c] S-lansoprazole is a sensitive substrate in CYP2C19 extensive metabolizer subjects
[d] Strong inhibitor of CYP1A2 and CYP2C19, and moderate inhibitor of CYP2D6 and CYP3A.
[e] Strong inhibitor of CYP2C8, weak inhibitor of CYP2B6, and inhibitor of OATP1B1. The glucoronide metabolite is also an inhibitor for CYP2C8 and OATP1B1.
[f] Strong inhibitor of CYP2C8 and inhibitor of OATP1B1 and OAT3. The glucoronide metabolite is also an inhibitor for CYP2C8 and OATP1B1.
[g] Strong inhibitor of CYP2C19 and moderate inhibitor of CYP2C9 and CYP3A.
[h] Strong inhibitors of CYP2C19 and CYP2D6.
[i] Inhibitor of P-gp (defined as those increasing area under the curve (AUC) of digoxin to ≥1.25-fold).
[j] Strong inducer of CYP1A2, CYP2C19, CYP3A, and moderate inducer of CYP2B6, CYP2C8, CYP2C9.
[k] Strong inducer of CYP3A and moderate inducer of CYP1A2, CYP2C19.

Over the years, PBPK modelling of CYP-mediated DDIs has reached a considerable regulatory acceptance, however, transporter-mediated DDIs are still a less explored application field of PBPK modelling [15,16]. Prominent examples of transporters that play a critical role in the disposition of many drugs are P-glycoprotein (P-gp), breast cancer resistance protein (BCRP), organic anion transporting polypeptide (OATP)1B1 and OATP1B3 are, but the general level of confidence in PBPK models involving transporters is still lower than for enzyme-mediated drug interactions due to limitations in *in-vitro* assays and limited knowledge and experience (also see Section 8.4 'Variability and Uncertainty').

Similar to the list of CYP3A4 index drugs for DDI, an example list of clinical transporters substrates, inhibitors and inducers is provided by the FDA [14], but most of the listed drugs are not classified as index drugs for DDI studies as they lack specificity for one transporter and often, more specific alternatives are not known to date [2]. Furthermore, most transporter-mediated DDIs usually exhibit lower AUCRs than the ones reported for CYP-mediated DDIs.

8.2 INTERACTION MECHANISMS AND MODEL ASSUMPTIONS

8.2.1 Historic Perspective: Evolution of Mathematical DDI Prediction Models

Regulatory guidance documents on drug interaction studies usually refer to three different modelling approaches of different complexity to evaluate the DDI potential of a drug [3,5], i.e. the basic model approach, the mechanistic static model approach and mechanistic dynamic modelling approaches such as PBPK modelling. The following section provides a brief overview about the evolution of these mathematical prediction models to determine the magnitude of DDIs using the example of competitive inhibition (see Section 8.2.3). All these approaches are particularly developed for CYP enzymes.

The **basic model** is the simplest of the approaches and uses the ratio $[I]/K_i$ of a single *in-vivo* inhibitor concentration $[I]$ and the inhibitor potency, represented by the inhibition constant K_i for reversible inhibitors [17–20]. It exclusively considers liver metabolism and does not regard the renal elimination. The fold change in exposure of the substrate in the presence of an inhibitor (the FDA refers to this ratio as R_1 [3]) can be described as

$$R_1 = \frac{AUCi}{AUC} = 1 + \frac{[I]}{K_i}$$

where AUC is the area under the curve in the presence (AUCi) or absence (AUC) of the inhibitor and $[I]$ = maximal inhibitor concentration

A few assumptions are related to this approach such as the steady state of the inhibitor, competitive or non-competitive type of inhibition, exclusive clearance of the substrate by a single metabolic enzyme, which is inhibited by the inhibitor, well-stirred conditions in the liver compartment [21] and negligible metabolism in the gut wall or other organs. To ensure a conservative approach, inhibitor concentrations $[I]$ are assumed to be the maximal concentrations I_{max} observed *in-vivo*.

The **mechanistic static model** is an extension of the basic model and also uses the ratio $[I]/K_i$ as well as similar assumptions, but additionally considers other clearance pathways apart from the inhibited pathway by employing the f_m for the metabolic enzyme. In general, this approach is less conservative than the basic model approach and the predicted substrate exposure increase may turn out smaller. However, this approach also applies static inhibitor concentrations to calculate a point estimate of the exposure increase of the substrate [17,22]. For reversible inhibition and assuming metabolization exclusively in the liver through a single enzyme, the mechanistic static model approach is given by the following Equation (8.3):

$$AUCR = \frac{AUCi}{AUC} = \frac{1}{\dfrac{f_m}{1 + \dfrac{[I]}{K_i}} + (1 - f_m)},$$

and

$$[I] = f_{u,p} * \left(C_{max} + \frac{\left(F_a \times F_g \times k_a \times \text{Dose} \right)}{Q_h / R_B} \right),$$

where

F_a is the fraction absorbed after oral administration,

F_g is the fraction escaping gut wall metabolism,

k_a is the first order absorption rate constant in vivo,

Q_h is the hepatic blood flow,

R_B is the blood-to-plasma concentration ratio,

$f_{u,p}$ is the unbound fraction in the plasma,

$C_{\max}$ is the maximum total inhibitor concentration in the plasma at steady state.

This approach can be extended to include gut wall metabolism. Both approaches, the basic and the mechanistic static approach, can be also adjusted to irreversible inhibition and induction, further information is provided e.g. in the FDA guidance for in-vitro drug interaction studies [3].

Dynamic modelling approaches like **PBPK modelling** use as well a $1 + \dfrac{[I]}{K_i}$ term for the description of reversible interactions, but in contrast to the previously described 'static' approaches, the PBPK models employ the temporal profile of the perpetrator and the substrate drug, hence, steady-state conditions of the inhibitor are not required for the calculation of the interaction. This even allows to calculate the magnitude of interaction over time as well as the calculation of the ratio of peak concentrations ($C_{\max}$R) in contrast to static models, which only enable the calculation of the integral exposure change (AUCR). In particular, this feature allows to inform the design of clinical studies, e.g., by identifying the optimal lag time between perpetrator and substrate administration, or informative sampling time-points for the substrate and perpetrator drugs.

8.2.2 Overview of Interaction Mechanisms and General Assumptions

In general, PBPK modelling of DDIs is conducted through coupling two PBPK models by insertion of an interaction term that operates on the substrate's clearance or disposition and contains both, dynamic substrate and perpetrator concentrations, and, if applicable, a change of enzyme or transporter abundance/activity over time.

Typically, the following interaction mechanisms can be distinguished:

1. Inhibition

    a. Reversible inhibition (see Section 8.2.3):

        i. Competitive inhibition

        ii. Uncompetitive inhibition

        iii. Mixed inhibition (incl. non-competitive inhibition as special case of the mixed inhibition)

    b. Irreversible inhibition, i.e., mechanism-based inactivation (see Section 8.2.4)

2. Induction and suppression (see Section 8.2.5)

    The underlying mathematical equations which are commonly used to describe these mechanisms in the context of PBPK DDI modelling are further detailed in the following sections.

    A basic assumption for these equations is that the clearance and disposition processes follow Michaelis–Menten kinetics of the form:

$$v = \frac{V_{\max} * [S]}{K_m + [S]},$$

where

v represents the reaction rate

$V_{\max}$ represents the maximum reaction rate

$[S]$ represents the substrate concentration

K_m represents the substrate concentration at half of $V_{\max}$

Furthermore, the presence of a single active site for the interaction of the substrate with the enzyme/transporter is assumed [23].

In a strict sense, perpetrator and substrate are influencing each other, but in a lot of cases, the influence of the substrate on the pharmacokinetics of the perpetrator is negligible, and, hence, is frequently not represented in the equations. This is the case for K_m values of the substrate that are much higher than the K_i values of the inhibitor. For lower K_m values in the range of the K_i values of the inhibitor, it might be appropriate to include mutual inhibition in the equations. In the following sections, the influence of the substrate on the pharmacokinetics of the perpetrator is assumed to be negligible, and, hence, is not regarded in the equations.

8.2.3 Reversible Inhibition

In the case of reversible inhibition, the inhibitor reversibly binds to the enzyme. In general, reversible inhibition can be distinguished into four types of mechanisms: competitive, uncompetitive and mixed inhibition as well as the non-competitive inhibition as a special case of mixed inhibition (see e.g. [24]).

The most prominent example of reversible inhibition is the **competitive inhibition** where the inhibitor and the substrate compete for the same binding site of the enzyme, represented in the following as

E=Enzyme, S=Substrate, ES=Enzyme-Substrate complex, I=Inhibitor, EI=Enzyme-Inhibitor complex, P=Product:

$$E + S \leftrightarrow ES \rightarrow E + P$$

and

$$E + I \leftrightarrow EI$$

The reaction rate can be described as

$$v = \frac{V_{\max} * [S]}{K_{m,\text{app}} + [S]}$$

in which the apparent K_m, i.e. $K_{m,\text{app}}$ is given by

$$K_{m,\text{app}} = K_m \left(1 + \frac{[I]}{K_i}\right)$$

where $[I]$ is the inhibitor concentration and K_i the dissociation constant between inhibitor and enzyme.

In particular, the K_i value is assumed to be independent of the substrate and exclusively a property of the competitive inhibitor with respect to a specific enzyme. Therefore, it can be applied to other substrates in combination with the same competitive inhibitor and enzyme. The formula above implies that the apparent K_m increases in comparison to the original K_m, $V_{\max}$ remains unaffected such that the reaction rate is slowed.

An example of competitive inhibition is the interaction of itraconazole, a strong CYP3A4 inhibitor with midazolam, a sensitive CYP3A4 substrate shown in Figure 8.1.

In the case of **uncompetitive inhibition**, the inhibitor binds to the enzyme-substrate complex meaning that the binding of the inhibitor requires prior binding of the substrate to the enzyme. This can be represented as

$$E + S \leftrightarrow ES \rightarrow E + P$$

and

$$ES + I \leftrightarrow ESI \quad \text{with } ESI = \text{Enzyme-Substrate-Inhibitor complex}$$

the reaction rate can be described as

$$v = \frac{V_{\max,\text{app}} * [S]}{K_{m,\text{app}} + [S]}$$

$$\text{with } V_{\max,\text{app}} = \frac{V_{\max}}{1 + [I]/K_i} \text{ and } K_{m,\text{app}} = \frac{K_m}{1 + [I]/K_i}$$

in which both, apparent K_m and apparent V_{max} decrease.

Mixed inhibition is a combination of competitive and uncompetitive inhibition in which the inhibitor binds to both enzyme and enzyme-substrate complex, as shown in the following:

$$E+S \leftrightarrow ES \rightarrow E+P \text{ and}$$

$$E+I \leftrightarrow EI \text{ with } K_{i,c} \text{ being the dissociation constant of enzyme and inhibitor (competitive)}$$

$$ES+I \leftrightarrow ESI \text{ with } K_{i,u} \text{ being the dissociation constant of the}$$
enzyme-substrate complex and the inhibitor (uncompetitive), and

$$EI+S \leftrightarrow ESI$$

The reaction rate can be described as

$$v = \frac{V_{max,app} * [S]}{K_{m,app} + [S]}$$

$$\text{with } V_{max,app} = \frac{V_{max}}{1+[I]/K_{i,u}}$$

$$\text{and } K_{m,app} = K_m \frac{1+[I]/K_{i,c}}{1+[I]/K_{i,u}}$$

The formulas reveal that the apparent V_{max} decreases and the apparent K_m changes. The inhibitor binding site is different from substrate binding site.

The **non-competitive inhibition** is a special case of the mixed inhibition, in which the inhibitor binds to the enzyme and the enzyme-substrate complex with same K_i, i.e., $K_{i,c}=K_{i,u}$

In this context, V_{max} decreases, and K_m is unaffected.

8.2.4 Irreversible Inhibition

This type of inhibition is called **mechanism-based inactivation (MBI)**, as the inhibitor (inactivator) irreversibly inactivates its target, i.e., the enzyme mediating the interaction, by covalent bonding and forming an irreversible complex. Thereby, it reduces the target's baseline level. Due to the irreversible nature of this inhibition, interaction may persist even when the inactivating drug is washed out. The duration of inhibition in that case is mainly determined by target turnover. This also means that the present magnitude of interaction is not only dependent on the actual drug concentrations but also depends on the elapsed time after administration. Therefore, this type of interaction is also called time-dependent inhibition (TDI). In contrast to reversible inhibition, MBI can also cause an auto-inactivation of an enzyme. E.g., a drug that is both, mechanism-based inactivator and substrate of the particular enzyme that it inactivates may auto-inactivate its own metabolization leading to time non-linear pharmacokinetics.

The return to baseline levels of the inactivated target requires endogenous de-novo synthesis.

In brief:

$$E+I \leftrightarrow EI \rightarrow EI' \rightarrow E_{inact}, \text{ where } E_{inact} \text{ is the inactivated enzyme and}$$

$$EI' \rightarrow E+P$$

The enzyme inactivation rate can be described as [25–27]

$$\frac{k_{inact} * [I]}{K_I + [I]} * [E]$$

where

k_{inact} is the inactivation rate constant and

K_I is the inhibition constant

$[E]$ is the enzyme concentration over time

For

$$v = \frac{V_{max,app} * [S]}{K_{m,app} + [S]},$$

the apparent V_{max} and K_m can be described as

$$V_{max,app} = k_{cat} * [E] \text{ and } K_{m,app} = K_m \left(1 + \frac{[I]}{K_i} \right)$$

MBIs are also competitive inhibitors which is reflected in the apparent K_m.

An example of MBI is the interaction of erythromycin, a moderate CYP3A4 inhibitor, with alfentanil, a sensitive CYP3A4 substrate, shown in Figure 8.1.

8.2.5 Induction and Suppression

Enzyme inducers cause an increased *de-novo* synthesis of the enzyme leading to a decrease of the area under the curve (AUC) of substrates of the enzyme. This upregulation primarily goes back on two molecular mechanisms depending on the involved enzyme. In the case of many CYP enzymes including CYP3A4, the pregnane X receptor (PXR) mediates this upregulation, in the case of e.g. CYP2B10 and CYP3A11, it is mediated by the constitutive androstane receptor (CAR) [28]. In contrast to inducers, suppressors lead to a decreased *de-novo* synthesis, and hence, may increase AUC.

Induction and suppression are modelled through a relative induction factor (RIF) on the endogenous production rate of the enzyme, which can be expressed as

$$RIF = \frac{E_{max} * [IND]}{EC_{50} + [IND]}$$

see e.g. [29,30]

where

E_{max} is the maximum induction ratio and

EC_{50} is the concentration at half maximum induction

[IND] is the unbound concentration of the inducer over time

If $E_{max} > 0$, RIF is positive and the production rate will increase resulting in an induction, for $-1 \le E_{max} < 0$, the production rate decreases resulting in a suppression of the enzyme and $E_{max} = 0$ yields no effect on the production rate.

The metabolic reaction velocity

$$v = \frac{V_{max,app} * [S]}{K_m + [S]}$$

The maximum reaction velocity can be expressed as

$$V_{max,app} = k_{cat} * [E],$$

with k_{cat} being the turnover number and [E] being the enzyme concentration over time.

Inducers can also be subject of auto-induction if they induce an enzyme or transporter, which is involved in the inducer's metabolization or disposition.

An example of induction is the interaction of rifampicin, a strong CYP3A4 inducer with midazolam, a sensitive CYP3A4 substrate shown in Figure 8.1.

8.2.6 Dynamic Enzyme Abundance

The abundance of an enzyme is the available amount of the enzyme. The enzyme turnover can be expressed as the synthesis rate (R_{syn}) minus the degradation rate defined by the degradation constant k_{deg} and the enzyme concentration over time [E]

$$\frac{d[E]}{dt} = R_{syn} - k_{deg} * [E]$$

$$= k_{deg} * E_0 - k_{deg} * [E],$$

E_0 is the baseline enzyme level.

In the case of a MBI with one Michaelis-Menten substrate, it yields

$$\frac{d[E]}{dt} = k_{deg} * E_0 - \left(k_{deg} + \frac{k_{inact} * [MBI]}{K_I + [MBI]} \right) * [E]$$

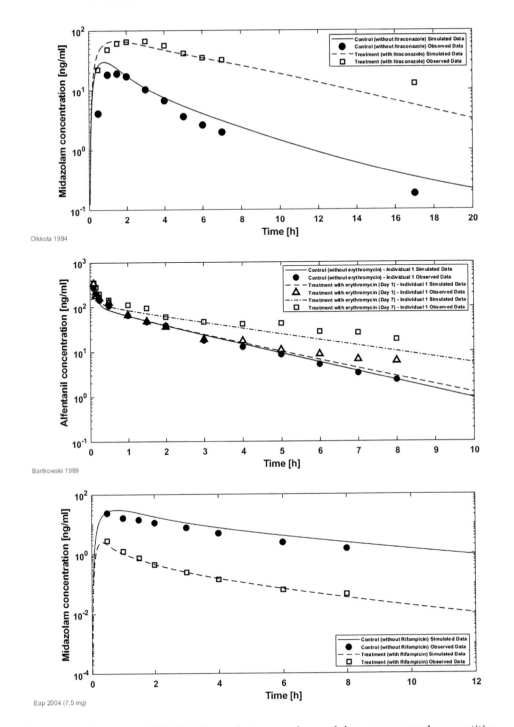

Figure 8.1 Examples of PBPK DDI simulations vs. observed data, upper panel: competitive inhibition, concentration-time profiles of orally administered midazolam alone (solid line) and under co-administration of the strong CYP3A4 inhibitor itraconazole (dashed line), observed data are taken from Olkkola et al. [31], middle panel: mechanism-based inactivation, concentration-time profiles of intravenously administered alfentanil alone (solid line), under co-administration of the moderate CYP3A4 inhibitor erythromycin on day 1 (dashed line) and on day 7 (dashed-dotted line), observed data are taken from Bartkowski et al. [32], lower panel: induction, concentration-time profiles of orally administered midazolam alone (solid line) and under co-administration of the strong CYP3A4 inducer rifampicin (dashed line), observed data are taken from Eap et al. [33].

with [MBI] being the unbound concentrations of the mechanism-based inactivator over time
In case of induction or suppression, this term extends to

$$\frac{d[E]}{dt} = k_{\text{deg}} * E_0 * (1 + \text{RIF}) - k_{\text{deg}} * [E]$$

$$= k_{\text{deg}} * E_0 * \left(1 + \frac{E_{\text{max}} * [\text{IND}]}{EC_{50} + [\text{IND}]}\right) - k_{\text{deg}} * [E]$$

with [IND] being the unbound concentrations of the inducer over time.

This results in a metabolic reaction velocity of the substrate expressed by the following equation:

$$v = \frac{k_{\text{cat}} * [E]}{K_m * \left(1 + \dfrac{[\text{MBI}]}{K_i}\right) + [S]} * [S]$$

The formulas for the different mechanisms can also be combined. This is illustrated in the following example. Assuming a Michaelis–Menten substrate (S) combined with a competitive inhibitor (CI), a mechanism-based inactivator (MBI), and an inducer (IND), the enzyme turnover can be derived as:

$$\frac{d[E]}{dt} = k_{\text{deg}} * E_0 * \left(1 + \frac{E_{\text{max}} * [\text{IND}]}{EC_{50} + [\text{IND}]}\right) - \left(k_{\text{deg}} + \frac{k_{\text{inact}} * [\text{MBI}]}{K_I * \left(1 + \dfrac{[\text{CI}]}{K_{i,\text{CI}}}\right) + [\text{MBI}]}\right) * [E]$$

The metabolic reaction velocity of the substrate can be expressed as

$$v = \frac{k_{\text{cat}} * E(t)}{K_m * \left(1 + \dfrac{[\text{CI}]}{K_{i,\text{CI}}} + \dfrac{[\text{MBI}]}{K_{i,\text{MBI}}}\right) + [S]} * [S]$$

8.2.6.1 Case Example

Rifampicin is known to be a strong inducer of CYP3A4, but it also competitively inhibits this enzyme. These two processes act on different time scales. Induction involves de-novo synthesis of enzyme and therefore takes days to fully reach the highest levels, whereas the competitive inhibitory effect is related to actual drug concentrations at the site of action, and, therefore, is strongest at the time of highest exposure, usually 1–2 hours after oral administration [34]. CYP3A4 induction and de-induction as well as midazolam PK under rifampicin co-administration is shown in Figure 8.2.

8.3 DEVELOPMENT AND VERIFICATION OF INTERACTION MODELS

This subchapter refers to the development of specific PBPK models for the simulation of DDIs with a particular emphasis on f_m and/or the fraction of drug transported (f_t) for substrates and integration of interaction parameters in perpetrator models. A general introduction to PBPK model development can be found in previous chapters of this book as well as publications, see e.g. [36].

8.3.1 Integration of *in-vitro* (IVIVE) and *in-vivo* Data

As a prerequisite for the PBPK modelling of DDIs, the type of interaction (see Section 8.2) and the involved enzyme or transporter must be known. Depending on the type, parameters listed in Table 8.3 should be available. In case these parameters are not available, these can be estimated if a sufficiently large PK data set of clinical interaction studies is available.

In case of K_i is not available for modelling of inhibition, IC_{50} can be used to calculate or estimate this parameter by the Cheng-Prusoff equation [37]:

$$K_i = \frac{IC_{50}}{1 + \dfrac{[S]}{K_m}}.$$

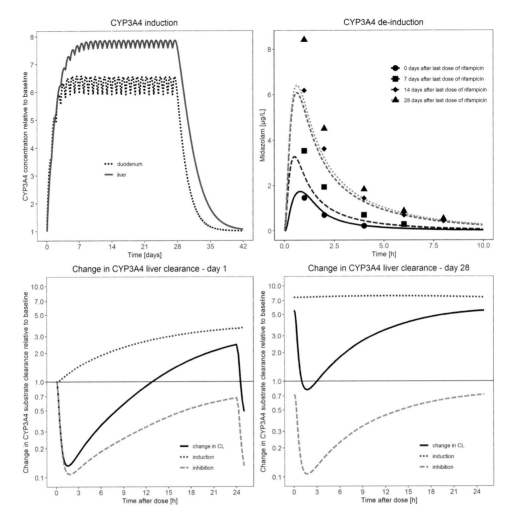

Figure 8.2 CYP3A4 induction by rifampicin, de-induction and resulting change in substrate clearance after a 600 mg rifampicin QD. Upper left panel: predicted CYP3A4 enzyme concentrations relative to baseline values in liver (solid) and duodenum (dashed) after a 600 mg rifampicin QD over 28 days, upper right panel: simulated (lines) and observed (symbols) midazolam plasma concentration-time profiles after administration of 2 mg midazolam 0 h (sim: solid line, obs: circles), 7 (sim: long dashed line, obs: squares), 14 (sim: short dashed line, obs: diamonds) and 28 days (sim: dotted line, obs: triangles) after the last dose of a 600 mg rifampicin QD treatment, simulations were adapted from Hanke et al. [34], observed data are from Reitman et al. [35], lower left panel: change in CYP3A4 substrate liver clearance on day 1 relative to baseline and on day 28 (lower right panel), induction calculated as in upper left panel, change in substrate liver clearance due to competitive inhibition of rifampicin is calculated independently of the substrate as

$$\frac{1}{1+\dfrac{[\text{Rifampicin}]}{K_i}},$$ change in CYP3A4 liver clearance is calculated as the product of induction and inhibition.

In general, all concentration constants, i.e., K_m, K_i, IC_{50} and EC_{50} always refer to unbound concentrations.

For modelling of induction, *in-vitro* measured values for EC_{50} and E_{max} of a potential inducer usually depend on the used cell lines and experimental setting ($EC_{50, \text{in vitro, test}}$ and $E_{max, \text{in vitro, test}}$). Caution is needed when transferring these values for *in vivo* PBPK predictions. It is generally

Table 8.3: Types of Interaction and Corresponding Parameters

Type of Interaction	Parameter
Reversible inhibition (competitive, non-competitive, uncompetitve and mixed inhibition)	K_i
Mechanism-based inactivation	K_I, K_i, k_{inact} (if K_i is not available, set $K_i = K_I$)
Induction and Suppression	E_{max}, EC_{50}

K_i is the inhibition constant for the reversible inhibition
K_I is the inhibition constant for the mechanism-based inactivation
k_{inact} is the inactivation rate constant
E_{max} is the maximum induction ratio
EC_{50} is the concentration at half maximum induction

recommended to perform a simple calibration (if possible) using already qualified *in vivo* EC_{50} and E_{max} values of an index inducer (like Rifampicin) for which a verified PBPK model is available ($EC_{50, in vivo, index}$ and $E_{max, in vivo, index}$). A prerequisite is that in the *in vitro* experiment this index inducer has also been tested (e.g., as a positive control) next to the potential inducer ($EC_{50, in vitro, index}$ and $E_{max, in vitro, index}$). The calibrated values ($EC_{50, in vivo, test}$ and $E_{max, in vivo, test}$) are calculated as follows:

$$EC_{50, in vivo, test} = EC_{50, in vitro, test} * \frac{EC_{50, in vivo, index}}{EC_{50, in vitro, index}}$$

$$E_{max, in vivo, test} = E_{max, in vitro, test} * \frac{E_{max, in vivo, index}}{E_{max, in vitro, index}}$$

For modelling of MBI and induction, the turnover rates of enzymes and transporters are critical. These turnover rates can be estimated from the recovery of the metabolic clearance of a probe drug enzyme after MBI or the kinetics of de-induction, i.e., the return to baseline clearance levels of the substrate, after the administration of inducers is discontinued. Using de-induction data of verapamil as a substrate of CYP3A4 induction of rifampicin, a half-life of approximately 36 hours is calculated for hepatic CYP3A4 turnover [38,39]. Turnover rates in other organs may differ from the estimated hepatic values. Based on the recovery of oral midazolam clearance following specific CYP3A4 inactivation in the gut wall by grapefruit juice, a half-life of approximately 23–24 hours can be estimated for the intestinal tissues [39–41]. A potential reason for the faster turnover in the gut might be the desquamation of the intestinal mucosa.

In general, active ADME processes such as metabolization through enzymes or disposition by transporters may occur at multiple sites depending on the expression pattern of the underlying affected enzyme or transporter. For example, CYP3A4 is mainly expressed in the liver and to a smaller extent in the gut wall. In the case of oral administration of a CYP3A4 substrate, a relevant portion of the drug is metabolized in the gut wall and, hence, inhibition or induction of CYP3A4 in the gut wall may dramatically affect the substrate's pharmacokinetics [38]. For example, Greenblatt et al. [40] showed that the PK of midazolam, a sensitive CYP3A4 substrate, is strongly altered when taken together with grapefruit juice, a specific inhibitor of CYP3A4 in the gut wall. So, PBPK models should aim to include enzyme/transporter at all relevant expression sites such that interaction processes take place at all these locations and properly reflect the *in-vivo* situation.

8.3.2 Development of PBPK Interaction Models

The development of a coupled interaction model requires the previous development of at least a substrate and a perpetrator model. As illustrated in Figure 8.3, such substrate and perpetrator models are developed in the first instance as all other PBPK models by integration of drug-dependent information such as physicochemical and *in-vitro* ADME data as previously described (e.g. [36]). In case of a substrate DDI model, the emphasis should be on f_m and f_t of the affected enzyme and transporter, respectively, in case of a perpetrator DDI model, the emphasis should be on the interaction parameters and the unbound concentrations at the sites of interaction. The primary goal of the PBPK model development and evaluation process is to describe, analyze and understand the drug's own pharmacokinetics. Essentially, this implies ensuring consistency with all available observed data, ideally over different dosing regimens and through different administration routes (intravenous and oral) and, if applicable, across different populations. For this purpose, a subset of the clinical data may also be used as a training set to estimate or optimize model parameters.

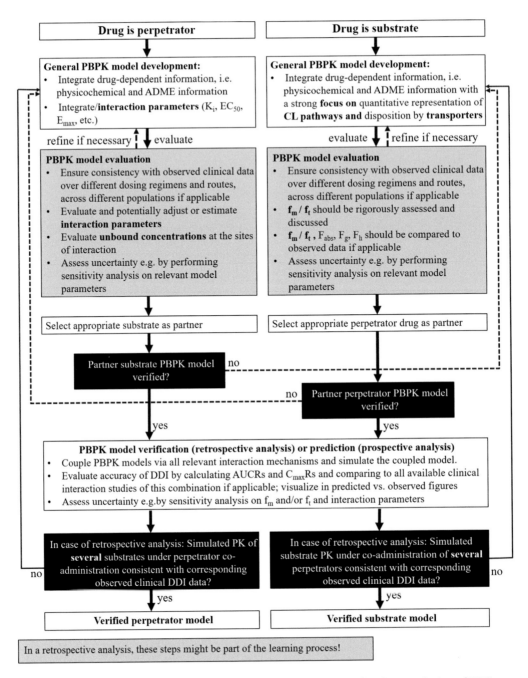

Figure 8.3 Workflow for developing and verifying PBPK models for the simulation of DDIs.

To evaluate substrate PBPK models, f_m and f_t should be rigorously assessed and f_m/f_t, the fraction absorbed (F_{abs}), the fraction escaping gut wall metabolism (F_g), and the fraction escaping hepatic elimination (F_h) should be compared to the corresponding values derived from observed clinical data if available. If auto-inhibition or -induction might play a relevant role, it is necessary to include these interaction processes in the stand-alone perpetrator model. It is highly recommended to evaluate a model not only against data from single-dose studies but also against data from multiple dose studies, given that these can help detecting changes in enzyme- or transporter-mediated mechanisms caused by auto-induction or inhibition [16]. For both PBPK models, a sensitivity analysis should be performed to assess uncertainty in input parameters on relevant model output parameters of the stand-alone models.

8.3.3 Retrospective and Prospective Analyses

In the following, two general DDI application scenarios are distinguished: A retrospective analysis where observed data from a clinical DDI study are available, and the PBPK model approach is used for learning and interpreting these data, and a prospective analysis where the simulated DDI study is used for predicting and informing or even replacing a clinical DDI study.

In the case of a retrospective analysis, the PBPK model for the drug of interest does not necessarily need to be fully verified. The idea here is to learn about f_m and/or f_t in the case of a substrate drug and learn about interaction parameters (e.g., K_i, EC_{50}, E_{max}, etc.) in the case of perpetrator drugs by coupling the model to a verified interaction partner substance model.

8.3.4 Verification of Interaction Models

Before using the PBPK model of interest in DDI predictions, the model should be verified for this intended use. In this context, verification refers to a retrospective analysis where observed data from a clinical DDI study are available, and, hence, can be used to verify or falsify the predictivity of the model. Obviously, the process of verifying a PBPK model for the use in a DDI study requires an interaction partner model. To increase confidence in the predictivity of the PBPK model in DDI simulations, preferably, a set of several interaction partner models of well-characterized substrates and perpetrators with different underlying interaction mechanisms (see Table 8.2) should be selected. As these partner models should be verified as well, the verification process initially comes down to establishing a network of substrate and perpetrator models of a specific enzyme in which all substrate-perpetrator combinations are reasonably in line with the corresponding observed PK data [42].

Because of a general lack of index perpetrators for transporter-mediated pathways, the choice of transporter perpetrators is typically based on the likelihood of concomitant use e.g., to obtain clinically relevant DDI data that can inform labeling regarding the management of a DDI [2].

As shown in Figure 8.3, the PBPK model verification of both, substrate and perpetrator models, is always based on the extent of PK changes of the substrate and comprises different steps. First the PBPK model of interest is coupled to an interaction partner model and the concentration-time profiles (of at least the substrate) are simulated and compared to observed data. Second, the accuracy of this DDI simulation is further evaluated by calculating AUCR and C_{max}R and comparing these values to the corresponding data of all available clinical interaction studies of this substrate-perpetrator combination. This can be visualized in simulated vs. observed plots, as shown in Section 8.3.6. Third, uncertainty in input parameters such as f_m, f_t, and interaction parameters on relevant model output parameters should be assessed in a sensitivity analysis of the coupled model (see Section 8.4).

Finally, a perpetrator model can be considered verified if the simulated pharmacokinetics of several substrates under perpetrator co-administration are consistent with the corresponding observed data. Conversely, a substrate model can be considered verified if the simulated pharmacokinetics under co-administration of several perpetrators are consistent with the corresponding observed data (see Figure 8.3).

8.3.5 Regulatory Recommendations and Requirements for the Verification of PBPK DDI Models and the Qualification of the PBPK Platform

When PBPK models are used for regulatory purposes, it is crucial to demonstrate that the model is verified for its intended use [43]. Regulatory agencies such as the US Food and Drug Administration (FDA) or the European Medicines Agency (EMA) demand to demonstrate the predictive performance of PBPK models as well as the PBPK platform for a specific context of use such as DDI. The FDA, for example, requires demonstrating that the PBPK model, firstly, is appropriate for the intended use, i.e. predicting DDIs in the current context and, secondly, that the uncertainties in the predictions are acceptable regarding the safety and efficacy profile of the involved drugs [1]. Considering that, the FDA proposes a workflow for the development of substrate and perpetrator models, coupling of the PBPK models and simulation of the resulting DDI which is reflected in Figure 8.3. In detail, model evaluation is required to ensure consistency to the available clinical data, to ensure that the elimination pathways quantitatively capture available *in-vitro* and *in-vivo* data (for substrates) and that inhibition and induction mechanisms are separately considered (for perpetrators) [3,44–46]. Moreover, sensitivity analyses for parameters with high levels of uncertainty are recommended (further detailed in Section 8.4).

The concept of establishing verified PBPK models is further detailed in the EMA Guideline for PBPK modelling [4]. Particularly for modelling purposes with a high regulatory impact such as the use of a PBPK model in lieu of a clinical study, the whole PBPK platform using a set of dedicated interaction models should be qualified for the intended purpose of predicting DDI. Ideally, this set of interaction models comprises a series of PBPK models for well characterized substrates eliminated to a significant portion by this enzyme as well as a series of PBPK models for perpetrators of different potency, and ideally, different mechanisms of interaction. As depicted in the previous section, this set of substrate and perpetrator models can be interpreted as a network, in which pairs of substrates and perpetrators are simulated and compared to observed data. Figure 8.4 (upper panel) shows such a CYP3A4 interaction network, and the same approach can be applied to other enzymes and transporters. Established PBPK modelling software tools such as GastroPlus®, PK-Sim® and Simcyp™, provide model libraries that include PBPK models which are verified for the use in e.g., CYP3A4 DDIs [42,47]. The quality of the prediction of interactions can be assessed, for example, by visualizing predicted vs. observed data in specific plots (see Section 8.3.6).

8.3.6 Visualizing the Predictive Performance of PBPK DDI Models

A common way of assessing and visualizing the predictive performance of a network of interaction models is to compare observed and predicted AUCR and C_{max}R as well as residuals vs. observed AUC- and C_{max} ratios for a specific enzyme as shown in Figure 8.4.

DDI prediction success is widely associated with the predictions falling within a two-fold range of the observed data. However, this acceptance criterion has some limitations at lower interaction levels for weak inhibitors and inducers; therefore, an alternative criterion was proposed by Guest et al. [48]. The idea is to evaluate the prediction success with a variable prediction margin dependent on the AUC ratio by employing a stricter success criterion around predicted vs. observed DDI ratios of 1. The outer limits of the Guest-criterion resemble the propeller-shaped area visualized in Figure 8.4.

8.3.7 Prediction of DDIs (Prospective Analysis)

Once substrate and perpetrator PBPK models are verified, qualified DDI predictions can be performed. For a conservative DDI evaluation as recommended by regulatory authorities, it is important to consider using the highest recommended clinical dose of the perpetrator to achieve the maximum inhibitory or inductive effect [3]. Furthermore, sufficiently long pre-dosing of the perpetrator and an optimal time lag of substrate administration after perpetrator dosing should be taken into account.

8.3.7.1 Case Example: The Ibrutinib Modelling Approach as a Blueprint for a DDI (Modelling) Strategy Accepted by Regulatory Authorities

In their guidance for clinical drug interaction studies, the FDA explicitly lists PBPK modelling to be used in lieu of prospective clinical DDI studies [2]. Moreover, if a clinical DDI study with strong index inhibitors or inducers indicates that there is a clinically significant interaction, the agency recommends evaluating the impact of moderate inhibitors or inducers to gain a full understanding of the investigational drug's DDI potential. In the pharmaceutical industry, this approach has frequently been performed using PBPK modelling in the last few years. In this context, the example of the ibrutinib PBPK model approach has developed to a blueprint for a PBPK modelling strategy in the field of DDI modelling that has been accepted by regulatory authorities [49].

This approach consists of a verification step with strong perpetrators representing the extremes of PK changes and an interpolation step to predict the effect of moderate and weak perpetrators in between. This approach is graphically summarized in Figure 8.5.

As a basis, clinical interaction studies of ibrutinib, a sensitive CYP3A4 substrate, with a strong CYP3A4 inhibitor (ketoconazole) and a strong CYP3A4 inducer (rifampicin) were conducted. In the verification step, PBPK models of ibrutinib coupled with ketoconazole and with rifampicin were simulated and the predicted AUCR and C_{max}R were compared to the corresponding values of the clinical study. A good agreement between predicted and observed PK parameter ratios was shown. This also demonstrates that the fraction metabolized through CYP3A4 of ibrutinib is adequately captured by the model, and, hence, the model is suited to predict drug interactions with

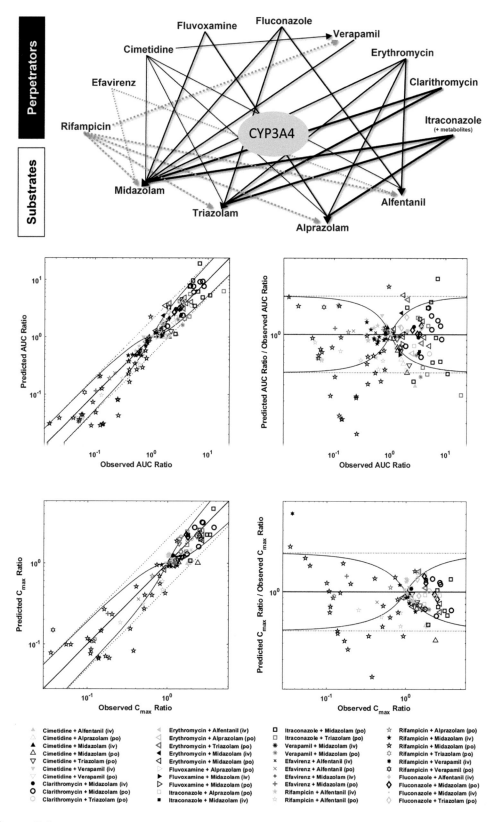

Figure 8.4

(*Continued*)

Figure 8.4 (Continued)   Upper panel: Network of CYP3A4 substrates and perpetrator substances, dotted lines indicate induction studies with available observed data, solid lines indicate inhibition studies with available observed data. Middle and lower panel: graphical representation of the performance of the CYP3A4 network, each symbol represents a single study of a specific combination, left panels: Predicted vs. observed plots, right panels: Predicted/observed vs. observed plots, the dotted lines denote 0.50–2.00 (2-fold) criterion, the solid lines denote the limits as suggested by Guest et al. [48], bold solid line denotes the unity line, observed pharmacokinetic data of interaction studies are publicly available and the study setups can be used to tailor the PBPK simulations to predict the corresponding outcome in comparison. (Taken from Open Systems Pharmacology, https://github.com/Open-Systems-Pharmacology/OSP-Qualification-Reports/blob/v10.0.1/DDI_Qualification_CYP3A4/report.md, with permission.)

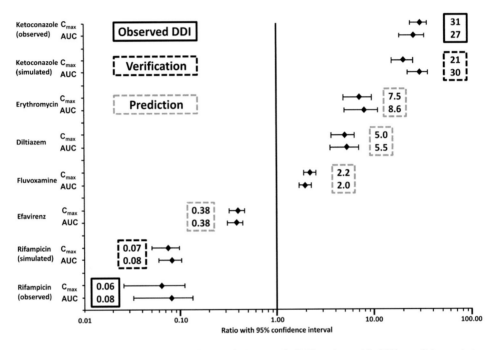

Figure 8.5   Simulated and observed ibrutinib C_{max} and AUC ratios with 95% confidence intervals of weak, moderate and strong inhibitors and moderate and strong inducers of CYP3A4. Observed DDI ratios were available for strong perpetrators (ketoconazole and rifampicin; ratios in solid black frames), these ratios were verified with corresponding PBPK DDI models (ratios in dashed black frames). The verified ibrutinib PBPK model was then used to predict the ratios with weak and moderate perpetrators (erythromycin, diltiazem, fluvoxamine and efavirenz; ratios in grey dashed frames). (Figure modified from Simcyp with permission.)

other perpetrators. These predictions are performed in the next step. Here, the PBPK model for ibrutinib was simulated in combination with erythromycin (a moderate MBI), diltiazem (a moderate inhibitor), fluvoxamine (a weak to moderate inhibitor), and efavirenz (a moderate inducer).

8.4 VARIABILITY AND UNCERTAINTY

PBPK models usually include model parameters from diverse sources (*in-vitro* and *in-vivo* studies, parameter estimation, databases, etc.) with different levels of uncertainty. Once a model is considered acceptable, uncertainty is often neglected and all model parameters are assumed to be fixed or just assessed by one-dimensional sensitivity analyses [48,50]. For a robust uncertainty assessment, quantifying, and propagating uncertainty in model parameters into DDI simulations is highly recommended. For this purpose, the aim is to distinctively quantify (i) population variability due to interindividual variability in physiology and enzyme/transporter abundances with the construction of population prediction intervals and (ii) the impact of uncertainty in model parameters on the substrate's AUC and C_{max} ratios with the construction of confidence intervals around a desired population statistic of interest (e.g., geometric mean, coefficient of variation, population quantiles, etc.).

8.4.1 Population Variability

Current knowledge suggests handling of interaction parameters (i.e., K_i, E_{max}, EC_{50}, etc.) as drug-dependent properties of the perpetrator without population variability. This assumption is well established in case of inhibition processes. Concerning induction, *in-vitro* experiments with hepatocytes from different donors show often high interindividual variability. However, these induction parameters are also treated drug-dependent without population variability. Reasons for this include (i) that *in-vivo* interindividual variability in these parameters is not well characterized and (ii) when merely looking at common CYP3A4 substrates (e.g. midazolam) in combination with common inducers (e.g. rifampicin), there is no obvious evidence that the relative variability in AUC before and after induction substantially differs.

So, population variability in DDI simulations is predominantly related to variability in anatomy and physiology, which may impact, e.g., the unbound concentrations at the sites of interaction and, thereby, may cause variability in AUCR and C_{max}R.

8.4.2 Uncertainty in Input Parameters and the PBPK Platform

PBPK model parameters usually originate from different sources, e.g., interaction parameters like inhibition constants (K_i) or induction parameters (EC_{50} and E_{max}) from *in-vitro* experiments, clearance parameters from e.g., parameter optimization using *in-vivo* clinical data, physiological parameters and their respective distributions in the population from dedicated databases, and other parameters simply might be assumed. These model parameters possess a varying degree of uncertainty and a sensitive analysis may help identify the parameters, which most likely contribute to misprediction [50]. Using this information, the measured or estimated uncertainty in these parameters as well as alternatives to the assumptions can be propagated to DDI simulations, e.g., as confidence intervals around the population median, and, potentially, around the 5th and 95th percentiles of the population prediction.

Confidence in the PBPK platform, i.e., the software/computer program including the library compound model files, can also be assessed. For example, when establishing a network of substrates and perpetrators for a specific enzyme as interaction partners, the predicted AUCRs and C_{max}Rs can be compared to the corresponding observed values, as e.g., shown in Figure 8.4. The predicted/observed ratio can be calculated for each study of the network of compounds and the geometric mean fold error (GMFE) of the ratios can be calculated as:

$$GMFE = 10^{\frac{\sum \left| \log\left(\frac{Pred}{Obs}\right) \right|}{n}}$$

The GMFE of AUCR and C_{max}R derived from the simulated combinations of the established DDI network can serve as a measure of mean uncertainty, and thus can be propagated to predictions. Depending on the quantity of the available DDI study data, these GMFEs can also be calculated per interaction mechanism or per perpetrator in the same way.

8.4.2.1 Case Example: Propagating the GMFE for DDI Predictions

The GMFE for all simulated combinations of the CYP3A4-DDI network on Open Systems Pharmacology (OSP, see https://github.com/Open-Systems-Pharmacology/OSP-Qualification-Reports/blob/v10.0.1/DDI_Qualification_CYP3A4/report.md) was calculated to be approximately 1.40 on AUCR and 1.35 on C_{max}R [42,51]. Stratified by mechanism, the GMFEs for induction are 1.43 and 1.47 for AUCR and C_{max}R, respectively, for mechanism-based inactivation, it yields 1.28 and 1.24 for AUCR and C_{max}R, respectively, and for reversible inhibition, it yields 1.43 and 1.25 for AUCR and C_{max}R, respectively. As a result of that, deviations for DDI predictions with models of this network may be expected in this range meaning that this error can be propagated to AUCR and C_{max}R.

8.4.3 Regulatory Perspective on Uncertainty

Regulatory guidance documents such as the ones from the FDA [1–3] and the EMA [4,5] mainly propose to address uncertainty by sensitivity analyses and basically recommend conservative approaches for the handling of uncertainties in DDI predictions. The EMA recommends in their

PBPK modelling guideline that a sensitivity analysis should be performed for parameters that are key to the model, i.e., parameters that are likely to noticeably influence the outcome or parameters that are uncertain. Examples of parameters that are considered uncertain are (see [4]):

- Parameters related to important assumptions
- Key experimentally determined parameters
- Parameters reported with broad value range in literature
- Parameters optimized during the model development process
- Parameters that are difficult to experimentally determine.

In DDI modelling practice, f_m or f_t for substrate models and the interaction parameters for perpetrator models fall into these categories. The EMA specifically suggests to prespecify the range of parameter values to be tested based on a scientific rationale, published data or known variability. For some parameters, the EMA recommends a 'worst-case' approach of e.g., 10-fold for CYP enzymes, and 30-fold for transporters [4].

8.4.3.1 Case Example: Sensitivity Analysis on f_m for the Sensitive CYP3A4 Substrate Finerenone Agreed with the FDA

Finerenone was investigated as a substrate of CYP3A4 ($f_{m,liver}=90\%$) and CYP2C8 ($f_{m,liver}=10\%$) using a PBPK modelling approach [51]. As finerenone was considered for contra-indication with strong CYP3A4 inhibitors and inducers early on, clinical DDI studies were exclusively performed with moderate CYP3A4 inhibitors. After a retrospective analysis and verification of the moderate inhibition with a PBPK modelling approach, predictions with several index inhibitors and inducers were performed to evaluate the DDI potential. For a proper understanding of the impact of f_m on AUCR and $C_{max}R$, a sensitivity analysis was performed using three scenarios:

- The reference scenario according to the established PBPK model, i.e., 90% CYP3A4 and 10% CYP2C8 in the liver
- Scenario 1 i.e., 85% CYP3A4 and 15% CYP2C8 in the liver
- Scenario 2 i.e., 95% CYP3A4 and 5% CYP2C8 in the liver

The results of this sensitivity analysis are summarized in Table 8.4. Overall, the differences between the three scenarios are small, and the reference scenario describes the evaluated interactions in a better way than scenario #1 or #2.

8.4.4 Confidence and Limitations in PBPK DDI Applications

Owing to limitations in *in-vitro* assays and limited knowledge and experience in different areas of PBPK DDI modelling, there is a varying level of confidence in DDI predictions. Experimental challenges regarding accurate *in-vitro* estimation of key parameters for the prediction of DDIs such as f_m, f_t and inhibition constants as well as limitations in the translation of *in-vitro* data to *in-vivo* apply to most areas in the field of DDI modelling. On the other hand, a high number of reported f_m and interaction parameter measurements, as well as a variety of published modelling approaches for particularly CYP substrates and perpetrators may outweigh these limitations and give confidence to other DDI models where the same enzymes are involved. Jones et al. [13] analyzed different PBPK DDI applications and proposed a classification of confidence levels on the basis of the type of interaction and the involved enzymes and/or transporters. PBPK DDI predictions involving reversible CYP inhibition alone or CYP induction alone are considered to have a high to moderate level of confidence, and, thus, represent the most reliable application in the field. DDI predictions involving apical active transporter such as OATP influx transporters or P-gp like efflux transporter are deemed to have a moderate level of confidence. Mechanism-based CYP inactivation and inhibition or induction of non-CYP pathways have a lower to moderate confidence level, whereas prediction of combined reversible, MBI and induction of CYPs as well as prediction of basolateral transport possess a low level of confidence.

It can be assumed that more experience in areas with limited knowledge is gathered, knowledge gaps are closed, and more DDI modelling approaches are performed and published in the future such that the level of confidence also rises in these application fields.

Table 8.4: Comparison of Observed and Simulated AUCR and C_{max}R and their CV for Finerenone-Drug Interactions in Different Scenarios, Reference Scenario: 90% CYP3A4 and 10% CYP2C8 in the Liver, Scenario #1: 85% CYP3A4 and 15% CYP2C8 in the Liver, Scenario #2: 95% CYP3A4 and 5% CYP2C8 in the Liver

Modulator	Scenario	AUCR geo. mean	AUCR geo. CV	C_{max}R geo. mean	C_{max}R geo. CV
Gemfibrozil	Observed in clinical study	1.10	0.18	1.16	0.31
	Simulated reference scenario	1.11	0.08	1.06	0.04
	Simulated scenario #1	1.19	0.11	1.09	0.06
	Simulated scenario #2	1.06	0.04	1.03	0.02
Erythromycin	Observed in clinical study	3.48	0.22	1.88	0.22
	Simulated reference scenario	3.46	0.25	2.00	0.16
	Simulated scenario #1	3.19	0.25	1.93	0.16
	Simulated scenario #2	3.74	0.25	2.07	0.17
Verapamil	Observed in clinical study	2.70	0.15	2.22	0.24
	Simulated reference scenario	2.91	0.29	1.86	0.15
	Simulated scenario #1	2.73	0.28	1.80	0.15
	Simulated scenario #2	3.09	0.30	1.91	0.16
Itraconazole	Simulated reference scenario	6.31	0.39	2.37	0.20
	Simulated scenario #1	5.23	0.39	2.24	0.19
	Simulated scenario #2	7.76	0.40	2.50	0.20
Clarithromycin	Simulated reference scenario	5.28	0.40	2.25	0.17
	Simulated scenario #1	4.52	0.38	2.14	0.16
	Simulated scenario #2	6.27	0.45	2.36	0.17
Fluvoxamine	Simulated reference scenario	1.57	0.16	1.38	0.10
	Simulated scenario #1	1.54	0.15	1.36	0.10
	Simulated scenario #2	1.59	0.16	1.39	0.10
Cimetidine	Simulated reference scenario	1.59	0.17	1.40	0.11
	Simulated scenario #1	1.56	0.17	1.39	0.11
	Simulated scenario #2	1.61	0.18	1.42	0.11
Efavirenz	Simulated reference scenario	0.19	0.21	0.32	0.18
	Simulated scenario #1	0.20	0.22	0.33	0.18
	Simulated scenario #2	0.18	0.21	0.31	0.18
Rifampicin	Simulated reference scenario	0.071	0.25	0.14	0.20
	Simulated scenario #1	0.074	0.26	0.15	0.21
	Simulated scenario #2	0.068	0.24	0.14	0.20

Dark grey background: study used to inform f_m in the model, light grey background: studies used to confirm f_m in a retrospective analysis, white background: studies used to predict in a prospective analysis.
Abbreviations: AUCR, AUC ratio; C_{max}R, C_{max} ratio; geo., geometric; CV, coefficient of variation.

REFERENCES

1. US Food and Drug Administration. Physiologically Based Pharmacokinetic Analyses - Format and Content Guidance for Industry.

2. US Food and Drug Administration. Clinical Drug Interaction Studies - Cytochrome P450 Enzyme- and Transporter-Mediated Drug Interactions Guidance for Industry.

3. US Food and Drug Administration. In Vitro Drug Interaction Studies - Cytochrome P450 Enzyme- and Transporter-Mediated Drug Interactions Guidance for Industry.

4. European Medicines Agency. Guideline on the Reporting of Physiologically Based Pharmacokinetic (PBPK) Modelling and Simulation.

5. European Medicines Agency. Guideline on the Investigation of Drug Interactions.

6. Frechen S., Rostami-Hodjegan A. Quality assurance of PBPK modeling platforms and guidance on building, evaluating, verifying and applying PBPK models prudently under the umbrella of qualification: Why, when, what, how and by whom? *Pharm Res.* 2022;39(8):1733–48.

7. Zhao P, Zhang L, Grillo JA, Liu Q, Bullock JM, Moon YJ, et al. Applications of physiologically based pharmacokinetic (PBPK) modeling and simulation during regulatory review. *Clinical Pharmacology and Therapeutics.* 2011;89(2):259–67.

8. Grimstein M, Yang Y, Zhang X, Grillo J, Huang SM, Zineh I, et al. Physiologically based pharmacokinetic modeling in regulatory science: An update from the U.S. Food and Drug Administration's Office of Clinical Pharmacology. *Journal of Pharmaceutical Sciences.* 2019;108(1):21–5.

9. Luzon E, Blake K, Cole S, Nordmark A, Versantvoort C, Berglund EG. Physiologically based pharmacokinetic modeling in regulatory decision-making at the European Medicines Agency. *Clinical Pharmacology and Therapeutics.* 2017;102(1):98–105.

10. Zhang X, Yang Y, Grimstein M, Fan J, Grillo JA, Huang SM, et al. Application of PBPK modeling and simulation for regulatory decision making and its impact on US prescribing information: An update on the 2018–2019 submissions to the US FDA's Office of Clinical Pharmacology. *Journal of Clinical Pharmacology.* 2020;60(Suppl 1):S160–S78.

11. Hsueh CH, Hsu V, Zhao P, Zhang L, Giacomini KM, Huang SM. PBPK modeling of the effect of reduced kidney function on the pharmacokinetics of drugs excreted renally by organic anion transporters. *Clinical Pharmacology and Therapeutics.* 2018;103(3):485–92.

12. Wagner C, Zhao P, Pan Y, Hsu V, Grillo J, Huang SM, et al. Application of physiologically based pharmacokinetic (PBPK) modeling to support dose selection: Report of an FDA public workshop on PBPK. *CPT: Pharmacometrics & Systems Pharmacology.* 2015;4(4):226–30.

13. Jones HM, Chen Y, Gibson C, Heimbach T, Parrott N, Peters SA, et al. Physiologically based pharmacokinetic modeling in drug discovery and development: A pharmaceutical industry perspective. *Clinical Pharmacology and Therapeutics.* 2015;97(3):247–62.

14. US Food and Drug Administration. Drug Development and Drug Interactions | Table of Substrates, Inhibitors and Inducers [Available from: https://www.fda.gov/drugs/drug-interactions-labeling/drug-development-and-drug-interactions-table-substrates-inhibitors-and-inducers].

15. International Transporter C, Giacomini KM, Huang SM, Tweedie DJ, Benet LZ, Brouwer KL, et al. Membrane transporters in drug development. *Nature Reviews Drug discovery.* 2010;9(3):215–36.

16. Taskar KS, Pilla Reddy V, Burt H, Posada MM, Varma M, Zheng M, et al. Physiologically-based pharmacokinetic models for evaluating membrane transporter mediated drug-drug interactions: Current capabilities, case studies, future opportunities, and recommendations. *Clinical Pharmacology and Therapeutics.* 2020;107(5):1082–115.

17. Einolf HJ. Comparison of different approaches to predict metabolic drug-drug interactions. *Xenobiotica; the fate of foreign compounds in biological systems.* 2007;37(10–11):1257–94.

18. Tucker GT. The rational selection of drug interaction studies: Implications of recent advances in drug metabolism. *International Journal of Clinical Pharmacology, Therapy, and Toxicology.* 1992;30(11):550–3.

19. Tucker GT, Houston JB, Huang SM. Optimizing drug development: Strategies to assess drug metabolism/transporter interaction potential--towards a consensus. *British Journal of Clinical Pharmacology.* 2001;52(1):107–17.

20. Vieira ML, Kirby B, Ragueneau-Majlessi I, Galetin A, Chien JY, Einolf HJ, et al. Evaluation of various static in vitro-in vivo extrapolation models for risk assessment of the CYP3A inhibition potential of an investigational drug. *Clinical Pharmacology and Therapeutics.* 2014;95(2):189–98.

21. Yang J, Jamei M, Yeo KR, Rostami-Hodjegan A, Tucker GT. Misuse of the well-stirred model of hepatic drug clearance. *Drug Metabolism and Disposition*: the biological fate of chemicals. 2007;35(3):501–2.

22. Fahmi OA, Hurst S, Plowchalk D, Cook J, Guo F, Youdim K, et al. Comparison of different algorithms for predicting clinical drug-drug interactions, based on the use of CYP3A4 in vitro data: Predictions of compounds as precipitants of interaction. *Drug Metabolism and Disposition*: the biological fate of chemicals. 2009;37(8):1658–66.

23. Houston JB, Galetin A. Modelling atypical CYP3A4 kinetics: Principles and pragmatism. *Archives of Biochemistry and Biophysics.* 2005;433(2):351–60.

24. Ito K, Iwatsubo T, Kanamitsu S, Ueda K, Suzuki H, Sugiyama Y. Prediction of pharma-cokinetic alterations caused by drug-drug interactions: Metabolic interaction in the liver. *Pharmacological Reviews.* 1998;50(3):387–412.

25. Tatsunami S, Yago N, Hosoe M. Kinetics of suicide substrates. Steady-state treatments and computer-aided exact solutions. *Biochimica et Biophysica Acta.* 1981;662(2):226–35.

26. Waley SG. Kinetics of suicide substrates. *The Biochemical Journal.* 1980;185(3):771–3.

27. Walsh C, Cromartie T, Marcotte P, Spencer R. Suicide substrates for flavoprotein enzymes. *Methods in Enzymology.* 1978;53:437–48.

28. Ueda A, Hamadeh HK, Webb HK, Yamamoto Y, Sueyoshi T, Afshari CA, et al. Diverse roles of the nuclear orphan receptor CAR in regulating hepatic genes in response to phenobarbital. *Molecular Pharmacology.* 2002;61(1):1–6.

29. Almond LM, Yang J, Jamei M, Tucker GT, Rostami-Hodjegan A. Towards a quantitative framework for the prediction of DDIs arising from cytochrome P450 induction. *Current Drug Metabolism.* 2009;10(4):420–32.

30. Fahmi OA, Ripp SL. Evaluation of models for predicting drug-drug interactions due to induction. *Expert Opinion on Drug Metabolism & Toxicology.* 2010;6(11):1399–416.

31. Olkkola KT, Backman JT, Neuvonen PJ. Midazolam should be avoided in patients receiving the systemic antimycotics ketoconazole or itraconazole. *Clinical Pharmacology and Therapeutics.* 1994;55(5):481–5.

32. Bartkowski RR, Goldberg ME, Larijani GE, Boerner T. Inhibition of alfentanil metabolism by erythromycin. *Clinical Pharmacology and Therapeutics.* 1989;46(1):99–102.

33. Eap CB, Buclin T, Cucchia G, Zullino D, Hustert E, Bleiber G, et al. Oral administration of a low dose of midazolam (75 microg) as an in vivo probe for CYP3A activity. *European Journal of Clinical Pharmacology.* 2004;60(4):237–46.

34. Hanke N, Frechen S, Moj D, Britz H, Eissing T, Wendl T, et al. PBPK models for CYP3A4 and P-gp DDI prediction: A modeling network of rifampicin, itraconazole, clarithromycin, midazolam, alfentanil, and digoxin. *CPT: Pharmacometrics & Systems Pharmacology.* 2018;7(10):647–59.

35. Reitman ML, Chu X, Cai X, Yabut J, Venkatasubramanian R, Zajic S, et al. Rifampin's acute inhibitory and chronic inductive drug interactions: Experimental and model-based approaches to drug-drug interaction trial design. *Clinical Pharmacology and Therapeutics.* 2011;89(2):234–42.

36. Kuepfer L, Niederalt C, Wendl T, Schlender JF, Willmann S, Lippert J, et al. Applied concepts in PBPK modeling: How to build a PBPK/PD model. *CPT: Pharmacometrics & Systems Pharmacology.* 2016;5(10):516–31.

37. Cheng Y, Prusoff WH. Relationship between the inhibition constant (K1) and the concentration of inhibitor which causes 50 per cent inhibition (I50) of an enzymatic reaction. *Biochemical Pharmacology.* 1973;22(23):3099–108.

38. Fromm MF, Busse D, Kroemer HK, Eichelbaum M. Differential induction of prehepatic and hepatic metabolism of verapamil by rifampin. *Hepatology.* 1996;24(4):796–801.

39. Obach RS, Walsky RL, Venkatakrishnan K. Mechanism-based inactivation of human cytochrome p450 enzymes and the prediction of drug-drug interactions. *Drug Metabolism and Disposition: The Biological Fate of Chemicals.* 2007;35(2):246–55.

40. Greenblatt DJ, von Moltke LL, Harmatz JS, Chen G, Weemhoff JL, Jen C, et al. Time course of recovery of cytochrome p450 3A function after single doses of grapefruit juice. *Clinical Pharmacology and Therapeutics.* 2003;74(2):121–9.

41. Venkatakrishnan K, Obach RS, Rostami-Hodjegan A. Mechanism-based inactivation of human cytochrome P450 enzymes: Strategies for diagnosis and drug-drug interaction risk assessment. *Xenobiotica*; the fate of foreign compounds in biological systems. 2007;37(10–11):1225–56.

42. Frechen S, Solodenko J, Wendl T, Dallmann A, Ince I, Lehr T, et al. A generic framework for the physiologically-based pharmacokinetic platform qualification of PK-Sim and its application to predicting cytochrome P450 3A4-mediated drug-drug interactions. *CPT: Pharmacometrics & Systems Pharmacology.* 2021;10(6):633–44.

43. Kuemmel C, Yang Y, Zhang X, Florian J, Zhu H, Tegenge M, et al. Consideration of a credibility assessment framework in model-informed drug development: Potential application to physiologically-based pharmacokinetic modeling and simulation. *CPT: Pharmacometrics & Systems Pharmacology.* 2020;9(1):21–8.

44. Vieira MD, Kim MJ, Apparaju S, Sinha V, Zineh I, Huang SM, et al. PBPK model describes the effects of comedication and genetic polymorphism on systemic exposure of drugs that undergo multiple clearance pathways. *Clinical Pharmacology and Therapeutics.* 2014;95(5):550–7.

45. Wagner C, Pan Y, Hsu V, Grillo JA, Zhang L, Reynolds KS, et al. Predicting the effect of cytochrome P450 inhibitors on substrate drugs: Analysis of physiologically based pharmacokinetic modeling submissions to the US Food and Drug Administration. *Clinical Pharmacokinetics.* 2015;54(1):117–27.

46. Wagner C, Pan Y, Hsu V, Sinha V, Zhao P. Predicting the effect of CYP3A inducers on the pharmacokinetics of substrate drugs using physiologically based pharmacokinetic (PBPK) modeling: An analysis of PBPK submissions to the US FDA. *Clinical Pharmacokinetics.* 2016;55(4):475–83.

47. Marsousi N, Desmeules JA, Rudaz S, Daali Y. Prediction of drug-drug interactions using physiologically-based pharmacokinetic models of CYP450 modulators included in Simcyp software. *Biopharmaceutics & Drug Disposition*. 2018;39(1):3–17.

48. Guest EJ, Aarons L, Houston JB, Rostami-Hodjegan A, Galetin A. Critique of the two-fold measure of prediction success for ratios: Application for the assessment of drug-drug interactions. *Drug Metabolism and Disposition*: the biological fate of chemicals. 2011;39(2):170–3.

49. US Food and Drug Administration. Clinical Pharmacology and Biopharmaceutics Review, Application Number 205552Orig1s000.

50. Almond LM, Mukadam S, Gardner I, Okialda K, Wong S, Hatley O, et al. Prediction of drug-drug interactions arising from CYP3A induction using a physiologically based dynamic model. *Drug Metabolism and Disposition*: the biological fate of chemicals. 2016;44(6):821–32.

51. Wendl T, Frechen S, Gerisch M, Heinig R, Eissing T. Physiologically-based pharmacokinetic modeling to predict CYP3A4-mediated drug-drug interactions of finerenone. *CPT: Pharmacometrics & Systems Pharmacology*. 2021;11(2):199–211.

9 Applying PBPK Modeling to Predict Drug Exposure in Special Populations

*Mariana Guimarães, Mubtasim Murshed, Janny Pineiro-Llanes,
Rodrigo Cristofoletti, and Nikoletta Fotaki*

9.1 INTRODUCTION

The use of physiologically-based pharmacokinetic (PBPK) modeling in the pharmaceutical industry began in the early 2000s with its growth increasing significantly in both industrial and academic applications since 2010 [1]. This has led to the release of draft guidance documents from the FDA and the EMA in 2017 [2,3]. The initial accepted application of PBPK was for the evaluation of metabolism-related drug–drug interaction potential [4]. However, over recent years, PBPK applications have expanded, especially in its use for the prediction of pharmacokinetics (PK) in special populations. A deep understanding of physiology and anatomy stands as one of the pivotal requirements in the development of PBPK models. PBPK models can be tailored to discern the effects on PK by integration of insights on how diseases and age affect physiology and anatomy. During drug development, pharmacokinetic evaluations are traditionally made in healthy volunteers or specific disease populations. PBPK modeling allows leveraging the existing pharmacokinetics knowledge gathered during drug development to make extrapolations for specialized demographics such as pediatrics and patients with gastrointestinal (GI) diseases. Several PBPK models have been described in the literature predicting pharmacokinetics in special populations such as patients with hepatic impairment, renal impairment, children, elderly, pregnancy, obesity, bariatric surgery, and oncology patients [5–14]. Some of these special population PBPK models have been integrated into commercial and/or open-source software platforms and applied by multiple pharmaceutical industry scientists for internal decision support as well as for regulatory interactions. From 2008 to 2017, the FDA Office of Clinical Pharmacology received 130 investigational new drug (IND) and 94 new drug application (NDA) submissions containing PBPK modeling; in total the application of PBPK models to special populations (i.e., hepatic and renal impairment and pediatric patients) made up 25% of the total submissions [15].

So far, the impact and reliability of these special population predictions have only been partially assessed. For example, a recent publication by a consortium of pharmaceutical industry scientists has evaluated predictions in patients with hepatic and renal impairment [16]. For a set of 29 development compounds in patients with hepatic and renal impairment, the agreement of predictions with clinical study data was sufficient to recommend that such population predictions could be used prospectively to determine the need and timing of organ impairment studies.

While there has been progress for some populations over the last few years, the existing PBPK models are still limited with several gaps, especially considering the wide number of populations of interest, some of which are very poorly characterized. When it comes to oral absorption, most of these models incorporate limited capabilities due to ongoing challenges in gathering relevant anatomical and physiological data to fully parameterize a patient population (including characterization of patient inter and intra-subject variability). A review of pediatric oral drug absorption using Simcyp™ (Certara®) noted gaps in knowledge related to the ontogeny of the GI tract [17]. Traditionally during drug development, clinical trials in special populations may not be performed, and thus limited data is available in pediatric, elderly, pregnant patients, and/or patients with severe hepatic/renal impairment, GI diseases, and other disease states. PBPK models offer the unique opportunity to perform an informed risk assessment of the impact of population-related changes on drug exposure and guide clinicians for a better use of medicines. This chapter will describe a typical approach for building a PBPK model for special populations.

9.2 BUILDING A PBPK MODEL FOR SPECIAL POPULATIONS

The most common approach in constructing a PBPK model for special populations is to first build a PBPK model in a reference population which will often be healthy volunteers (Figure 9.1, **Step 1**). After validation of the intravenous (IV) model, the model for oral administration can be developed (Figure 9.1, **Step 2**). The validation of PBPK models involves a stepwise approach (from step 1 to step 2) that ideally starts with the IV pharmacokinetics before verifying oral absorption models, however, this might not always be possible due to data availability.

DOI: 10.1201/9781003031802-9

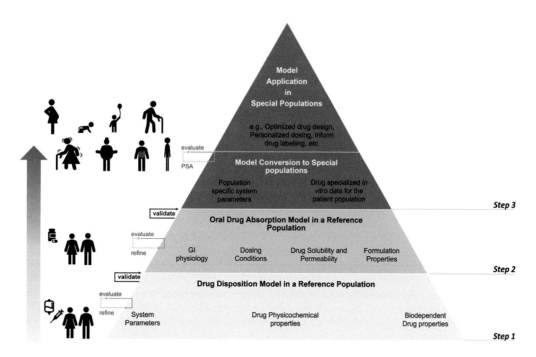

Figure 9.1 Strategy for building a PBPK model to predict drug exposure after oral administration in special populations. PSA: parameter sensitivity analysis; bio-dependent drug properties: drug parameter values that depend on the drug and the system physiology.

9.2.1 Step 1 – Building a Drug Disposition PBPK Model for a Reference Population

The development of a PBPK model is heavily dependent on the data available for model building. A model will require system-dependent data (i.e., organ sizes, blood flow, and tissue composition) and compound-dependent parameters (i.e., physicochemical properties like pKa and log$P$ but also bio-dependent parameters such as fraction unbound, plasma/blood-partitioning, and intrinsic clearance).

The PBPK model uses these input parameters within mathematical equations to represent the system (human or animal) as compartments representing organs and tissues linked by arterial and venous blood flow. The disposition model will be based on differential equations that describe drug movement in and out of the tissue and organ compartments. A dosing scenario should be defined, by informing the model on the population (human or animal and if human specify if healthy volunteers or a special population), key demographics such as age, sex, and dosing conditions. In the case of a disposition model, a simulation will try to predict the plasma concentration-time profiles after an IV bolus or infusion dosing. To validate/verify the PBPK model, IV data will be needed. A model is predictive of an *in vivo* simulation if it can recover closely the observed PK profile. If the PK simulations of the model mismatch the observed clinical IV data, model optimization (e.g., volume distribution and clearance) can be performed. Optimization of parameters should be informed by clinical data and appropriately justified. When there is good prediction between the simulated and the observed data for an IV administration, the modeling of oral drug absorption can be initiated.

9.2.2 Step 2 – Building Oral Absorption PBPK Model for a Reference Population

Mechanistic oral absorption modeling can be accomplished by using complex oral absorption models that divide the gastrointestinal tract in several sequentially connected compartments (i.e., the stomach, duodenum, upper and lower jejunum, and upper and lower ileum and colon). Examples of these models are available in commercial software such as the advanced compartmental absorption and transit (ACAT) model (GastroPlus®) or the advanced dissolution and absorption and metabolism (ADAM) model (Simcyp™).

In these models, each compartment will be characterized by its own surface area, fluid composition, volumes, etc. Similar to the disposition model, differential equations will describe the movement of the drug in its many states (solid, dissolved) through the GI compartments. Drug permeation from the GI tract to the enterocytes can be informed by *in vivo* or *in vitro* permeability studies or estimated with models via the utilized software. The models also incorporate mathematical equations that allow the user to predict the solubility and the dissolution of the drug in the GI compartments (based on physicochemical properties such as the Henderson-Hasselbalch equation and dissolution equations such as Noyes-Whitney and Wang Flanagan, etc.). At this stage, information on the drug formulation is crucial (e.g., immediate release *vs* modified release formulation). Biorelevant solubility and dissolution data from *in vitro* tests can be used to inform the model by either direct incorporation or modeled with software (i.e. SIVA) to deconvolute key drug properties such as intrinsic solubility, precipitation parameters, etc. [18]. The more mechanistic incorporation of the data, the higher the model flexibility to explore 'what-if' scenarios. Drug dissolution, precipitation, and/or the supersaturation phenomenon can be considered relevant for the drug substance and drug product. Fraction of drug absorbed, degraded, or metabolized can be considered in the model. To validate/verify the PBPK model, oral PK data will be required. If the oral PK simulations of the model mismatch the observed *in vivo* oral data, model rational optimization (e.g., permeability, solubility) can be performed. If oral solution PK data is available in the literature, this data can be used prior to moving on to the simulation of exposure after the administration of solid dosage forms. Sequential model development can help identify the critical variables of absorption, as validation of the model after the administration of a solution, which is independent of drug release and dissolution, increases the confidence in the model prediction of intestinal permeability and/or gut wall metabolism. When there is a good prediction between the simulated and the observed data for an oral administration in the reference population, the modeling of other populations can proceed.

9.2.3 Step 3 – PBPK Model Conversion to Special Populations

If the PBPK model in the reference population provides an adequate prediction of the available clinical data, the scaling to the special population can be carried out by either:

i. selecting a default special population available in a software platform that contains default information on age-dependent changes and scaling of anatomy and physiology (further details will be presented in the following subsections)

ii. creating a new virtual population from scratch by applying relevant anatomical and physiological changes in comparison to healthy volunteers/reference population. The building of a virtual special population from scratch will involve data collection and meta-analysis of the literature available to characterize the key changes in anatomy/physiology for that special patient population.

The following sections of this book chapter will explore how a PBPK model can be converted into special populations, including a description of recently published case studies.

9.2.3.1 *PBPK Model Conversion to the Pediatric Population*

The anatomy and physiology between adult and pediatric populations are substantially different and therefore require a change in many of the key components of a PBPK model. Model conversion commonly begins by selecting the appropriate pediatric population option within the PBPK software package, or if a dedicated module does not exist, designing a tailored pediatric population using the software's input functions.

The pediatric modules take into consideration multiple age-dependent changes in physiology that impact pharmacokinetic outcomes of a drug. Other factors such as specific ethnic populations (e.g., American/Western, Japanese, and Chinese), gender (male/female), gestational age (including pre-mature newborns), body weight, height, body-mass index and percent body fat are also taken into account as tissue volumes and perfusion rates are adjusted based on these values [19].

Prediction of oral absorption within pediatric populations is defined by the ontogeny of the GI tract. PBPK models use intestinal growth data or body-surface area (BSA) functions to calculate intestinal length and radius, while GI organs, blood perfusion rates, fluid secretion volumes, and small intestinal transit times (SITT) are changed dependent on age [20–22]. Using discrete values, such as BSA, to define multiple anatomical features can introduce inaccuracies within pediatric models as they do not take into consideration any adjustments to surface area due to villi and microvilli growth with age [23]. Other uncertainties can also arise from the assumption that growth occurs proportionally across the small intestine (SI) with age.

Due to the lack of quality data in pediatric populations, many adult parameter values are still widely used within pediatric PBPK modeling software. Currently, adult values are adopted for GI tract pH (all regions), gastric emptying, bile salt composition, and site of reabsorption. The Simcyp™ platform does provide an exception, as it employs a higher gastric pH in the fasted state of newborns and infants. Higher values are considered for these subpopulations as they exist in a constant fed-state due to the frequency of their meals causing an absence of a 'true' fasted-state [17]. The adoption of adult values can lead to further uncertainties in the model; estimation of passive drug absorption can be affected while solubility and permeability of compounds with higher dependencies on bile salts can be inaccurate. These uncertainties are further skewed for younger populations (< 3 years) where there is a greater physiological difference from adults [21].

As the CYP3A4 enzyme is well-defined in pediatrics, expression and density of other metabolic enzyme families are either calculated based on the CYP3A4s change with ontogeny or the default adult values are used depending on the specific software. Intestinal transport proteins are less investigated and therefore the adult values are adopted [24,25]. User modification to the default values for enzymes and transporters can be implemented in the PBPK modeling software. The Simcyp™ platform gives the user more choices by allowing the selection of meal type as it can simulate the effects of liquid, semi-solid or solid meal ingestion. Selection of a meal type will change the gastric emptying (GE) time input; however, the SITT values remain independent from age and are directly adopted from the adult values [24].

9.2.3.1.1 Model Development Process

When conducting simulations within pediatric subpopulations, it is usually advised to begin with the older age groups i.e., adolescents or children, before gradually moving toward the younger subpopulations [26]. This can help evolve the model parameterization as older pediatric groups have fewer physiological differences compared to adults than infants and newborns. Similarly to building the adult model, steps to confirm, validate, and refine (if necessary) the pediatric model are undertaken. Gradually adapting the model between each subpopulation can also allow easier identification of areas that may require refinement [26]. Differences between predicted and observed clinical data should be investigated through parameter sensitivity analysis (PSA) [17,21,25]. PSA can also be used to explore "what-if" scenarios where the uncertainties and assumptions within the model can be tested.

9.2.3.1.2 Integration of New Pediatric Anatomical and Physiological Findings within a PBPK Model

Various adult physiological values are still used within their PBPK software pediatric modules due to the lack of verified values from pediatric populations. More research is continuously being conducted to fill these gaps; however, the large variability in results from pediatrics often makes it difficult to set a specific value for each model parameter. The section below describes recent advances in pediatric research and how they may be considered in future PBPK models.

9.2.3.1.3 Metabolic Enzymes and Transporters

Extensive research has been recently conducted in the investigation of the abundance of metabolic enzymes and transporters within pediatric populations. The CYP3A4 family has been well characterized previously for pediatric age groups and a recent publication has quantified a wider variety of drug metabolism enzymes and transporter proteins (DMET) [27]. Using pinch biopsies, 36 samples were collected from a pediatric population aged from 11 months to 15 years. 21 intestinal DMET of interest were investigated with a major focus being on CYP enzymes, as they are known to metabolize approximately 70% of drugs administered in children [28]. Results confirmed that CYP3A4 was the most abundant CYP enzyme, followed by CYP3A5, CYP2C9, CYP2D6 and CYP2C19. These results were true across all the pediatric age groups tested. Within the UGT enzymes, UGT2B17 was the most expressed followed by UGT1A1 and UGT2B7. Among transporter proteins SLC22A1 protein was the most expressed; however, a rank-order thereafter was less clear with multiple transporters showing similar expression levels. Results from this study support the current extrapolation method of DMET abundancy values from adults to pediatrics in the PBPK modeling software for ages above 2 years.

Another study provided a comprehensive characterization of neonatal microbiome [29]. The study collected umbilical cord blood, gastric liquid, and meconium samples from 178 neonates, while also collecting vaginal discharge and amniotic fluid from their mothers. Microbial DNA was isolated from the samples and sequencing data was generated and cataloged. Microbiome in neonate gastric liquid was similar to that of their mothers (but not identical) and results suggested that microbiome colonization within neonates must begin during pregnancy as a distinct bacterial composition was found in the meconium. This extensive library of microbiome data created from this research may not have an immediate impact on determining drug absorption in pediatrics, however, the data can be used to ascertain the patterns and extent of microbiota present in the gut, especially at the beginning of the ontogeny cycle.

9.2.3.1.4 Gastric Emptying Time (GET)

GET describes the time required for the stomach to release its content into the SI. GET in pediatrics has shown to be widely variable and heavily affected by the prandial state of the individual. GET determined by ultrasound in 48 healthy formula-fed neonates ranged from 45 to 150 minutes with an average of 92.9 minutes [30]. This value was slightly higher than the $GET_{1/2}$ reported in Guimarães et al. [31]; however, this could potentially be due to the results being specific to formula-fed neonates, as breast milk has been shown to empty faster [32]. This further exemplifies the difficulties associated with assigning a set GET to a specific age group since factors such as feeding schedule, fed type, and amount given can impact this characteristic. This variability can be modeled using PBPK modeling software. GET values can be used as input in the modeling software, usually under their population tabs. Often, software allows the input of the mean gastric residence times, mean drug residence times, and options to establish a food staggering model. Using the PBPK modeling software, it is possible to assess a range of GETs using the PSA option. PSA allows the user to change one parameter over a set range at a time while keeping other parameters constant. Some software also allow the performance of global sensitivity analysis (GSA) where the impact of multiple parameters can be assessed simultaneously including their potential interactions. These tools are extremely useful in pediatric populations as they allow interrogation of the model and quick understanding of the critical variables in drug absorption.

9.2.3.1.5 GI Tract Fluid Volumes

Fluid volumes within the individual GI tract sections are important factors for determining the overall absorption from a specific drug formulation. Previous pediatric research focused on fasted gastric volumes with no information found on intestinal volumes. A recent study (2022) [33] retrospectively used magnetic resonance imaging (MRI) to capture 140 images from all the sections of the GI tract of pediatric subpopulations (except neonates). The study only selected fasted patients, but the authors conceded that they could not guarantee that all young infants had adhered to the required 6 hours fasting period. The median (fasted) gastric volume in infants (aged 0.1–1 year) was reported to be 5 mL while total small intestinal volume was calculated at 23.57 mL. An increase in all fluid volume in majority of the GI tract sections was observed with age, conversely, fluid volume within the ileum remained stable throughout the age groups. A statistically significant linear correlation was found between fluid volume and body characteristics such as weight and height, confirming that the common method within PBPK software of extrapolating fluid volume directly from weight or height is accurate. Deeper analysis of the regression also showed that even though extrapolation from body measurements was deemed correct, the reliability of a direct prediction is low, and therefore, other inputs should be taken into consideration when making estimates. The values reported within this study can inform PBPK modeling, similar to that discussed for GET. PBPK software allows the input of basal (steady state) fluid volumes that have been split into the stomach, SI, and colon, or the user can define the volumes within individual sections of the GI tract i.e., duodenum, jejunum I, jejunum II, etc. Modeling a variety of different fluid volumes through the GI tract can allow for a better understanding of how drug absorption is impacted. To analyze this, the study used PBPK modeling and sensitivity analysis to predict the % fraction absorbed with a change in SI volume. The results confirmed that SI volume majorly impacts lower solubility drugs, especially those without high permeability.

9.2.3.1.6 Intestinal Length

The intestinal length is a key factor in calculating the intestinal surface area available for oral drug absorption. An increase in surface area commonly correlates with an increase in drug absorption, and therefore it is vital to have data corroborating the physical size of the intestine. This is usually difficult in pediatric populations due to ethical concerns; however, post-mortem samples have allowed for some measurements, albeit the studies can be decades old. Recently, small and large intestinal linear lengths from 131 post-mortem fetus and neonate samples were measured [34]. The individuals were both preterm and term with gestational ages ranging from 13 to 41 weeks. The study reported an average length of the SI to be 147.7 ± 82.7 cm, while for the colon it was 30.6 ± 17.7 cm. The study also confirmed the positive linear relationship between age and intestinal length in this specific pediatric population. The researchers further broke down their findings into gestational ages, allowing a precise understanding of some of the most vulnerable preterm neonates. The values reported are higher than those given as general SI reference values (80 cm for newborns) but less than the other values reported in an original study by Weaver et al. [35] (275 cm at birth). SI length can usually be directly inputted into the modeling software. The large variability of the results seems to be a constant in pediatric physiology, and as discussed before, this variability can be effectively tested using the PSA function within PBPK modeling software.

9.2.3.1.7 Use of Biorelevant Media during *in vitro* Experiments

Typically, PBPK software applies release/dissolution models to predict the release/dissolution of a formulation based on key model inputs, but they also allow for the input of discrete *in vitro* release/dissolution profiles to better understand how differences in formulations can impact the overall drug absorption. Quality control release/dissolution studies are usually conducted using set USP buffers and apparatus; the application of biorelevant media allows for a more physiologically relevant understanding of drug release/dissolution kinetics, especially for poorly soluble compounds. Biorelevant media for the pediatric population were first proposed by Maharaj et al. [36], with the established adult biorelevant media being used as a reference during their development [37–39]. Solubility of seven compounds was tested in the age-specific media with the results showing that six out of seven compounds fell outside the 80%–125% range when compared against their adult media counterparts, highlighting the variance of drug behavior between the adult and pediatric GI fluid [36]. Applying age-dependent biorelevant *in vitro* release/dissolution profiles into pediatric PBPK models will increase their robustness. The current iteration of pediatric biorelevant media will continue to evolve as updates on the characterization of pediatric GI tract fluids become available [40,41].

Pawar et al. [40] characterized intestinal and gastric fluid from 55 children aged between 11 months to 15 years, while a study conducted by de Waal et al. [41] collected GI tract fluid from 21 neonate and infant patients from a variety of locations within the SI and colon. Both studies characterized the pH, buffer capacity, osmolality, and bile salts concentrations, with total protein, phospholipids, cholesterol, and lipid digestion products also quantified in the de Waal et al. [41] study. The new studies reiterate the large variability in results seen in pediatric populations where a single mean value may not accurately represent the whole age group. The samples collected for the studies originated from a small number of participants and therefore the results should be seen as guideline figures rather than absolute values. As majority of the values and ranges reported in the two new studies were similar to those established initially by Maharaj et al. [36], definitive changes to media composition are not proposed.

Acquiring additional physiological and clinical data from pediatric populations is imperative for creating robust PBPK models, however, it is becoming ever more difficult as strong regulation and ethical concerns must be adhered to when conducting research. Of the research which has been published, on many occasions the results have come from children which are already in hospital for other ailments, that could skew the results and are usually of a singular demographic and ethnic group. Extrapolating these types of results to a general pediatric PBPK model may produce bias within the algorithm which could mask incorrect predictions as appropriate results. Predicting pediatric responses to medication is a difficult task but the advancements in technology, especially computing, may allow scientists to overcome many of these limitations in the future.

9.2.3.1.8 Example of Pediatric PBPK Absorption Models

9.2.3.1.8.1 Paracetamol The successful extrapolation of paracetamol exposure from adults to infants using a PBPK model built using GastroPlus® V9.7 (Simulations Plus, USA) has been described [42]. The aim of the research was to ascertain whether dosing conditions in adult clinical trials substantially affected the extrapolation to infant populations. The development of the PBPK model utilized a 'middle-out' approach where model parameterization was guided by both literature values and clinical observations in humans. The overall model-building strategy was similar to that described in this chapter (Figure 9.1). A disposition model was first developed, optimized, and verified for healthy adults using the clinical studies where paracetamol was administered intravenously. An oral absorption model was then built in healthy adults using the ACAT module with optimization and verification being completed using the liquid drug formulation (i.e., solution, suspension) data. The model was first scaled to pediatric age groups where IV data was available, and a disposition model could be developed, optimized, and verified. Finally, prandial states and dosing conditions were explored in a pediatric absorption model where the administration of the pediatric suspension was extrapolated from adults to infants and compared with data observed in this pediatric population. The study concluded that when building a PBPK model, it is more favorable to use age-relevant formulation and dosing conditions prior to extrapolation, rather than just using the default software settings [42].

9.2.3.1.8.2 Montelukast *In vitro* dissolution data was coupled with PBPK modeling to study the performance between adult and pediatric formulations of montelukast (case-study 1) and the effect delivery vehicles (i.e., apple sauce, formula) had on drug exposure in infants (case-study 2) [43]. Dissolution studies were performed in multiple USP apparatus using both adult and pediatric biorelevant media [44]. Simcyp™ software V18.2 (Certara®, UK) was used to build the PBPK models with the Simcyp™ pediatric module utilized for pediatric simulations. In case-study 1, dissolution profiles (adult and pediatric) from Singulair® chewable tablets (Merck Sharp & Dohme Ltd, UK) were obtained using a μDISS profiler™ and incorporated into the PBPK model as direct dissolution profiles. The models were able to successfully predict the plasma concentration-time profiles in adults and children. The focus of the case-study 2 was how co-administration of medicine with different vehicles would affect drug exposure in infants. Dissolution was conducted using a USP IV apparatus where small amounts of applesauce or formula were mixed with Singulair® granules (Merck Sharp & Dohme Ltd, UK). The resulting simulated fasted gastric to fed intestinal dissolution profiles were directly applied to a fed-state PBPK model, achieving a good prediction of the *in vivo* performance of the formulation. The type of dissolution input within a model can have a large effect on the outputs, suggesting that the 'best' input may be different depending on drug physiochemical properties and formulation properties. Ultimately, these case studies demonstrate how the addition of *in vitro* dissolution profiles into a PBPK absorption modeling strategy can facilitate the prediction of drug formulation performance in pediatrics.

9.2.3.2 PBPK Model Conversion to the Cystic Fibrosis Population

Cystic fibrosis (CF) is the most common life-threatening recessively inherited disease in Caucasians. The disease is caused by genetic lesions in the *CFTR* (CF transmembrane conductance regulator) gene that encodes a protein that mainly functions as the most predominant chloride channel in exocrine epithelia [45]. Under normal circumstances, the *CFTR* gene undergoes transcription and is translated into a CFTR protein that traffics to the cell membrane where it fully functions as a chloride channel. In CF, the majority of CFTR mutations involve changes in three or fewer nucleotides and result in amino acid substitutions, frameshifts, splice site, or nonsense mutations. The most common and first identified mutation, the F508del, corresponds to a three-base pair deletion that codes for phenylalanine at position 508 of the CFTR protein. It is the presence of the F508del mutation that increases the frequency of CF in the Caucasian population relative to other races. Yet, presently over 1,900 different CFTR mutations have been identified [46]. CF mutations can disrupt CFTR function through a variety of mechanisms, ranging from complete loss of protein synthesis to normal apical membrane expression of a protein with poor chloride conductance [47]. The basic defect in CF cells is the faulty chloride transport which causes dehydration of secretions with hyper-viscous mucus and leads to chronic airway obstruction, pancreatic insufficiency, and intestinal malabsorption [46]. Owing to early referral to specialized, multidisciplinary reference centers for CF, and more comprehensive care, survival has improved over time [46]. Therefore, they may face other comorbidities during their lifetime, like inflammatory conditions and infections. However, patients with CF are excluded from clinical trials because of concerns about potential adverse impacts arising from comorbidities and concomitant medications, even though they may use the new drug under evaluation if it is approved. In other words, CF patients are underrepresented in clinical trials for new drugs not targeting CF. Much attention has been paid to the internal validity of a clinical trial, i.e., the extent to which the design and conduct of a trial eliminates the possibility of bias. High internal validity is necessary to unequivocally link observed clinical responses to the tested intervention but it does not address the generalizability (i.e., external validity) of the causal relationship to patients other than those in the original study population [48].

This is further complicated when the comorbidities also affect the GI tract and, thus, oral drug absorption. CF does alter the intraluminal environment of the SI [49]. For example, a significant delay in the small intestinal transit and a deficient buffering capacity required to neutralize gastric acid in the proximal small bowel of CF patients has been demonstrated [50]. These deficiencies have the potential to impair the intraluminal dissolution rate of modified-release formulations and immediate-release formulations containing poorly soluble drugs [51], with a consequent impact on oral absorption. Since there might be endless permutations of physiological and disease-related conditions to be studied *in vivo*, integrating *in vitro* to *in vivo* extrapolation (IVIVE) techniques and PBPK modeling to investigate drug- or formulation-disease interactions would be a useful approach to optimize drug therapy in underrepresented patient populations.

9.2.3.2.1 Example of CF PBPK Model

9.2.3.2.1.1 Ibuprofen In this context, an *in vitro-in silico-in vivo* framework to investigate the feasibility of extrapolating the safety and efficacy profiles of ibuprofen (as summarized in the approved therapeutic dosing recommendations) to febrile children with CF has been applied [52]. In this proof-of-concept research, first, an IVIVE-PBPK model was developed for oral ibuprofen in healthy adults. After confirming that the model was able to recapitulate the oral ibuprofen PK in adults, all drug-specific parameters in the model were kept and the system-parameters were changed to represent a pediatric population (8 and 11 years old). The system component of the pediatric PBPK model was set using the Simcyp™ Pediatric population database. For the mechanistic absorption model, pediatric age-specific parameters were included for salivary flow, gastric pH, GE (and associated food effects), and duodenal bile salt concentrations. For other parameters, there was either evidence of no age-related changes or a lack of data, so adult values were applied instead. Allometric scaling was applied based on a reference body weight of 70 kg and with exponents for clearance and organ blood flow as 0.75 and 1.0, respectively. After verifying the model performance, the drug-specific parameters were kept and the system component was adjusted to better predict the pathogenesis of CF. Briefly, duodenal and proximal jejunum pH values ranging from 4 to 5.5 are the most prevalent GI symptoms in patients with CF, as opposed to pH values of 6.4 to 6.8 in healthy subjects [50]. Also, a 10-fold lower duodenal bicarbonate concentration was observed in patients with CF in comparison to healthy subjects [53]. Drug metabolism mediated by uridine 5′-diphospho-glucuronosyltransferase (UGT) seems to increase in CF patients, but a mechanistic understanding of this observation is still lacking [54]. All these disease-related components were factored into the model. The resulting CF-PBPK model was able to predict the oral ibuprofen PK in CF pediatric patients, with simulated to observed AUC and C_{max} ratios falling within a 1.25-fold error. The CF-PBPK model was further linked to an antipyretic model and simulations suggested that changing dosing rate rather than the dose may lead to an improved antipyretic response in CF children [54]. This proof-of-concept research illustrates the usefulness of using disease-based PK/PD modeling to assess drug efficacy in underrepresented populations. Since enrolling all possible patient subsets in controlled clinical trials seems unfeasible, shifting the regulatory paradigm from empirical one-size-fits-all criteria toward model-informed approaches, leveraging tailored *in vitro* DMPK studies and clinical knowledge may play a key role to extrapolate the efficacy and safety to underrepresented populations.

9.2.3.3 PBPK Model Conversion to the Down Syndrome Population

Down Syndrome (DS) is the most common chromosomal condition associated with intellectual disability and is characterized by a variety of additional clinical findings. It occurs in approximately 1 of 800 births worldwide. A gene dosage hypothesis, which includes both the direct effects of overexpressed human chromosome 21 genes (HSA21) and the downstream consequences of this overexpression has been proposed to explain the phenotypic manifestations of DS [55]. The simplest effect of trisomy 21 (Ts21) is the direct effect of an increased dosage on a single HSA21 gene. For example, an increased dosage of APP, an HSA21 gene that encodes amyloid precursor protein (APP), increases susceptibility to early-onset Alzheimer's disease in individuals with DS. Although APP is clearly an 'effector' gene, whether only the direct and downstream effects of APP overexpression affect the penetrance and severity of Alzheimer's disease, or whether other aspects of Ts21 also have a role, remains to be determined. Furthermore, Ts21 may also affect global transcription, either directly if an HSA21 gene functions in transcription regulation or indirectly as a by-product of the additional genetic material [56]. Differential gene expression in a pair of monozygotic twins discordant for Ts21 (post-mortem) was assessed and it was identified that genes related to phase II

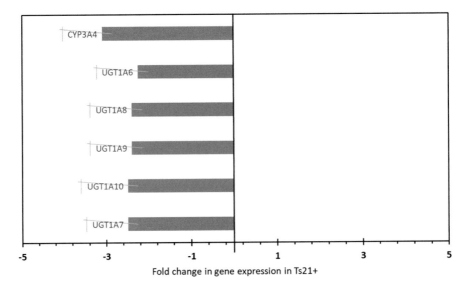

Figure 9.2 Fold change in gene expression in a pair of monozygotic twins discordant for Ts21. (Plot generated from reported supplementary data [56].)

drug-metabolizing UDP glucuronosyltransferases (e.g., UGT1A6, UGT2B7, UGT1A8, UGT1A9, etc.) and even CYP3A4 enzyme are significantly down-regulated in DS (Figure 9.2), which may affect drug metabolism and exposure in such patients.

However, at present, there is no clear understanding whether alterations in gene expression measured at the transcript level might reflect alterations in protein levels and enzyme functionality [57].

9.2.3.3.1 Prediction of Intestinal and Hepatic Metabolic Clearance

Currently, there is scant research that considers pharmacotherapy in subjects with DS and many chronic conditions they commonly face, especially as they age [58]. Guiding patient stratification and individual dosing will therefore crucially require quantitative characterization, beyond genetics, of hepatic and intestinal enzymes in individual patients [59]. As access to tissue biopsies is limited [60], integrating human stem cell technology (e.g., human induced pluripotent stem cell (iPSC) lines derived from minimally invasive skin biopsy) and organotypic modeling may offer an alternative pathway to inform precision dosing (Figure 9.3).

The caveat of this approach is that deriving liver organoids from human iPSCs remains rather challenging as a harmonized differentiation protocol is still not available and current reports describe a rather immature phenotype of induced pluripotent stem cell (iPSC)-derived hepatocytes [61]. Since many hepatic drug-metabolizing enzymes are also expressed by enterocytes, one may use intestinal organoids as a surrogate model to assess patient-specific enzyme activity. Current approaches for bottom-up prediction of intestinal and hepatic metabolic clearance, including biologically associated variability, are based on the assumption that enzyme activity is proportional to specific protein abundance. Enzyme kinetics can be described by the following equation:

$$E + S \xleftrightarrow{\ k_{diss}\ } ES \xrightarrow{\ k_{cat}\ } E + P$$

where E=enzyme concentration, S=substrate concentration, k_{diss}=dissociation constant, k_{cat}=catalytic efficiency of a given enzyme and P=product of the enzymatic reaction. In this context, $k_{cat}=V_{max}/E$ and thus, Michaelis-Menten parameters (V_{max} and K_m) derived using certain gut enzyme(s) can be used together with respective enzyme abundance to estimate intestinal and liver metabolism by the same enzyme(s) and vice versa. This relationship has been demonstrated in a study using matched human liver and intestinal microsomes [62]. A linear correlation between hepatic and intestinal intrinsic clearance values for CYP3A4 was found (Figure 9.4) [62].

Therefore, it is hypothesized that the ratio between intestinal V_{max} estimated in DS intestinal organoids/non-DS intestinal organoids could be useful to calibrate/scale enzyme protein

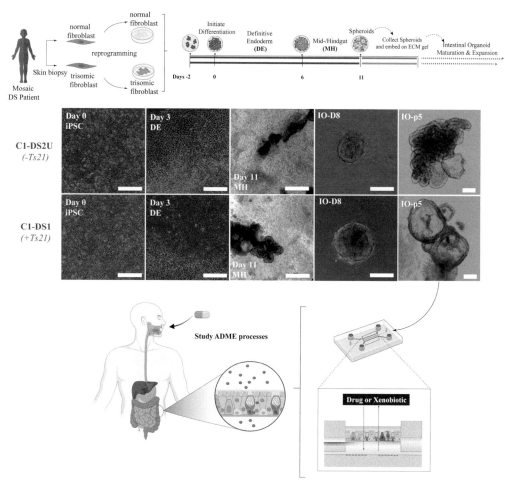

Figure 9.3 Generation of Intestinal Organoids from iPSCs emulating monozygotic twins discordant for Ts21.

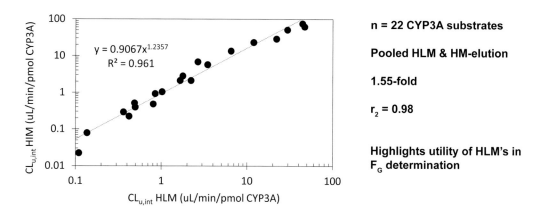

Figure 9.4 Comparison of CL_{uint} (µL/min/pmol of CYP3A) from HLM (mean±S.D., $n=3$) and HIM for 22 drugs. Dashed line indicates a bias of 1.55-fold deviation from unity. (Plot generated from reported data [62].)

171

abundance in DS patients compared to non-DS individuals. Since liver and intestinal enzymes are encoded by the same master transcription factor, the pregnane X-receptor (PXR), the estimated scaling factor in intestinal organoids could be used to calibrate the respective enzyme protein abundance in the liver. Then, hepatic metabolism/clearance could be calculated using PBPK modeling [63]. If successful, this approach can establish a translational tool to inform precision dosing of metabolically cleared drugs in DS patients as long as the enzyme is expressed in the gut and liver.

When a robust protocol to derive hepatocytes from iPSCs is developed, translational research would be able to develop matched liver and intestinal organoids, which could be of paramount importance to move toward individualized dosing in special populations using IVIVE-PBPK modeling.

9.3 EMERGING TOOLS TO STUDY DRUG TRANSPORT AND METABOLISM IN SPECIAL POPULATIONS

Evaluating the pharmacological characteristics of a drug candidate is critical during lead selection and optimization. The unique physiological, developmental, and pathological differences in populations such as pediatric, geriatric, or individuals with rare genetic disorders complicate studying drug absorption, distribution, metabolism, and excretion (ADME). Obtaining biological samples from these populations is extremely difficult for several reasons, including the invasive nature of procedures required for sample collection and the rarity of the disorder. While animal models have traditionally been used in pharmaceutical research to study drug transport and metabolism, they fail to adequately replicate human genetics, developmental stages, and the wide inter-individual phenotypic variability in humans [64]. These challenges have fueled the utilization of alternative *in vitro* platforms for studying ADME in special populations.

9.3.1 Defining Microphysiological Systems (MPS) and Organoids

Organoids and MPS are becoming promising avenues to study ADME in special populations. Both organoids and MPS are three-dimensional *in vitro* models that closely mimic the physiological conditions of human organs. Organoids are 3D miniature tissues generated *in vitro* from stem cells or tissue samples, and they mimic the structure and functionality of the organ of interest. MPS are a fusion of cell biology with bio-electromechanical systems (BioMEMs) engineering, surface chemistry, and mechatronics, to replicate basic organ functions within a microfluidic device often called 'organ-on-a-chip.' In other words, the final platforms commonly incorporate cells cultured on advanced electronic tools such as microelectrode arrays, and mechanical systems like microcantilever arrays, that enable non-invasive functional assessments of cell or drug response and toxicity. The complexity of the system varies according to the research questions. Organoids can be either integrated into microfluidic devices to create MPS that model specific tissue/organs or these two technologies can be used separately. Also, MPS can be designed to incorporate various tissue/organ systems to investigate the impact of drugs or disease conditions on multiple organs in a controlled setting [65]. Integrating organoids, MPS, and iPSC technology to generate patient-specific *in vitro* models provides cost-effective and disease-specific platforms for ADME studies.

9.3.2 Designing Accurate Biomimetic MPS for ADME Studies

MPS design aspects such as fluid movement, shear stress, and biomaterial properties are crucial to achieve an accurate biomimetic representation of native tissue/organ. For instance, surface modification and coating with extracellular matrix (ECM) are key factors in the replication of the cellular microenvironment. The composition of the ECM, the mechanical properties, and the source (e.g., animal, human, synthetic) affect cellular behavior. Several biomaterial systems are used in MPS including decellularizing animal tissue, hydrogel systems, and cell-derived matrices [66,67]. All these biomaterial systems have advantages and disadvantages. While decellularized animal tissues preserve the complex composition of native ECM, the impact of xenogenic material on human cells is a frequent concern regarding the clinical translation of the results. On the other side, hydrogel systems are not xenogeneic and offer great flexibility to match tissue stiffness and viscosity, yet they might require higher supplementation of growth factors for an efficient cell culture microenvironment. Altogether, MPS is a promising tool in pharmaceutical research, and it represents an even more powerful tool when talking about special populations.

9.3.3 Examples of MPS and Organoid Models

9.3.3.1 *Example of MPS and Organoids Model of Genetic Disorders*

MPS and organoids are also beneficial for ADME studies in populations affected by genetic disorders. Specifically, combining MPS with iPSCs and gene editing technology is particularly useful to generate isogenic cells from the same disease patient but with the corrected genetic variant as a control group. MPS made using these isogenic control iPSCs help to better distinguish the contribution of the pathogenic genetic variants to the disease progression and therapeutic effect of new molecules. For disorders associated with several pathogenic genetic variants, it is difficult to recruit patients who are representative of all these variants during clinical studies; however, it is feasible to generate *in vitro* MPS and organoid models representing a wider range of genetic variants which can significantly improve the ability to predict ADME characteristics in these populations. For instance, given that there are over 1,000 pathogenic variants in the CFTR gene leading to cystic fibrosis, it is not feasible to enroll all groups of patients in clinical trials. However, the *in vitro* efficacy of Kalydeco® (ivacaftor) was assessed using an MPS representative of a wide range of the variants and it supported the drug approval and label indications [68] which proves the impactful potential of MPS and organoids for ADME studies.

9.3.3.2 *Example of MPS and Organoids for Liver Toxicity Studies*

The metabolic clearance, frequently assayed during ADME studies, is a critical parameter for predicting human dosing projections, which are used to move a compound from pre-clinical testing to early clinical trial plans. Primary cells like hepatocytes are widely used to study metabolism-based clearance; however, hepatocytes lose the metabolic function capacity over time in culture [69]. MPS platforms capable of replicating liver functions have been developed and have been used to obtain critical parameters of ADME studies and additional toxicity investigations. For instance, a liver-on-chip platform with bio-printed hepatic spheroids that remained functional during 30 days of continuous culture has been developed. The utility of the platforms was validated by testing acetaminophen toxicity and comparing the results with previous animal studies [70]. Additionally, a multi-organ human-on-a-chip system that recapitulates primary aspects of the *in vivo* crosstalk between heart and liver enables evaluation of drug's cardiotoxicity, hepatotoxicity, and their metabolites [71].

9.3.3.3 *Potentials of Organotypic Model of DS*

The combination of organoid, MPS, and iPSC technologies could help to tackle the challenges associated with DS pre-clinical studies. For instance, as shown in Figure 9.3, human iPSC derived from mosaic DS patients can be leveraged to generate *in vitro* intestinal organoids emulating monozygotic twins discordant for Ts21 (+Ts21, Line C1-DS1 and isogenic control C1-DS2U). Then, these organoids could be used to investigate the impact of Ts21 on gut development (e.g., malformations) and homeostasis (e.g., drug-metabolizing enzyme activity, intestinal epithelium integrity, and secretion of endogenous antimicrobial peptides and inflammatory cytokines). Also, DS organoids could be integrated into an MPS with modules replicating multi-organ interaction, such as the gut-brain axis. A gut-brain MPS representative of DS can facilitate not only answering mechanistic questions related to the gut-brain axis in DS, but also studying ADME characteristics of therapeutic molecules.

9.3.4 MPS for Drug Transport, Metabolism, and Toxicity Studies: Current Challenges

Currently, a challenge that hinders MPS adoption includes the widespread use of polydimethylsiloxane (PDMS), which is known to bind to some classes of molecules [72]. Several other polymers are currently being explored, and some, like oly(methyl methacrylate) PMMA show promise as the small molecules cannot infiltrate the material [73,74]. Another challenge is associated with the diversity of design and formats of current academically generated chips, which makes it difficult to incorporate them into automated platforms and industry workflows [75]. As commercial providers of these technologies drive an increase in availability and easy-to-operate designs, end-users will speed up the validation of these models for ADME studies.

9.4 FUTURE PERSPECTIVES

Improvement of physiological relevance using *in vitro* systems such as MPS and organoids is expected to improve the predictive capabilities for efficacy and toxicity of test compounds.

Ensuring the reliability, reproducibility, and relevance of MPS is paramount to "gaining confidence" in the drug development industry for ADME studies.

While the combination of *ex vivo* methodology with PBPK modeling is a promising tool to predict oral drug disposition in special populations, the validation of these models using *in vivo* PK and/or phenotyping studies is needed. Validation of a wide range of compounds might be able to establish a workflow for successful *in vitro* to *in vivo* translation.

In recent years, progress has been made in coupling simple biorelevant *in vitro* methods with PBPK modeling to evaluate the impact of the physiology of GI tract of special populations on the performance of oral medicines. In some scenarios, these methods can be limited, for example in the prediction of the performance of complex formulations, where factors such as hydrodynamics and food digestion need to be considered. Limited work has been performed so far using more complex *in vitro* systems such as the TNO model (e.g., TIM-1 and tiny-TIM) in special populations. These compartmental, dynamic *in vitro* models mimic closely the GI tract and can provide assessment of oral drug absorption in special populations if adapted with patient-specific information on the GI tract. As these complex *in vitro* models become more widely applied toward predicting drug absorption in patient-specific populations, there will be an opportunity for coupling this knowledge toward enhancing the predictive capability of PBPK models.

Overall, conducting high-quality clinical studies in special populations will be crucial to further characterize the specific physiological traits encumbered to each population. This additional knowledge will pin-point the development and optimization of the *in vitro* and the *in silico* models (i.e., PBPK models) for a higher accuracy in prediction.

ACKNOWLEDGMENT

Funding has been received from Horizon 2020 Marie Sklodowska-Curie Innovative Training Networks programme (grant agreement No. 674909) and the Bill and Melinda Gates Foundation.

REFERENCES

1. Rowland M, Peck C, Tucker G. Physiologically-based pharmacokinetics in drug development and regulatory science. *Annual Review of Pharmacology and Toxicology.* 2011;51(1):45–73.

2. Administration US FDA. Clinical pharmacology. Guidance for Industry. Physiologically based pharmacokinetic analyses-format and content, 2018 [Available from: https://www.fda.gov/downloads/drugs/guidancecomplianceregulatoryinformation/guidances/ucm531207.pdf].

3. Agency EM. Guideline on the reporting of physiologically based pharmacokinetic (PBPK) modelling and simulation, 2018 [Available from: https://www.ema.europa.eu/en/documents/scientific-guideline/guideline-reporting-physiologically-based-pharmacokinetic-pbpk-modelling-simulation_en.pdf].

4. Wagner C, Zhao P, Pan Y, Hsu V, Grillo J, Huang SM, et al. Application of physiologically based pharmacokinetic (PBPK) modeling to support dose selection: Report of an FDA public workshop on PBPK. *CPT: Pharmacometrics & Systems Pharmacology.* 2015;4(4):226–30.

5. Cheeti S, Budha NR, Rajan S, Dresser MJ, Jin JY. A physiologically based pharmacokinetic (PBPK) approach to evaluate pharmacokinetics in patients with cancer. *Biopharmaceutics & Drug Disposition.* 2013;34:141–54.

6. Johnson TN, Boussery K, Rowland-Yeo K, Tucker GT, Rostami-Hodjegan A. A semi-mechanistic model to predict the effects of liver cirrhosis on drug clearance. *Clinical Pharmacokinetics.* 2010;49(3):189–206.

7. Edginton AN, Willmann S. Physiology-Based Simulations of a Pathological Condition Prediction of Pharmacokinetics in Patients with Liver Cirrhosis. *Clinical Pharmacokinetics.* 2006;47(11):743–52.

8. Rowland-Yeo K, Aarabi M, Jamei M, Rostami-Hodjegan A. Modeling and predicting drug pharmacokinetics in patients with renal impairment. *Expert Review of Clinical Pharmacology.* 2011;4(2):261–74.

9. Edginton AN, Schmitt W, Willmann S. Development and evaluation of a generic physiologically based pharmacokinetic model for children. *Clinical Pharmacokinetics*. 2006;45(10):1013–34.

10. Chetty M, Johnson TN, Polak S, Salem F, Doki K, Rostami-Hodjegan A. Physiologically based pharmacokinetic modelling to guide drug delivery in older people. *Advanced Drug Delivery Reviews*. 2018;135:85–96.

11. Schlender JF, Meyer M, Thelen K, Krauss M, Willmann S, Eissing T, et al. Development of a whole-body physiologically based pharmacokinetic approach to assess the pharmacokinetics of drugs in elderly individuals. *Clinical Pharmacokinetics*. 2016;55(12):1573–89.

12. Dallmann A, Solodenko J, Ince I, Eissing T. Applied Concepts in PBPK modeling: How to extend an open systems pharmacology model to the special population of pregnant women. *CPT: Pharmacometrics & Systems Pharmacology*. 2018;7(7):419–31.

13. Ghobadi C, Johnson TN, Aarabi M, Almond LM, Allabi AC, Rowland-Yeo K, et al. Application of a systems approach to the bottom-up assessment of pharmacokinetics in obese patients. *Clinical Pharmacokinetics*. 2011;50(12):809–22.

14. Darwich AS, Pade D, Ammori BJ, Jamei M, Ashcroft DM, Rostami-Hodjegan A. A mechanistic pharmacokinetic model to assess modified oral drug bioavailability post bariatric surgery in morbidly obese patients: Interplay between CYP3A gut wall metabolism, permeability and dissolution. *Journal of Pharmacy and Pharmacology*. 2012;64(7):1008–24.

15. Grimstein M, Yang Y, Zhang X, Grillo J, Shiew-Mei Huang, Zineh I, et al. Physiologically based pharmacokinetic modeling in regulatory science: An update from the U.S. Food and Drug Administration's Office of Clinical Pharmacology. *Journal of Pharmaceutical Sciences*. 2019;108:21–5.

16. Heimbach T, Chen Y, Chen J, Dixit V, Parrott N, Peters SA, et al. Physiologically-based pharmacokinetic modeling in renal and hepatic impairment populations: A pharmaceutical industry perspective. *Clinical Pharmacology & Therapeutics*. 2021;110(2):297–310.

17. Johnson TN, Bonner JJ, Tucker GT, Turner DB, Jamei M. Development and applications of a physiologically-based model of paediatric oral drug absorption. *European Journal of Pharmaceutical Sciences*. 2018;115:57–67.

18. Jamei M, Abrahamsson B, Brown J, Bevernage J, Bolger MB, Heimbach T, et al. Current status and future opportunities for incorporation of dissolution data in PBPK modeling for pharmaceutical development and regulatory applications: OrBiTo consortium commentary. *European Journal of Pharmaceutics and Biopharmaceutics*. 2020;155:55–68.

19. GastroPlus - PBPK modeling software...from discovery through development, 2016.

20. Maharaj AR, Barrett JS, Edginton AN. A workflow example of PBPK modeling to support pediatric research and development: Case study with lorazepam. *The AAPS Journal*. 2013;15(2):455–64.

21. Cristofoletti R, Charoo NA, Dressman JB. Exploratory investigation of the limiting steps of oral absorption of fluconazole and ketoconazole in children using an in silico pediatric absorption model. *Journal of Pharmaceutical Sciences*. 2016;105(9):2794–803.

22. SimulationsPlus. Applications and Considerations of Drug Exposure Predictions in Pediatric Populations Using GastroPlus. In: Lukacova V, editor. GastroPlus User Group Webinar. YouTube, 2015.

23. Kohlmann P, Stillhart C, Kuentz M, Parrott N. Investigating oral absorption of carbamazepine in pediatric populations. *The AAPS Journal*. 2017;19(6):1864–77.

24. Edginton AN, Ritter L. Predicting plasma concentrations of bisphenol A in children younger than 2 years of age after typical feeding schedules, using a physiologically based toxicokinetic model. *Environmental Health Perspectives.* 2009;117(4):645–52.

25. Villiger A, Stillhart C, Parrott N, Kuentz M. Using physiologically based pharmacokinetic (PBPK) modelling to gain insights into the effect of physiological factors on oral absorption in paediatric populations. *The AAPS Journal.* 2016;18(4):933–47.

26. Reflection paper on the use of extrapolation in the development of medicines for paediatrics - Draft. London, United Kingdom: European Medicines Agency; 2017.

27. Goelen J, Farrell G, McGeehan J, Titman CM, Rattray NJW, Johnson TN, et al. Quantification of drug metabolising enzymes and transporter proteins in the paediatric duodenum via LC-MS/MS proteomics using a QconCAT technique. *European Journal of Pharmaceutics and Biopharmaceutics.* 2023;191:68–77.

28. Batchelor HK, Marriott JF. Paediatric pharmacokinetics: Key considerations. *British Journal of Clinical Pharmacology.* 2015;79(3):395–404.

29. Park JY, Yun H, Lee S-b, Kim HJ, Jung YH, Choi CW, et al. Comprehensive characterization of maternal, fetal, and neonatal microbiomes supports prenatal colonization of the gastrointestinal tract. *Scientific Reports.* 2023;13(1):4652.

30. Lee JJ, Price JC, Duren A, Shertzer A, Hannum III R, , Akita FA, et al. Ultrasound evaluation of gastric emptying time in healthy term neonates after formula feeding. *Anesthesiology.* 2021;134(6):845–51.

31. Guimarães M, Statelova M, Holm R, Reppas C, Symilllides M, Vertzoni M, et al. Biopharmaceutical considerations in paediatrics with a view to the evaluation of orally administered drug products - a PEARRL review. *Journal of Pharmacy and Pharmacology.* 2019;71(4):603–42.

32. Bonner JJ, Vajjah P, Abduljalil K, Jamei M, Rostami-Hodjegan A, Tucker GT, et al. Does age affect gastric emptying time? A model-based meta-analysis of data from premature neonates through to adults. *Biopharmaceutics & Drug Disposition.* 2015;36(4):245–57.

33. Van der Veken M, Aertsen M, Brouwers J, Stillhart C, Parrott N, Augustijns P. Gastrointestinal fluid volumes in pediatrics: A retrospective MRI study. *Pharmaceutics.* 2022;14(9):1935.

34. Bardwell C, Demellawy DE, Oltean I, Murphy M, Agarwal A, Hamid JS, et al. Establishing normal ranges for fetal and neonatal small and large intestinal lengths: Results from a prospective postmortem study. *World Journal of Pediatric Surgery.* 2022;5(3):e000397.

35. Weaver LT, Austin S, Cole TJ. Small intestinal length: A factor essential for gut adaptation. *Gut.* 1991;32(11):1321.

36. Maharaj AR, Edginton AN, Fotaki N. Assessment of age-related changes in pediatric gastrointestinal solubility. *Pharmaceutical Research.* 2016;33(1):52–71.

37. Galia E, Nicolaides E, Hörter D, Löbenberg R, Reppas C, Dressman JB. Evaluation of various dissolution media for predicting in vivo performance of class I and II drugs. *Pharmaceutical Research.* 1998;15(5):698–705.

38. Jantratid E, Janssen N, Reppas C, Dressman JB. Dissolution media simulating conditions in the proximal human gastrointestinal tract: An update. *Pharmaceutical Research.* 2008;25(7):1663–76.

39. Vertzoni M, Dressman J, Butler J, Hempenstall J, Reppas C. Simulation of fasting gastric conditions and its importance for the in vivo dissolution of lipophilic compounds. *European Journal of Pharmaceutics and Biopharmaceutics.* 2005;60(3):413–7.

40. Pawar G, Papadatou-Soulou E, Mason J, Muhammed R, Watson A, Cotter C, et al. Characterisation of fasted state gastric and intestinal fluids collected from children. *European Journal of Pharmaceutics and Biopharmaceutics.* 2021;158:156–65.

41. de Waal T, Brouwers J, Mols R, Hoffman I, Rayyan M, Augustijns P. Characterization of neonatal and infant enterostomy fluids. *International Journal of Pharmaceutics.* 2023;639:122943.

42. Statelova M, Holm R, Fotaki N, Reppas C, Vertzoni M. Successful extrapolation of paracetamol exposure from adults to infants after oral administration of a pediatric aqueous suspension is highly dependent on the study dosing conditions. *The AAPS Journal.* 2020;22(6):126.

43. Guimarães M, Vertzoni M, Fotaki N. Performance evaluation of montelukast pediatric formulations: Part II - a PBPK modelling approach. *The AAPS Journal.* 2022;24(1):27.

44. Guimarães M, Somville P, Vertzoni M, Fotaki N. Performance evaluation of montelukast pediatric formulations: Part I-age-related in vitro conditions. *The AAPS Journal.* 2022;24(1):26.

45. Kerem BS, Rommens JM, Buchanan JA, Markiewicz D, Cox TK, Chakravarti A, et al. Identification of the cystic fibrosis gene: Genetic analysis. *Science.* 1989;245(4922):1073–80.

46. Lubamba B, Dhooghe B, Noel S, Leal T. Cystic fibrosis: Insight into CFTR pathophysiology and pharmacotherapy. *Clinical Biochemistry.* 2012;45(15):1132–44.

47. Welsh MJ, Smith AE. Molecular mechanisms of CFTR chloride channel dysfunction in cystic fibrosis. *Cell.* 1993;73(7):1251–54.

48. Juhi P, Altman DG, Egger M. Systematic reviews in health care: Assessing the quality of controlled clinical trials. *British Medical Journal.* 2001;323(7303):42–46.

49. De Lisle RC, Borowitz D. The cystic fibrosis intestine. *Cold Spring Harbor Perspectives in Medicine.* 2013;3(9).

50. Gelfond D, Ma C, Semler J, Borowitz D. Intestinal ph and gastrointestinal transit profiles in cystic fibrosis patients measured by wireless motility capsule. *Digestive Diseases and Sciences.* 2013;58(8):2275–81.

51. Cristofoletti R, Hens B, Patel N, Esteban VV, Schmidt S, Dressman J. Integrating drug- and formulation-related properties with gastrointestinal tract variability using a product-specific particle size approach: Case example ibuprofen. *Journal of Pharmaceutical Sciences.* 2019;108(12):3842–47.

52. Cicali B, Long T, Kim S, Cristofoletti R. Assessing the impact of cystic fibrosis on the antipyretic response of ibuprofen in children: Physiologically-based modeling as a candle in the dark. *British Journal of Clinical Pharmacology.* 2020;86(11):2247–55.

53. Engjom T, Erchinger F, Lrum BN, Tjora E, Aksnes L, Gilja OH, et al. Diagnostic accuracy of a short endoscopic secretin test in patients with cystic fibrosis. *Pancreas.* 2015;44(8):1266.

54. Rey E, Tréluyer JM, Pons G. Drug disposition in cystic fibrosis. *Clinical Pharmacokinetics.* 1998;35(4):313–29.

55. Korenbergab JR, Chena XN, Schippera R, Suna Z, Gonskya R, Gerwehra S, et al. Down syndrome phenotypes: The consequences of chromosomal imbalance. *Proceedings of the National Academy of Sciences*. 1994;91(11):4997–5001.

56. Letourneau A, Santoni FA, Bonilla X, Sailani MR, Gonzalez D, Kind J, et al. Domains of genome-wide gene expression dysregulation in Down's syndrome. *Nature*. 2014;508(7496):345–50.

57. Greenbaum D, Colangelo C, Williams K, Gerstein M. Comparing protein abundance and mRNA expression levels on a genomic scale. *Genome Biology*. 2003;4(9):1–8.

58. Hefti E, Blanco JG. Pharmacotherapeutic considerations for individuals with Down syndrome. *Pharmacotherapy*. 2017 Feb;37(2):214–20.

59. Polasek TM, Shakib S, Rostami-Hodjegan A. Precision dosing in clinical medicine: Present and future. *Expert Review of Clinical Pharmacology*. 2018;11(8):743–6.

60. Prasad B, Achour B, Artursson P, Hop CECA, Lai Y, Smith PC, et al. Toward a consensus on applying quantitative liquid chromatography-tandem mass spectrometry proteomics in translational pharmacology research: A white paper. *Clinical Pharmacology and Therapeutics*. 2019;106(3):525–43.

61. Ardisasmita AI, Schene IF, Joore IP, Kok G, Hendriks D, Artegiani B, et al. A comprehensive transcriptomic comparison of hepatocyte model systems improves selection of models for experimental use. *Communications Biology*. 2022;5(1):1094.

62. Gertz M, Harrison A, Houston JB, Galetin A. Prediction of human intestinal first-pass metabolism of 25 CYP3A substrates from in vitro clearance and permeability data. *Drug Metabolism and Disposition*. 2010;38(7):1147–58.

63. Rostami-Hodjegan A, Tucker GT. Simulation and prediction of in vivo drug metabolism in human populations from in vitro data. *Nature Reviews Drug Discovery*. 2007;6(2):140–8.

64. Greek R, Menache A. Systematic reviews of animal models: Methodology versus epistemology. *International Journal of Medical Sciences*. 2013;10(3):206–21.

65. Skardal A, Murphy SV, Devarasetty M, Mead I, Kang HW, Seol YJ, et al. Multi-tissue interactions in an integrated three-tissue organ-on-a-chip platform. *Scientific Reports*. 2017;7(1):8837.

66. Hong Y, Koh I, Park K, Kim P. On-chip fabrication of a cell-derived extracellular matrix sheet. *ACS Biomaterials Science & Engineering*. 2017;3(12):3546–52.

67. Cao UMN, Zhang Y, Chen J, Sayson D, Pillai S, Tran SD. Microfluidic organ-on-A-chip: A guide to biomaterial choice and fabrication. *International Journal of Molecular Sciences*. 2023;24(4):3232.

68. Dekkers JF, Wiegerinck CL, De Jonge HR, Bronsveld I, Janssens HM, De Winter-De Groot KM, et al. A functional CFTR assay using primary cystic fibrosis intestinal organoids. *Nature Medicine*. 2013;19(7):939–45.

69. Smith CM, Nolan CK, Edwards MA, Hatfield JB, Stewart TW, Ferguson SS, et al. A comprehensive evaluation of metabolic activity and intrinsic clearance in suspensions and monolayer cultures of cryopreserved primary human hepatocytes. *Journal of Pharmaceutical Sciences*. 2012;101(10):3989–4002.

70. Bhise NS, Manoharan V, Massa S, Tamayol A, Ghaderi M, Miscuglio M, et al. A liver-on-a-chip platform with bioprinted hepatic spheroids. *Biofabrication*. 2016;8(1):014101.

71. Oleaga C, Riu A, Rothemund S, Lavado A, McAleer CW, Long CJ, et al. Investigation of the effect of hepatic metabolism on off-target cardiotoxicity in a multi-organ human-on-a-chip system. *Biomaterials*. 2018;182:176–90.

72. Toepke MW, Beebe DJ. PDMS absorption of small molecules and consequences in microfluidic applications. *Lab on a Chip*. 2006;6(12):1484–6.

73. Nguyen T, Jung SH, Lee MS, Park TE, Ahn SK, Kang JH. Robust chemical bonding of PMMA microfluidic devices to porous PETE membranes for reliable cytotoxicity testing of drugs. *Lab on a Chip*. 2019;19(21):3706–13.

74. Galateanu B, Hudita A, Biru EI, Iovu H, Zaharia C, Simsensohn E, et al. Applications of polymers for organ-on-chip technology in urology. *Polymers*. 2022;14(9):1668.

75. Junaid A, Mashaghi A, Hankemeier T, Vulto P. An end-user perspective on Organ-on-a-Chip: Assays and usability aspects. *Current Opinion in Biomedical Engineering*. 2017;1:15–22.

10 PBPK-Based Virtual Bioequivalence Trials to Guide Drug Development

Amitava Mitra, Jim Mullin, and Siri Kalyan Chirumamilla

10.1 INTRODUCTION

Bioequivalence (BE) studies are an integral part of clinical pharmacology strategy for drug development such as to support formulation changes in late-stage development (i.e. preapproval changes), manufacturing site change, dissolution specification changes, and to support SUPAC requirements during post-approval changes in a new drug application (NDA) [1–3] or abbreviated new drug application (ANDA) [4]. There are some differences in BE requirements from different regulatory agencies for immediate release (IR) products. According to European Medicines Agency BE guidance [5], a BE study should be conducted under fasting conditions as this is considered to be the most sensitive condition to detect a potential difference between formulations. For products that are recommended to be taken with food, the BE study should be conducted only under fed conditions [5]. In the US FDA guidance [4], fasting and fed studies might be needed for IR products. Exceptions can be made when the product is recommended to be taken only on an empty stomach. If the product is to be taken only with food, fasting and fed studies are recommended, except when there is safety concern with fasting administration. However, a review of BE guidelines from the regulatory agencies in Australia, Brazil, Canada, China, Chinese Taipei, the European Medicines Agency, Japan, Mexico, Singapore, South Korea, Switzerland, US FDA, and the World Health Organization show that by-and-large the approaches are similar [6]. The recommended bioequivalence study design is a randomized, single-dose, two-way crossover in healthy normal subjects.

Owing to the importance of BE studies in drug product development, successful application of physiological models, such as Physiologically-Based Biopharmaceutics Modelling (PBBM), to predict BE outcome (i.e. virtual BE or VBE) will be helpful in guiding formulation development based on mechanistic understanding of factors impacting drug absorption, streamline product development, design BE studies, and support biowaiver argument on a case-by-case basis. VBE is a powerful technique whereby a validated PBPK model can be applied to a population of virtual subjects that reflect the real-world variability of all physicochemical, physiologic, and formulation/dissolution input parameters. The result is a prediction of each subject's plasma and tissue concentration vs. time profiles, and population pharmacokinetic endpoints such as maximum concentration (C_{max}), exposure (AUC), and bioequivalence [7].

Biowaivers for BCS class I and III drugs have been a specific target application for virtual BE. Virtual BE provides a framework where one can utilize biopredictive dissolution, IVIVC, and validated PBPK models to predict whether or not a generic formulation is bioequivalent with a reference innovator product. The approach is now commonplace in the industry and is referenced in FDA guidance [8]. The main research now is to extend the VBE approach to poorly soluble drugs such as BCS class II. For acidic drugs with high solubility in the intestine, the WHO and EMA will accept virtual BE as evidence for biowaivers. Furthermore, published studies showing the usefulness of VBE for class II weakly basic drugs with precipitation in cases where stomach pH was modified have shown promise [9].

Setting clinically relevant dissolution specifications, developing a dissolution safe space, or supporting manufacturing or site-based transfers are some of the key applications of VBE. The concept of safe space has been described in detail in previous publications [10–12]. Safe space is defined as the boundaries demarcated by in vitro specifications (i.e., dissolution or, when applicable, other relevant drug product quality attributes), within which drug product variants are anticipated to be bioequivalent to one another [8,12].

In fact, recently published draft guidance references these applications and when and how they can be utilized [8]. The setting of dissolution specification using VBE allows one to mechanistically and rationally determine whether a tightened specification is necessary or if a less stringent specification is warranted based on the totality of the data and the bioequivalence prediction. The method has been shown valuable for many drug products [13,14]. Additionally, virtual BE has been shown to be predictive of site manufacturing changes [15]. For example, the outcome of bioequivalence of two different site batches of Etoricoxib tablets was demonstrated against a clinical BE study [16].

VBE is most valuable in later half of the development stages of a drug product to determine the likelihood of bioequivalence between different drug formulations or drug product manufacturing variants in Phase II, Phase III, and post approval. It is also a key tool used by many generic

DOI: 10.1201/9781003031802-10

companies to reverse engineer innovator products. The most common application of the method is to predict or assess the statistical likelihood of whether a specific pilot or full-scale pharmaceutical trial will pass/fail in showing bioequivalence between two or more formulation variants in parallel or crossover trials. Additionally, it is utilized to determine whether clinical studies are sufficiently powered to assess the question of bioequivalence given a specific sample size of a given population. One such example for ibuprofen shows how VBE can be applied to determine the likelihood of pass/fail and power of the study based on the number of subjects [17]. VBE is a key tool for rationally defining dissolution specifications or creating dissolution safe space for a formulation which can aid in regulatory submissions when submitting an NDA to regulatory agencies. This can give flexibility in manufacturing and show regulatory agencies you understand the link between the product's in vitro dissolution and the resulting in vivo exposure. VBE allows a framework to compare new formulations to a reference. As such, there are a few issues of utmost importance when performing VBE using PBPK models.

VBE is an important tool to look at various aspects of drug-drug interaction (DDI); this could be due to gastric pH mediated such as effect of proton pump inhibitor (PPI) or H2 receptor antagonist (H2RA), as well as CYP mediated DDI. The utility of VBE in the case of differing stomach pHs has been demonstrated with respect to weakly basic precipitating compounds such as ketoconazole and Posaconazole [9]. VBE for CYP mediated DDI is well positioned to help determine dosage adjustments necessary to provide bioequivalence with product in the absence of inhibitors or inducers. Recently, Hong et al. used virtual populations and bioequivalence to determine dosing regimens for codosing of ritonavir or nirmatrelvir-ritonavir with elexacaftor, tezacaftor, and ivacaftor for treatment of COVID-19 [18]. A study by Stader showed that virtual trials could be used to predict the DDI magnitudes in elderly patients with age-related comorbidities for midazolam, amilodipine, atorvastatin, rosuvastatin, and dolutegravir in combination with different perpetrators [19]. However, the accuracy of predictions for C_{max} and AUC was not always within the 1.25-fold bioequivalence limits, which again shows that challenges remain in accurately describing populations for various DDI applications [20]. The success of VBE depends on some key modelling aspects including but not limited to the choice of either mechanistic dissolution or IVIVC correlation, generation of realistic subjects and populations, application of physiologic variability from both inter- and intrasubject variabilities, and specific modifications for disease states. Therefore, we will discuss all these at length and provide details behind the various treatments in some commercial software packages. Once mechanistic modelling details are discussed, we will then get into the specific applications of VBE namely dissolution specification justification, formulation switch, biowaiver, and paediatric VBE.

Finally, we will discuss the gaps in VBE. There are currently limitations inherent in the PBPK approach given the lack of measured physiological variability especially related to intrasubject variability but also to a lesser extent intersubject variability. The current approach is to calibrate some of the unknown variabilities to clinical data. However, with improved physiological parameters for a multitude of intestinal and PBPK tissues, a priori predictions of these variabilities will improve. Additionally, advances in the field of paediatric and special population PBPK will accelerate effective exposure predictions for children and disease state patients within the industry. Improvements in the modelling approaches will lead to increasing acceptance and guidance from regulatory agencies. Currently, there is no harmony in the review or acceptance of VBE submissions among the different regulatory agencies. But as more knowledge and confidence in gained, this should be rectified which would significantly advance the field of VBE.

10.2 BUILDING VBE MODEL

10.2.1 Dissolution Input for Virtual BE

Dissolution data is an important aspect of virtual BE. The end goal of virtual BE is to determine if a reference formulation is bioequivalent with another formulation variant or a manufacturing variant in a clinically relevant population. Therefore, an accurate description of dissolution is key for the virtual BE simulation to be accurate. Dissolution of IR formulations can be predicted using mechanistic models like the Lu et al. [21] or Wang and Flannagan [19,22] models which are based on Noyes-Whitney model for the dissolution of solid drugs. While these models consider the impact of particle size distribution, diffusion layer thickness, solubility, fluid volume, diffusivity, density, and shape factor on the dissolution of drug along the intestinal tract, the changing of fluid volumes, pH, and bile salt concentrations, as the particles transit through the intestine effect the solubility of the drug and in turn the drug dissolution.

In vitro dissolution data can also be utilized to calculate the in vivo dissolution within the virtual BE framework for IR formulations. The z-factor model is a dissolution model that lumps all the relevant transport terms such as diffusivity, particle size, diffusion layer thickness, density, and particle shape into a fitted parameter, z [23], and its value is fit to in vitro dissolution data. Similarly, the diffusion layer model (DLM) scalar can be optimized to recover observed in vitro dissolution in cases where the Wang Flannagan dissolution model cannot predict the observed dissolution profile. This then begs the question: what type of in vitro dissolution data in what type of media should one use? The answer is complicated and is drug product/property-dependent. For neutral compounds and acids, the safe bet would be to use biorelevant media like FaSSIF because the solubility profiles of these molecules dictate that an IR drug product would dissolve in the upper intestine. If the drug is a base and the solubility is high in the gastric fluids at low pH, a gastric buffer dissolution may be sufficient to determine the z-factor and may be most indicative of the drug products dissolution. However, these generalizations should be treated with caution, and a case-by-case decision should be made depending on the properties of the drug substance and product. While excipients can also affect the dissolution, their effect could change with the pH of the medium; therefore, dissolution should be evaluated across a physiologically relevant pH range to determine what provides the most biorelevant dissolution. If excipients change the dissolution behaviour of a formulation at different pH values, one can define a z-factor vs. pH profile in most PBPK software packages. Therefore, one can account for pH-dependent dissolution of the IR formulation in more complex cases.

Weakly basic molecules and enabled formulations can exhibit supersaturation and crystallization in vivo. Precipitation is often the cause of clinical variability in exposure. Precipitation can be modelled as a first-order process or with a thermodynamics approach like a mechanistic nucleation and growth model [24]. Precipitation kinetics can be incorporated by fitting precipitation kinetics to in vitro data or vivo data. Many complex in vitro experiments have been devised to try to determine precipitation kinetics more accurately. Membrane dissolution, biphasic dissolution, TIM, and transfer dissolution experiments, like the artificial stomach duodenum (ASD), have all been devised to try to account for some of the aspects that affect precipitation such as absorption and transit/dilution. In vitro software tools like DDDPlus™ and SIVA from Simulations Plus, Inc. and Certara, Inc., respectively, exist to aide modellers in the determination of precipitation kinetics from in vitro experiments. Once precipitation kinetics are known, random variability can be added to the precipitation kinetic parameters in the population simulations to account for the variability introduced due to crystallization and high variability is often observed in these cases. While in vitro dissolution can be used as direct input by using empirical models such as Weibull function for VBE model development, the input dissolution will not be sensitive to the regional (between GI segments), between subject and within subject differences in the GI physiological parameters, thereby could lead to underestimation of intrasubject variability in the plasma PK parameters (C_{max} and AUC). Therefore, it is recommended to use semi-mechanistic models such as DLM or z-factor model to input dissolution data. However, for complex dosage forms where semi-mechanistic models are not yet available, the empirical models can be used. Figure 10.1 shows the considerations for selecting the dissolution input into VBE models.

Controlled release formulations present a different set of problems for virtual BE. Dissolution models in PBPK platforms are generally non-mechanistic in the case of controlled release. Dissolution is either defined directly as tabulated in vitro data or using a Weibull function that is fit to the in vitro data to calculate the release vs. time in the intestinal tract. Unfortunately, this usually doesn't work unless in vitro dissolution is the same as in vivo dissolution or the in vitro-in vivo correlation (IVIVC) is 1:1. This is usually not the case. Therefore, IVIVC is a necessary and a key step that needs to be considered. PBPK software packages provide different types of IVIVC models, but the mechanistic method is the recommended method as it has been shown to be superior to traditional methods like Wagner [25]. The mechanistic model consists of three main steps: deconvolution of in vivo dissolution, correlation between in vivo dissolution and in vitro dissolution, and convolution or prediction of plasma concentration using the IVIVC correlation. Deconvolution is the process of determining the in vivo dissolution that accurately represents the observed concentration time profile. This is typically performed by optimizing Weibull function parameters to approximate the best fit in vivo dissolution that predicts the plasma concentration profile. Correlation is then performed to find a transformation function of the form $y=f(x)$ where $f(x)$ is a function that takes the input x (in vitro dissolution) and calculates the corresponding in vivo dissolution y. This function can be linear, polynomial, power law, or a time shifting/scaling function. The development of the mechanistic IVIVC requires a validated PBPK model that incorporates

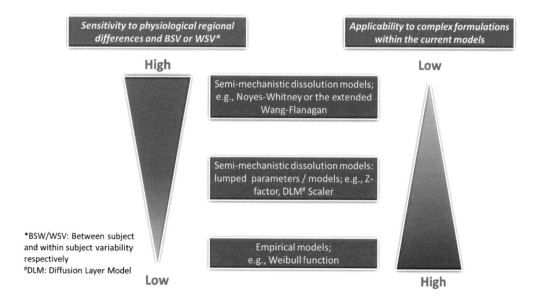

Figure 10.1 Factors effecting selecting dissolution data input for VBE. (Adapted from Ref. [26].)

all important absorption and disposition mechanisms. This generally requires some combination of IV, IR solution, or IR tablet PK data to ensure the model accounts for all mechanisms. Of course, all physicochemical properties are necessary at the outset of the model development process.

10.2.2 Generating Populations

For virtual BE to be utilized effectively, the population generation algorithms must be realistic and accurately describe clinical populations and subjects. Therefore, a population generator is necessary that can generate realistic subjects but also allows the user to constrain the generated population to match clinical demographics such as sex, height, weight, BMI, and age. There are two main approaches to define a population. The population can be sampled from a preexisting fixed database of real subjects, or they can be generated via statistical sampling algorithms that are tuned specifically to reproduce the global average and variance of a given population subject attributes. Once the age, weight, gender, disease state of the subject have been generated, the physiologic parameters such as tissue weights, blood flows, intestinal transit times, fluid volume, pH, bile salt concentrations, and enzyme expressions can be generated by the software. The physicochemical properties such as Fup, Rbp, permeability; and formulation parameters such as dose, particle size and/or dissolution rate must be determined based on all available literature information. The variability in all these parameters can be described by normal, log-normal, or uniform distribution and can be sampled with Monte Carlo approaches. The Population Estimates for Age-Related (PEAR) distribution method does consider covariation of parameters in the algorithm when they can be characterized based on literature information. Intrasubject variability can be applied to crossover trails to describe additional variability within the same subject after two subsequent doses of the same or different formulation.

In the Simcyp Simulator, with the exception of the Simcyp Population Representative (PopRep) option, all Simcyp simulations require the generation of a sample population which consists of a user-defined number of virtual individuals, divided into trial groups, exhibiting a range of physical and physiological characteristics and genotypes, the physical and physiological characteristics of the simulated population are described by the parameter values stored in the population libraries. Details of a trial population in terms of the number of individuals to include, their ages, gender and other demographic parameters are all specified by the user. Simcyp also provides the means to generate mixed populations whereby user-defined proportions of a trial population are made up of individuals generated from more than one population library. Thus, for example, a trial population may consist of 75% North European Caucasians and 25% Japanese – the disease libraries may also be sampled in this way if required. The virtual subjects are generated

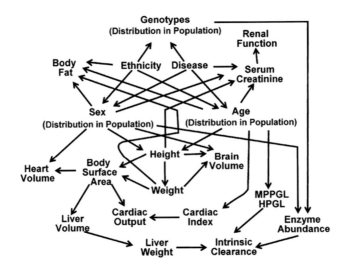

Figure 10.2 Inter-relationship between covariates used to generate virtual subjects in Simcyp Simulator. (Adapted from Ref. [28].)

considering complex framework of inter-relationship between covariates and variability between physiological parameters observed in populations. Figure 10.2 shows a part of the inter-relationship between covariates as incorpraoted in the Simcyp simulator. Any of the existing available population libraries can be used for virtual bioequivalence. This ability to select different populations in VBE studies to the healthy volunteers (which is generally used in clinical BE studies) helps in understanding the effect of populations on the BE outcome [27].

In a parallel VBE simulations, however, subjects are generated from the same population library, the subjects differ between each period and within period due to intersubject variability in the physiological parameters. However, it should be noted that intersubject variability should always be accounted for in BE simulations. Users can define the proportion of males and females and also the age range specific to the simulated period in line with the clinical BE protocol. The effect of population differences on the bioequivalence can also be simulated by selecting different populations in each period.

In a crossover VBE simulation, the subjects generated for the first period are reused in the following periods to be in line with the clinical BE where the same subjects are dosed across periods. However, the physiological parameters which usually change across periods in each subject are changed between periods using intrasubject (within subject) variability.

The generated population can either have fed (varying meal calories and fat content) or fasted state gut physiologies, these could be used for simulating either fed state or fasted state VBE studies. To simulate food effect BE study, fasted state physiology can be selected for the first period and fed state for the second period. In a fasted state clinical BE study though, subjects are fasted overnight food is provided to the subjects about 4 hours after dosing, the food intake after 4 hours of dosing could also have an impact on the systemic concentrations of the drug, these scenarios could be handled using the food staggering model where physiology changes from fasted to fed and fed to fasted can be simulated.

10.2.2.1 Algorithmic/Statistical Sampling Approach for Population Generation

The algorithmic approach for generating populations in GastroPlus is known as the Population Estimates for Age-Related (PEAR®) physiology method which leverages demographic data from government databases or literature papers, measured organ weights and perfusions, intestinal physiology data, and enzyme expression data to define a process for calculating virtual subjects from the bottom up. Other similar methods exist such as PopGen which uses similar frameworks [29]. The subjects generated are unique in that if the generator is run multiple times with the same input parameters, new subjects/populations will be generated each time. Subjects are not sampled from a predefined fixed database of subjects. There is an infinite set of populations that can be generated with the PEAR algorithm. The process the PEAR method utilizes follows the following steps.

■ User defines the population for the trial

- Gender (% male vs. female), age range, weight range, BMI range, ethnicity, and disease state.

■ Age and gender of the subject are randomly sampled from population specifications.

■ Based on the ethnicity, age, and gender, a bivariate height/weight distribution is sampled to determine realistic height and weight combination for each subject.

- If the subject defined is outside the defined population weight and BMI range the user selected, it is thrown out and a new subject is sampled from the distribution.

- There are separate bivariate distributions defined for male/female adults, adolescents, and paediatrics based on ethnicity.

■ Tissue weights and perfusions are calculated based on correlations with various parameters like age, body weight, height, body surface area, and BMI.

- Additional random variability is added based on a distribution (normal, log-normal, and uniform) and coefficient of variation (CV%).

■ Gastrointestinal model parameters are calculated based on subject parameters

- Additional random variability is added based on a distribution and coefficient of variation (CV%).

■ Formulation and drug parameters are sampled based on distribution and CV%.

Demographic data for subjects of various ethnicity comes from multiple sources. For Caucasian subjects, demographic data is from the NHANES 2003/2004 database [30]. Japanese subject populations are constructed based on the work of Ogiu et al. [31]. Chinese population data was collected from a multitude of sources including the China Health and Nutrition Survey [32]. Specific equations that produce each tissue weight or gastrointestinal parameter have not been published. However, it is important to give some level of validation for the population generation. As such, Figure 10.3 shows overlay of the bivariate height and weight distribution sampling algorithm in GastroPlus for male subjects of 20–67 years old with the real-world subject data from the NHANES database. The sampling algorithms produce populations that are highly realistic and reproduce real word data which make it a solid foundation for the calculation of all additional subject physiologic parameters.

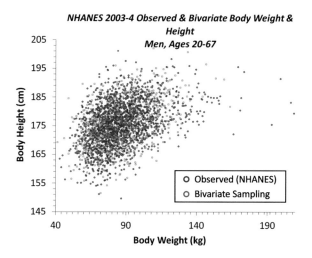

Figure 10.3 GastroPlus virtual population generation for male subjects 20–67 years age for $N = 1668$ subjects. (Dark blue circles correspond to NHANES observed data and light blue circles are bivariate population generator)

With an accurate reproduction of the most basic aspects of a population such as body height and weight, all other subject parameters such as tissue weights, perfusions, intestinal physiology and enzyme expression levels can be calculated. The GastroPlus population generator will use various covariates such as age, weight, height, body surface area, BMI, etc. to calculate specific aspects of the physiology like tissue sizes to ensure that the different tissues have realistic covariation. For instance, it is not possible for the population generator to create a tall subject which has small lungs or a small lean subject with a large liver. This fallacy keeps being reported in literature and podium presentations by uninformed researchers. One tissue that is very important toward predicting volume of distribution is the adipose. There is a wealth of dual energy X-ray absorbance measurements (DXA) in the NHANES database which can be used to calculate the body fat. When the DXA data is compared against GastroPlus PEAR population generation algorithm, very reasonable results are obtained as shown in Figure 10.4.

Liver weight is a very important tissue as it ultimately determines the amount of metabolic enzymes for a given subject. The GastroPlus PEAR population generator is able to recapitulate literature measurements of liver weight accurately as shown in Figure 10.5 [33]. This liver data is from the 1960s and 1970s and the GastroPlus algorithm at first glance would seem to be slightly overpredicting the liver weight but this is simply due to the increase in body weight in modern day American populations.

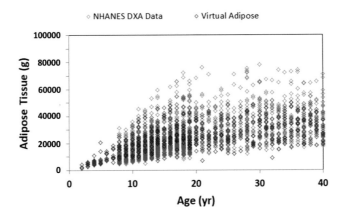

Figure 10.4 GastroPlus PEAR physiology adipose sampling vs. NHANES DXAm adipose measurements. (Blue circles correspond to NHANES DXA data and red circles the PEAR population generator)

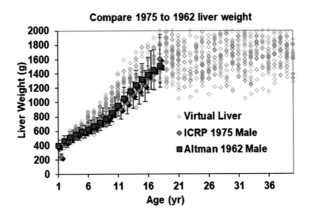

Figure 10.5 GastroPlus PEAR physiology liver weight sampling vs. literature measurements. (Green open diamonds correspond to GastroPlus PEAR population generator, red squares are data from Altman, and solid green diamonds are from ICRP measurements)

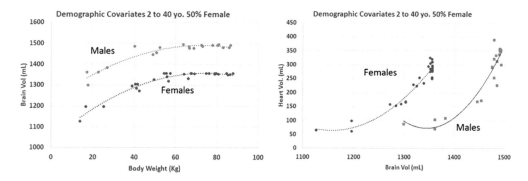

Figure 10.6 Example of GastroPlus virtual subject generated by PEAR algorithm showing physiologic covariates for body weight vs. brain volume and brain volume vs. heart volume for 2–40 year old 50/50% male/female subjects which shows it is not possible to generate non-realistic covariates like a large brain volume and low body weight or large brain volume and small heart volume.

Covariation of tissue sizes in the past has been a key point of contention with respect to Monte Carlo-based population sampling. The algorithm in GastroPlus does not simply randomly sample tissue sizes. Tissues are generated based on various equations which utilize covariate relationships and variability is added on top of these tissue weight calculations. Therefore, subjects generated with the PEAR population have the expected covariation present between different tissues with realistic variability. The covariation of brain volume, body weight and resulting covariation between heart volumes and brain volume are shown in Figure 10.6 for male and female subjects. Indeed, there are no subjects generated with large heart volumes and small brain sizes or even large brain size and small body weight. Again, this historic criticism is not well founded.

In the Simcyp Simulator, the patient population libraries have been built from public health databases, particularly the US NHANES database and census data produced by UK and Japanese government bodies, together with exhaustive meta-analyses of numerous literature sources. They incorporate numerical and statistical information on physiological parameters that impact upon drug disposition and effect. Many of these physiological variables are related to gender, age, body size, ethnicity, environmental effects – such as dietary habits or smoker/non-smoker status – and genetic differences in the enzymes and transporters responsible for drug handling. Simcyp includes the demographics of healthy populations and disease populations, such as those with renal disease or liver cirrhosis, so that simulations based on these virtual populations will be more reflective of the target patient population for relevant drugs. In addition to adult populations, Simcyp has a paediatric population database that allows predictions of pharmacokinetics in neonates, infants and children.

To generate a trial population with inter-individual differences, Monte-Carlo statistical sampling of a user-specified population library (e.g. Healthy Volunteer, General North European Caucasian, Renally Impaired, etc.) is undertaken. Thus, the initial step is the random selection of individuals by age. Age is then linked to height, weight, body surface area (BSA) and cardiac output, for example, and then from some of these values to further parameters such as organ volumes and so on, thus propagating covariation in a rational manner – thus Correlated-Monte Carlo methods are being used considering complex framework of inter-relationship between covariates and variability between physiological parameters observed in populations as shown in Figure 10.2. It is important to reiterate that physiological parameters are not varied independently. Rather the covariation of parameters is accounted for where they are known to exist and where such can be quantified. An example of the complexity of covariate effects involved in the calculation of hepatic drug clearance by Simcyp is given in Figure 10.7. At the base level, for example, there is a clear, strong correlation between age and height and also height and body weight.

While some relationships such as age-weight maybe intuitive, this is not always the case. For example, there are more complex temporal changes in liver weight with respect to body weight. Thus, wherever robust data are available, which may include relationships with low but statistically significant correlation, account is taken of the covariation of physiological parameters and variability is propagated across a population in a rational manner. This means that impossible combinations of parameters are not generated and virtual individuals match real people as closely

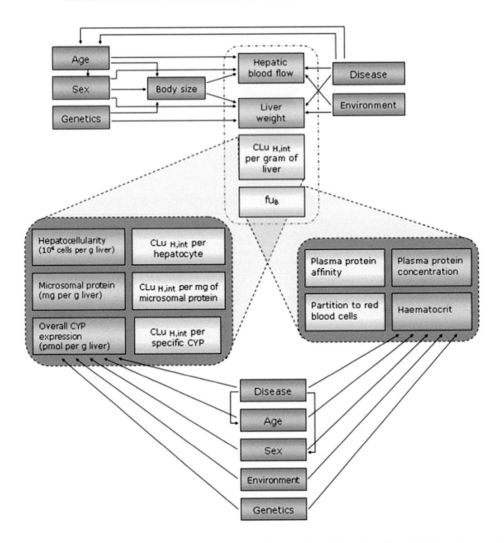

Figure 10.7 Influence of patient characteristic on chosen drug behaviour (hepatic drug clearance). (Adapted from Ref. [34].)

as possible. In addition, in the Simcyp Simulator, to reproduce an executed clinical BE study, the fixed individual trial option provides the flexibility to define each subject covariates such as age, weight, height, sex, serum creatinine, human serum albumin, haematocrit, CYP2D6 phenotype and smoking status which are measured in the clinical study, when these parameters are defined, virtual subjects are generated with the defined covariates.

10.2.3 Intrasubject Variability

Human physiology changes with time, while some physiological parameters change slowly over time, few change more frequently within the time frame of BE study duration. This change in the physiological parameters from one period to another may lead to a change in the way formulation dissolves and absorbs. For formulations that are sensitive to these physiological parameters, this could lead to differences in systemic exposure and PK parameters (C_{max}, AUC) in a crossover (non-replicate, partial replicate and full replicate) BE study, where formulation is dosed more than once in the same subject. This variability in PK parameters determines the extent of confidence intervals of Test/Reference (T/R) ratios in statistical BE analysis, therefore, accounting for intra-subject (within subject) variability in the physiological parameters is an essential aspect of VBE model development. Few of the physiological parameters relevant for oral dosage forms that could change between periods are listed below:

- GI tract fluid transit times

- GI tract formulation transit times

- Baseline Luminal pH - fasted and fed states

- Stomach fed pH - Time to return to fasted pH

- Luminal Bile Salts - fasted and fed states

- Baseline fluid Volumes - fasted and fed states

- Liver Enterohepatic Recirculation parameters

Intrasubject variability can be accounted for in virtual BE simulations by either resampling model input parameters that are known to vary upon dosing occasions, or randomly resampling the C_{max} and AUC of the BE simulation results according to the population intrasubject CV%. The first method is a mechanistic description that utilizes literature data to impart additional variability. In GastroPlus, parameters such as stomach and intestinal transit time, intestinal pH, luminal fluid volume, and bile salt concentration can be automatically resampled during a population simulation to account for physiological intrasubject variability that has been reported in the literature [35–38]. Gastroplus also includes Within-Batch Variability (WBV) for the formulation variables. Variability of particle size, dose, or in vivo dissolution via Weibull function is added to account for changes in dissolution within the same subject across multiple dosing occasions. Physiological parameters that should not be changing rapidly or that do not have any available literature data that can be used to specify distribution parameters such as tissue sizes, partition coefficients, intestinal length/radius, expression levels on enzymes and transporters, fraction unbound in plasma, and blood to plasma ratio are not adjusted between occasions. In the future, as more data becomes available in the literature, additional parameters will be incorporated with relevant distribution and CV% parameters so that more accurate representations of intrasubject variability can be predicted. This method can be used as a predictive tool when there is no clinical information regarding the intrasubject variability available. Or, the CV% parameters for intrasubject variables can be adjusted to match observed clinical intrasubject variability. Much the same as one modifies the CV% of population generation parameters to match observed variability.

The second method to account for intrasubject variability within GastroPlus is the resampling method. In this method you run a crossover study with two formulations and the software will resample the output (C_{max} and AUC) of the second formulation or simulation in the crossover study with user-defined variability or CV%. The CV% can be assumed or, more optimally, determined based on previous clinical data. In GastroPlus you can simulate the variability of C_{max} and AUC separately if your estimated intrasubject CV% is not constant between the two metrics. This method would be applicable if you have measured intrasubject variability data for both C_{max} and AUC.

In Simcyp simulator, the intrasubject variability is incorporated in addition to intersubject variability, where the physiological parameter value for an individual (τ_i) is generated from population mean and intersubject variability CV%, and parameter value for a particular period ($\tau_{i,k}$) is generated from individual mean (τ_i) and WSV CV% through sampling from the relevant distribution. Figure 10.8 shows the process of generating parameters in a VBE simulation.

The main challenge of incorporating intrasubject variability in the physiological parameters is the availability of observed intrasubject variability CV% values to use in the simulations. Some software platforms like the Simcyp Simulator provide a database of intersubject variability CV% for key GI tract parameters determined from meta-analysis of literature data where measurements are performed in subjects on more than one occasion. These values are currently not available for many GI tract parameters. Intrasubject variability CV% can also be estimated using population estimation algorithms in the Simcyp Simulator. In this approach, clinical PK profiles from replicated (partial or full) crossover studies are required. Other approaches to estimate plausible intrasubject variability in physiology parameters have been proposed in the literature, for example, Bego et al. established a pragmatic workflow that would describe more realistically the observed variation in the PK parameters [39]. In the absence of intrasubject variability CV% values, users can either follow a worst-case scenario (for the sponsor) where intrasubject variability values are set to be equal to respective BSV values of the physiological parameters or a blanket value of 30% [40].

Another source of variability leading to intrasubject variability in the test or reference formulations PK parameters (C_{max}, AUC) is the WBV in the formulations. This is the difference between dosage units (e.g., tablets or capsules) resulting from drug content differences (reflected

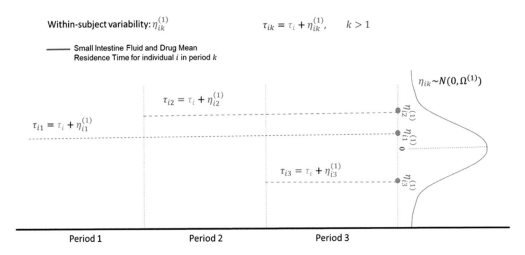

Figure 10.8 Example showing the generation of Small Intestinal Mean Residence Time (a GI tract parameter in the ADAM model), over various periods. τ_i- the individual mean value of subject i is added to $\eta_{ik} \sim N\left(0, \Omega^{(1)}\right)$ to get the individual value for period k. The correlation between parameters are not taken into account, hence $\Omega^{(1)}$ is a diagonal matrix.

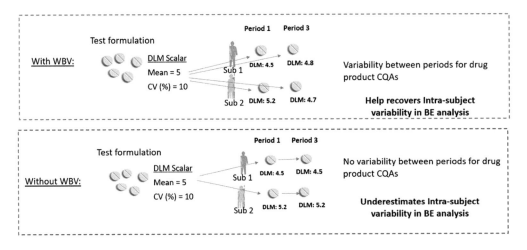

Figure 10.9 Schematic showing handling of within batch variability (WBV) in replicate crossover studies in Simcyp Simulator using test formulation as an example.

in uniformity of dosage units test), excipient content differences or process parameters resulting in for example hardness differences, this could lead to variability in dissolution between dosage units or precipitation differences between dosage units. In Simcyp simulator, this WBV is considered between periods in replicate (partial or full) VBE designs and between subjects in all BE designs (Figure 10.9).

10.3 APPLICATIONS OF VBE

10.3.1 Dissolution Specification Justification

The rate and extent of drug release from the drug product (e.g. tablet or capsule) in the body resulting in consistent in vivo performance (i.e. bioperformance) is an important critical quality attribute (CQA). Since measuring the rate and extent of drug release in vivo (i.e. in vivo dissolution) is impractical, this CQA is assessed via in vitro dissolution methods. Both FDA and EMA guidances [41,42] clearly mention the need for dissolution methods to be able to assess the in vivo performance, in addition to quality control, of the drug products. This goal leads to the concept of defining dissolution specification, which should be sensitive towards any product and/or manufacturing variables that could impact the in vivo performance of the drug product. Further, the dissolution specifications are typically only based on the release data from the products used in pivotal clinical trials, to ensure every commercial product batch performs according to the product label. However, sponsors also need to be careful to not develop overly sensitive dissolution methods and define unnecessarily tight specifications which could lead to unjustified dissolution failures and rejection of product batches. To overcome these seemingly discordant goals, the concept of clinically relevant dissolution specification (CRDS) [8] has been developed with the goal to support the dissolution specification by studying drug products with different in vitro dissolution profiles, representing a range of product variants, that may impact in vivo performance. Subsequently, a link between the clinical performance of the drug products, and dissolution specifications can be developed, and then the dissolution method is deemed 'clinically relevant'.

The development of CRDS for poorly soluble drugs (BCS 2 and BCS 4) can be particularly challenging, as several material attributes and process parameters might play a critical role in ensuring the appropriate drug product quality. In addition, the complex behaviour of poorly soluble drugs in the gastrointestinal tract requires the development of sensitive and often complicated dissolution methodologies to be able to correlate the in vitro data to in vivo performance. Mechanistic modelling approaches such as PBPK (or physiologically-based biopharmaceutics modelling, PBBM), is an indispensable toolset to build the in vitro to in vivo correlation for poorly soluble drugs. Once the PBPK model is appropriately built and verified, VBE approach can be used in the setting and justification of CRDS through the establishment of a dissolution safe space (Figure 10.10) [43], within which in vitro dissolution changes have no clinically relevant impact on in vivo performance i.e. PK, and subsequently on safety and/or efficacy of the product.

Alternatively, through PBPK the edge of dissolution failure can also be established, i.e. in vitro dissolution changes beyond which an unacceptable impact on PK is expected. A typical step-by-step approach to developing and verifying a PBPK model for VBE application is shown in Figure 10.11.

The dissolution profiles of the drug products generated using an adequately developed dissolution method are used as an input to the PBPK model to estimate in vivo dissolution in the various parts of the GI tract and predict human exposure. A model is usually set up to account for differences of dosage form transit, dissolution, local pH and bile salt concentrations in the GI tract, and fluid volumes available for dissolution. The inclusion of a human IV data enables the estimation

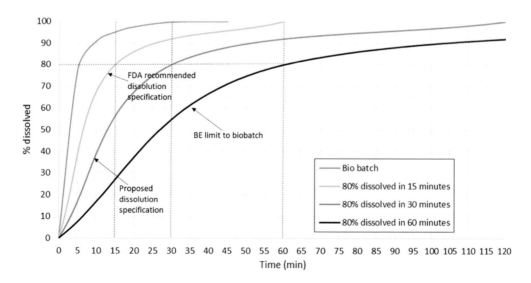

Figure 10.10 Dissolution specification justification using oral absorption modelling. Virtual BE modelling can be used to support the expansion of dissolution specification from 80% dissolved in 15 minutes to 80% dissolved in 30 minutes. (From Ref. [43].)

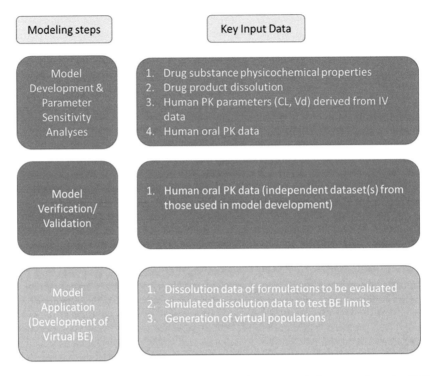

Figure 10.11 Schematic of PBPK/PBBM model development, validation and use in VBE.

of distribution and elimination parameters. The predictive ability of the model is demonstrated by confirming that it can reproduce the observed PK data for independent clinical trial, which is typically the reference and test batches evaluated in the clinic using a crossover design. The model should be able to predict that the drug product test batches that pass the proposed dissolution specification are bioequivalent to the clinical reference batch, as observed in the clinical trial. This is achieved by running virtual trials with a predefined number of virtual subjects to compare test and reference formulations. Subsequently, bioequivalence is calculated using simulated PK parameters.

To explore the dissolution space, additional VBE simulations are performed using the theoretical dissolution profile below the proposed specification. The goal of these simulations is to demonstrate that the proposed dissolution specification would be within a region of dissolution performance where bioequivalence is anticipated and define the edge of failure for dissolution, providing additional confidence to the proposed specifications. Several examples of applications of VBE for dissolution specification setting and justification have been published such as lesinurad [44], fevipiprant [45] and naproxen [40].

10.3.2 Formulation Switch

During drug development lifecycle, there are often changes in the formulation with respect to type (i.e. capsule to tablet), composition, process and/or manufacturing conditions. A common scenario is that usually in early development (e.g. phase 1 clinical trial) a fit-for-purpose drug in capsule formulation can be used, which is subsequently changed to a film coated tablet for late stage clinical trial (e.g. phase 3) and for commercialization. In these instances, the existing formulation is usually used as the reference formulation, to which the new formulation should be compared with regard to dissolution and bioperformance. To avoid unnecessary clinical studies, it is important to understand the potential impact of any formulation changes to PK, such that formulation changes are avoided that would result in significant PK changes and thus affect safety and efficacy profiles in patients. In this aspect the use of PBPK modelling via VBE, can play a very important role in defining a safe space within which formulation changes would not be expected to have clinically

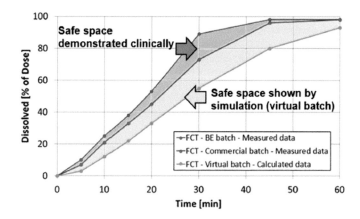

Figure 10.12 Dissolution safe space for BE of ribociclib tablets. (From Ref. [47].)

meaningful impact on the bioperformance. Using the VBE approach is superior to f2 dissolution similarity criteria since f2 calculation can be overly conservative and f2 criteria have little or no rationale for its ability to predict similar or unacceptable changes in bioperformance [46]. The overall model development and VBE technique remain the same as described in the above section on Dissolution Specification Justification, where PBPK is used to link dissolution to formulation bioperformance (i.e. PK) and then to define a 'bioequivalence safe-space' for dissolution, using VBE approach, as shown in Figures 10.10 and 10.11.

The use of VBE to create a formulation safe space to enable formulation switch has been demonstrated for ribociclib [47]. PBPK was used to simulate PK of a capsule formulation in healthy volunteers. The modelling demonstrated rapid and complete dissolution in the human stomach without intestinal precipitation and with permeation-controlled absorption. VBE simulations predicted bioequivalence between capsule and tablet in healthy volunteers, despite f2 calculation showing non-similar (i.e. f2<50) dissolution kinetics between capsule and tablet. Subsequently BE was demonstrated in a clinical study. Thus, proving the f2 criteria to be overly conservative. VBE simulations also predicted comparable PK in cancer patients between capsule and commercial tablet formulation, which was also confirmed in a clinical study. Finally, virtual trial simulations were conducted using virtual dissolution profiles to define a BE safe space within which formulation changes would not result in BE failure (Figure 10.12). Such a safe space can be used to predict BE study outcomes for formulation changes and supersede the dissolution similarity f2 criteria.

10.3.3 Biowaiver

Once a safe space has been developed, it can be used to support biowaiver (i.e. waiver of in-vivo relative bioavailability or bioequivalence studies). An example of such application was to support the biowaiver of a lower strength (20 mg) dasatinib tablet, based on the observed BE data for the higher (100 mg) strength tablet and PBPK modelling of the bioperformance of the lower strength tablet [15]. Biowaiver was granted by regulatory agency.

VBE approach to support biowaiver to support manufacturing site change, even when there is failure to show dissolution similarity per US FDA SUPAC guidance, was demonstrated for etoricoxib tablets [9]. The guidance recommends conducting BE study when the dissolution similarity factor for the two products, F2, is less than 50 in multimedia dissolution tests. VBE simulations demonstrated that tablets manufactured at the two sites would be bioequivalent, even though dissolution testing at pH 4.5 and pH 6.8 media failed to show comparability (F2 was <50) of the tablets manufactured at the two sites.

Biowaiver has been granted by US FDA for commercial elagolix capsule formulation which has slower dissolution compared to the elagolix tablet formulation used in the Phase 3 clinical studies [48]. While the agency recommended performing a BE study, sponsors utilized a PBPK model developed for DDI submissions and incorporated dissolution data of capsule and tablet formulations to perform VBE study in the Simcyp Simulator. The sponsors were able to show bioequivalence using virtual healthy female population using simulations, in lieu of exposing healthy menopausal women to the drug [48].

Similarly, biowaiver has been granted by EMA for lower strength of a BCS class III IR generic drug product which failed F2 when compared to the higher strength [13]. Agency recommends performing BE study for lower strengths when F2 is less than 50 in multimedia dissolution tests when compared to higher strength drug product for which pivotal BE study has been conducted. However, sponsors were able to obtain biowaiver for lower strength by developing a mechanistic oral absorption model integrating in vitro dissolution data and validating against observed test-to-reference ratio of higher strength BE study. The sponsors were able to show that higher strength can still pass the BE by using lower strength dissolution (which failed F2) as input using VBE study [13].

The examples shown here are all for oral drugs, but it should be noted that similar VBE applications have been successful used for other routes of administration like dermal where ANDA has been approved by waiving clinical PD endpoint study [49].

10.4 PAEDIATRIC VBE

10.4.1 Paediatric Virtual Population Generation

Paediatric populations present a real challenge but are arguably one of the most crucial use cases for virtual BE. Paediatric subjects are probably the most vulnerable population. It is much harder to carry out clinical studies on more fragile paediatric populations. Ethical issues are also often at the forefront as it isn't possible for a child to consent or understand the decision to take a medication. More recently, due to enhancements in the science and initiatives by the FDA, drug research in paediatric populations has accelerated. There are big benefits in de-risking these clinical trials by predicting the likely outcome a priori with mechanistic PBPK modelling and virtual BE. As such, paediatric PBPK models have been developed by multiple vendors and the goal for this section is to describe the key physiologic parameters that require adjustment in paediatric patients to give the reader an understanding of the complex physiological adjustments necessary to implement a PBPK model for paediatric subjects. Once the physiological aspects are discussed, we will then highlight some case studies utilizing paediatric virtual BE to answer key questions like dose scaling where successful application of these models has been applied.

Paediatric PBPK models require several key adjustments to account for changes to their unique physiological parameters. A list of the most key physiological and physicochemical parameter adjustments are:

- Tissue sizes
- Blood volume and cardiac output
- Changes to plasma protein concentrations (AAG and Albumin)
- Changes to blood to plasma concentration ratio Rbp due to hematocrit
- Tissue composition (water, lipid content)
  - Total body water and extracellular water changes with age
- Renal function – glomerular filtration rate (GFR) increases with age.
- Enzyme expression levels.
- Changes in intestinal physiology
  - Intestinal length, radius, surface area, fluid volume

In GastroPlus, the algorithms for human physiologies were extended to cover children of all ages, including infants less than 1 year old and newborns born up to 16 weeks premature. All ages of adolescents are included when scaling physiologies in GastroPlus, but the neonates and infants below 1 year old are more complex due to rapid changes in the physiology and so we will focus on these aspects and ontogenies described in this section. The core information for individual parameters (body height and weight, tissue sizes, etc.) was obtained from ICRP publication 23 supplemented by data from additional publications (details are listed below) [50]. For the total body height and weight, as well as majority of tissue sizes, there seems to be a continuous progression of growth from fetus to neonate and infant. Birth does not appear to be a significant event and the rate of development is dependent only on post-menstrual age (PMA = gestational age + postnatal age).

For these cases, smooth relationships between the size and PMA covering the entire range of ages from a sixteen-week-premature newborn to a term-born 1-year-old infant were found and implemented in the program (Figures 10.13–10.15).

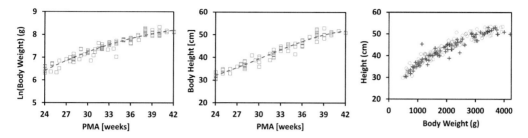

Figure 10.13 Plots of body weight and height for preterm/term infants up to 42 weeks old. Plot on the left and in the middle show Ln body weight and body height, respectively, vs postmenstrual age (PMA). Points represent experimental data [50–60], lines show tissue weights and heights calculated using equations implemented in GastroPlus. The plot on the right compares the observed distribution of body weights and heights (cross) in these infants with the distribution of body weights and heights generated by bivariate distribution function implemented in GastroPlus (circles).

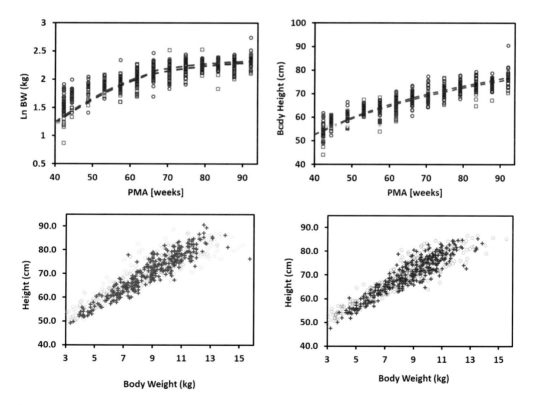

Figure 10.14 Plots of body weight and height for term infants up to 1 year old. The plots on the top show ln body weight (left) and body height (right) vs post-menstrual age (PMA). Points represent NHANES 2003–2004 survey data [30], lines show body weights and heights calculated using equations implemented in GastroPlus. The data for males and females are shown in blue and red, respectively. The plots on the bottom compare the observed distributions of body weights and heights (cross) in these infants with the distribution of body weights and heights generated by bivariate distribution function (see Section 10.2.2.1) implemented in GastroPlus (circles) for males (left) and females (right).

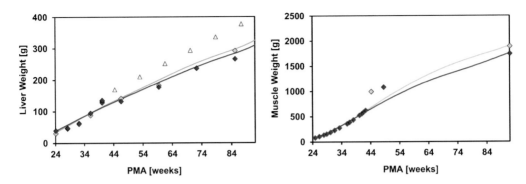

Figure 10.15 Plots of tissue weight vs post-menstrual age (PMA) for infants up to 1 year old for liver (left) and kidneys (right). Points represent experimental data [50], lines show tissue weights calculated using equations implemented in GastroPlus. The data for males and females are shown in blue and red, respectively. Tissue weights calculated using previously published equations for healthy Danish infants [61] are shown (yellow triangles) for comparison.

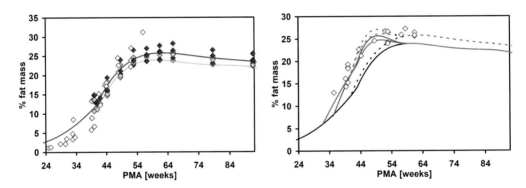

Figure 10.16 Plots of percent fat mass vs post-menstrual age (PMA) for term-born (left) and preterm (right) infants up to 1 year old. Points represent experimental data [50,54,57,62–71], lines show % fat mass calculated using equations implemented in GastroPlus. On the left, the data for males and females are shown in blue and red, respectively. The data from publications which did not specify the gender are shown in yellow. On the right, the solid and dotted lines show calculated percent fat mass for males and females, respectively. The black lines show calculated percent fat mass for term-born infants (these are the same as blue and red lines on the left). The green and magenta lines represent percent fat mass calculated for infants born after 31 and 35 weeks of gestation, respectively. Gender information was not included in the data for preterm infants.

Some of the physiological parameters are, however, dependent separately on gestational age and postnatal age. For example, premature neonates and infants appear to go through a "catch-up" period during the first few weeks and the percent of fat mass in their bodies increases faster (Figure 10.16) than in their term-born counterparts (neonates and infants of the same post-menstrual age born at term). Similarly, the hematocrit and GFR ontogeny change at birth, so the values need to be estimated considering gestational age and postnatal age separately.

Majority of the observed physiological parameters used to derive the algorithms for infant physiologies were for infants from western populations. For the time being, the same equations are being used also for infants from Japanese and Chinese populations. As we continue the research in this area, the infant physiologies for these two populations may be updated in future versions. Individual organ physiology models have not been published, but example plots of experimental data and relationships implemented in GastroPlus for some of the tissue sizes, compositions and some of the physiological parameters are provided in the next section to give the reader an understanding of the physiological changes that occur.

10.4.1.1 Body and Tissue Sizes

For infants with PMA ≤ 39 weeks, the weight and height data were not available from survey data. Instead, they were extracted from multiple publications, which included both Chinese and Caucasian infants. The same bivariate distribution function for weight and height is used across Chinese, Caucasian and Japanese infants (both females and males) in this age range.

10.4.1.2 Blood Parameters

Several key blood-related parameters such as cardiac output, blood volume, fraction bound to plasma proteins and blood to plasma ratio must be adjusted with age for any virtual BE PBPK simulations. Blood volume and cardiac output are continuously increasing as paediatric and adolescent subjects increase in age and body size. As such, GastroPlus has several relationships for different age ranges to calculate the blood volume and cardiac output as shown in Figures 10.17 and 10.18.

GastroPlus also accounts for differences in fraction unbound in plasma (Fup) and blood/plasma concentration ratio (Rbp) between children and adults due to different levels of protein and hematocrit, respectively. The Fup scaling is based on the previously published Equation 10.1 [80] and

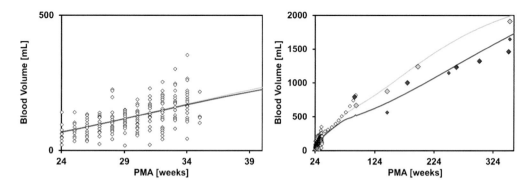

Figure 10.17 Plot of blood volume vs post-menstrual age (PMA) for neonates born after 24–40 weeks of gestation (left) and infants and children up to 3 year old (right). Points represent experimental data [50,72,73]. The lines show blood volumes calculated using equations implemented in GastroPlus. The data for males and females are shown in blue and red, respectively. The data from publications that did not specify the gender are shown in yellow.

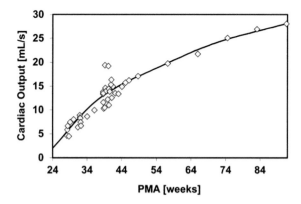

Figure 10.18 Plot of cardiac output vs post-menstrual age (PMA) for infants up to 1 year old. Points represent experimental data [74–79], line shows cardiac output calculated in GastroPlus. Gender information was not included in the data.

assumes that the input experimental percent unbound in plasma is representative of nonspecific drug-protein binding in adult plasma:

$$\text{Fup}_{ped} = \cfrac{1}{1 + \cfrac{P_{ped}}{P_{adult}} \times \cfrac{\left(1 - \text{Fup}_{adult}\right)}{\text{Fup}_{adult}}} \qquad (10.1)$$

where P_{ped} and P_{adult} represent protein concentrations in paediatric and adult plasma, respectively; Fup_{ped} and Fup_{adult} represent fraction unbound in paediatric and adult plasma respectively.

The ratio of paediatric to adult plasma protein (P_{ped}/P_{adult}) is based on the ontogeny of the two major drug-binding proteins in plasma: αl-acid glycoprotein (AAG) and albumin (Figure 10.19).

McNamara also pointed out the propensity of different compounds to bind preferentially to plasma albumin or to plasma AAG [80] As such, the binding to albumin and AAG in paediatrics requires continued research to determine the structural features that cause this binding preference, and a more detailed binding model may need to be implemented in the future. For now, we are combining the ontogeny of albumin and AAG to calculate the changes in the total drug-binding plasma protein with age and using the total drug-binding protein (albumin+AAG) to scale Fup values. Predictions using total drug-binding protein were compared to predictions based on the major binding protein for each compound and the performance of both approaches is similar as summarized in Figure 10.20 [80]. The similar performance of both approaches may be due to similar ontogenies when expressed as percent of adult level for these two proteins (Figure 10.19).

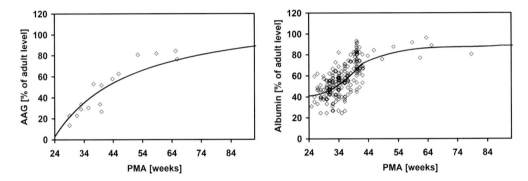

Figure 10.19 Plot of AAG (left) and albumin (right) concentration in plasma (shown as % of adult levels) vs post-menstrual age (PMA) for infants up to 1 year old. Points represent experimental data [81–89], lines show values calculated using equations implemented in GastroPlus.

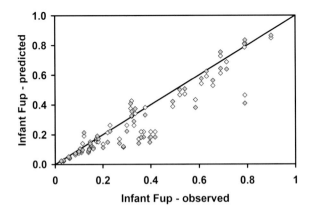

Figure 10.20 Comparison of predicting infant Fup using the major binding protein (yellow diamonds) as proposed by McNamara and Alcom [80] and using the total drug-binding protein (green diamonds) as currently implemented in GastroPlus. Observed data are used as compiled by McNamara et al. Identity line is shown for reference.

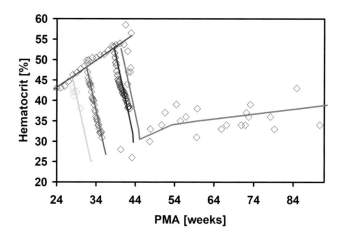

Figure 10.21 Plot of hematocrit vs post-menstrual age (PMA) for infants up to 1 year old. Points represent experimental data [79,90,91], lines show values calculated using equations implemented in GastroPlus. Individual colours represent fetus (red), neonates born after 28 (cyan), 31.5 (light blue), 38.5 (dark blue), and 40 (green) weeks of gestation. The experimental data shown in green were not accompanied by exact specification of gestation age for each subject [91] but based on the reported body weights for the youngest subjects and the authors description of the subjects as "normal well children" we assumed these to be term-born infants.

Infant Rbp scaling utilizes a derived equation (Equation 10.2) assuming the input experimental Rbp value represents binding to red blood cells in adult blood (hematocrit=0.45).

$$\text{Rbp}_{\text{ped}} = \frac{\text{Hct}_{\text{ped}}}{0.45} \times \left(\text{Rbp}_{\text{adult}} - (1 - 0.45) \right) + \left(1 - \text{Hct}_{\text{ped}} \right) \tag{10.2}$$

where Hct_{ped} and $\text{Hct}_{\text{adult}}$ represent hematocrit (expressed as fraction) in paediatric and adult blood, respectively; Rbp_{ped} and $\text{Rbp}_{\text{adult}}$ represent Blood/Plasma Concentration Ratio in paediatric and adult blood, respectively. The changes in hematocrit with age are shown in Figure 10.21.

10.4.1.3 Tissue Compositions

|||For accurate prediction of tissue partition coefficients in paediatric subjects, it is necessary to know the ontogeny of the tissue compositions. The amount of tissue water and lipids changes quite drastically and will affect how lipophilic drugs will partition in the tissues. Lipid content increases with post-menstrual age and thus would lead to increased partition coefficients for lipophilic drugs. At the same time, tissue water decreases which would decrease the partition coefficients for hydrophilic drugs with post-menstrual age. Figure 10.22 shows the composition of two tissues adipose and liver with post-menstrual age. Age dependency for extracellular volume fraction was not found for individual tissues and is estimated from changes in total body water (TBW) and total extracellular water (ECW). TBW vs. post-menstrual age which is used to estimate extracellular water is shown in Figure 10.23.

10.4.1.4 Renal Function

The development of GFR (as well as tubular secretion rate) has been extensively studied, and a number of reports on changes in GFR in fetus as well as after birth were found in the literature. In general, it was observed that GFR development is slower *in utero* and a sharp increase in GFR was observed in the first few days after birth or after reaching 33–35 weeks PMA, whichever occurred later. This would correspond to nephrogenesis being completed at ~35–36 weeks of gestational age. Equations incorporated into GastroPlus account for the effects of gestational age and postnatal age on GFR in the first few weeks after birth. After ~12 weeks of age, the effect of gestational age does not seem to be as dominant, and GFR is estimated based on postnatal age alone (Figure 10.24).

Similarly, the Simcyp Paediatric population databases (Sim-Paediatric, Sim-Paediatric-Japanese, Sim-Paediatric-Chinese, Sim-Paediatric-Cancer-Haem and Sim-Paediatric-Cancer-Solid) allow

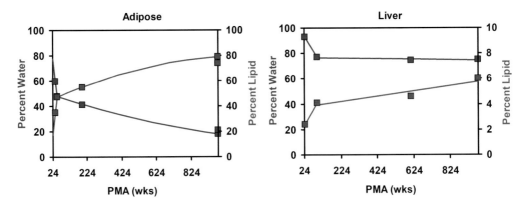

Figure 10.22 Plots of tissue compositions vs post-menstrual age (PMA) for adipose and liver. Points represent experimental data [92], lines show values calculated using equations implemented in GastroPlus. Data for percent of water and total lipid in each tissue are shown in blue and magenta, respectively. Only sparse experimental data is available for these tissue compositions so the entire range of ages from newborn born after 24 weeks of gestation up to an 18-year-old adult (PMA=976 weeks) is shown.

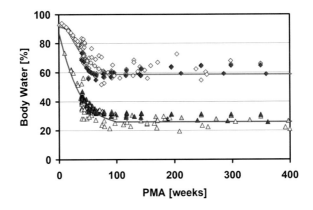

Figure 10.23 Plot of total body water and extracellular water vs post-menstrual age (PMA). Diamonds and triangles represent experimental data for total body water [65, 93–95] and extracellular water [65, 93–95], respectively. Data for males and females are shown in blue and red, respectively. The data from publications which did not specify the gender are shown in yellow.

the prediction of pharmacokinetics in neonates, infants and children [103]. The Paediatric Population Libraries have been built in a similar way to other populations in the Simcyp simulator. However, an extra level of complexity is introduced to account for the age-related changes in many of the system parameters such as organ sizes, organ blood flows and ontogeny of drug metabolizing enzymes. Physiological variability is accounted for in the Paediatric Simulator at different ages. The systems information, when linked to drug-specific physicochemical and *in vitro* data on absorption and disposition in Simcyp algorithms, allows the prediction of drug behaviour in the virtual paediatric population from birth until adulthood. The systems information, when linked to drug-specific physicochemical and *in vitro* data on absorption and disposition in Simcyp algorithms, allows the prediction of drug behaviour in the virtual paediatric population from birth until adulthood.

The Simcyp Preterm Population Library has been built in a similar way to the paediatric population library. However, an extra level of complexity is introduced to account for the post-menstrual, gestational and postnatal age-related changes in many of the system parameters such as organ blood flows, binding proteins, haematocrit and ontogeny of drug metabolizing enzymes.

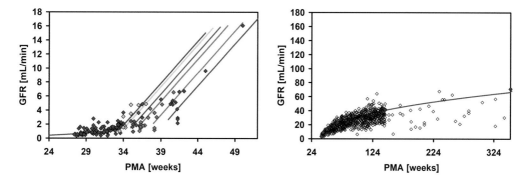

Figure 10.24 Plot of GFR vs post-menstrual age (PMA) for neonates up to 12 weeks old (left) and born after 27–33 (dark blue), 34 (light blue), 35 (magenta), 36 (green), 38 (orange) and 40 (red) weeks of gestation (left). Plot of GFR vs post-menstrual age (PMA) for infants and children up to 6 years old (right). (Left plot) Points represent experimental data [96–98] lines show GFR calculated in GastroPlus. (Right plot) Points represent experimental data [99–102] line shows GFR calculated in GastroPlus for infants and children from 12 weeks to 6 years.

Physiological variability is accounted for at different ages [104]. The Preterm population database, when linked to drug-specific physicochemical and *in vitro* data on absorption and disposition in Simcyp algorithms, allows the prediction of pharmacokinetics and pharmacodynamics in the virtual preterm population between 25 and 44 weeks of post-menstrual age [105].

In addition, Simcyp Simulator also considers time-based changes in the systems parameters during a simulation. The development of physiological and biochemical processes occurs rapidly in the first few months of life, consequently the pharmacokinetics of drugs may also change rapidly during this period. These changes in the physiological and biochemical process (systems parameters in Simcyp) need to be accounted for in order to achieve an accurate prediction of the time course of drug concentrations in paediatric populations. This feature allows, for example, a one-day-old neonate to grow physiologically and biochemically (ontogeny) during the time course of a 28-day drug study so that they will have the size and drug elimination characteristics of a 1-month-old neonate on completion [106] of simulation. As within Simcyp all parameters are directly, or indirectly, related to age and so it is possible to redefine each subject by age at given relevant time points during development. One of the key elements of introducing the time-based physiological changes into Simcyp is the frequency of re-defining/sampling individuals within a simulation. This depends on the starting age and duration of the study.

10.4.2 Case Studies Demonstrating Paediatric Virtual BE

Unfortunately, very few case studies have been published in the literature utilizing virtual BE for paediatric populations. However, there are several applications where virtual BE can answer questions specific to drug product manufacturing and reduction of in vivo testing. Miao and colleagues at the FDA recently published in 2020 a virtual BE analysis of dissolution specifications for Oseltamivir in adult and paediatric populations [107]. Oseltamivir is an antiviral neuraminidase inhibitor for the treatment or prevention of flu symptoms in adult and paediatric subjects. Oseltamivir is a borderline BCS class I weakly basic drug that is metabolized via carboxylesterase 1 (CES1). Oseltamivir phosphate (OP) and primary metabolite Oseltamivir carboxylate (OC) were studied in adults and four different paediatric populations including neonates 0–2 months age, neonates 3–12 months age, children 1–5 years, and adolescents 9–18 year. As such this is a good validation of how commercial software platforms can automatically scale physiology across a wide age range and generate populations that are realistic and produce the observed clinical variability. In this study, default population parameters were utilized from GastroPlus and they were able to reproduce the population variability adequately against clinical data as shown in Figure 10.25. The model was then used to identify a dissolution safe space for the different paediatric subject populations to determine if dissolution-release specifications would need to be tightened for the paediatric subjects. They found that for 0–2 month patients, anything greater than +-4% dissolution rate from baseline would lead to failed bioequivalence whereas adult and adolescent populations were bioequivalent at ±10% and ±7% dissolution specifications as shown in Table 10.1.

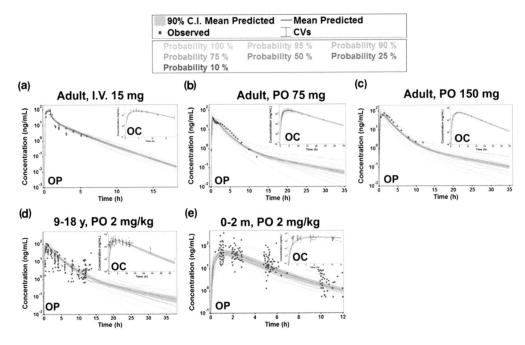

Figure 10.25 Predicted and observed plasma concentration time profiles of OP and OC following IV and PO administration in adults and different paediatric groups reproduced from the literature [103]. (a) Population simulation of IV OP and OC in adults (n=50), (b) and (c) population simulation of oral OP and OC in adults (n=50) after the oral administration of 75 and 150 mg OP using PBPK. (d) population simulation (n=25) and observed data for adolescents (9–18 years) after the administration of OP 2 mg/kg oral suspension. (e) Population simulation (n=25) and observed data in neonates (0–2 months) after 2 mg/kg oral suspension. The black line is the mean predicted concentration, green band the 90% CI, and blue curves are the population probability contours. (From Ref. [107].)

Table 10.1: Geometric Mean Ratio (GMR) and 90% CI for Reference OP Products for Lower Dissolution Profiles for Virtual BE Study in Adults, Adolescent, and Neonates (0–2 Months)

	GMR% (T/R) (90% CI)	
Low Dissolution Profiles	C_{max}	AUC
Adults		
10%	91.4 (80.7–103.5)	93.8 (83.8–105.1)
12%	88.2 (78.1–99.7)	90.7 (81.1–101.4)
Adolescent		
6%	93.7 (81.9–107.2)	95.8 (83.1–110.4)
7%	92.1 (75.3–112.6)	94.3 (79.2–112.2)
0–2 Months		
4%	98.3 (80.2–120.6)	100.1 (82.4–121.5)
6%	94.9 (75.7–118.9)	96.4 (77.3–120.2)

Source: Reproduced from Ref. [107].
GMR, geometric mean ration; 90% CI, 90% confidence interval.

In a similar application, Virtual BE was performed to look at dissolution specifications for Adderall XR® vs. and a test product (Product Y) by Babiskin and Zhang from the FDA [108]. Adderall is approved for use in children over 6 years for treatment for ADHD. It is a BCS class I molecule with high solubility and permeability. In this study, paediatric PBPK simulations were used to predict the pharmacokinetics of amphetamine salts in paediatric (ages 6–12), adolescents (ages 13–17), and adult subjects based on in vitro dissolution profiles for commercial extended release (ER) product vs. a test product. First an in vitro to in vivo relationship (IVIVR) was developed to relate the in vitro dissolution to in vivo dissolution in the intestinal lumen. Then baseline simulations of the reference and test product were performed, and theoretical dissolution profiles were generated that span the hypothetical dissolution acceptance range as shown in Figure 10.26 [108]. These dissolution profiles were then subjected to virtual BE simulations with 12–72 subjects

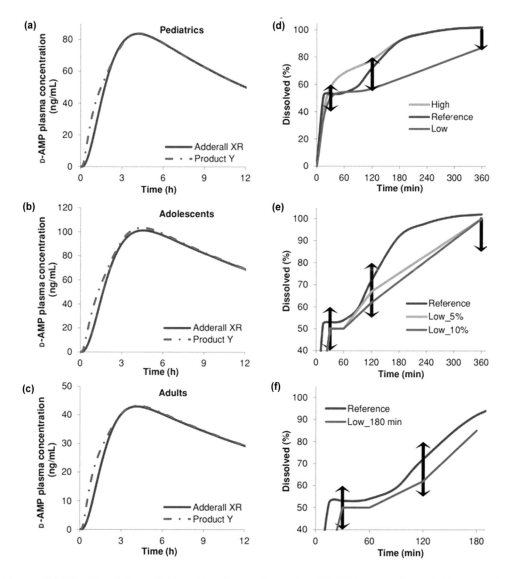

Figure 10.26 Simulation of PK profiles for amphetamine (AMP) drug products (left) and various in vitro dissolution profiles and hypothetical dissolution safe space ranges or hypothetical acceptance criteria for virtual BE analysis from reference [108]. (Left) simulated profiles for two drug products in the virtual BE analysis for dissolution specifications for Adderall XR and Product Y in paediatrics (a), adolescents (b), and adults (c). (Right) dissolution profiles and proposed specifications for drug product Y in paediatrics (d), adolescents (e), and adults (f).

to determine the passing ratios for Product Y vs. the reference. In Table 10.2 from the publication, the reference and low formulations were inequivalent with any number of subjects in the virtual BE simulations while other formulations "Low_10%" and "Low_5%" were non-bioequivalent in small populations but as subjects are increased, the formulations are bioequivalent with the reference if 48 and 24 subjects are simulated respectively. This highlights another key aspect of virtual BE, it doesn't just tell you whether or not the formulations are equivalent but what type of study or what power study you would need to ensure passage of bioequivalence.

Another application of virtual bioequivalence for reference dasatinib formulation vs. two suspension formulations was published by Vaidhyanathan et al. [109]. This study didn't aim to predict bioequivalence but instead retrospectively predict the results from the bioequivalence study to prove the potential for using VBE in a prospective manner. Mechanistic dissolution buoyed by biorelevant in vitro dissolution data was used with PBPK model of paediatric subjects to do an assessment of their clinical bioequivalence study with three formulations. Table 10.3 shows the observed and predicted geometric mean ratios for C_{max} and AUC for these formulations were all less than 1.13. This again gives evidence for the prospective usage of these tools in predicting outcomes of bioequivalence trials a priori.

10.5 GAPS IN VBE AND FUTURE STATE

There has been significant interest in recent years in the application of PBPK in drug product quality and growing evidence of the application of PBPK in VBE projection. Several such applications have been described in this chapter.

Demonstrating BE can be challenging, especially for poorly soluble drugs (*i.e.* BCS 2 or 4), as the absorption-related parameters of poorly soluble drugs may change randomly between subjects (*i.e.* inter-individual variability) and study occasions (i.e. inter-occasion or intrasubject variability) due to the highly variable conditions within the human gastrointestinal tract [110]. Single simulations might provide misleading information about the outcome of a BE study, hence a properly verified VBE model should be used to predict the BE outcome. In addition, VBE trials can be used to select the appropriate number of subjects in a BE trial, without the need to run many pilot studies. In this context, VBE concept has gained attraction and evolved from an academic nicety to a regulatory necessity. VBE approach has been used to support regulatory submissions on justification of the proposed specifications [40,44,45,111], assessing bioequivalence [7,43], justifying biowaiver [15,47] and manufacturing site change [16]. Also, VBE is listed among the research priorities of US FDA's Generic Drug User Fee Amendments (GDUFA) to modernize generic drug development and review under the umbrella of model-informed drug development [112].

Although the focus of this chapter is VBE projection, it is imperative that the model is built and verified against available independent clinical datasets prior to embarking on any BE simulations. As part of the model development, input parameters should be guided based on experimental data and physiological plausibility. Additionally, appropriate sensitivity analyses should be considered to demonstrate robustness of the model and any significant changes in inputs to fit the observed data should be adequately rationalized. Model verification should be carried out against sufficient number of independent clinical datasets to ensure that the model is able to accurately predict the clinical observations.

For VBE modelling, there are specific considerations that needs to be accounted for –

1. Intrasubject CV (ISCV) on the PK and physiological (*e.g.* gastrointestinal transit time, gastrointestinal fluid volume, etc.) parameters is one of the key inputs in the model, since ISCV is one of the key determinants of sample size for BE study and hence the study power [113–115]. The ISCV for PK parameters can be calculated from previous clinical data such as single ascending dose, relative BA and/or BE study. However, ISCV for physiological parameters is not readily available, although there are some publications in this area [116–119], and is a gap that is an area of active research [39]. Mechanistic incorporation of ISCV in VBE assessment, but propagation in the simulations have been reported [40]. It should be clarified that appropriate assignment of both inter- and intrasubject CV is essential to accurately describe population variability, in order to avoid biased simulation of BE due to misrepresentation of the overall variability.

2. The number of subjects used in the population simulations. It is recommended that the number of subjects in the model is similar to the number of subjects that will be used in the BE study, so that the model is not over-powered and hence would result in false-positive prediction, or that the model is under-powered resulting in false negative prediction. It is typical to calculate the sample size for a BE study based on the known or expected GMR for the test and reference products and the ISCV [120].

Table 10.2: Summary of Passing Ratios for Product Y Virtual BE Trails in Paediatric, Adolescent, and Adult Populations

Number of Subjects	Reference Versus Reference	Low Versus Low	High Versus High	Reference Versus Low	Reference Versus High	Reference Versus Low_10%	Reference Versus Low_5%	Reference Versus Low_180 minutes
12	99.1	89.0	97.0	0.4	92.4	34.9	56.9	84.9
24	100	99.9	100	0.1	100	57.3	86.3	98.6
36	100	100	100	0.1	100	76.5	97.7	99.9
48	100	100	100	0	100	85.4	99.4	100
72	100	100	100	0	100	96.6	100	100

Source: From Ref. [108].

Table 10.3: PBPK Virtual Trial Population Simulations Vs. Clinical Outcomes for 100 mg Reference Tablet of Dasatinib Vs. Two Suspensions

Treatment	Geometric Mean AUC (0–24) (ng-h/mL)		GMR (Sim/Obs)	Geometric Mean C_{max} (ng/mL)		GMR (Sim/Obs)	Median T_{max} (hours)	
	Obs	Sim		Obs	Sim		Obs	Sim
Reference tablet	374	398	1.06	114	97	0.86	1.0	1.2
PFOS	327	369	1.13	106	96	0.91	0.5	0.8
Dispersed tablet	342		1.08	110		0.88	0.5	

Source: From Ref. [109].
GMR, geometric mean ratio.

3. The number of VBE trials that should be conducted is an area of vigorous discussion. A survey of the literature shows a wide range of number of virtual trials being used for safe space determination from one [45] to ten [47] to twenty [7] to twenty-five [44]. It is unlikely that a generalized recommendation can be made at this time and must be decided on a case-by-case basis, depending on the biopharmaceutics and clinical pharmacology knowledge of the drug substance and the drug product.

4. Regarding the overall strategy of VBE application, the need to include a product batch that is non-bioequivalent to the clinical reference in the clinical trial and subsequently in the model development has been a topic of intense debate [121]. While it might be ideal to have a batch that is not BE to reference clinical batch to validate the model, it might be technically and/or logistically improbable to make and test such a product batch. Hence, from a practical standpoint VBE can still be applied for the purpose of building a safe space even if all available clinical variants are BE to the clinical reference. However, in this case, the safe space can be defined based on the variant level changes studied. This would still bring manufacturing flexibility while maintaining product quality if the variants tested are fit for purpose (i.e., a specification could be justified within the evaluated dissolution range).

5. Finally, harmonization on evidentiary standards from regulatory agencies across the world will significantly advance VBE applications. By finding and agreeing on commonalities, identifying critical requirements, and providing common standards will minimize redundant or conflicting standards. Such efforts will go a long way to minimize the burden on modellers and expediting drug product development.

REFERENCES

1. U.S. Department of Health and Human Services, Food and Drug Administration (FDA). Center for Evaluation and Research (CDER). Bioavailability and Bioequivalence Studies Submitted in NDAs or INDs - General Considerations. Guidance for Industry; Draft guidance. Available at: https://www.fda.gov/media/88254/download. Accessed November 28, 2019.

2. U.S. Department of Health and Human Services, Food and Drug Administration (FDA). Center for Evaluation and Research (CDER). Immediate Release Solid Oral Dosage Forms. Scale-Up and Postapproval Changes: Chemistry, Manufacturing, and Controls, *In Vitro* Dissolution Testing and *In Vivo* Bioequivalence Documentation. Guidance for Industry. Available at: https://www.fda.gov/media/70949/download. Accessed November 28, 2019.

3. U.S. Department of Health and Human Services, Food and Drug Administration (FDA). Center for Evaluation and Research (CDER). SUPAC-MR: Modified Release Solid Oral Dosage Forms. Scale-Up and Postapproval Changes: Chemistry, Manufacturing, and Controls; *In Vitro* Dissolution Testing and *In Vivo* Bioequivalence Documentation. Guidance for Industry. Available at: https://www.fda.gov/media/70956/download. Accessed November 28, 2019.

4. U.S. Department of Health and Human Services, Food and Drug Administration (FDA). Center for Evaluation and Research (CDER). Bioequivalence Studies with Pharmacokinetic Endpoints for Drugs Submitted Under an ANDA. Guidance for Industry; Draft guidance. Available at: https://www.fda.gov/media/87219/download. Accessed November 28, 2019.

5. European Medicines Agency (EMA). Committee for Proprietary Medicinal Products (CPMP). Guideline on the investigation of bioequivalence. Available at: https://www.ema.europa. eu/en/documents/scientific-guideline/guideline-investigation-bioequivalence-rev1_en.pdf. Accessed November 12, 2019.

6. Davit, B., Braddy, A.C., Conner, D.P. and Yu, L.X. (2013). "International guidelines for bio-equivalence of systemically available orally administered generic drug products: A survey of similarities and differences." *AAPS J* 15(4): 974–90. doi: 10.1208/s12248-013-9499-x.

7. Mitra, A., Petek, B., Bajc, A., Velagapudi, R. and Legen, I. (2019). "Physiologically based absorption modeling to predict bioequivalence of controlled release and immediate release oral products." *Eur J Pharm Biopharm* 134: 117–25. doi: 10.1016/j.ejpb.2018.11.019.

8. US FDA (CDER). "The Use of Physiologically Based Pharmacokinetic Analyses - Biopharmaceutics Applications for Oral Drug Product Development, Manufacturing Changes, and Controls Guidance for Industry", Oct. 2020.

9. Cristofoletti, R., Patel, N. and Dressman, J.B. (2017). "Assessment of bioequivalence of weak base formulations under various dosing conditions using physiologically based pharmacokinetic simulations in virtual populations. Case examples: Ketoconazole and posaconazole." *J Pharm Sci* 106(2): 560–9.

10. Dickinson, P.A., Lee, W., Stott, P.W., Townsend, A.I., Smart, J.P., Ghahramani, P., Hammett, T., Billett, L., Behn, S., Gibb, R.C. and Abrahamsson, B. (2008). "Clinical relevance of dissolution testing in quality by design." *AAPS J* 10(2):380–90.

11. Heimbach, T., Suarez-Sharp, S., Kakhi, M., Holmstock, N., Olivares-Morales, A., Pepin, X., Sjogren, E., Tsakalozou, E., Seo, P., Li, M., Zhang, X., Lin, H.P., Montague, T., Mitra, A., Morris, D., Patel, N. and Kesisoglou, F. (2019). "Dissolution and translational modeling strategies toward establishing an *in vitro-in vivo* link-a workshop summary report." *AAPS J* 21: 29.

12. Abend, A., Heimbach, T., Cohen, M., Kesisoglou, F., Pepin, X. and Suarez-Sharp, S. (2018). "Dissolution and translational modeling strategies enabling patient-centric drug product development: The M-CERSI workshop summary report." *AAPS J* 20: 60.

13. Wu, D., et al. (2023). "Physiologically based pharmacokinetics modeling in biopharmaceutics: Case studies for establishing the bioequivalence safe space for innovator and generic drugs." *Pharm Res* 40: 337–57.

14. Mukherjee, D., et al. (2022). "Physiologically based pharmacokinetic modeling and simulations to inform dissolution specifications and clinical relevance of release rates on elagolix exposure." *Biopharm Drug Dispos* 43(3): 98–107.

15. Heimbach, T., et al. (2021). "Establishing the bioequivalence safe space for immediate-release oral dosage forms using physiologically based biopharmaceutics modeling (PBBM): Case studies." *J Pharm Sci* 110(12): 3896–906.

16. Mitra, A., et al. (2015) "Application of absorption modeling to predict bioequivalence outcome of two batches of etoricoxib tablets." *AAPS PharmSciTech* 16(1): 76–84.

17. Loisios-Konstantinidis, I., et al. (2020). "Using physiologically based pharmacokinetic modeling to assess the risks of failing bioequivalence criteria: A tale of two ibuprofen products." *AAPS J* 22: 1–9.

18. Hong, E., et al. (2022). "Physiologically-based pharmacokinetic-led guidance for patients with cystic fibrosis taking elexacaftor-tezacaftor-ivacaftor with nirmatrelvir-ritonavir for the treatment of COVID-19." *Clin Pharmacol Therapeut* 111(6): 1324–33.

19. Wang, J. and Flanagan, D.R. (1999). "General solution for diffusion-controlled dissolution of spherical particles. 1. Theory." *J Pharm Sci* 88(7): 731–8.

20. Stader, F., et al. (2021). "Clinical data combined with modeling and simulation indicate unchanged drug-drug interaction magnitudes in the elderly." *Clin Pharmacol Therapeut* 109(2): 471–84.

21. Lu, A.T., Frisella, M.E., et al. (1993). "Dissolution modeling: Factors affecting the dissolution rates of polydisperse powders." *Pharm Res* 10(9): 1308–14.

22. Wang, J. and Flanagan, D.R. (2002). "General solution for diffusion-controlled dissolution of spherical particles. 2. Evaluation of experimental data." *J Pharm Sci* 91(2): 534–42.

23. Takano, R., Sugano, K., et al. (2006). "Oral absorption of poorly water-soluble drugs: Computer simulation of fraction absorbed in humans from a miniscale dissolution test." *Pharm Res* 23(6): 1144–56.

24. Lindfors, L., et al. (2008). "Nucleation and crystal growth in supersaturated solutions of a model drug." *J Colloid Interface Sci* 325(2): 404–13.

25. Wagner, J.G. (1983). "Pharmacokinetic absorption plots from oral data alone or oral/intravenous data and an exact Loo-Riegelman equation." *J Pharm Sci* 72(7): 838–42.

26. Jamei, M., Abrahamsson, B., Brown, J., Bevernage, J., Bolger, M.B., Heimbach, T., Karlsson, E., Kotzagiorgis, E., Lindahl, A., McAllister, M. and Mullin, J.M (2020). "Current status and future opportunities for incorporation of dissolution data in PBPK modeling for pharmaceutical development and regulatory applications: OrBiTo consortium commentary." *Eu J Pharm Biopharm* 155: 55–68.

27. Doki, K., Darwich, A.S., Patel, N. and Rostami-Hodjegan, A. (2017). "Virtual bioequivalence for achlorhydric subjects: The use of PBPK modelling to assess the formulation-dependent effect of achlorhydria." *Eur J Pharm Sci* 109: 111–20.

28. Jamei, M., Dickinson, G.L. and Rostami-Hodjegan, A. (2009). "A framework for assessing inter-individual variability in pharmacokinetics using virtual human populations and integrating general knowledge of physical chemistry, biology, anatomy, physiology and genetics: A tale of 'bottom-up' vs 'top-down' recognition of covariates. *Drug Metab Pharmacokinet* 24(1): 53–75.

29. McNally, K., et al. (2014). "PopGen: A virtual human population generator." *Toxicology* 315: 70–85.

30. NHANES Database: https://www.cdc.gov/nchs/nhanes/index.htm.

31. Ogiu, N., Nakamura, Y., et al. (1997). "A statistical analysis of the internal organ weights of normal Japanese people." *Health Phys* 72(3): 368–83.

32. (CHNS) "China Health and Nutrition Survery". https://www.cpc.unc.edu/projects/china/.

33. Altman, P.L. and Dittmer, D.S. (1962). "*Growth: Including Reproduction and Morphological Development.*" Washington, DC: Federation of American Societies for Experimental Biology, 608 pages.

34. Rostami-Hodjegan, A. and Tucker, G.T. (2007). "Simulation and prediction of in vivo drug metabolism in human populations from in vitro data." *Nat Rev Drug Discov* 6(2): 140–8.

35. Abuhelwa, A.Y., Foster, D.J. and Upton, R.N. (2016). "A quantitative review and meta-models of the variability and factors affecting oral drug absorption-part I: Gastrointestinal pH." *AAPS J* 18(5): 1309–21.

36. Abuhelwa, A.Y., Foster, D.J. and Upton, R.N. (2016). "A quantitative review and meta-models of the variability and factors affecting oral drug absorption-part II: Gastrointestinal transit time." *AAPS J* 18(5): 1322–33.

37. Mikolajczyk, A.E., et al. (2015). "Assessment of tandem measurements of pH and total gut transit time in healthy volunteers." *Clin Transl Gastroenterol* 6(7): e100.

38. Fuchs, A. and Dressman, J.B. (2014). "Composition and physicochemical properties of fasted-state human duodenal and jejunal fluid: A critical evaluation of the available data." *J Pharm Sci* 103(11): 3398–411.

30. Bego, M., Patel, N., Cristofoletti, R. and Rostami-Hodjegan, A. (2022). "Proof of concept in assignment of within-subject variability during virtual bioequivalence studies: Propagation of intra-subject variation in gastrointestinal physiology using physiologically based pharmacokinetic modeling." *AAPS J* 24(1): 21.

40. Loisios-Konstantinidis, I., Cristofoletti, R., Fotaki, N., Turner, D.B. and Dressman, J. (2020). "Establishing virtual bioequivalence and clinically relevant specifications using *in vitro* biorelevant dissolution testing and physiologically-based population pharmacokinetic modeling. Case example: Naproxen." *Eur J Pharm Sci* 143: 105170.

41. U.S. Food and Drug Administration. Guidance for Industry: Dissolution Testing of Immediate Release Solid Oral Dosage Forms. 1997.

42. EMA, European Medicines Agency (EMA). Reflection Paper on the Dissolution Specification for Generic Solid Oral Immediate Release Products with Systemic Action (EMA/CHMP/CVMP/QWP/336031/2017); EMA: London, UK, 2017.

43. Mitra, A (2019). "Maximizing the role of physiologically based oral absorption modeling in generic drug development." *Clin Pharmacol Ther* 105: 307–9.

44. Pepin, X.J.H., et al. (2016). "Justification of drug product dissolution rate and drug substance particle size specifications based on absorption PBPK modelling for lesinurad immediate release tablets." *Mol Pharm* 13(9): 3256–69.

45. Kourentas, A., et al. (2023). "Establishing the safe space via physiologically based biopharmaceutics modeling. Case study: Fevipiprant/QAW039." *AAPS J* 25(1): 25.

46. Muselik, J., et al. (2021). "A critical overview of FDA and EMA statistical methods to compare in vitro drug dissolution profiles of pharmaceutical products." *Pharmaceutics* 13: 1703.

47. Laisney, M., et al. (2022). "Physiologically based biopharmaceutics modeling to demonstrate virtual bioequivalence and bioequivalence safe-space for ribociclib which has permeation rate-controlled absorption." *J Pharm Sci* 111: 274–84.

48. Mukherjee, D., et al. (2023). "Virtual bioequivalence assessment of elagolix formulations using physiologically based pharmacokinetic modeling." *AAPS J* 25: 30.

49. Tsakalozou, E., et al. (2021). "Physiologically-based pharmacokinetic modeling to support bioequivalence and approval of generic products: A case for diclofenac sodium topical gel, 1%." *CPT: Pharm Syst Pharmacol* 10: 399–411.

50. Snyder, W.S., Cook, M.J., et al. (1975). "*Report of the Task Group on Reference Man* (ICRP Publication 23)." Elsevier Science Inc., pp. 480.

51. Bertino, E., Coscia, A., et al. (2009). "Weight growth velocity of very low birth weight infants: Role of gender, gestational age and major morbidities." *Early Hum Dev* 85(6): 339–47.

52. Chen, T.H. (1998). "A further discussion on fetal organ growth model." *Chinese J Med Phys* 15(4): 217–20.

53. Cooke, R.J. and Griffin, I. (2009). "Altered body composition in preterm infants at hospital discharge." *Acta Paediatr* 98(8): 1269–73.

54. Enzi, G., Zanardo, V., et al. (1981). "Intrauterine growth and adipose tissue development." *Am J Clin Nutr* 34(9): 1785–90.

55. Gao, S.Y., Xiang, S.R., et al. (1990). "Evaluation of organ weights of 150 fetuses in Jiangxi province." *Chinese J Anat* 13(2): 148–53.

56. Hammarlund, K. and Sedin, G. (1979). "Transepidermal water loss in newborn infants. III. Relation to gestational age." *Acta Paediatr Scand* 68(6): 795–801.

57. Iob, V. and Swanson, W.W. (1934). "Mineral growth of the human fetus." *Am J Dis Child* 47(2): 302–6.

58. Usher, R. and McLean, F. (1969). "Intrauterine growth of live-born Caucasian infants at sea level: Standards obtained from measurements in 7 dimensions of infants born between 25 and 44 weeks of gestation." *J Pediatr* 74(6): 901–10.

59. Wang, Q., Hu, P., et al. (1989). "An approach to the rules of fetal growth through organometry." *Acta Acad Med Jiangxi* 29(3): 19–25.

60. Zhang, Z.Y., Zhang, J.P., et al. (1994). "The analysis of liver weight, age and body weight in 189 fetuses." *J Jining Medical College* 17(3): 45.

61. Kock, K.F., Lammert, O., et al. (1997). "Organ weights in healthy and apparently healthy Danish infants." *Am J Hum Biol* 9(1): 35–8.

62. Anderson, A.K. (2009). "Association between Infant Feeding and Early Postpartum Infant Body Composition: A Pilot Prospective Study." *Int J Pediatr* 2009: 648091.

63. Deierlein, A.L., Thornton, J., et al. (2012). "An anthropometric model to estimate neonatal fat mass using air displacement plethysmography." *Nutr Metab (Lond)* 9: 21.

64. Fields, D.A., Gilchrist, J.M., et al. (2011). "Longitudinal body composition data in exclusively breast-fed infants: A multicenter study." *Obesity* 19(9): 1887–91.

65. Fomon, S.J., Haschke, F., et al. (1982). "Body composition of reference children from birth to age 10 years." *Am J Clin Nutr* 35(5 Suppl): 1169–75.

66. Gianni, M.L., Roggero, P.M., et al. (2012). "Postnatal catch-up fat after late preterm birth." *Pediatr Res* 72(6): 637–40.

67. Gianni, M.L., Roggero, P.M., et al. (2009). "Adiposity in small for gestational age preterm infants assessed at term equivalent age." *Arch Dis Child Fetal Neonatal Ed* 94(5): F368–72.

68. Ramel, S.E., Gray, H.L., et al. (2011). "Body composition changes in preterm infants following hospital discharge: Comparison with term infants." *J Pediatr Gastroenterol Nutr* 53(3): 333–8.

69. Roggero, P.M., Gianni, M.L., et al. (2008). "Postnatal growth failure in preterm infants: Recovery of growth and body composition after term." *Early Hum Dev* 84(8): 555–9.

70. Roggero, P.M., Gianni, M.L., et al. (2011). "Rapid recovery of fat mass in small for gestational age preterm infants after term." *PLoS One* 6(1): e14489.

71. Schmelzle, H.R. and Fusch, C. (2002). "Body fat in neonates and young infants: Validation of skinfold thickness versus dual-energy X-ray absorptiometry." *Am J Clin Nutr* 76(5): 1096–100.

72. Haddad, S., Restieri, C., et al. (2001). "Characterization of age-related changes in body weight and organ weights from birth to adolescence in humans." *J Toxicol Environ Health A* 64(6): 453–64.

73. Smith, G.C. and Cameron, A.D. (2002). "Estimating human fetal blood volume on the basis of gestational age and fetal abdominal circumference." *BJOG* 109(6): 721–2.

74. Alverson, D.C., Aldrich, M., et al. (1987). "Longitudinal trends in left ventricular cardiac output in healthy infants in the first year of life." *J Ultrasound Med* 6(9): 519–24.

75. Coskun, S., Yüksel, H., et al. (2001). "Non-invasive evaluation of the adaptations of cardiac function in the neonatal period: A comparison of healthy infants delivered by vaginal route and caesarean section." *Acta Med Okayama* 55(4): 213–8.

76. Seppänen, M.P., Kääpä, P.O., et al. (1994). "Doppler-derived systolic pulmonary artery pressure in acute neonatal respiratory distress syndrome." *Pediatrics* 93(5): 769–73.

77. Walther, F.J., Siassi, B., et al. (1985). "Pulsed Doppler determinations of cardiac output in neonates: Normal standards for clinical use." *Pediatrics* 76(5): 829–33.

78. Winberg, P. and Lundell, B.P. (1990). "Left ventricular stroke volume and output in healthy term infants." *Am J Perinatol* 7(3): 223–6.

79. Yanowitz, T.D., Yao, A.C., et al. (1999). "Postnatal hemodynamic changes in very-low-birth-weight infants." *J Appl Physiol* 87(1): 370–80.

80. McNamara, P.J. and Alcorn, J. (2002). "Protein binding predictions in infants." *AAPS PharmSci* 4(1): E4.

81. Cartlidge, P.H. and Rutter, N. (1986). "Serum albumin concentrations and oedema in the newborn." *Arch Dis Child* 61(7): 657–60.

82. Colón, A.R. (1990). "*Textbook of Pediatric Hepatology.*" Chicago: Year Book Medical Publishers, Inc., pp. 353.

83. Darrow, D.C. and Cary, M.K. (1933). "The serum albumin and globulin of newborn, premature and normal infants." *J Pediatr* 3: 573–9.

84. Ehrnebo, M., Aqurell, S., et al. (1971). "Age differences in drug binding by plasma proteins: Studies on human foetuses, neonates and adults." *Eur J Clin Pharmacol* 3(4): 189–93.

85. Kanakoudi, F., Drossou, V., et al. (1995). "Serum concentrations of 10 acute-phase proteins in healthy term and preterm infants from birth to age 6 months." *Clin Chem* 41(4): 605–8.

86. Lerman, J., Strong, H.A., et al. (1989). "Effects of age on the serum concentration of alpha 1-acid glycoprotein and the binding of lidocaine in pediatric patients." *Clin Pharmacol Ther* 46(2): 219–25.

87. Philip, A.G. and Hewitt, J.R. (1983). "Alpha 1-acid glycoprotein in the neonate with and without infection." *Biol Neonate* 43(3–4): 118–24.

88. Rane, A., Lunde, P.K., et al. (1971). "Plasma protein binding of diphenylhydantoin in normal and hyperbilirubinemic infants." *J Pediatr* 78(5): 877–82.

89. Reading, R.F., Ellis, R., et al. (1990). "Plasma albumin and total protein in preterm babies from birth to eight weeks." *Early Hum Dev* 22(2): 81–7.

90. Jopling, J., Henry, E., et al. (2009). "Reference ranges for hematocrit and blood hemoglobin concentration during the neonatal period: Data from a multihospital health care system." *Pediatrics* 123(2): e333–7.

91. Rubin, M.I., Bruck, E., et al. (1949). "Maturation of renal function in childhood; clearance studies." *J Clin Invest* 28(5 Pt 2): 1144–62.

92. White, D.R., Widdowson, E.M., et al. (1991). "The composition of body tissues (II). Fetus to young adult." *Br J Radiol* 64(758): 149–59.

93. Butte, N.F., Hopkinson, J.M., et al. (2000). "Body composition during the first 2 years of life: An updated reference." *Pediatr Res* 47(5): 578–85.

94. Flexner, L.B. and Wilde, W.S. (1947). "The estimation of extracellular and total body water in the newborn human infant with radioactive sodium and deuterium oxide." *J Pediatr* 30(4): 413–5.

95. Friis-Hansen, B. (1983). "Water distribution in the foetus and newborn infant." *Acta Paediatr Scand Suppl* 305: 7–11.

96. Coulthard, M.G. (1985). "Maturation of glomerular filtration in preterm and mature babies." *Early Hum Dev* 11(3–4): 281–92.

97. DeWoskin, R.S. and Thompson, C.M. (2008). "Renal clearance parameters for PBPK model analysis of early lifestage differences in the disposition of environmental toxicants." *Regul Toxicol Pharmacol* 51(1): 66–86.

98. Fawer, C.L., Torrado, A., et al. (1979). "Maturation of renal function in full-term and premature neonates." *Helv Paediatr Acta* 34(1): 11–21.

99. Bird, N.J., Henderson, B.L., et al. (2003). "Indexing glomerular filtration rate to suit children." *J Nucl Med* 44(7): 1037–43.

100. Kearns, G.L., Abdel-Rahman, S.M., et al. (2003). "Developmental pharmacology-Drug disposition, action, and therapy in infants and children." *N Engl J Med* 349(12): 1157–67.

101. Peters, A.M., Gordon, I., et al. (1994). "Normalization of glomerular filtration rate in children: Body surface area, body weight or extracellular fluid volume?" *J Nucl Med* 35(3): 438–44.

102. Stevens, L.A. and Levey, A.S. (2007). *"Frequently Asked Questions about GFR Estimates."* New York: National Kidney Foundation, pp. 17.

103. Johnson, T.N., Rostami-Hodjegan, A. and Tucker, G.T. (2006). "Prediction of the clearance of eleven drugs and associated variability in neonates, infants and children." *Clin Pharmacokinet* 45: 931–56.

104. Abduljalil, K., Pan, X., Pansari, A., Jamei, M. and Johnson, T.N. (2020). "A preterm physiologically based pharmacokinetic model. Part I: Physiological parameters and model building." *Clin Pharmacokinet* 59: 485–500.

105. Abduljalil, K., Pan, X., Pansari, A., Jamei, M. and Johnson, T.N. (2020). "Preterm physiologically based pharmacokinetic model. Part II: Applications of the model to predict drug pharmacokinetics in the preterm population." *Clin Pharmacokinet* 59: 501–18.

106. Abduljalil, K., Jamei, M., Rostami-Hodjegan, A. and Johnson, T.N., 2014. "Changes in individual drug-independent system parameters during virtual paediatric pharmacokinetic trials: Introducing time-varying physiology into a paediatric PBPK model. *AAPS J* 16: 568–76.

107. Miao, L., et al. (2020). "Using a physiologically based pharmacokinetic absorption model to establish dissolution bioequivalence safe space for oseltamivir in adult and pediatric populations." *AAPS J* 22(5): 1–10.

108. Babiskin, A.H. and Zhang, X. (2015). "Application of physiologically based absorption modeling for amphetamine salts drug products in generic drug evaluation." *J Pharm Sci* 104(9): 3170–82.

109. Vaidhyanathan, S., et al. (2019). "Bioequivalence comparison of pediatric dasatinib formulations and elucidation of absorption mechanisms through integrated PBPK modeling." *J Pharm Sci* 108(1): 741–9.

110. Grimm, M., Koziolek, M., Kühn, J.P. and Weitschies W. (2018). "Interindividual and intraindividual variability of fasted state gastric fluid volume and gastric emptying of water." *Eur J Pharm Biopharm* 127: 309–17. doi: 10.1016/j.ejpb.2018.03.002.

111. Pepin, X., et al. (2023). "Acalabrutinib maleate tablets: The physiologically based biopharmaceutics model behind the drug product dissolution specification." *Mol Pharmaceut*. doi: 10.1021/acs.molpharmaceut.3c00005.

112. Fang, L., Kim, M.J., Li, Z., et al. (2018). "Model-informed drug development and review for generic products: Summary of FDA public workshop." *Clin Pharmacol Ther* 104(1): 27–30. doi: 10.1002/cpt.1065

113. Ring, A., Lang, B., Kazaroho, C., Labes, D., Schall, R. and Schütz, H. (2019). "Sample size determination in bioequivalence studies using statistical assurance." *Br J Clin Pharmacol* 85(10): 2369–77. doi: 10.1111/bcp.14055.

114. Sugihara, M., Takeuchi, S., Sugita, M., Higaki, K., Kataoka, M. and Yamashita, S. (2015). "Analysis of intra- and intersubject variability in oral drug absorption in human bioequivalence studies of 113 generic products." *Mol Pharm* 12(12): 4405–13. doi: 10.1021/acs.molpharmaceut.5b00602.

115. Karalis, V., Symillides, M. and Macheras, P. (2004). "Novel scaled average bioequivalence limits based on GMR and variability considerations." *Pharm Res* 21(10): 1933–42. doi: 10.1023/b:pham.0000045249.83899.ae.

116. Mudie, D.M., Murray, K., Hoad, C.L., Pritchard, S.E., Garnett, M.C., Amidon, G.L., Gowland, P.A., Spiller, R.C., Amidon, G.E. and Marciani, L. (2014). "Quantification of gastrointestinal liquid volumes and distribution following a 240 mL dose of water in the fasted state." *Mol Pharm* 11(9):3039–47. doi: 10.1021/mp500210c.

117. Koziolek, M., Grimm, M., Schneider, F., et al. (2016). "Navigating the human gastrointestinal tract for oral drug delivery: Uncharted waters and new frontiers." *Adv Drug Deliv Rev* 101:75–88. doi: 10.1016/j.addr.2016.03.009.

118. Murray, K., Hoad, C.L., Mudie, D.M., Wright, J., Heissam, K., Abrehart, N., Pritchard, S.E., Al Atwah, S., Gowland, P.A., Garnett, M.C., Amidon, G.E., Spiller, R.C., Amidon, G.L. and Marciani, L. (2017). "Magnetic resonance imaging quantification of fasted state colonic liquid pockets in healthy humans." *Mol Pharm* 14(8): 2629–38. doi: 10.1021/acs.molpharmaceut.7b00095.

119. Reppas, C., Karatza, E., Goumas, C., Markopoulos, C. and Vertzoni, M. (2015). "Characterization of contents of distal ileum and cecum to which drugs/drug products are exposed during bioavailability/bioequivalence studies in healthy adults." *Pharm Res* 32(10): 3338–49. doi:10.1007/s11095-015-1710-6.

120. Potvin, D., DiLiberti, C.E., Hauck, W.W., Parr, A.F., Schuirmann, D.J. and Smith, R.A. (2008). "Sequential design approaches for bioequivalence studies with crossover designs." *Pharm Stat* 7(4): 245–62. doi: 10.1002/pst.294.

121. Mitra, A., et al. (2021). "Applications of physiologically based biopharmaceutics modeling (PBBM) to support drug product quality: A workshop summary report." *J Pharm Sci* 110(2): 594–609.

11 Application of PBPK Modeling to Support Clinical Pharmacology Regulatory Decision-Making

*Xinyuan Zhang, Yuching Yang, Sreedharan Sabarinath,
Ramana Uppoor, and Mehul Mehta*

11.1 UTILITY OF PBPK IN CLINICAL PHARMACOLOGY REVIEWS

Clinical pharmacology covers a broad scope of science ranging from basic pharmacology to study the effects of drugs in humans. It is inherently a translational science. In the regulatory setting, clinical pharmacology focuses on the impact of intrinsic and extrinsic factors on inter-patient and intra-subject variability in drug exposure and response [1]. Physiologically-based pharmacokinetic (PBPK) modeling and simulation is a tool that has been used in clinical pharmacology reviews evaluating the impact of intrinsic (such as age, organ dysfunction, pharmacogenetic, etc.) and extrinsic (such as food, concomitant medications, etc.) factors on drug exposure [2–6], and consequently on the safety and efficacy. In the following subsections, we will discuss each specific area with examples that were submitted to the US FDA.

11.2 MODEL-INTEGRATED EVIDENCE APPROACH

A PBPK model is built based on the mechanistic understanding of a drug's absorption, distribution, metabolism, and excretion (ADME) properties. It integrates cumulative knowledge of the human anatomy, physiology, and a drug's property to predict its vivo PK [7]. In theory, a PBPK model can be built based on physiochemical properties, in vitro, and in silico data, which is also known as the 'bottom up' approach. At the early phase of drug development when in vivo human data are limited, a PBPK model can predict the PK profile and aid in dose selection prior to the first in human study [8]. The predictive performance of bottom-up PBPK models was evaluated systemically in the oral biopharmaceutics tools (OrBiTo) project [9–12]. In this project, approximately 52.9% and 37.2% of predicted AUC was within twofold of observed following i.v., and oral administration, respectively, suggesting predictive performance declining with the increasing complexity of drug's ADME process [10]. Nevertheless, the initial PBPK model serves as a basis for future model applications after model refinement when more information/data become available for the investigational drug.

For many oncology drugs, first-in-human studies are conducted in patient populations instead of healthy volunteers. Therefore, early assessment of potential drug–drug interaction (DDI) is necessary to inform protocol development regarding concomitant medication uses. PBPK modeling and simulation have been extensively used to predict DDI potentials. PBPK models can also be used to predict the effect of organ impairment on the exposure. A recent study by a working group under the International Consortium for Innovation and Quality in Pharmaceutical Development (IQ Consortium) suggested that PBPK models could predict the AUC ratios within twofold of the observed ratios for >90% (47/50) treatment groups in renal impairment for compounds that are mainly eliminated via metabolism. The AUC ratios of hepatic impairment to healthy subjects were predicted within twofold of the observed ratios for >70% (43/56) treatment groups [13]. The model predictive performance declines with the increasing severity of hepatic impairment. Nevertheless, the PBPK models could provide a rough estimation of the effect of organ impairment and inform protocol development regarding the inclusion, and exclusion criteria, or dose justification and appropriate PK sampling schemes.

In many pediatric programs, PBPK models have been used to predict the exposures in pediatric populations especially in patients less than 2 years of age prior to first in pediatric studies [14]. A staggered enrollment from older to younger children and integrated PBPK modeling approach are generally adapted to build and refine the models.

When the program advances to the stage of New Drug Application (NDA) or Biologics License Application (BLA), comprehensive PBPK analyses are submitted to inform regulatory decisions such as supporting dose adjustment recommendation for DDI conditions, evaluating complex clinical conditions that are infeasible to study, and informing the United States Prescribing Information (USPI) [4,5]. In this chapter, we will focus on the PBPK applications in regulatory submissions.

DOI: 10.1201/9781003031802-11

11.3 PBPK SUBMISSIONS TO THE OFFICE OF CLINICAL PHARMACOLOGY BETWEEN 2008 AND 2022

The FDA's Office of Clinical Pharmacology (OCP) has been providing periodic updates on the submissions that contain PBPK analyses [4,5,15]. From 2008 to 2017, in a total of 254 submissions that OCP received, the majority of PBPK analyses were applied to address DDI related questions, where enzyme-mediated DDIs accounted for 60%, and transporter-mediated DDIs accounted for 7%. Approximately 15% of the PBPK analyses were applied in pediatric-related programs. PBPK applications were relatively low in the areas of evaluating the effects of hepatic impairment, renal impairment, pharmacogenetics, absorption and/or food effect, and other intrinsic and extrinsic factors on PK. From 2018 to 2021, among the total of 293 submissions that OCP received, enzyme-mediated DDIs accounted for 44%, transporter-mediated DDIs accounted for 17%, and pediatrics accounted for 12% (Figure 11.1).

Comparing the number of PBPK submissions between 2018 and 2021 ($N=293$ in 4 years), and between 2008 and 2017 ($N=254$ in 10 years), the average submissions per year increased by approximately threefold. With regard to the areas of application of PBPK analyses, DDIs and pediatrics are the two major areas. There are more transporter- mediated DDI PBPK analyses in recent years compared to the previous 10 years. We also see more PBPK applications in absorption/food effect/acid-reducing agents (ARAs)-mediated DDI predictions. The percentages of PBPK applications in the areas of evaluating the effects of hepatic impairment, renal impairment, and pharmacogenetics remain relatively low. Of note, the statistics summarized in this section were based on the PBPK analyses submitted to the regulatory agency (OCP/FDA), which may not represent how PBPK analyses are being used during the drug development process, which includes pre-clinical, first-in-human dose projection, phase 1/2/3 protocol development, regulatory submissions, post-market evaluations, and life cycle management. Examples of PBPK analyses from novel drug approvals between 2008 and 2019 are summarized in previous publications [4,5]. PBPK analyses in novel drug approvals between 2020 and 2022 are summarized in Table 11.1.

2018-2021, N=293

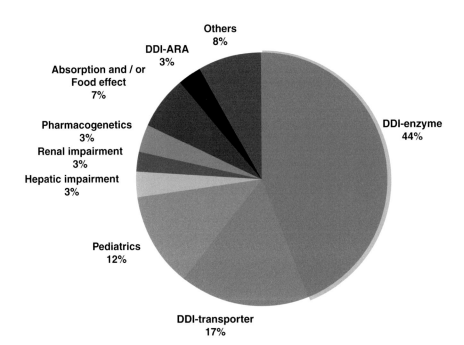

Figure 11.1 PBPK submissions to the Office of Clinical Pharmacology (OCP) at the US Food and Drug Administration (FDA) and distribution of PBPK application areas from 2018 to 2021. (Pie charts are regenerated based on the data published in Ref. [15].) ARA, acid-reducing agent; DDI, drug-drug interaction.

Table 11.1: Summary of PBPK Analyses in Novel Drug Approvals between 2020 and 2022

NDA/BLA	Generic Name	Intended Use of the PBPK Modeling Analysis	FDA's Assessment for Intended Use of the Models	Review Reference
212608	Avapritinib	To evaluate the effect of CYP3A inhibitors and inducers on the PK of avapritinib at steady state	Adequate	[16]
212801	Osilodrostat	To predict the effect of osilodrostat on the steady-state PK of caffeine (CYP1A2), midazolam (CYP3A4), omeprazole (CYP2C19), dextromethorphan (CYP2D6), warfarin (CYP2C9)	Adequate	[17]
		To predict the effect of osilodrostat on the steady-state PK of bupropion (CYP2B6)	Inadequate	
213756	Selumetinib	To evaluate the effect of CYP3A inhibitors (erythromycin and diltiazem) on the PK of selumetinib	Adequate	[18]
		To evaluate the effect of CYP3A inducers (efavirenz and dexamethasone) on the PK of selumetinib	Adequate	
		To evaluate the effect of CYP2C19 inhibitor (fluoxetine) on the PK of selumetinib	Adequate	
213411	Tucatinib	To predict the effect of itraconazole (a strong CYP3A4 inhibitor), gemfibrozil (a strong CYP2C8 inhibitor), carbamazepine (a strong CYP3A4 inducer), and phenytoin (a strong CYP3A4 inducer) on the steady-state PK of tucatinib	Adequate	[19]
		To predict the effect of tucatinib on the PK of raltegravir (a UGT1A1 substrate) and rosuvastatin (an OATP1B1/3 substrate)	Adequate	
213736	Pemigatinib	To evaluate the effect of strong CYP3A inhibitor (clarithromycin), moderate CYP3A inhibitors (erythromycin, diltiazem, and fluconazole), and a weak CYP3A inhibitor (fluvoxamine), and a strong (rifampin), and moderate (efavirenz) CYP3A inducer on the PK of pemigatinib	Adequate	[20]
		To evaluate the effect of a weak (dexamethasone) CYP3A inducer on the PK of pemigatinib	Inadequate	
		To assess the potential effect of pemigatinib as an inhibitor of P-gp, OCT2, and MATE1	Inadequate	
213591	Capmatinib	To assess the effect of a moderate CYP3A4 inhibitor or inducer on the exposure of multiple-dose capmatinib in the fasted state	Adequate	[21]
		To assess the effect of capmatinib on the exposures of repaglinide (CYP2C8), rosiglitazone (CYP2C8), warfarin (CYP2C9), and CYP2C19 (omeprazole)	Adequate	
		To assess the effect of capmatinib on the exposures of bupropion (CYP2B6)	Inadequate	
213246	Selpercatinib	To predict the effect of strong (itraconazole, ketoconazole, ritonavir, and clarithromycin) and moderate (diltiazem, fluconazole, verapamil) CYP3A inhibitors, strong (rifampin), moderate (bosentan, efavirenz), and weak (modafinil) CYP3A inducers on selpercatinib PK	Adequate	[22]
210730	Oliceridine	To assess the impact of inhibitors of CYP3A4 or CYP2D6 on oliceridine exposure in CYP2D6 poor metabolizers (PM) and non-PM subjects	Inadequate	[23]

(Continued)

Table 11.1: (Continued) Summary of PBPK Analyses in Novel Drug Approvals between 2020 and 2022

NDA/BLA	Generic Name	Intended Use of the PBPK Modeling Analysis	FDA's Assessment for Intended Use of the Models	Review Reference
213535	Risdiplam	To evaluate the effect risdiplam on the PK of a sensitive CYP3A substrate (midazolam) in children 2 months to 18 yrs of age	Adequate	[24]
761149	Satralizumab-mwge	To investigate the potential of satralizumab to reverse IL-6 mediated suppression of CYP enzymes	Exploratory	[25]
213721	Pralsetinib	To evaluate the effect of repeat doses of a moderate CYP3A inhibitor, and a combined P-gp and moderate CYP3A inhibitor on the PK of pralsetinib	Issued as a PMR, review is N/A	[26]
214787	Remdesivir	To predict the PK of remdesivir and its metabolites (GS-704277 and GS-441524) in pediatric patients 12 years of age and older and weighing at least 40 kg	adequate	[27]
214377	Vericiguat	To evaluate the effect of mefenamic acid (an UGT1A9 inhibitor) on vericiguat PK	Adequate	[28]
		To evaluate the effect of atazanavir (an UGT1A1 inhibitor) on vericiguat PK	Adequate	
212888	Cabotegravir and rilpivirine	To evaluate the effect of cabotegravir on the PK of OAT1 and OAT3 substrates	Adequate	[29]
		To evaluate the effect of UGT1A1/9 inhibitors on the PK of cabotegravir	Adequate	
213716	Voclosporin	To evaluate the effect of moderate (diltiazem and fluconazole), and weak (fluvoxamine and cimetidine) CYP3A inhibitors and moderate CYP3A inducer (efavirenz) on the PK of voclosporin	Adequate	[30]
		To evaluate the effect of voclosporin on the PK of an OATP1B substrate (e.g. rosuvastatin and pravastatin)	Inadequate	
214096	Tepotinib	To assess the effect of tepotinib treatment on the exposures of warfarin (CYP2C9)	Adequate	[31]
		To assess the effect of tepotinib treatment on the exposures of bupropion (CYP2B6)	Inadequate	
213176	Umbralisib	To predict the effect of umbralisib on the PK of midazolam (CYP3A4), repaglinide (CYP2C8), tolbutamide (CYP2C9), and S-mephenytoin (CYP2C19)	Inadequate	[32]
213498	Ponesimod	To assess the effect of ponesimod on the exposures of midazolam (CYP3A), warfarin (CYP2C9), tolbutamide (CYP2C9) and omeprazole (CYP2C19).	Adequate	[33]
213378	Olanzapine and samidorphan	To evaluate the effect of a strong CYP3A inhibitor (itraconazole) on samidorphan exposure	Adequate	[34]
		To evaluate the effect of hepatic impairment on the exposure of orally administered samidorphan (a different formulation)	Adequate	

(Continued)

Table 11.1: (Continued) Summary of PBPK Analyses in Novel Drug Approvals between 2020 and 2022

NDA/ BLA	Generic Name	Intended Use of the PBPK Modeling Analysis	FDA's Assessment for Intended Use of the Models	Review Reference
214665	Sotorasib	To evaluate the effect of sotorasib on the PK of a CYP2D6 substrate (desipramine)	Adequate	[35]
		To evaluate the effect of sotorasib as an inducer on the PK of CYP2C8, CYP2C9, and CYP2B6 substrates	Inadequate	
215341	Finerenone	To evaluate the effect of various CYP3A4 perpetrators (itraconazole, clarithromycin, fluvoxamine, efavirenz, rifampin)	Adequate	[36]
214783	Belumosudil	To assess the effect of CYP3A moderate inhibitors and inducers on the PK of belumosudil	Adequate	[37]
		To evaluate the effect of belumosudil on the PK of a substrate of CYP2C8, CYP2C9, and CYP3A4	Adequate	
		To evaluate the effect of belumosudil on the PK of a substrate of P-gp, OATP1B1, BCRP, and MATEs	Inadequate	
215383	Belzutifan	To evaluate the effect of UGT2B17 and CYP2C19 phenotype on the PK of belzutifan	Adequate	[38]
		To evaluate the effect of belzutifan on the PK of a CYP3A substrate (midazolam)	Adequate	
215310	Mobocertinib	To assess the effect of strong, moderate, and weak CYP3A inhibitors, and strong and moderate CYP3A inducers, on the single- and multiple-dose PK of mobocertinib and its active metabolites	Adequate	[39]
		To assess the effect of mobocertinib and its metabolites on the PK of CYP2B6 (bupropion), CYP2C8 (repaglinide), CYP2C9 (warfarin), CYP3A4 (midazolam, and alprazolam) substrates	Adequate	
		To assess the effect of mobocertinib on the PK of P-gp substrates (digoxin, and dabigatran)	Adequate	
		To assess the effect of mobocertinib on the PK of a BCRP substrate (sulfasalazine)	Inadequate	
215206	Atogepant	To predict the effect of a strong CYP3A inhibitor or a strong CYP3A inducer on the PK of atogepant if only considering CYP-mediated DDI in healthy subjects.	Adequate	[40]
		To predict the effect of a moderate CYP3A inhibitor (i.e., fluconazole) and a weak CYP3A inhibitor (i.e., cimetidine) on the PK of atogepant in healthy subjects	Adequate	
		To predict the PK of atogepant with and without complete knockout of P-gp or breast cancer resistance protein (BCRP) transporter function in healthy subjects.	Adequate	
214662	Maralixibat	To predict the potential drug interactions of maralixibat with intestinal CYP3A at the proposed dosing regimen	Not reviewed	[41]

(Continued)

Table 11.1: (Continued) Summary of PBPK Analyses in Novel Drug Approvals between 2020 and 2022

NDA/ BLA	Generic Name	Intended Use of the PBPK Modeling Analysis	FDA's Assessment for Intended Use of the Models	Review Reference
215358	Asciminib	To predict the effect of strong CYP3A modulators on the exposure of asciminib	Inadequate	[42]
		To predict the changes in exposure of asciminib, at higher dose levels, in the presence of food	Inadequate	
		To predict the changes in exposure of asciminib due to hepatic impairment or renal impairment	Inadequate	
		To confirm a negative DDI potential of asciminib with a BCRP/OATP1B substrate	Inadequate	
		To predict the effect of asciminib on the PK of a P-gp substrate	Adequate	
		To predict the effect of asciminib on the PK of a CYP1A2, UGT1A1, CYP3A, CYP2C8, CYP2C9, and CYP2C19 substrates	Adequate	
		To evaluate the effect of elevated gastric pH on the PK of asciminib at a higher dose level	Adequate	
215596	Maribavir	To predict the effect of ritonavir (strong CYP3A inhibitor), diltiazem and erythromycin (moderate CYP3A inhibitors), carbamazepine and phenytoin (strong CYP3A inducers), and phenobarbital and efavirenz (moderate CYP3A inducers) on the PK of maribavir in healthy subjects	Adequate	[43]
		To predict the effect of maribavir on the PK of rosuvastatin (a BCRP substrate).	Adequate	
214985	Daridorexant	To evaluate the effect of strong (intraconazole, ketoconazole), moderate (verapamil, erythromycin, and fluconazole), and weak (cimetidine and ranitidine) CYP3A inhibitors, and strong (carbamazepine and rifampin), and moderate (efavirenz) CYP3A inducer on the PK of daridorexant	Adequate	[44]
216196	Mitapivat	To evaluate the effect of strong (intraconazole, ketoconazole), moderate (verapamil, erythromycin, and fluconazole) CYP3A inhibitors, and strong (rifampin), and moderate (efavirenz) CYP3A inducer on the PK of mitapivat at steady state	Adequate	[45]
		To evaluate the effect of mitapivat on the PK of a sensitive CYP3A substrate (midazolam)	Adequate	
		To evaluate the induction effect of mitapivat on CYP2B6, CYP2C8, CYP2C9, and CYP2C19 substrates	Inadequate	
		To evaluate the effect of mitapivat on the PK of substrates of the transporters OATP1B, MATE2, and OCT1	Inadequate	
		To evaluate the effect of mitapivat on the PK of a OAT3 substrate	Adequate	
		To evaluate the effect of elevated gastric pH on the exposure of mitapivat	Adequate	
208712	Pacritinib	To predict the DDI effect of clarithromycin on pacritinib under a more conservative scenario (such as a longer clarithromycin treatment).	Inadequate	[46]
		To predict the DDI effect of a moderate CYP3A inducer, such as efavirenz.	Inadequate	

(Continued)

Table 11.1: (Continued) Summary of PBPK Analyses in Novel Drug Approvals between 2020 and 2022

NDA/ BLA	Generic Name	Intended Use of the PBPK Modeling Analysis	FDA's Assessment for Intended Use of the Models	Review Reference
214998	Mavacamten	To evaluate the effect of CYP2C19 phenotype on the PK of mavacamten	Adequate	[47]
		To evaluate the effect of CYP2C19 and CYP3A4 inhibitors and inducers on the PK of mavacamten	Adequate	
		To evaluate the effect of mavacamten on the PK of CYP3A and CYP2C19 substrates	Adequate	
215152	Vonoprazan, amoxicillin, and clarithromycin	To evaluate the effect of combo on the PK of CYP2C19 substrates (omeprazole and lansoprazole)	Adequate	[48]
		To evaluate the effect of CYP2D6 polymorphism on the PK of vonoprazan	Suggested additional study	
		To evaluate the effect of strong CYP3A inducers on the PK of vonoprazan	Inadequate	
215866	Tirzepatide	To provide a qualitative assessment of the effect of tirzepatide-mediated delayed gastric emptying on the PK of acetaminophen, atorvastatin, digoxin, lisinopril, metformin, metoprolol, sitagliptin, and S-warfarin	Adequate	[49]
761261	Olipudase alfa	To describe the distribution and clearance of olipudase alfa in plasma and in tissues of interest	Adequate	[50]
214801	Futibatinib	To evaluate the effect of CYP3A modulators on the PK of futibatinib	Inadequate	[51]
		To evaluate the effect of futibatinib as a perpetrator of P-gp and BCRP substrates	Supportive	
761291	Teclistamab-cqyv	To evaluate IL-6 effects on CYP activity	Not reviewed	[52]

Adequate: the PBPK analysis is adequate for the specific intended use and conclusions can support relevant regulatory decisions; inadequate: the PBPK analysis is inadequate for the specific intended use and cannot support relevant regulatory decisions; suggested additional study or supportive: additional studies were recommended based on PBPK analysis; not reviewed: PBPK model was not reviewed in detail.

11.4 PBPK-RELATED GUIDANCES

In 2020, the FDA guidance for industry on in-vitro and clinical DDI studies to promote a consistent approach in designing, conducting, and interpreting enzyme- or transporter-mediated in vitro and clinical DDI studies was finalized. Regulatory agencies (such as EMA and PMDA) and ICH also published guidances on DDI interactions. A similar workflow was proposed in this guidance to support the identification and evaluation of the DDI potential of a drug using in-vitro and in-vivo data. The first step is to identify the DDI potential for a drug as a victim (effect of other drugs on the investigational drug, including relevant metabolites) and as a perpetrator (effect of the investigational drug on concomitant drugs). If in vitro studies suggest the investigational drug is a substrate of a metabolic enzyme or transporter, dedicated clinical DDI studies are recommended. If in vitro data suggest the investigational drug as a perpetrator on the major enzymes or transporter pathways, the applicant may use the mechanistic models such as PBPK modeling to further evaluate the DDI potential of the investigational drug or conduct an in vivo DDI study. For the latter part, there are some discrepancies between FDA and EMA/PMDA guidances regarding the applicability of PBPK modeling as a screening tool to identify the DDI potential of a drug as a transporter perpetrator based on in-vitro data.

The utility of PBPK modeling to inform the design of clinical trials and DDI studies at all stages of drug development program is well recognized by regulatory agencies and industries. It is also agreed that a PBPK model, after validation using additional data from clinical and/or DDI studies that used strong index perpetrators, can be used to predict the effect of a less potent inhibitor or in a different dosage regimen. While all the guidelines recommend the use of modeling and simulation tools, e.g. mechanistic static, and dynamic PBPK models to support DDI assessment, discrepancies were noted on the applicability of PBPK modeling on CYPs induction and transporter-based DDI (Table 11.2). FDA considers PBPK modeling to screen the DDI potential for drugs as inhibitors or inducers of CYP enzymes based on in-vitro data. For transporter, FDA noted that there are knowledge gaps in transporter biology and limited experience in determining and modeling the kinetics of transporters. Compared to CYP enzymes, the predictive performance of PBPK modeling for transporter-based DDIs has not been established.

In comparison, EMA's guidance did not mention the applicability of PBPK modeling to predict the DDI potential of a drug as an inducer of CYP enzymes or perpetrator of transporters. EMA uses a relative induction score (RIS) approach to identify the drug's induction potential. Both PMDA and ICH recognized the applicability of PBPK models to evaluate CYP induction potential. Similar to EMA, PMDA did not discuss the applicability of PBPK modeling for assessing transporter-based DDI. However, ICH considered the PBPK modeling to support negative DDI prediction when the drug is an in vitro inhibitor for a basolateral uptake transporter.

As the number of regulatory submissions including PBPK models grows, it becomes challenging for regulators to interpret the modeling analyses in various contexts and formats within a short review timeline. To facilitate efficient assessment, FDA, EMA and PMDA have issued guidances for industries for reporting PBPK analyses in regulatory submissions [57–59]. In general, the FDA guidance does not intend to define what are best practices for conducting PBPK analyses or evaluating PBPK approaches for regulatory applications; rather, it outlines standardized content and format for PBPK analysis reports submitted to the FDA [57]. In the EMA guideline, special emphasis has been given to the expectation on qualifying a PBPK platform for the intended use and evaluating the predictive performance of the model. PMDA guidance is generally in-line with

Table 11.2: Comparison of Recommendations of using PBPK Analyses for DDI Evaluation by Various Guidances

Area of Application	FDA [53]	EMA [54]	PMDA [55]	ICH [56]
Describe enzyme-mediated ADME process	Applicable	Applicable	Applicable	Applicable
CYP interactions for drugs (as victims or perpetrators) once verified with clinical DDI data	Applicable	Applicable	Applicable	Applicable
CYP interactions for drugs as inhibitors based on in-vitro data	Applicable	Applicable	Applicable	Applicable
CYP interactions for drugs as inducers based on in-vitro data	Applicable	Not mentioned	Applicable	Applicable
Describe transporter-mediated ADME process	Applicable	Not mentioned	Not mentioned	Applicable
Transporter-mediated DDI	The predictive performance has not been established.	Not mentioned	Not mentioned	PBPK models can be used to support negative DDI prediction when the drug is an in vitro inhibitor for a basolateral uptake transporter.
Predict the magnitude of DDI in specific population (s)	Yes, such as in patients with renal impairment or patients with genetic deficiencies in certain metabolizing enzymes.	Yes, such as DDI in genetic subgroups and in pediatrics	Yes, can be used to evaluate DDI in special population or populations with specific diseases	Not mentioned

FDA's guidance but includes some recommendations on a model's performance similar to those discussed in EMA's guidance, e.g. tendency of concentration-time profiles, and inter-individual variability. All guidances emphasize that it is critical for the applicant to clearly state the purpose, context of use of the modeling analysis, its relevance to regulatory decisions and demonstrate how the model has been adequately validated for its intended purpose. These concepts have been discussed in a recently proposed credibility assessment framework for general model evaluation which could potentially be applied to PBPK model assessment [60]. Sensitivity analysis is recommended to evaluate the impact of uncertainties of the model parameters on the simulation results. The decision to accept results from PBPK analyses is made on a case-by-case basis by considering its intended uses. Table 11.3 provides an overview of the reporting template among three guidance documents.

Table 11.3: Summary and Comparison of FDA, EMA, and PMDA Guidances on PBPK Analyses Reporting Template

	FDA [57]	EMA [58]	PMDA [59]
A. Content of an PBPK Analysis Report Submitted for Regulatory Review			
Summary/ Objective	• State the objectives and rationales of the analyses • Provide an overview and key conclusions of the report • State how the analyses can address a clinical concern and to support a regulatory decision	• State the objectives and the intended regulatory purposes of the PBPK modelling, and it's proposed impact on Summary of Product Characteristics (SmPC)	• Summarize the objectives of the PBPK analyses, methods, results, discussions and important conclusions
Introduction/ Background	• Drug's physicochemical, PK and PD properties • Summary of exposure-response relationship for efficacy and safety • A PBPK-related regulatory history • Cross-reference to PBPK reports of the same drug substance or product	• Drug's physicochemical properties; -In-vitro and in-vivo ADME information • A quantitative mass-balance diagram • Summary of clinical studies related to the intended purpose of the model • Summary of exposure-response relationship for efficacy and safety	• Clinical development strategies related to PBPK model analysis • Drug's physicochemical and pharmacogenetic properties, in-vitro and in vivo ADME information and a quantitative mass-balance diagram. • Summary of exposure-response relationship for efficacy and safety • Summary of results obtained from prior PBPK model analysis
Materials and Methods	• Detail step-wise description of modeling development and strategy • Model parameters and assumptions • Simulation conditions and details • Justification of using previous developed models (e.g., a virtual population)	• Model parameter • Model development • Modeling assumptions • Simulation trials and scenario • Approaches used to test the modeling assumptions and uncertainties	• Workflow of the model analysis • Modeling assumptions • Simulation • Model validation (compared to observed data) and sensitivity analyses
Results	• Include results of model verification, validation and sensitivity analysis • Present the results to address a clinical concern/question in text, tabulated and figures format	• Present in tabulated and figures format • Include descriptive statistics of pharmacokinetic parameters • Include results of sensitivity analysis	• Demonstrate model's predictive performance and robustness of the model relevant to model's objective • Include results of model validation and sensitivity analysis • Present the results visually (e.g., overlay plots) and/or as tabular data (descriptive statistics, etc)

(Continued)

Table 11.3: (Continued) Summary and Comparison of FDA, EMA, and PMDA Guidances on PBPK Analyses Reporting Template

	FDA [57]	EMA [58]	PMDA [59]
Discussion	• Demonstrate the adequacy of the PBPK analysis to address the proposed scientific, regulatory, or clinical questions. • Discuss and justify the validity of the proposed application in the context of the totality of evidence and the level of confidence for the intended uses of the model	• Discuss the contribution and uncertainty of the PBPK analysis to the regulatory decision-making	• Discuss the scientific validity of the PBPK model as well as its uncertainty and limitations. • Describe the validity of the simulation results according to the purpose of use.

B. Comments on Evaluation and Acceptance of a Model

	FDA	EMA	PMDA
Sensitivity analysis	• Used to assess the uncertainties of model parameters • Used to evaluate the robustness of the models • Mentioned in the methods and results sections	• Used to evaluate the key model parameters that are likely to impact the simulation results or are highly uncertain • Should be performed both during the development and application of the drug model • Used to evaluate the uncertainty regarding the ontogeny and allometry for pediatric application	• Used to evaluate the key model parameters that are likely to impact the simulation results or are highly uncertain • Need to justify the range of each parameter employed in sensitivity analysis • Used to evaluate the uncertainty regarding the ontogeny for pediatric application
Acceptance/ Predictive performance	• The decision is made on a case-by-case basis considering the intended uses and other factors	• Acceptance criteria (adequacy of prediction) depend on the regulatory impact and needs to be considered • Additional example available in Appendix	• The evaluation criteria may vary depending on the purpose of analysis
PBPK platform/ modeling files	• FDA does not endorse a particular software for PBPK modeling • Schematic view of the model structure and mathematical equations • Submit all the files related to modeling, simulation, datasets • Documentations to aid the reviewer to execute the model	• Include information to support platform qualification • Additional examples are available in the Appendix to support qualification of a PBPK platform based on its intended purpose, and regulatory impact of the modeling • The models need to be in an executable format	• Accepting commercially available or proprietarily built PBPK platforms • Modeling files should be submitted along with the PBPK report

11.5 DDI PREDICTIONS

PBPK analysis for DDIs is the largest portion of PBPK submissions to OCP/FDA. There are extensive research and studies for model building, development, and validation for DDI assessments. Within the spectrum of DDIs, the complexity also varies from less complicated scenarios with high confidence in model prediction to more complex scenarios with low confidence in model prediction.

Figure 11.2 is a schematic diagram of model validation involving one specific pathway. Using the CYP3A pathway as an example, models are developed for CYP3A probe substrates (such as midazolam, triazolam, alprazolam, and alfentanil), strong (such as itraconazole and clarithromycin), moderate (such as erythromycin, and verapamil), and weak (fluvoxamine and cimetidine) CYP3A inhibitors, and strong (rifampin), and moderate (efavirenz) CYP3A inducers. Each substrate drug

224

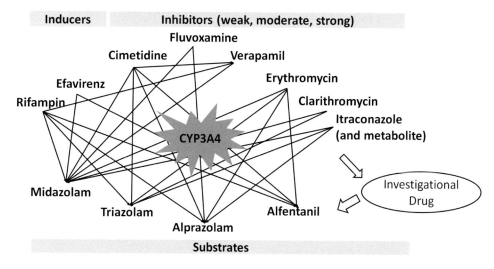

Figure 11.2 A general scheme of PBPK model validation for DDI predictions. (Modified from Ref. [61].)

was validated against several modulators, and each modulator was validated against several substrates. Each line in the diagram represents a DDI study. Following model validation, the modulator models then can be used to predict their effects on an investigational drug, which is a CYP3A substrate. The probe substrate models can be used to predict the effect of an investigational drug on the PK of a CYP3A substrate. CYP3A is one of the extensively studied pathways as it is involved in the metabolism of many drugs. The DDI model development and validation for other pathways follow similar principles but may face challenges including less number of available studies, less reliable in vitro systems, lack of suitable probe substrates, and specific inhibitors. The readers are referred to the DDI chapter in this book for more details regarding PBPK analyses for DDI predictions. In this chapter, we will use case examples to illustrate the utility of PBPK analyses for DDI predictions in regulatory decision-making.

11.5.1 Enzyme-Mediated DDIs

The enzymes that are evaluated in the PBPK analyses include both CYP and non-CYP enzymes. A comprehensive list of examples can be found in previous publications [4,5] and Table 11.1. Here, we highlight a few interesting examples.

Ibrutinib (initial US approval in 2013) is one of the early examples where PBPK analyses were used to inform labeling. Ibrutinib is a small-molecule inhibitor of Bruton's tyrosine kinase (BTK). The recommended dosages of ibrutinib are 420 or 560 mg once daily depending on the disease types.

The absolute bioavailability of ibrutinib in fasted condition was 2.9% in healthy subjects. Following oral administration, the median Tmax of ibrutinib was 1–2 hours. Food increased ibrutinib Cmax and AUC by approximately 2 to 4- and 2-fold, respectively, compared with the fasted condition [62]. Ibrutinib binding to human plasma protein in vitro was 97.3% with no concentration dependence in the range of 50–1,000 ng/mL. The volume of distribution (V_d) was 683 L, and the apparent volume of distribution at steady state ($V_{d,ss}/F$) was approximately 10,000 L [62]. Ibrutinib is mainly eliminated via metabolism primarily by CYP3A and to a minor extent by CYP2D6. The clearance following intravenous administration was 62 and 76 L/h in the fasted and fed conditions, respectively. The apparent oral clearance is approximately 2,000 and 1,000 L/h in the fasted and fed conditions, respectively. The half-life of ibrutinib is 4–6 hours [62]. In vivo DDI studies suggested that ketoconazole (a strong CYP3A inhibitor) increased ibrutinib dose-normalized Cmax and AUC by 29-fold and 24-fold, respectively; rifampin (a strong CYP3A inducer) decreased ibrutinib Cmax and AUC by more than 13- and 10-fold [62].

During the initial approval, the applicant conducted PBPK analyses to evaluate the effects of moderate CYP3A inhibitors and inducers on the PK of ibrutinib. Specifically, the effects of moderate CYP3A inhibitors (diltiazem, erythromycin), weak CYP3A inhibitor (fluvoxamine), and

Table 11.4: Predicted Pharmacokinetic Parameter Ratios for Ibrutinib Following Interactions with CYP3A4 Inhibitors under Fasted Condition

Modulator	AUCR	$C_{max}R$
Itraconazole	19	15
Voriconazole	9.1	8.4
Clarithromycin	14	12
Erythromycin	7.5	6.7
Diltiazem	4.9	4.7
Fluvoxamine	1.9	2.0

Source: Modified from Ref. [67].
AUCR and $C_{max}R$ are the geometric mean ratios of ibrutinib AUC and C_{max} in the presence and absence of an inhibitor.

moderate CYP3A inducer (efavirenz) were predicted by PBPK modeling and simulation [63]. The PBPK analyses predicted that erythromycin, diltiazem, and fluvoxamine increased the geometric mean AUC of ibrutinib by 7.5, 4.9, and 1.9-fold, respectively (Table 11.4). Efavirenz was predicted to decrease the AUC of ibrutinib by approximately 60%. The PBPK prediction results are reflected in the labeling [64]. Based on the PBPK simulations, the consideration that exposures observed in the dose range between 140 and 840 mg are safe and efficacious, and the limitation that only one dosage strength (140 mg) was available, a dose of 140 mg was recommended when ibrutinib must be co-administered with a moderate CYP3A inhibitor [63,64].

After the original approval, the applicant continued to expand the indications and refine the dosage strengths for ibrutinib. Voriconazole and posaconazole are commonly used concomitant medications. Both drugs may increase the exposure of ibrutinib by more than fivefold. PBPK modeling and simulation suggested that the effect of posaconazole was dose and formulation-dependent [65], and avoid using was recommended when posaconazole was given as immediate-release dosage form at 400 mg twice daily. Later, when a lower strength of 70 mg capsules became available, dosage adjustment could be recommended when ibrutinib is co-administered with posaconazole suspensions [66].

This case example illustrated the impact of PBPK analyses not only on the initial labeling but also on the continuous drug product development into life cycle management. There are many other CYP enzyme-mediated DDI PBPK analyses examples in regulatory submissions as listed in Table 11.1 and previous publications [4,5] which are not discussed here.

In recent years, PBPK analyses have also made progress in non-CYP enzyme-mediated DDIs for the investigational drug as a perpetrator (asciminib and tucatinib), and a substrate (ertugliflozin, cabotegravir, and vericiguat). As these cases are relatively recent and have not been extensively discussed previously, we provide a summary for each case.

In the asciminib and tucatinib programs, PBPK analyses were applied to evaluate their inhibition effects on the PK of a UGT substrate (Table 11.5). Both drugs are inhibitors of UGT1A1. Raltegravir is the substrate in both PBPK analyses. In vitro inhibition constant (K_i) values were first applied to predict the AUC change of raltegravir in the presence and absence of an inhibitor. Sensitivity analyses were performed using 10- to 20-fold lower K_i values. Currently, there is no consensus regarding the range of sensitivity analysis for the K_i value due to limited experience. For asciminib, the inhibition potential on a UGT1A substrate cannot be ruled out based on a 10-fold decrease in in vitro K_i value [42]. For tucatinib, the weak inhibition effect (> 1.25 and <2-fold) was concluded based on a 20-fold decrease in in vitro K_i value [19].

Ertugliflozin, a sodium glucose co-transporter 2 (SGLT2) inhibitor indicated as an adjunct to diet and exercise to improve glycemic control in adults with type 2 diabetes mellitus, is a UGT1A9 and UGT2B7 substrate [68]. PBPK analyses were performed to evaluate the effect of a UGT inhibitor on the PK of ertugliflozin. To develop the ertugliflozin model, PK data following intravenous administration, oral administration, and human ADME (absorption, distribution, metabolism, and excretion) studies were used to calibrate the metabolism via the UGT pathways. Further, an

Table 11.5: Summary of PBPK Analyses Evaluating the Investigational Drug as a UGT Inhibitor in Regulatory Submissions

Perpetrator	Dose (mg)	Pathway	Substrate	K_i (μM)	Source	Pred. AUCR of Substrate	Conclusion
Asciminib	40 mg BID	UGT1A1	Raltegravir	0.35	In vitro	1.16	The inhibition potential on a UGT1A substrate cannot be excluded.
				0.175	SA	1.28	
	200 mg BID			0.35	In vitro	1.62	
				0.175	SA	2.14	
Tucatinib	300 mg BID			1.81	In vitro	1.04	The effect of tucatinib on a UGT1A1 substrate is expected to be weak.
				0.181	SA	1.27	
				0.09	SA	1.45	

Source: Data are extracted from Refs. [19,42].
SA, sensitivity analysis.

in vitro inhibition of UGT activity in human liver microsomes (HLM) study and an in vitro UGT reaction phenotyping study were used to calibrate the kidney and liver UGT metabolism, and estimate the f_m (fractional metabolism) values via UGT1A9 and UGT2B7 [69]. The estimated f_m values are shown in Table 11.6. The mefenamic acid (an inhibitor of UGT1A9 and UGT2B7) model was developed and validated against available PK and DDI data with dapagliflozin (a UGT1A9 and UGT2B7 substrate) [69,70]. The inhibition constants (K_i) of mefenamic acid for both UGT1A9 and UGT2B7 pathways were reduced by approximated threefold (from 0.11 to 0.038 μM for UGT1A9, and from 0.15 to 0.051 μM for UGT2B7) to capture the observed effects of mefenamic acid on the PK of dapagliflozin (Table 11.6). The inhibition constants (K_i) of mefenamic acid were further reduced by approximately 50%, 0.019 μM for UGT1A9, and 0.026 μM for UGT2B7, to account for a worst-case scenario, which suggested that the predicted increase in ertugliflozin AUC was less than twofold (Table 11.6). The simulation results are reflected in the ertugliflozin 2017 labeling "Physiologically based PK (PBPK) modeling suggests that co-administration of mefenamic acid (UGT inhibitor) may increase the AUC and C_{max} of ertugliflozin by 1.51- and 1.19-fold, respectively." [68]

Cabotegravir, a human immunodeficiency virus type-1 (HIV-1) integrase strand transfer inhibitor (INSTI), is a substrate of UGT1A1 and UGT1A9 [71]. In the cabotegravir program, one of the PBPK analyses aims was to evaluate the effect of a UGT1A1 inhibitor on the PK of cabotegravir. In the cabotegravir model, the UGT1A1 contribution to cabotegravir metabolism ($f_{m,UGT1A1}=0.62$) was

Table 11.6: Summary of PBPK Analyses Evaluating an Investigational Drug as a UGT Substrate in Regulatory Submissions

Substrate	Metabolism Fraction	Inhibitor (Interaction Pathway)	In vitro K_i (μM)	Model K_i (μM)	AUCR
Ertugliflozin	$f_{m,CYP}=0.12, f_{m,UGT1A9}=0.70, f_{m,UGT2B7}=0.16$	Mefenamic acid (UGT1A9/UGT2B7)	UGT1A9: 0.11 UGT2B7: 0.15	UGT1A9: 0.038 UGT2B7: 0.051	1.19
				UGT1A9: 0.019 UGT2B7: 0.026	1.27
Cabotegravir	$f_{m,UGT1A1}=0.62, f_{m,UGT1A9}=0.37$	Atazanavir (UGT1A1)	1.9	1.9	1.1
	$f_{m,UGT1A1}=0.96$			1.9	1.2
	$f_{m,UGT1A1}=0.62, f_{m,UGT1A9}=0.37$			0.19	1.5
	$f_{m,UGT1A1}=0.92$			0.19	1.9
Vericiguat	$f_{m,UGT1A1}=0.19, f_{m,UGT1A9}=0.67$	Atazanavir (UGT1A1)	0.19	0.19	1.12
		Mefenamic acid (UGT1A9)	0.3	0.3	
	$f_{m,UGT1A1}=0.34, f_{m,UGT1A9}=0.52$	Atazanavir (UGT1A1)	0.19	0.05	1.27
		Mefenamic acid (UGT1A9)	0.3	0.15	

Source: Data are extracted from Refs. [28,29,69,70,72,74].

verified against clinical PK data from UGT1A1 poor metabolizers (PMs) [29,72]. Atazanavir model was developed as the UGT1A1 inhibitor and validated against the DDI study with raltegravir (a UGT1A1 substrate). Using the in vitro UGT1A1 K_i of 1.9 μM, the PBPK analysis was able to capture the observed effect of atazanavir on raltegravir. To capture uncertainties in the f_m and K_i values, sensitivity analyses were performed on $f_{m,UGT1A1}$ and K_i (Table 11.6), and results suggested that the effect of atazanavir on the PK of cabotegravir is less than twofold. The PBPK simulation results were reflected in the cabotegravir 2021 labeling "Simulations using PBPK modeling show that no clinically significant interaction is expected during co-administration of cabotegravir with drugs that inhibit UGT1A1." [71]

Vericiguat, a soluble guanylate cyclase (sGC) stimulator, is a substrate of UGT1A1 and UGT1A9. PBPK analyses were performed to evaluate the effect of UGT1A1 inhibitor (atazanavir) and UGT1A9 inhibitor (mefenamic acid) on the PK of vericiguat. Atazanavir and mefenamic acid models were validated against the DDI studies with raltegravir and dapagliflozin, respectively, using the in vitro K_i values (Table 11.6). However, using a set of lower K_i values (0.05 μM for atazanavir (UGT1A1) and 0.15 μM for mefenamic acid (UGT1A9)), the model estimation was numerically closer to the observed AUC ratios of raltegravir and dapagliflozin in the presence and absence of atazanavir and mefenamic acid, respectively. A different set of f_m values were also explored ($f_{m,UGT1A1}=0.34, f_{m,UGT1A9}=0.52$). Overall, the predicted increase in vericiguat AUC is lower than twofold in the presence of UGT1A1 and UGT1A9 inhibitors. The PBPK simulations are reflected in the vericiguat 2021 labeling "No clinically significant differences on vericiguat pharmacokinetics were predicted with co-administration of atazanavir (UGT1A1 inhibitor)." [73]

The magnitude of UGT enzymes mediated inhibition rarely exceeds threefold and is often around twofold or less as recognized by the International Council for Harmonisation of Technical Requirements for Pharmaceuticals for Human Use (ICH) M12 Drug Interaction Studies guideline [56]. As such, the models appear to be insensitive to the changes in fractional metabolism (f_m) or inhibition constant (K_i). In addition, the "middle-out" approach, a model building approach based on both mechanistic knowledge and clinical observations, is commonly used in the PBPK analyses evaluating UGT enzyme-mediated DDIs.

11.5.2 Transporter-Mediated DDIs

We have seen more PBPK analyses evaluating transporter-mediated DDIs in recent years compared to the period between 2008 and 2017. Table 11.7 is a list of examples that consisted of PBPK analyses evaluating transporter-mediated DDIs or transporter's involvement in a drug's ADME. More PBPK analyses were used for evaluating the investigational drug as a perpetrator compared to evaluating the investigational drug as a substrate.

To quantitatively evaluate an investigational drug as a substrate, typically, the substrate model is quantified for the specific pathway. It could be challenging to validate a transporter substrate model because transporters are often located at multiple organs, and plasma PK may not be the most relevant and sensitive metric. To validate the substrate model, a pathway-specific DDI

Table 11.7: Examples of PBPK Analyses to Evaluate Transporter-Mediated DDIs or Transporter's Involvement in a Drug's ADME in Regulatory Submission

Pathway	Drug as a Substrate	Drug as a Perpetrator
P-gp	rivaroxaban, ceritinib, prucalopride, upadacitinib, neratinib, naloxegol, atogepant	ibrutinib, prucalopride, elagolix, fosnetupitant, ivosidenib, lasmiditan, erdafitinib, fedratinib, lefamulin, pemigatinib, belumosudil, mobocertinib, asciminib, futibatinib
BCRP	prucalopride, upadacitinib, atogepant	osimertinib, pexidartinib, fedratinib, belumosudil, mobocertinib, asciminib, maribavir, futibatinib
OATP1B1/3	simeprevir, letermovir	fosnetupitant, ivosidenib, pexidartinib, fedratinib, lefamulin, tucatinib, voclosporin, belumosudil, asciminib, mitapivat
OAT1/3	baricitinib	apalutamide, ivosidenib, cabotegravir, mitapivat
OCT2/ MATEs		prucalopride, apalutamide, pexidartinib, erdafitinib, fedratinib, lefamulin, pemigatinib, belumosudil, mitapivat

Source: Drugs@FDA, [4,5].

study is commonly needed due to the lack of in vitro to in vivo extrapolation for transporters. To evaluate the effect of an investigational drug as a perpetrator, a robust substrate model is needed. Ideally, the substrate model should be specific and be able to describe all available PK, pharmacogenetics (if relevant), and DDI studies [56]. Our current experience with transporter-mediated DDI PBPK modeling showed that the in vitro K_i values need to be decreased significantly (often by more than 10-fold) to capture the observed in vivo DDI magnitude. Therefore, the PBPK analyses evaluating an investigational drug as a transporter perpetrator are generally used to rule out or identify potential DDI liabilities. In this section, we use two examples, mobocertinib and baricitinib, to illustrate the key considerations when using PBPK analyses to evaluate an investigational drug as a perpetrator and substrate, respectively. Of note, for different transporters, key considerations could be different due to their properties.

Mobocertinib is a P-gp inhibitor in vitro. Comparing the systemic exposure with the in vitro K_i, the effect of mobocertinib on systemic P-gp is unlikely, based on the basic model calculation. Therefore, the evaluation focused on the interaction via the gut P-gp. The two substrate models, digoxin and dabigatran, were validated against multiple perpetrator models, including clarithromycin, quinidine, ritonavir, verapamil/norverapamil, and ketoconazole [39]. The sensitivity range for K_i was obtained by comparing the model K_i with in vitro K_i values reported in the University of Washington Drug Interaction Database (https://www.druginteractionsolutions.org/). P-gp is an efflux transporter. Therefore, the K_i value should be estimated based on intracellular concentration. There is a large range of in vitro K_i values for the same pair of perpetrator and substrate in the literature due to different experimental conditions, and data analysis methods. Ideally, when comparing the model K_i with in vitro K_i values, the in vitro K_i estimated using the same analysis method should be applied to minimize the variability. In the mobocertinib PBPK analysis, evaluating its effect on the PK of a P-gp substrate, the importance of using a mechanistic oral absorption model instead of a first-order absorption model was also illustrated. Mobocertinib has high solubility. Using a first-order absorption may significantly underestimate the gut concentration which is the concentration at the site of interaction. After applying a mechanistic oral absorption model and based on sensitivity analysis on K_i, it was concluded that no clinically relevant increase in the exposure of digoxin and dabigatran when they were co-administered with mobocertinib.

Baricitinib, a Janus kinase (JAK) inhibitor, is a substrate of OAT3. In vivo, probenecid (an OAT3 inhibitor) increased baricitinib AUC by approximately twofold. One of the purposes of PBPK analyses was to evaluate the effect of other OAT3 inhibitors on the PK of baricitinib. Figure 11.3 illustrated the modeling strategy evaluating the effect of OAT3 inhibitors on the PK of baricitinib [75,76]. Briefly, baricitinib substrate model was developed and validated against available plasma and urine PK, and DDI study with probenecid. OAT3 inhibitor models, diclofenac and ibuprofen, were developed and validated against available PK, and ibuprofen and pemetrexed DDI study [77]. The diclofenac and ibuprofen models were then used to predict their effects on the PK of

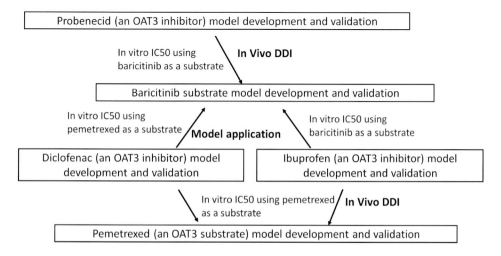

Figure 11.3 PBPK modeling and simulation strategy evaluating the effect of OAT3 inhibitors on the PK of baricitinib.

baricitinib. The modeling and simulation result informed labeling "simulations with diclofenac and ibuprofen (OAT3 inhibitors with less inhibition potential) predicted minimal effect on the PK of baricitinib." In this example, in vitro IC50 values using the same pair of inhibitor and substrate generally provided reasonable DDI predictions suggesting a potential for in vitro to in vivo extrapolation. More examples of this type will increase our confidence in broadly using the PBPK analyses for assessing OAT3-mediated DDIs.

11.5.3 DDIs Via Other Mechanisms

In addition to enzyme- and transporter- mediated DDIs, PBPK analyses have also been used to evaluate DDIs via pharmacodynamic (PD) effect-mediated mechanisms such as elevated gastric pH-mediated DDIs, the investigational drug as a cytokine (such as IL-6) modulator and consequently affecting CYP enzyme activity and the metabolism of concomitant medications, or the investigational drug affecting gastric emptying time and consequently the absorption of concomitant medications. In this section, we provide a few examples of PBPK analyses in those areas in the regulatory submissions.

11.5.3.1 Gastric pH-Mediated DDIs

Gastric ARAs such as proton pump inhibitors (PPIs) are commonly used medications to reduce stomach acid. They increase the stomach pH to approximately above 4. Many drugs have pH-dependent solubility and therefore, the absorption could be impacted by co-administration with an ARA. PPIs are widely prescribed and available over the counter. Recently, FDA published a draft guidance entitled 'Evaluation of Gastric pH-Dependent Drug Interactions With Acid-Reducing Agents: Study Design, Data Analysis, and Clinical Implications' to facilitate the evaluation of gastric pH-mediated DDI evaluation during product development [78]. In the guidance, PBPK modeling and simulations are identified as a tool to assess the potential for gastric pH-mediated DDIs. Many examples have been published in the literature [79–84] applying PBPK analyses evaluating the effect of elevated gastric pH on the drug's absorption. Here, we provide a few such examples in regulatory submissions.

Panobinostat, a histone deacetylase inhibitor, has non-linear and pH-dependent solubility. Overall, the solubility is high according to the definition by Biopharmaceutics Classification System (BCS) (i.e., highest single therapeutic dose completely soluble in 250 mL or less of aqueous media over the pH range of 1.2–6.8) except in pH 7.6 where the amount that can be completely dissolved in 250 mL medium was less than the recommended highest single dose [85]. In the submission, the applicant provided PBPK simulations to evaluate if a pH modifying agent may impact the absorption of panobinostat. The model appeared to be able to describe the effect of food on T_{max} and C_{max}. The simulations suggested that elevated gastric pH does not impact the absorption of panobinostat [85]. The simulation results were used to inform labeling "Coadministration of FARYDAK with drugs that elevate the gastric pH was not evaluated in vitro or in a clinical trial; however, altered panobinostat absorption was not observed in simulations using physiologically based pharmacokinetic (PBPK) models." [86]

Mitapivat, a pyruvate kinase activator, has pH-dependent solubility and high solubility at pH ≤ 5.5 for all strengths [87]. A mechanistic PBPK absorption model was developed to evaluate the effect of elevated gastric pH on the exposure of mitapivat. The model was validated against PK data following administration of single dose ranging from 30 to 700 mg and multiple-dose ranging from 15 to 120 mg BID (twice daily). Elevated gastric pH up to 5 did not have significant impact on mitapivat PK and fraction absorbed. Sensitivity analyses were performed to evaluate the impact of particle size, critical supersaturation ratio, and solubility factor on the predicted PK under various gastric pH conditions. Based on the totality of evidence, it was concluded that elevated gastric pH may have no clinically relevant impact on the absorption and PK of mitapivat [45].

11.5.3.2 Glucagon-Like Peptide-1 (GLP-1) Receptor Agonist Mediated DDIs

Glucagon-like peptide-1 (GLP-1) receptor agonists are known to prolong gastric emptying [88], which consequently may affect the absorption of concomitant medications. DDI studies were performed in a few GLP-1 receptor agonist programs, such as exenatide [89], liraglutide [90], lixisenatide [91], and dulaglutide [92]. Tirzepatide is a glucose-dependent insulinotropic polypeptide (GIP) receptor and GLP-1 receptor agonist [93]. In the tirzepatide program, mechanistic PBPK absorption model were developed to evaluate the effect of tirzepatide on the absorption of concomitant medications [49]. Based on the previous experience with other GLP receptor agonists, and PBPK simulation results, it was concluded that 'Tirzepatide-mediated delayed gastric emptying is not expected to result in clinically meaningful impact on the PK of acetaminophen, atorvastatin, digoxin, lisinopril, metformin, metoprolol, sitagliptin, and S-warfarin.' [49]

11.5.3.3 Cytokine Modulator Mediated DDIs

Therapeutic proteins that are proinflammatory cytokines or that may increase the proinflammatory cytokine levels can inhibit the expression of CYP enzymes and consequently decrease the metabolism of CYP enzyme substrates [94]. On the other side, therapeutic proteins that reduce cytokine levels can relieve the CYP downregulation and thereby increase CYP expression and activity and reduce exposure of CYP enzyme substrates. In the guidance entitled "Drug-Drug Interaction Assessment for Therapeutic Proteins", PBPK modeling has been recognized as a potential tool to evaluate the therapeutic protein-mediated DDI. There are literature reports applying PBPK analyses evaluating the effect of changes in interleukin (IL)-6 on the PK of concomitant medications [95–97].

Blinatumomab is a bispecific CD19-directed CD3 T-cell engager indicated for the treatment of certain CD19-positive acute lymphoblastic leukemia [98]. In the original submission package (2014), a PBPK model was used to evaluate the potential indirect effect of blinatumomab on the CYP enzymes due to the transient cytokine elevation. FDA review concluded that "the PBPK model prediction cannot adequately address the drug interaction potential of blinatumomab, as an exposure-response relationship between plasma IL-6 levels and changes in CYP activities in humans has not been established." However, the details cannot be provided as many details have been redacted in the FDA review [99]. Nevertheless, the PBPK model was published by the applicant [100]. Briefly, in vitro studies were conducted evaluating the effect of blinatumomab and a cocktail of cytokines (IL-2, IL-6, IL-10, interferon-gamma [IFN-γ], and tumor necrosis factor [TNF]-α) on CYP enzymes (CYP1A2, CYP2C9, CYP2D6, CYP2C19, and CYP3A4/5) in human hepatocytes [100]. The in vitro study suggested that the cytokine cocktail showed >50% suppression of CYP1A2 activity in cells from all donors, >50% suppression of CYP3A4/5 and CYP2C9 activities in cells from two of the three donors, and <50% suppression of suppression of CYP2C19 and CYP2D6 in cells from two of the three donors [100]. PBPK models were developed to evaluate the effect of IL-6 fluctuation on the activity of CYP3A4, CYP1A2, and CYP2C9. IL-6 was selected as the perpetrator among the three most relevant cytokines (IL-6, IL-10, and IFN-γ) because IL-10 had no effect on CYP450 in human, and no clinical data was available evaluating the effect of IFN-γ on CYP450 activity [100]. The model was validated by simulating the tocilizumab and simvastatin interaction where the IL-6 exposures were in the range of 50-100 pg/mL and resulted in 2- to 2.6-fold change in simvastatin AUC. Based on this model, the magnitude and duration of suppression of CYP enzymes, and effects on the exposures of CYP3A4 substrates (simvastatin and midazolam), CYP1A2 substrates (theophylline and caffeine), and CYP2C9 substrate ((S)-warfarin) were simulated [100].

Satralizumab is an IL-6 receptor antagonist indicated for the treatment of neuromyelitis optica spectrum disorder (NMOSD) in certain adult patients [101]. The applicant developed PBPK models evaluating the effect of the reversal of IL-6 mediated CYP enzyme suppression upon administration of satralizumab in patients with NMOSD [25]. The reviewer identified a few limitations in the modeling, including uncertainties in the in vitro to in vivo extrapolation of IL-6 suppression data, verification of the response curve of CYP suppression, and the disease effect. The reviewer concluded that the PBPK analysis was deemed exploratory [25]. Nevertheless, since the baseline IL-6 levels in the patient population are low, the IL-6-mediated suppression of CYP enzymes is expected to be low [25].

The examples illustrated here suggest that more research work is needed to prospectively predict the IL-6 or broadly cytokines-mediated effects on CYP enzymes.

11.6 EFFECTS OF INTRINSIC FACTORS

Compared with evaluating the effects of extrinsic factors (such as concomitant medications), evaluating the effects of intrinsic factors (such as age, organ impairment, disease state, pregnancy, and pharmacogenomics) by a PBPK approach can be more challenging for various reasons. This includes heterogeneity within each population category and uncertainties in extrapolating from established models based on a group of drugs to a new investigational drug. Nevertheless, there are examples in regulatory submissions where PBPK analyses were used to evaluate the effects of intrinsic factors on the PK of an investigational drug and will be discussed in this section.

11.6.1 Age

PBPK analysis in pediatrics is the second commonly used area following DDIs in regulatory submissions. One of the frequently asked questions is the dosage in neonates, infants and toddlers in phase 1/2 studies in pediatric programs. Besides pediatrics, PBPK modeling and simulation has also been used to address geriatric populations [102–105] although this category has not been specifically surveyed in the regulatory submissions. PBPK modeling and simulation has the ability to incorporate age-related changes in physiology that may potentially impact the drug's ADME, such as enzyme maturation in neonates and infants, and decrease in kidney function in elderly populations.

Entrectinib is a kinase inhibitor indicated for the treatment of ROS1-positive non-small cell lung cancer (NSCLC) and NTRK gene fusion-positive solid tumors [106]. PBPK analyses were used to address several clinical pharmacology-related questions including DDIs, and PK in pediatric populations of a formulation that were not studied in pediatrics [107]. In the entrectinib program, multiple formulations were developed to improve its biopharmaceutics properties, of which three formulations, namely F1, F2A, and F06, were most relevant to the model development and validation. Figure 11.4 is a schematic description of relative bioavailability, food effect, and effect of PPIs on each formulation. Briefly, the F1 formulation is an acidulant-free formulation and food may increase the exposure to entrectinib by approximately threefold following oral administration of F1 with a PPI [84]. F2A and F06 (the to-be-marketed formulation) are acidulant containing formulations and food has minimal impact on the exposure to entrectinib following oral administration of those two formulations [84,107]. Lansoprazole (a PPI) does not impact the exposure to entrectinib following oral administration of F2A under the fed condition and decreased the exposure to entrectinib by approximately 25% following oral administration of F06 under the fasting condition [107]. Bioequivalence was demonstrated between the F1 and F06 under a light meal condition, and between F2A and F06 under the fasting condition. Limited PK data were available in pediatric populations following oral administration of F1. The question was what dose in the F06 formulation should be given to pediatric populations. Entrectinib is a substrate of CYP3A4 with approximate 80% metabolism via CYP3A4. There are different CYP3A ontogeny profiles reported in the literature of which the CYP3A can differ by approximately 50% [108,109]. On the other hand, the aqueous solubility of entrectinib is low and pH-dependent [84], which complicated the modeling of oral absorption. The applicant developed two models using different platforms (Simcyp and GastroPlus). Both models integrated uncertainties in CYP3A ontogeny. The model developed in GastroPlus incorporated a mechanistic oral absorption model that can account for the impact of particle size, bile salt concentrations, gastric pH, and other GI physiology. Overall, the PBPK model with a mechanistic oral absorption model was able to capture the PK with the predicted vs. observed AUC ratios within 0.5–1.5 in 69% (11/16) patients (4–20 years of age) [107]. For patients less than 4 years of age, the model showed a tendency of overestimation of the observed exposure. After applying the Upreti ontogeny (higher CYP3A activity), C_{max} was over-predicted by more than twofold in two of the three non-obese subjects [107]. Of note, this observation was based on a very limited number of subjects. We believe that the PBPK modeling efforts in this area require

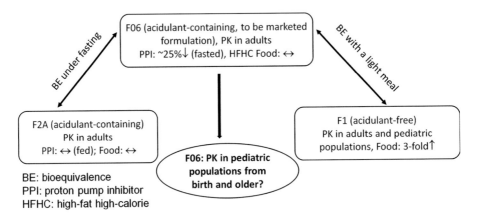

Figure 11.4 Schematic description of relative bioavailability, food effect, and effect of PPIs on each entrectinib formulation. BE, bioequivalence; PPI, proton pump inhibitor; HFHC, high-fat high-calorie.

further research and additional refinement. Nevertheless, this example demonstrated the potential utility of PBPK modeling and simulation in pediatric development programs.

11.6.2 Organ Impairment

Predicting the effect of organ impairment (specifically hepatic impairment and renal impairment) using the PBPK modeling approach has been considered valuable, but challenging. There are recent advancements in these areas [83] including a research paper published by industry scientists [13]. In the paper, the authors evaluated the predictive performance of PBPK models in subjects with renal impairment (RI) and hepatic impairment (HI) for 29 compounds, the majority of which were eliminated predominantly via metabolism [13]. Overall, the AUC ratios of RI to healthy subjects were predicted within twofold of the observed ratios for >90% (47/50) of the treatment groups. The AUC ratios of HI to healthy subjects were predicted within twofold of the observed ratios for >70% (43/56) of the treatment groups [13]. In the regulatory setting, PBPK analyses in renal and HI accounted for approximately less than 10% of total PBPK submissions as PK data are generally needed for model validation. However, PBPK modeling and simulation can be a valuable tool in evaluating complex scenarios or for reducing the need for additional clinical studies.

Duvelisib, a kinase inhibitor, is a substrate and inhibitor of CYP3A. Ketoconazole (a strong CYP3A inhibitor) increased single dose of duvelisib C_{max} by 1.7-fold and AUC by 4-fold. Duvelisib increased single dose of midazolam (a sensitive CYP3A substrate) AUC by 4.3-fold and C_{max} by 2.2-fold [110]. Extensive PBPK analyses were performed in duvelisib program to address multiple clinical pharmacology-related questions. In this section, we focus on the application of PBPK modeling and simulation in predicting the effect of HI on duvelisib PK at steady state. Briefly, a base PBPK model for duvelisib and IPI-656 (major metabolite) was developed and refined based on in vitro, human ADME, and single ascending dose (SAD) PK data. The PBPK model was validated for healthy volunteers (HVs) and oncology patients following single-dose (1–25 mg) and multiple-dose (1–10 mg) administration, as well as data from DDI studies with ketoconazole, midazolam, and rifampin. The base PBPK model was extended to subjects with HI. The PBPK model was refined based on a single dose clinical PK study in subjects with HI. In the HI PBPK model, CYP3A enzyme abundance and the fraction absorbed (f_a) values were modified to fit the clinical HI study. The fup (unbound fraction in plasma) values in HI populations were measured in the clinical HI study. In general, the revised model was able to describe the observed duvelisib total and unbound AUC ratios of HI relative to HVs (Figure 11.5). To simulate duvelisib exposures

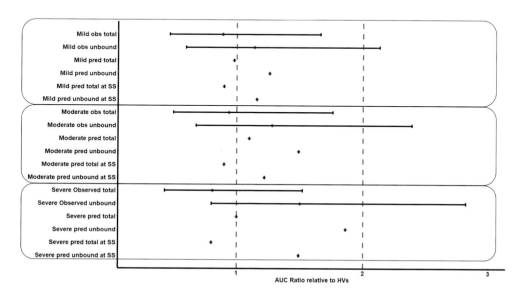

Figure 11.5 Observed and predicted duvelisib AUC ratios of HI relative to HVs. (Replotted based on data reported in Ref. [111].) diamond: observed geometric mean ratio of HI relative to HVs; error bars: 90% confidence interval; diamond with a central black dot: predicted geometric mean ratio of HI relative to HVs.

Table 11.8: Predicted and Observed Samidorphan PK Ratios of HI Relative to HVs

	Mild HI		Moderate HI		Severe HI	
	A Single Sublingual of 1 mg SAM					
	$C_{max}R$	AUCR	$C_{max}R$	AUCR	$C_{max}R$	AUCR
Pred.	1.08	1.29	1.23	1.94	1.34	2.58
Obs.	1.14	1.26	1.50	1.88	1.47	2.15
	Multiple Oral Doses of 10 mg SAM					
Pred.[a]	1.47	1.26	1.79	2.02	2.10	2.55
Pred.[b]	1.47	1.23	1.79	1.90	2.10	2.32

Source: Summarized based on data from Ref. [34].
$C_{max}R$ and AUCR are ratios of C_{max} and AUC comparing subjects with hepatic impairment to healthy volunteers.
SAM, samidorphan; HI, hepatic impairment.
[a] fup = 0.69; [b] fup = 0.71, 0.76, and 0.81 for mild, moderate, and severe HI.

in subjects with HI at steady state, the model assumes that the time-dependent inhibition (TDI) parameters were the same in HVs and in subjects with HI. The predicted unbound AUC ratios of HI relative to HVs at steady state were generally less than twofold and smaller than the single dose AUC ratios due to the autoinhibition effect and therefore were not considered clinically significant [110,111].

Samidorphan (SAM) is an opioid antagonist, in combination with olanzapine for the treatment of schizophrenia and bipolar I disorder [112]. In the olanzapine and samidorphan fixed dose combination program, PBPK analyses were used to leverage historical clinical data in subjects with HI and evaluate the effect of HI on the PK of SAM. Briefly, SAM models were developed based on in vitro, human ADME, and PK data. The models were validated against PK data following intravenous, sublingual, and oral administration, and DDI studies. The SAM PBPK models were expanded to subjects with HI and validated against PK data following single dose of SAM in subjects with mild, moderate, and severe HI. Physiology parameter changes in subjects with HI relative to HVs included decrease in liver volume, CYP abundance, albumin, hematocrits, and plasma glycoprotein, and slightly prolonged gastric emptying time. In addition, the absorption rate (K_a) for the subjects with moderate HI was increased, and fup was increased for subjects with mild, moderate, and severe HI. The HI PBPK model was able to describe the observed Cmax and AUC ratios between subjects with HI and HVs following a single sublingual administration of 1 mg of SAM (Table 11.8). The HI PBPK models were used to simulate the impact of HI on the PK following multiple oral doses of 10 mg of SAM. The models used two sets of fup values. As shown in Table 11.8, the model predicted similar AUC changes in subjects with HI relative to HVs following multiple oral doses of 10 mg of SAM compared to a single dose of 1 mg of SAM.

The two case examples discussed here demonstrated the utility of PBPK modeling and simulation to leverage available clinical data and evaluate complex and difficult-to-be-studied scenarios.

11.6.3 Diseases

Disease status may change physiological parameters that impact PK. For example, the cancer population may have different age and body weight distribution compared to a healthy volunteer population. The kidney function, plasma volume and protein levels, and enzymes and transporters' abundance may also be changed in cancer populations. As such, a cancer population may be created to capture the observed differences in PK between the patient population and HVs by incorporating the changes in physiology. In the erdafitinib program, different fup (unbound fraction in plasma) values were incorporated for cancer and healthy populations to describe the observed PK differences [113]. Similarly, reduced albumin levels were incorporated in the avapritinib PBPK model for patients with gastrointestinal stromal tumor (GIST) to simulate higher fup compared to that in healthy subjects [16]. The increase in fup resulted in a higher apparent clearance (CL/F) for the patients with GIST. Both models were considered exploratory as other physiology factors that may impact PK were not considered [16,113]. In the capmatinib program, the Application further reduced the hepatic and intestinal CYP3A4 abundance by 20% based on a previously developed cancer patient population to reduce the predictive error [21,114].

In the baricitinib program, a PBPK model was developed for patients with rheumatoid arthritis (RA) by incorporating decreased OAT3 activity. However, the Application was not able to provide data showing decreased expression or function of OAT3 in patients or animal models with RA or any other inflammatory conditions [76]. Therefore, although the downregulation of OAT3 could be a mechanism causing the apparent reduced active renal secretion of baricitinib in subjects with RA, there is lack of evidence supporting the hypothesis [76].

The examples illustrated here suggest that PBPK models for patient populations have been developed by incorporating known physiology changes in the patient populations with supporting evidence. Due to the complexity of physiology changes, the PBPK model may only incorporate a few key relevant parameters that impact PK.

11.6.4 Pharmacogenomics

It is known that enzyme polymorphisms may impact the PK of a substrate. In regulatory submissions, PBPK analyses have been used to evaluate the effects of enzyme polymorphisms and relevant DDIs for substrates of CYP2D6 (eliglustat), CYP2C9 (siponimod and erdafitinib), CYP2C19 (mavacamten), and UGT (belinostat and belzutifan) enzymes. In many of programs, PBPK analyses were conducted to evaluate the effects of concomitant medications on the PK of an investigational drug in populations with different enzyme polymorphisms. The complex effects by DDI and pharmacogenetics that led to dose adjustment based on PBPK analyses will be discussed in Section 11.8.1. In this section, we focus on PBPK analyses to evaluate the effect of enzyme polymorphism on PK.

A common approach when modeling the PK in populations with different enzyme polymorphisms is to estimate the relative enzyme activity (or abundance) in each sub-population. In theory, the relative enzyme activity of each polymorphism can be obtained from other drugs sharing the same metabolic pathway. In reality, such analyses are rarely conducted potentially due to the lack of specific substrates for model development and validation. To model the impact of enzyme polymorphisms on the PK of an investigational drug, both approaches have been applied, i.e., obtaining the relative enzyme activity from other substrates, or obtaining the relative enzyme activity by measuring the PK of the investigational drug in each sub-population.

Eliglustat is a glucosylceramide synthase inhibitor indicated for the long-term treatment of adult patients with Gaucher disease type 1 who are CYP2D6 extensive metabolizers (EMs), intermediate metabolizers (IMs), or PMs [115]. Eliglustat is not approved for CYP2D6 ultra-rapid metabolizers (UMs) due to the concern of not achieving adequate concentrations and therapeutic effect. Eliglustat is extensively metabolized mainly by CYP2D6 and to a lesser extent by CYP3A4. Following intravenous administration in HVs who are CYP2D6 EMs, the mean eliglustat total body clearance was 88 L/h approaching the hepatic blood flow, suggesting high hepatic extraction [115]. In the eliglustat PBPK model, for EMs and PMs, the platform default CYP2D6 abundance was used; for IM and UMs, the model was optimized against PK data to obtain the CYP2D6 abundance [116]. The PBPK model for CYP2D6 EMs tends to overestimate eliglustat exposure at a lower oral dose (50 mg) and underestimate at a higher oral dose (350 mg) [116]. The model overestimated eliglustat exposure by approximately twofold following 100 mg BID dosing [116]. For CYP2D6 PMs, the PBPK model was able to capture the observed PK with the simulated vs. observed C_{max} and AUC ratios within 0.5–2-fold [116]. For CYP2D6 PMs, the PBPK model overestimated the exposure of eliglustat in three out of four studies and underestimated the exposure in 1 out of 4 studies, suggesting large inter-study variability, and potentially wide range of CYP2D6 activity among IMs. The predictive performance of the PBPK model for UMs cannot be evaluated due to limited number ($N = 1$) of subjects [116]. Overall, it was concluded that the PBPK model for CYP2D6 EMs and IMs may need further refinement but can still be used to simulate the effect of various CYP modulators given the known safety margin [116].

Siponimod is a sphingosine 1-phosphate receptor modulator indicated for the treatment of relapsing forms of multiple sclerosis. Siponimod is a substrate of CYP2C9 (fmCYP2C9 ~ 79%) and CYP3A4 (fmCYP3A4 ~ 19%). PBPK models were developed for subjects carrying various CYP2C9 variants, *1/*1, *1/*2, *1/*3, *2/*2, *2/*3, and *3/*3. The intrinsic clearance of allelic CYP2C9 variants was calculated relative to wild-type value based on clearance values estimated from population PK analysis for each genotype [117]. Erdafitinib is a kinase inhibitor indicated for the treatment of certain urothelial carcinoma [118]. The elimination of erdafitinib involves multiple pathways. For subjects carrying CYP2C9 *1/*1 genotype, the estimated clearance via CYP2C9, CYP2A4, additional metabolism, renal, and biliary was approximately 41%, 18%, 7%, 14%, and 19%, respectively. There were no PK data in subjects with CYP2C9 *2/*2, *2/*3, and *3/*3 genotypes,

Table 11.9: CYP2C9 Mediated Clearance Relative to *1/*1 Genotype for CYP2C9 Substrates

Drugs	fm CYP2C9	*1/*1	*1/*2	*1/*3	*2/*2	*2/*3	*3/*3	Reference
		CYP2C9 Genotype						
S-flurbiprofen	0.96	1	0.73	0.56	NA	NA	NA	[119]
Losartan [E3174 formation]	0.84	1	0.52	0.64	0.68	0.23	0.01	
Phenytoin	0.83	1	0.70	0.71	0.62	0.40	0.70	
Tolbutamide	0.98	1	0.84	0.64	0.75	0.46	0.15	
Tolbutamide	0.94 (Simcyp default model)	1	0.91	0.64	0.72	0.49	0.17	[113]
Torsemide	0.97	1	0.98	0.54	0.94	0.44	0.33	[119]
S-warfarin	0.94	1	0.67	0.53	0.44	0.28	0.11	
S-warfarin	NA	1	0.58	0.52	0.32	0.23	0.09	[120]
Siponimod	0.79	1	0.91	0.66	0.50	0.38	0.06	Estimated from Ref. [117]
Erdafitinib	**0.39**	**1**	**0.89**	**0.65**	**0.71**	**0.46**	**0.11**	[113]

Source: Table is modified from Ref. [113]. The values extracted from Ref. [119] were mean values. Only substrates with fmCYP2C9 higher than 0.8 were included. Celecoxib was not included as large discrepancies were observed among the reported values. The number of subjects was less than two for phenytoin (*3/*3) and the data should be interpreted with caution. It was reported that genetic polymorphisms of both OATP1B1 and CYP2C9 affected the clearance of torsemide.

and PBPK analyses were conducted to simulate the PK of erdafitinib in those subjects. To estimate the relative enzyme activity of those genotypes, a literature survey was conducted by the applicant and reviewer. Table 11.9 is a summary of CYP2C9-mediated clearance relative to *1/*1 genotype for CYP2C9 different substrates. As shown in Table 11.9, the relative activity of CYP2C9 genotypes to *1/*1 is within similar range across CYP2C9 substrates. The applicant then selected a set of CYP2C9 activity to simulate the PK of erdafitinib in subjects carrying CYP2C9 *2/*2, *2/*3, and *3/*3 genotypes. Simulations suggested that the increase in erdafitinib exposure in subjects carrying CYP2C9 *3/*3 genotype was less than 60% compared to that in subjects with CYP2C9 *1/*1 genotype [113].

Mavacamten, a cardiac myosin inhibitor, is extensively metabolized, primarily through CYP2C19 (74%), CYP3A4 (18%), and CYP2C9 (8%) [121]. Mavacamten terminal half-life is 6–9 days in CYP2C19 normal metabolizers (NMs) and prolonged to 23 days in CYP2C19 PMs [121]. In the mavacamten program, PBPK modeling and simulation were conducted to evaluate the effect of CYP2C19 and CYP3A inhibitors on the PK of mavacamten in various CYP2C19 phenotypes. In the original submission, PBPK models were developed for CYP2C19 NMs and PMs but not for CYP2C19 IMs. During the review, the applicant developed a model for CYP2C19 IMs in response to FDA's information request. The IM model appeared underpredicting the Cmax and AUC of sensitive CYP2C19 substrates (such as omeprazole and lansoprazole) likely due to the small sample size and different formulations, but could reasonably predict the mavacamten PK [47].

Belinostat, a histone deacetylase inhibitor, is a substrate of UGT1A1 [122]. In the 2014 NDA review, it indicates that PBPK analysis was conducted by the FDA reviewer and concluded that subjects with homozygous for UGT1A1*28 may have 20% higher belinostat AUC than subjects with homozygous for UGT1A1*1. A dose reduction from 1,000 to 750 mg/m² is recommended for patients known to be homozygous for the UGT1A1*28 allele [122]. And a post-marketing requirement (PMR) was issued to evaluate the safety and PK in patients with homozygous UGT1A1*28 [123]. It is not clear how the reviewer conducted the PBPK modeling in the published review. Interestingly, in 2016, clinical study results and population PK analyses were published evaluating the effect of UGT1A polymorphisms on the PK of belinostat [124,125]. The results suggested that dose-normalized belinostat AUC in subjects with UGT1A1*28/*28 was approximately 30% higher than that in subjects with UGT1A1*1/*1 [124,125]. This case example demonstrated the predictability of the belinostat PBPK model.

Belzutifan, a hypoxia-inducible factor inhibitor, is a substrate of UGT2B17 and CYP2C19 [126]. In the belzutifan program, the effect of UGT2B17 and CYP2C19 phenotypes on the PK of belzutifan was analyzed by population PK and pharmacogenetic PK approaches. PBPK models for each sub-population were retrospectively developed. The CYP2C19 and UGT2B17 enzyme phenotype frequencies and relative enzyme abundance and activity were modified based on the observed belzutifan PK data [38]. The PBPK models were then used to simulate the exposure of belzutifan and evaluate the effects of belzutifan on the PK of midazolam in those subpopulations [38].

To summarize, the case examples discussed here demonstrated the utility of PBPK modeling and simulation in evaluating the effect of enzyme polymorphisms on PK. The relative enzyme activity for each genotype/phenotype population can be obtained by measuring the PK of the investigational drug or from other substrates sharing the same metabolism pathway. The PBPK models will be further utilized to evaluate the effect of concomitant medications (see Section 11.8.1).

11.6.5 Pregnancy/Fetus/Lactation

Predicting the drug exposure in pregnant women, fetus, and infants during lactation is an area that has attracted lot of interest in using PBPK modeling and simulation. There is a demanding need to understand the PK, safety and efficacy of a drug in those populations; on the other hand, studies are rarely conducted in those populations. Although there are not many regulatory PBPK submissions, research including publications from regulatory agencies in this area has been very active and the readers are referred to the publication for details about PBPK modeling and simulation advancement in pregnancy, fetus, and lactation [83,127–135].

11.7 DOSE SELECTION AND STUDY DESIGN

While many of the examples in this chapter are from the NDA/BLA reviews supporting the original drug approvals, the utility of PBPK modeling and simulation can start as early as the pre-clinical stage, throughout the drug development and life cycle management to address various clinical development questions. For example, the PBPK modeling approach has been used to predict the first-in-human dose for both large and small molecules [8,136,137]. The PBPK modeling approach has been recommended for dose selection in pediatric patients especially in younger children (< 2 years of age) as the models can incorporate the ontogeny of relevant enzymes [14]. Although there are ongoing debates regarding the predictive performance of PBPK models in pediatric populations, the focus should be on utilizing the available tool to address drug development questions. The efforts to systemically improve the predictive performance of these tools can be an ongoing process and may be done in parallel.

Other common questions that could be addressed by the PBPK approach during drug development are whether a DDI study is needed, and if so, what is the best study design (choices of inhibitors/inducers, single dose vs. multiple doses, and days needed to reach maximal inhibition/induction effect, etc.). A PBPK model linked to a pharmacodynamic model could also be used for phase 2/3 dose selection. A preliminary PBPK model can help design inclusion/exclusion criteria for clinical trial protocols. Understanding the limitations, defining the context of use and being innovative are the keys to successfully utilizing PBPK modeling during drug development.

11.8 PBPK MODELING TO EVALUATE COMPLICATED CLINICAL SCENARIOS

A valuable utility of PBPK modeling and simulation is its ability to evaluate clinical scenarios where conducting studies can be difficult. This often involves more than one factor that may impact the PK. For example, when both pharmacogenetics and concomitant medications may impact PK, it is time- and cost-consuming to conduct in vivo studies to include all potential combinations of pharmacogenetics (EMs, IMs, and PMs), and concomitant medications (strong, moderate, and weak inhibitors and inducers). Owing to the low prevalence of certain genotypes/phenotypes, the subject recruitment can be challenging. DDI studies are generally conducted in healthy adults. PBPK analyses can be used to evaluate if the DDI magnitude is the same in a different population (such as pediatric populations). DDI potential may also be different when comparing multiple-dose to single-dose administration for a drug that inhibits or induces its own metabolism. PBPK analyses have been used to simulate the DDI potential at steady state for auto-inhibitors or auto-inducers. In this section, we discuss several examples where PBPK analyses were used to address complex clinical situations in regulatory submissions.

11.8.1 The Effects of DDI and Pharmacogenetics

For a drug that is predominantly eliminated by a polymorphic enzyme (such as CYP2D6, CYP2C9, or CYP2C19), a minor metabolic pathway becomes the major pathway in PMs where the

Table 11.10: Summary of PBPK Simulated Eliglustat PK Changes Following 84 mg BID Oral Administration in CYP2D6 EMs, IMs, and PMs When Co-administered with CYP2D6 and/or CYP3A Inhibitors [115,116]

Perpetrator	CYP2D6 EMs			CYP2D6 IMs			CYP2D6 PMs		
	$C_{max}R$	$AUC_{0-12h}R$	Dosing	$C_{max}R$	$AUC_{0-12h}R$	Dosing	$C_{max}R$	$AUC_{0-24h}R$	Dosing
Paroxetine and ketoconazole	16.7	24.2	Contraindicated	7.48	9.81	Contraindicated	NA		
Terbinafine and fluconazole	10.2	13.6		4.16	4.99		NA		
Paroxetine	6.99[a]	8.41[a]	84 mg QD	2.12	2.31	84 mg QD	NA		
Terbinafine	3.80	4.49		1.55	1.64		NA		
Ketoconazole	3.98[a]	4.39[a]	84 mg BID	4.36	5.41	Contraindicated	4.27	6.22	Contraindicated
Fluconazole	2.77	3.21		2.53	2.85	Avoid use	2.38	2.95	Avoid use

Source: Data extracted from Refs. [115,116].
QD, once daily; BID, twice daily; $C_{max}R$ and AUCR, eliglustat $C_{max}R$ and AUC ratios in the presence and absence of an inhibitor in the same CYP2D6 phenotype population.
[a] Results from dedicated DDI study.

Table 11.11: Summary of Recommended Maintenance Dose for Siponimod Based on CYP2C9 Genotype

CYP2C9 Genotype	Siponimod Alone	Moderate CYP2C9 and Moderate / Strong CYP3A4 Inhibitor	Moderate CYP2C9 and Strong CYP3A4 Inducer	Moderate or Strong CYP3A4 Inducer
*1/*1	2 mg	Not recommended	Not recommended	2 mg
*1/*2	2 mg			
*2/*2	2 mg			Not recommended
*1/*3	1 mg			
*2/*3	1 mg			
*3/*3	Contraindicated			

elimination activity from the major pathway almost completely diminishes. In previous section, we discussed the utility of PBPK modeling and simulation in evaluating the effect of pharmacogenetics on the PK of a few drugs. Furthermore, PBPK modeling and simulation were used to evaluate the effect of concomitant medications on the PK for those drugs. In this section, we discuss a few examples where dose adjustment was recommended based on modeling and simulation for different subpopulations.

Following 84 mg twice daily oral administration of eliglustat, the mean AUC_{0-12h} in CYP2D6 PMs was approximately 6- to 14-fold higher than that in CYP2D6 EMs [116]. The recommended dosage is 84 mg twice daily in CYP2D6 EMs and IMs, and 84 mg once daily in CYP2D6 PMs considering the efficacy and safety window of eliglustat. DDI studies were conducted with paroxetine (a strong CYP2D6 inhibitor) and ketoconazole (a strong CYP3A inhibitor) in CYP2D6 EMs. Paroxetine increased eliglustat AUCtau and Cmax by approximately 8- and 7-fold, respectively, in CYP2D6 EMs. Ketoconazole increased eliglustat AUCtau and Cmax by approximately 4- and 4-fold, respectively, in CYP2D6 EMs. PBPK analyses were performed to predict the effects of strong CYP2D6 and CYP3A inhibitors in CYP2D6 IMs and PMs, the effects of moderate CYP2D6 (terbinafine) and CYP3A (fluconazole) inhibitors, and the combined effects from CYP2D6 and CYP3A inhibitors (Table 11.10). Dosing recommendations with CYP2D6 and CYP3A inhibitors in various CYP2D6 phenotype groups were largely based on PBPK analyses.

The siponimod AUC in subjects carrying CYP2C9 *3/*3 genotype was 3.8-fold higher than that in subjects carrying CYP2C9 *1/*1 genotype following a single dose of 0.25 mg oral administration. Dedicated DDI studies were conducted with fluconazole and rifampin in subjects carrying CYP2C9 *1/*1 genotype, and with itraconazole in subjects carrying CYP2C9 *1/*2 and *1/*3 genotypes [117]. The effect of CYP2C9 and CYP3A inhibitors and inducers on the PK of siponimod were simulated by PBPK models in subjects carrying various CYP2C9 genotypes [117,138]. Based on the PK, dedicated DDI studies, simulated DDIs, and considerations of the safety and efficacy profiles, dose adjustment is recommended based on CYP2C9 genotypes as summarized in Table 11.11.

The exposure (AUCinf) of mavacamten (a CYP2C19 and CYP3A substrate) in CYP2C19 PM was 3.4-fold of that in CYP2C19 NMs based on dedicated pharmacogenomic study. PBPK simulations were conducted to predict the effects of strong (ticlopidine), moderate (omeprazole, 20 mg BID), weak (omeprazole, 20 mg QD) CYP2C19 inhibitors, and strong (itraconazole), moderate (diltiazem), weak (cimetidine) CYP3A inhibitors, strong CYP3A4 and CYP2C19 inducer (rifampin), and moderate CYP3A and CYP2C19 inducer (efavirenz) on the PK of mavacamten to support dosing recommendations for various DDI scenarios. Considering the safety and efficacy profiles, the dosing posology and monitoring plan, there is no CYP2C19 genotyping assessment prior to the initiation of mavacamten treatment, contraindications are recommended for co-administration of mavacamten with moderate to strong CYP2C19 inhibitors or strong CYP3A4 inhibitors, and moderate to strong CYP2C19 inducers or moderate to strong CYP3A4 inducers regardless of CYP2C19 phenotypes [47,121].

11.8.2 The Effect of DDI in Specific Populations

Risdiplam is a survival of motor neuron 2 (SMN2) splicing modifier indicated for the treatment of spinal muscular atrophy (SMA) in patients 2 months of age and older [139]. In vitro, risdiplam and its metabolite showed TDI toward CYP3A. Understanding the effect of risdiplam on the PK

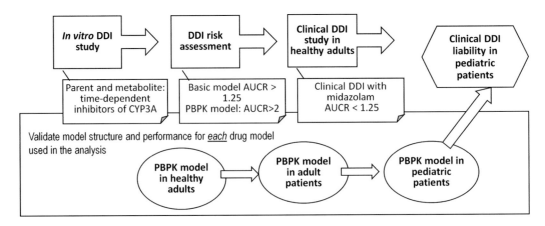

Figure 11.6 PBPK analyses workflow to evaluate the effect of risdiplam on the PK of CYP3A substrates in pediatric populations [140,141].

of CYP3A substrates in pediatric populations was needed but conducting a DDI study was not feasible. In the risdiplam program, PBPK analyses were conducted to evaluate its effect on the PK of CYP3A substrates in pediatric patients with SMA [140,141]. Figure 11.6 is workflow of PBPK analyses evaluating the effect of risdiplam on the PK of CYP3A substrates in pediatric populations. Briefly, risdiplam and midazolam (a sensitive CYP3A substrate) PBPK models were developed and validated against available PK data in both adults and pediatric populations. The PBPK model was also validated against a clinical DDI study evaluating the effect of risdiplam on the PK of midazolam in adults. The uncertainties in CYP3A ontogeny in both the intestine and the liver were also evaluated in the modeling exercises [24,140]. Based on extensive PBPK and sensitivity analyses, the label indicated that similar increase in midazolam exposure is expected in children and infants as young as 2 months of age as that observed in adults (AUC 11%; C_{max} 16%), and the increase is not considered clinically relevant [139].

11.8.3 CYP3A-Mediated Complex DDIs

When more than one mechanism and direction are involved, the DDIs can be complicated and one dedicated DDI study may not provide appropriate dosing recommendations. Figure 11.7 describes such as scenario. Briefly, in vitro studies suggest that an investigational drug is a substrate of CYP3A and P-gp. It also has TDI potential and induction potential toward CYP3A. The evaluation of the effects of CYP3A modulations becomes complicated in several ways. First, many CYP3A inhibitors and inducers are also P-gp inhibitors and inducers. Therefore, when an investigational drug is a dual CYP3A and P-gp substrate, the effect from each pathway could be difficult to

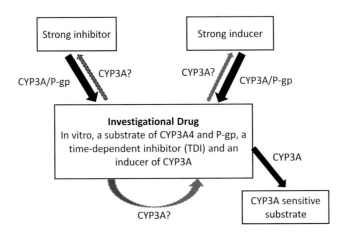

Figure 11.7 Schematic description of CYP3A mediated complex DDIs.

Table 11.12: Key Clinical Pharmacology Properties of Duvelisib and Ribociclib [110,142]

Drug	Dose (mg)	fmCYP3A	Effect on MDZ AUC	$T_{1/2}$ (h)[a]	CL/F (L/h) (CV%)[a]	V_{ss}/F (L) (CV%)
Duvelisib	25 mg BID	~0.7	↑ 4.3	4.7 (57%)[b]	4.2 (56%)	28.5 (62%)
Ribociclib	600 mg QD	~0.7	↑ 3.8 (400 mg)	32 (63%)[c]	25.5 (66%)	1,090

MDZ, midazolam; BID, twice daily; QD, once weekly.
[a] At steady state in patients; [b] Terminal half-life; [c] Effective half-life.

Table 11.13: Summary of Simulated Effect of CYP3A Inhibitors on the PK of Duvelisib or Ribociclib Following SD (Single Dose) and MD (Multiple Dose) Administration of the Substrate Drug [111,143]

Substrate Drug (Perpetrator)	Observed AUCR (SD of Substrate)	Predicted AUCR (MD of Substrate)
Duvelisib (w/ketoconazole)	~ 4	2.9 (1 mg BID), 2.3 (5 mg BID), 1.7 (25 mg BID)
Ribociclib (w/ritonavir or itraconazole)	3.2	2.7 (200 mg QD), 2.1 (400 mg QD), 1.8 (600 mg QD)

separate. Second, when an investigational drug is also a modulator of CYP3A, the effect of CYP3A inhibitors or inducers on the PK of the investigational drug could be different comparing single dose to multiple-dose administration of the investigational drug. Furthermore, if the concomitant CYP3A inhibitor or inducer is also a CYP3A substrate, its PK may be impacted by the investigational drug and consequently, its inhibition or induction may also be impacted. In this section, we will discuss several examples where PBPK modeling and simulation have been used to bridge gaps in complicated situations.

Duvelisib and ribociclib are CYP3A substrates with approximately 70% metabolism via CYP3A (Table 11.12). Both drugs are also inhibitors of CYP3A. Duvelisib increased midazolam AUC by approximately 4.3-fold, and ribociclib increased midazolam exposure by approximately 3.8-fold (Table 11.12). Duvelisib has relatively shorter half-life (4.7 hour) compared to ribociclib (32 hour) (Table 11.12).

Ketoconazole, a strong CYP3A inhibitor, increased the AUC of duvelisib by approximately fourfold following a single dose administration of duvelisib. Ritonavir (a strong CYP3A inhibitor) increased the AUC of ribociclib by approximately 3.2-fold following a single dose administration of ribociclib (Table 11.13). PBPK analyses were conducted for both drugs to evaluate the effect of CYP3A inhibitors on their PK at steady state and the results are summarized in Table 11.13. PBPK simulation predicted that ketoconazole increased the AUC of duvelisib by 2.9-, 2.3-, and 1.7- fold following 1, 5, and 25 mg twice daily administration of duvelisib, respectively. PBPK simulation predicted that itraconazole increased the AUC of ribociclib by 2.7-, 2.1-, and 1.8- fold following 200, 400, and 600 mg once daily administration of ribociclib, respectively. The PBPK simulation suggested that the effect of a strong CYP3A inhibitor is weaker at steady state compared to single dose because the substrate itself is also a CYP3A inhibitor. In addition, PBPK simulation also showed that the DDI potential is dependent on the dose of the substrate.

11.9 SUMMARY AND CONCLUSION

In this chapter, we provided an overview and case examples of PBPK modeling and simulation in supporting clinical pharmacology-related regulatory decision-making in the past 15 years. The case examples covered DDI prediction, PK prediction in specific populations, and complex clinical scenarios. We discussed how PBPK modeling and simulation can contribute during the product development stage. We provided many examples from the published reviews to illustrate the value of PBPK modeling and simulation to address complicated clinical pharmacology questions. Many of the PBPK predictions were used to inform drug labeling and offered potential benefits to larger groups of patient populations.

There are also examples where not all clinical pharmacology-related concerns were addressed during the original application review cycle, and PBPK analyses were recommended as part of PMR or post-marketing commitment (PMC) studies. For example, in the larotrectinib approval letter, a PMC was issued for conducting PBPK modeling to evaluate the effect of a moderate CYP3A4 inducer, and a PMR was issued for conducting PBPK modeling to evaluate the effect of a moderate CYP3A4 inhibitor on the PK of larotrectinib [144]. In the glasdegib approval letter, a PBPK modeling approach to determine the appropriate dose of glasdegib when co-administered with moderate CYP3A inducers was issued as a PMC [145]. In the pexidartinib approval letter, a PK trial or PBPK modeling to determine the effect of a moderate CYP3A4 inducer on the exposure of pexidartinib following single and multiple doses of pexidartinib was issued as a PMC [146]. In a PMR for fedratinib, a DDI study was requested with a dual CYP2C19 and CYP3A4 inhibitor following a single dose of fedratinib, and PBPK modeling was requested to simulate the effect following multiple doses of fedratinib based on the single dose study [147].

To conclude, the utility of PBPK modeling and simulations in regulatory settings has grown significantly in the past two decades. The growth was built upon several decades of research, knowledge accumulation and computational tool development. While many programs and broader patient populations have benefited, PBPK modeling and simulation have not reached their full potential. We believe that with active research in every scientific area, PBPK modeling and simulation, as an integrative tool, will play a larger role in the future in drug development and regulatory reviews.

DISCLAIMER

The views expressed in this paper are those of the authors and should not be construed to represent the views or policies of their employers (US FDA or Daiichi Sankyo, Inc).

REFERENCES

1. Liu Q, Ahadpour M, Rocca M, Huang SM. Clinical pharmacology regulatory sciences in drug development and precision medicine: Current status and emerging trends. *AAPS J.* 2021;23(3):54.

2. Zhao P, Zhang L, Grillo JA, Liu Q, Bullock JM, Moon YJ, et al. Applications of physiologically based pharmacokinetic (PBPK) modeling and simulation during regulatory review. *Clin Pharmacol Ther.* 2011;89(2):259–67.

3. Zhao P, Rowland M, Huang SM. Best practice in the use of physiologically based pharmacokinetic modeling and simulation to address clinical pharmacology regulatory questions. *Clin Pharmacol Ther.* 2012;92(1):17–20.

4. Grimstein M, Yang Y, Zhang X, Grillo J, Huang SM, Zineh I, et al. Physiologically based pharmacokinetic modeling in regulatory science: An update from the U.S. Food and Drug Administration's Office of Clinical Pharmacology. *J Pharm Sci.* 2019;108(1):21–5.

5. Zhang X, Yang Y, Grimstein M, Fan J, Grillo JA, Huang SM, et al. Application of PBPK modeling and simulation for regulatory decision making and its impact on US prescribing information: An update on the 2018–2019 submissions to the US FDA's Office of Clinical Pharmacology. *J Clin Pharmacol.* 2020;60(Suppl 1):S160–S78.

6. Jean D, Naik K, Milligan L, Hall S, Mei Huang S, Isoherranen N, et al. Development of best practices in physiologically based pharmacokinetic modeling to support clinical pharmacology regulatory decision-making-A workshop summary. *CPT Pharmacometrics Syst Pharmacol.* 2021;10(11):1271–5.

7. Jones H, Rowland-Yeo K. Basic concepts in physiologically based pharmacokinetic modeling in drug discovery and development. *CPT Pharmacometrics Syst Pharmacol.* 2013;2(8):e63.

8. Jones HM, Mayawala K, Poulin P. Dose selection based on physiologically based pharmacokinetic (PBPK) approaches. *AAPS J.* 2013;15(2):377–87.

9. Margolskee A, Darwich AS, Pepin X, Pathak SM, Bolger MB, Aarons L, et al. IMI - oral biopharmaceutics tools project - evaluation of bottom-up PBPK prediction success part 1: Characterisation of the OrBiTo database of compounds. *Eur J Pharm Sci.* 2017;96:598–609.

10. Margolskee A, Darwich AS, Pepin X, Aarons L, Galetin A, Rostami-Hodjegan A, et al. IMI - Oral biopharmaceutics tools project - Evaluation of bottom-up PBPK prediction success part 2: An introduction to the simulation exercise and overview of results. *Eur J Pharm Sci.* 2017;96:610–25.

11. Darwich AS, Margolskee A, Pepin X, Aarons L, Galetin A, Rostami-Hodjegan A, et al. IMI - Oral biopharmaceutics tools project - Evaluation of bottom-up PBPK prediction success part 3: Identifying gaps in system parameters by analysing In Silico performance across different compound classes. *Eur J Pharm Sci.* 2017;96:626–42.

12. Ahmad A, Pepin X, Aarons L, Wang Y, Darwich AS, Wood JM, et al. IMI - Oral biopharmaceutics tools project - Evaluation of bottom-up PBPK prediction success part 4: Prediction accuracy and software comparisons with improved data and modelling strategies. *Eur J Pharm Biopharm.* 2020;156:50–63.

13. Heimbach T, Chen Y, Chen J, Dixit V, Parrott N, Peters SA, et al. Physiologically-based pharmacokinetic modeling in renal and hepatic impairment populations: A pharmaceutical industry perspective. *Clin Pharmacol Ther.* 2021;110(2):297–310.

14. Johnson TN, Small BG, Rowland Yeo K. Increasing application of pediatric physiologically based pharmacokinetic models across academic and industry organizations. *CPT Pharmacometrics Syst Pharmacol.* 2022;11(3):373–83.

15. Chu X, Prasad B, Neuhoff S, Yoshida K, Leeder JS, Mukherjee D, et al. Clinical implications of altered drug transporter abundance/function and PBPK modeling in specific populations: An ITC perspective. *Clin Pharmacol Ther.* 2022;112(3):501–26.

16. FDA. NDA 212608 Avapritinib Review 2020 [Available from: https://www.accessdata.fda.gov/drugsatfda_docs/nda/2020/212608Orig1s000MultidisciplineR.pdf].

17. FDA. NDA 212801 Osilodrostat Review 2020 [Available from: https://www.accessdata.fda.gov/drugsatfda_docs/nda/2020/212801Orig1s000ClinPharmR.pdf].

18. NDA 213756 Selumetinib Review 2020 [Available from: https://www.accessdata.fda.gov/drugsatfda_docs/nda/2020/213756Orig1s000MultidisciplineR.pdf].

19. FDA. NDA 213411 Tucatinib Review 2020 [Available from: https://www.accessdata.fda.gov/drugsatfda_docs/nda/2020/213411Orig1s000MultidisciplineR.pdf].

20. FDA. NDA 213736 Pemigatinib Review 2020 [Available from: https://www.accessdata.fda.gov/drugsatfda_docs/nda/2020/213736Orig1s000MultidisciplineR.pdf].

21. FDA. NDA 213591 Capmatinib Review 2020 [Available from: https://www.accessdata.fda.gov/drugsatfda_docs/nda/2020/213591Orig1s000MultidisciplineR.pdf].

22. FDA. NDA 213246 Selpercatinib Review 2020 [Available from: https://www.accessdata.fda.gov/drugsatfda_docs/nda/2020/213246Orig1s000MultidisciplineR.pdf].

23. FDA. NDA 210730 Oliceridine Review 2020 [Available from: https://www.accessdata.fda.gov/drugsatfda_docs/nda/2020/210730Orig1s000MultidisciplineR.pdf].

24. FDA. NDA 213535 Risdiplam Review 2020 [Available from: https://www.accessdata.fda.gov/drugsatfda_docs/nda/2020/213535Orig1s000ClinPharmR.pdf].

25. FDA. BLA 761149 Satralizumab Review 2020 [Available from: https://www.accessdata.fda.gov/drugsatfda_docs/nda/2020/761149Orig1s000ClinPharmR.pdf].

26. FDA. NDA 213721 Pralsetinib Review 2020 [Available from: https://www.accessdata.fda.gov/drugsatfda_docs/nda/2020/213721Orig1s000MultidisciplineR.pdf].

27. FDA. NDA 214787 Remdesivir Review 2020 [Available from: https://www.accessdata.fda.gov/drugsatfda_docs/nda/2020/214787Orig1s000ClinpharmR.pdf].

28. FDA. NDA 214377 Vericiguat Review 2021 [Available from: https://www.accessdata.fda.gov/drugsatfda_docs/nda/2021/214377Orig1s000IntegratedR.pdf].

29. FDA. NDA 212887/212888 Cabotegravir Review 2021 [Available from: https://www.accessdata.fda.gov/drugsatfda_docs/nda/2021/212887Orig1s000,212888Orig1s000IntegratedR.pdf].

30. FDA. NDA 213716 Voclosporin Review 2021 [Available from: https://www.accessdata.fda.gov/drugsatfda_docs/nda/2021/213716Orig1s000MultidisciplineR.pdf].

31. FDA. NDA 214096 Tepotinib Review 2021 [Available from: https://www.accessdata.fda.gov/drugsatfda_docs/nda/2021/214096Orig1s000MultidisciplineR.pdf].

32. FDA. NDA 213176 Umbralisib Review 2021 [Available from: https://www.accessdata.fda.gov/drugsatfda_docs/nda/2021/213176Orig1Orig2s000MultidisciplineR.pdf].

33. FDA. NDA 213498 Ponesimod Review 2021 [Available from: https://www.accessdata.fda.gov/drugsatfda_docs/nda/2021/213498Orig1s000ClinPharmR.pdf].

34. FDA. NDA 213378 Olanzapine and Samidorphan Review 2021 [Available from: https://www.accessdata.fda.gov/drugsatfda_docs/nda/2021/213378Orig1Orig2s000MultidisciplineR.pdf].

35. FDA. NDA 214665 Sotorasib Review 2021 [Available from: https://www.accessdata.fda.gov/drugsatfda_docs/nda/2021/214665Orig1s000MultidisciplineR.pdf].

36. FDA. NDA 215341 Finerenone Review 2021 [Available from: https://www.accessdata.fda.gov/drugsatfda_docs/nda/2021/215341Orig1s000IntegratedR.pdf].

37. FDA. NDA 214783 Belumosudil Review 2021 [Available from: https://www.accessdata.fda.gov/drugsatfda_docs/nda/2021/214783Orig1s000MultidisciplineR.pdf].

38. FDA. NDA 215383 Belzutifan Review 2021 [Available from: https://www.accessdata.fda.gov/drugsatfda_docs/nda/2021/215383Orig1s000MultidisciplineR.pdf].

39. FDA. NDA 215310 Mobocertinib Review 2021 [Available from: https://www.accessdata.fda.gov/drugsatfda_docs/nda/2021/215310Orig1s000MultidisciplineR.pdf].

40. FDA. NDA 215206 Atogepant Review 2021 [Available from: https://www.accessdata.fda.gov/drugsatfda_docs/nda/2021/215206Orig1s000IntegratedR.pdf].

41. FDA. NDA 214662 Maralixibat Review 2021 [Available from: https://www.accessdata.fda.gov/drugsatfda_docs/nda/2021/214662Orig1s000IntegratedR.pdf].

42. FDA. NDA 215358 Asciminib Review 2021 [Available from: https://www.accessdata.fda.gov/drugsatfda_docs/nda/2021/215358Orig1s000,Orig2s000MultidisciplineR.pdf].

43. FDA. NDA 215596 Maribavir Review 2021 [Available from: https://www.accessdata.fda.gov/drugsatfda_docs/nda/2021/215596Orig1s000IntegratedR.pdf].

44. FDA. NDA 214985 Daridorexant Review 2022 [Available from: https://www.accessdata.fda.gov/drugsatfda_docs/nda/2022/214985Orig1s000IntegratedR.pdf].

45. FDA. NDA 216196 Mitapivat Review 2022 [Available from: https://www.accessdata.fda.gov/drugsatfda_docs/nda/2022/216196Orig1s000IntegratedR.pdf].

46. FDA. NDA 208712 Pacritinib Review 2022 [Available from: https://www.accessdata.fda.gov/drugsatfda_docs/nda/2022/208712Orig1s000IntegratedR.pdf].

47. FDA. NDA 214998 Mavacamten Clinical Pharmacology Review(s) 2022 [Available from: https://www.accessdata.fda.gov/drugsatfda_docs/nda/2022/214998Orig1s000ClinPharmR.pdf].

48. FDA. NDA 215152 / 215153 Vonoprazan, Clarithromycin, Amoxicillin / Vonoprazan, Amoxicillin Review 2022 [Available from: https://www.accessdata.fda.gov/drugsatfda_docs/nda/2022/215152Orig1s000,215153Orig1s000IntegratedR.pdf].

49. FDA. NDA 215866 Tirzepatide Clinical Pharmacology Review(s) 2022 [Available from: https://www.accessdata.fda.gov/drugsatfda_docs/nda/2022/215866Orig1s000ClinPharmR.pdf].

50. FDA. BLA 761261 Olipudase alfa Review 2022 [Available from: https://www.accessdata.fda.gov/drugsatfda_docs/nda/2022/761261Orig1s000IntegratedR.pdf].

51. FDA. NDA 214801 Futibatinib Review 2022 [Available from: https://www.accessdata.fda.gov/drugsatfda_docs/nda/2022/214801Orig1s000MultidisciplineR.pdf].

52. FDA. BLA 761291 Teclistamab Review 2022 [Available from: https://www.accessdata.fda.gov/drugsatfda_docs/nda/2022/761291Orig1s000MultidisciplineR.pdf].

53. FDA. In Vitro Drug Interaction Studies - Cytochrome P450 Enzyme- and Transporter-Mediated Drug Interactions Guidance for Industry 2020 [Available from: https://www.fda.gov/media/134582/download].

54. EMA EU. Guideline on the investigation of drug interactions 2012 [Available from: https://www.ema.europa.eu/en/documents/scientific-guideline/guideline-investigation-drug-interactions-revision-1_en.pdf].

55. PMDA. Guideline on drug interaction for drug development and appropriate provision of information 2019 [Available from: https://www.pmda.go.jp/files/000228122.pdf].

56. ICH. ICH M12 Drug Interaction Studies. 2022.

57. FDA. Physiologically Based Pharmacokinetic Analyses - Format and Content Guidance for Industry 2018 [Available from: https://www.fda.gov/media/101469/download].

58. EMA EU. Guideline on the reporting of physiologically based pharmacokinetic (PBPK) modelling and simulation 2018 [Available from: https://www.ema.europa.eu/en/documents/scientific-guideline/guideline-reporting-physiologically based-pharmacokinetic-pbpk-modelling-simulation_en.pdf].

59. PMDA. Guidelines for Analysis Reports Involving Physiologically based Pharmacokinetic Models 2020 [Available from: https://www.pmda.go.jp/files/000238192.pdf].

60. Kuemmel C, Yang Y, Zhang X, Florian J, Zhu H, Tegenge M, et al. Consideration of a credibility assessment framework in model-informed drug development: Potential application to physiologically-based pharmacokinetic modeling and simulation. *CPT Pharmacometrics Syst Pharmacol.* 2020;9(1):21–8.

61. Frechen S, Solodenko J, Wendl T, Dallmann A, Ince I, Lehr T, et al. A generic framework for the physiologically-based pharmacokinetic platform qualification of PK-Sim and its application to predicting cytochrome P450 3A4-mediated drug-drug interactions. *CPT Pharmacometrics Syst Pharmacol*. 2021;10(6):633–44.

62. FDA. NDA 205552 Ibrutinib SUPPL-7 Label 2016 [Available from: https://www.accessdata.fda.gov/drugsatfda_docs/label/2016/205552s007lbl.pdf].

63. FDA. NDA 205552 Ibrutinib Clinical Pharmacology Review 2013 [Available from: https://www.accessdata.fda.gov/drugsatfda_docs/nda/2014/205552Orig2s000ClinPharmR.pdf].

64. FDA. NDA 205552 Ibrutinib ORIG-1 Label 2013 [Available from: https://www.accessdata.fda.gov/drugsatfda_docs/label/2013/205552s000lbl.pdf].

65. FDA. NDA 205552/s017 Ibrutinib Review 2017 [Available from: https://www.accessdata.fda.gov/drugsatfda_docs/nda/2017/205552Origs1s017.pdf].

66. FDA. NDA 205552 Ibrutinib SUPPL-20 Label 2017 [Available from: https://www.accessdata.fda.gov/drugsatfda_docs/label/2017/205552s020lbl.pdf].

67. de Zwart L, Snoeys J, De Jong J, Sukbuntherng J, Mannaert E, Monshouwer M. Ibrutinib dosing strategies based on interaction potential of CYP3A4 perpetrators using physiologically based pharmacokinetic modeling. *Clin Pharmacol Ther*. 2016;100(5):548–57.

68. FDA. NDA 209803 Ertugliflozin Label 2017 [Available from: https://www.accessdata.fda.gov/drugsatfda_docs/label/2017/209803s000lbl.pdf].

69. Callegari E, Lin J, Tse S, Goosen TC, Sahasrabudhe V. Physiologically-based pharmacokinetic modeling of the drug-drug interaction of the UGT substrate ertugliflozin following co-administration with the UGT inhibitor mefenamic acid. *CPT Pharmacometrics Syst Pharmacol*. 2021;10(2):127–36.

70. FDA. NDA 209803 Ertugliflozin Review 2017 [Available from: https://www.accessdata.fda.gov/drugsatfda_docs/nda/2017/209803,209805,209806Orig1s000ClinPharmR.pdf].

71. FDA. NDA 212887 Cabotegravir Label 2021 [Available from: https://www.accessdata.fda.gov/drugsatfda_docs/label/2021/212887s000lbl.pdf].

72. Patel P, Xue Z, King KS, Parham L, Ford S, Lou Y, et al. Evaluation of the effect of UGT1A1 polymorphisms on the pharmacokinetics of oral and long-acting injectable cabotegravir. *J Antimicrob Chemother*. 2020;75(8):2240–8.

73. FDA. NDA 214377 Vericiguat Label 2021 [Available from: https://www.accessdata.fda.gov/drugsatfda_docs/label/2021/214377s000lbl.pdf].

74. Zhang D, Chando TJ, Everett DW, Patten CJ, Dehal SS, Humphreys WG. In vitro inhibition of UDP glucuronosyltransferases by atazanavir and other HIV protease inhibitors and the relationship of this property to in vivo bilirubin glucuronidation. *Drug Metab Dispos*. 2005;33(11):1729–39.

75. Posada MM, Cannady EA, Payne CD, Zhang X, Bacon JA, Pak YA, et al. Prediction of transporter-mediated drug-drug interactions for baricitinib. *Clin Transl Sci*. 2017;10(6):509–19.

76. FDA. NDA 207924 Baricitinib Review 2018 [Available from: https://www.accessdata.fda.gov/drugsatfda_docs/nda/2018/207924Orig1s000ClinPharmR.pdf].

77. Posada MM, Bacon JA, Schneck KB, Tirona RG, Kim RB, Higgins JW, et al. Prediction of renal transporter mediated drug-drug interactions for pemetrexed using physiologically based pharmacokinetic modeling. *Drug Metab Dispos.* 2015;43(3):325–34.

78. FDA. Evaluation of Gastric pH-Dependent Drug Interactions With Acid-Reducing Agents: Study Design, Data Analysis, and Clinical Implications Guidance for Industry: FDA; 2020 [Available from: https://www.fda.gov/regulatory-information/search-fda-guidance-documents/evaluation-gastric-ph-dependent-drug-interactions-acid-reducing-agents-study-design-data-analysis].

79. Dodd S, Kollipara S, Sanchez-Felix M, Kim H, Meng Q, Beato S, et al. Prediction of ARA/PPI drug-drug interactions at the drug discovery and development interface. *J Pharm Sci.* 2019;108(1):87–101.

80. Lu T, Fraczkiewicz G, Salphati L, Budha N, Dalziel G, Smelick GS, et al. Combining "bottom-up" and "top-down" approaches to assess the impact of food and gastric pH on pictilisib (GDC-0941) pharmacokinetics. *CPT: Pharmacometrics Syst Pharmacol.* 2017;6(11):747–55.

81. Samant TS, Dhuria S, Lu Y, Laisney M, Yang S, Grandeury A, et al. Ribociclib bioavailability is not affected by gastric pH changes or food intake: In silico and clinical evaluations. *Clin Pharmacol Therapeut.* 2018;104(2):374–83.

82. Dong Z, Li J, Wu F, Zhao P, Lee S-C, Zhang L, et al. Application of physiologically-based pharmacokinetic modeling to predict gastric pH-dependent drug-drug interactions for weak base drugs. *CPT: Pharmacometrics Syst Pharmacol.* 2020;9(8):456–65.

83. Lin W, Chen Y, Unadkat JD, Zhang X, Wu D, Heimbach T. Applications, challenges, and outlook for PBPK modeling and simulation: A regulatory, industrial and academic perspective. *Pharm Res.* 2022;39(8):1701–31.

84. Parrott N, Stillhart C, Lindenberg M, Wagner B, Kowalski K, Guerini E, et al. Physiologically based absorption modelling to explore the impact of food and gastric pH changes on the pharmacokinetics of entrectinib. *AAPS J.* 2020;22(4):78.

85. FDA. NDA 205353 Panobinostat Clinical Pharmacology and Biopharmaceutics Review(s) 2015 [Available from: https://www.accessdata.fda.gov/drugsatfda_docs/nda/2015/205353Orig1s000ClinPharmR.pdf.

86. FDA. NDA 205353 Panobinostat Label 2015 [Available from: https://www.accessdata.fda.gov/drugsatfda_docs/label/2015/205353s000lbl.pdf].

87. FDA. NDA 216196 Mitapivat Product Quality Review(s) 2022 [Available from: https://www.accessdata.fda.gov/drugsatfda_docs/nda/2022/216196Orig1s000ChemR.pdf].

88. Maselli DB, Camilleri M. Effects of GLP-1 and its analogs on gastric physiology in diabetes mellitus and obesity. *Adv Exp Med Biol.* 2021;1307:171–92.

89. FDA. NDA 021773 Exenatide ORIG-1 Label 2005 [Available from: https://www.accessdata.fda.gov/drugsatfda_docs/label/2005/021773lbl.pdf].

90. FDA. NDA 022341 Liraglutide ORIG-1 Label 2010 [Available from: https://www.accessdata.fda.gov/drugsatfda_docs/label/2010/022341lbl.pdf].

91. FDA. NDA 208471 Lixisenatide ORIG-1 Label 2016 [Available from: https://www.accessdata.fda.gov/drugsatfda_docs/label/2016/208471Orig1s000lbl.pdf].

92. FDA. BLA 125469 Dulaglutide ORIG-1 Label 2014 [Available from: https://www.accessdata.fda.gov/drugsatfda_docs/nda/2014/125469Orig1s000Lbl.pdf].

93. FDA. NDA 215866 Tirzepatide Label 2022 [Available from: https://www.accessdata.fda.gov/drugsatfda_docs/label/2022/215866s000lbl.pdf].

94. FDA. Guidance for Industry: Drug-Drug Interaction Assessment for Therapeutic Proteins FDA; 2020 [Available from: https://www.fda.gov/media/140909/download].

95. Jiang X, Zhuang Y, Xu Z, Wang W, Zhou H. Development of a physiologically based pharmacokinetic model to predict disease-mediated therapeutic protein-drug interactions: Modulation of multiple cytochrome P450 enzymes by interleukin-6. *AAPS J*. 2016;18(3):767–76.

96. Wang L, Chen Y, Zhou W, Miao X, Zhou H. Utilization of physiologically-based pharmacokinetic model to assess disease-mediated therapeutic protein-disease-drug interaction in immune-mediated inflammatory diseases. *Clin Transl Sci*. 2022;15(2):464–76.

97. Chen KF, Jones HM, Gill KL. PBPK modelling to predict drug-biologic interactions with cytokine modulators: Are these relevant and is IL-6 enough? *Drug Metab Dispos*. 2022 Oct; 50(10):1322–1331.

98. FDA. BLA 125557 SUPPL-21 Blinatumomab Label 2022 [Available from: https://www.accessdata.fda.gov/drugsatfda_docs/label/2022/125557s021lbl.pdf].

99. FDA. BLA 125557 Blinatumomab Clinical Pharmacology Review 2014 [Available from: https://www.accessdata.fda.gov/drugsatfda_docs/nda/2014/125557Orig1s000ClinPharmRedt.pdf].

100. Xu Y, Hijazi Y, Wolf A, Wu B, Sun YN, Zhu M. Physiologically based pharmacokinetic model to assess the influence of blinatumomab-mediated cytokine elevations on cytochrome P450 enzyme activity. *CPT: Pharmacometrics Syst Pharmacol*. 2015;4(9):507–15.

101. FDA. BLA 761149 Satralizumab Label 2020 [Available from: https://www.accessdata.fda.gov/drugsatfda_docs/label/2020/761149s000lbl.pdf].

102. Schlender JF, Meyer M, Thelen K, Krauss M, Willmann S, Eissing T, et al. Development of a whole-body physiologically based pharmacokinetic approach to assess the pharmacokinetics of drugs in elderly individuals. *Clin Pharmacokinet*. 2016;55(12):1573–89.

103. Stader F, Kinvig H, Penny MA, Battegay M, Siccardi M, Marzolini C. Physiologically based pharmacokinetic modelling to identify pharmacokinetic parameters driving drug exposure changes in the elderly. *Clin Pharmacokinet*. 2020;59(3):383–401.

104. Chetty M, Johnson TN, Polak S, Salem F, Doki K, Rostami-Hodjegan A. Physiologically based pharmacokinetic modelling to guide drug delivery in older people. *Adv Drug Deliv Rev*. 2018;135:85–96.

105. Wang Z, Chan ECY. Physiologically-based pharmacokinetic modelling to investigate baricitinib and tofacitinib dosing recommendations for COVID-19 in geriatrics. *Clin Pharmacol Ther*. 2022;112(2):291–6.

106. FDA. NDA 212725 / 212726 Entrectinib Label 2019 [Available from: https://www.accessdata.fda.gov/drugsatfda_docs/label/2019/212726s000lbl.pdf].

107. FDA. NDA 212725 / 212726 Entrectinib Review 2019 [Available from: https://www.accessdata.fda.gov/drugsatfda_docs/nda/2019/212725Orig1s000,%20212726Orig1s000 MultidisciplineR.pdf].

108. Upreti VV, Wahlstrom JL. Meta-analysis of hepatic cytochrome P450 ontogeny to underwrite the prediction of pediatric pharmacokinetics using physiologically based pharmacokinetic modeling. *J Clin Pharmacol*. 2016;56(3):266–83.

109. Johnson TN, Rostami-Hodjegan A, Tucker GT. Prediction of the clearance of eleven drugs and associated variability in neonates, infants and children. *Clin Pharmacokinet*. 2006; 45(9):931–56.

110. FDA. NDA 211155 Duvelisib Label 2018 [Available from: https://www.accessdata.fda.gov/drugsatfda_docs/label/2018/211155s000lbl.pdf].

111. FDA. NDA 211155 Duvelisib Review 2018 [Available from: https://www.accessdata.fda.gov/drugsatfda_docs/nda/2018/211155Orig1Orig2s000MultidisciplineR.pdf].

112. FDA. NDA 213378 Olanzapine and Samidorphan Label 2021 [Available from: https://www.accessdata.fda.gov/drugsatfda_docs/label/2021/213378s000lbl.pdf].

113. FDA. NDA 212018 Erdafinitib Review 2019 [Available from: https://www.accessdata.fda.gov/drugsatfda_docs/nda/2019/212018Orig1s000MultidisciplineR.pdf].

114. Schwenger E, Reddy VP, Moorthy G, Sharma P, Tomkinson H, Masson E, et al. Harnessing meta-analysis to refine an oncology patient population for physiology-based pharmacokinetic modeling of drugs. *Clin Pharmacol Ther*. 2018;103(2):271–80.

115. FDA. NDA 205494 Eliglustat Label 2014 [Available from: https://www.accessdata.fda.gov/drugsatfda_docs/label/2014/205494Orig1s000lbl.pdf].

116. FDA. NDA 205494 Eliglustat Clinical Pharmacology and Biopharmaceutics Review(s) 2014 [Available from: https://www.accessdata.fda.gov/drugsatfda_docs/nda/2014/205494Orig1s000ClinPharmR.pdf].

117. FDA. NDA 209884 Siponimod Clinical Pharmacology Biopharmaceutics Review(s) 2019 [Available from: https://www.accessdata.fda.gov/drugsatfda_docs/nda/2019/209884Orig1s000ClinPharmR.pdf.

118. FDA. NDA 212018 Erdafinitib Label 2019 [Available from: https://www.accessdata.fda.gov/drugsatfda_docs/label/2019/212018s000lbl.pdf].

119. Kusama M, Maeda K, Chiba K, Aoyama A, Sugiyama Y. Prediction of the effects of genetic polymorphism on the pharmacokinetics of CYP2C9 substrates from in vitro data. *Pharm Res*. 2009;26(4):822–35.

120. Scordo MG, Pengo V, Spina E, Dahl ML, Gusella M, Padrini R. Influence of CYP2C9 and CYP2C19 genetic polymorphisms on warfarin maintenance dose and metabolic clearance. *Clin Pharmacol Ther*. 2002;72(6):702–10.

121. FDA. NDA 214998 Mavacamten Label 2022 [Available from: https://www.accessdata.fda.gov/drugsatfda_docs/label/2022/214998s000lbl.pdf].

122. FDA. NDA 206256 Belinostat Label 2014 [Available from: https://www.accessdata.fda.gov/drugsatfda_docs/label/2014/206256lbl.pdf].

123. FDA. NDA 206256 Belinostat Approval Letter 2014 [Available from: https://www.accessdata.fda.gov/drugsatfda_docs/appletter/2014/206256Orig1s000ltr.pdf].

124. Goey AK, Sissung TM, Peer CJ, Trepel JB, Lee MJ, Tomita Y, et al. Effects of UGT1A1 genotype on the pharmacokinetics, pharmacodynamics, and toxicities of belinostat administered by 48-hour continuous infusion in patients with cancer. *J Clin Pharmacol*. 2016;56(4):461–73.

125. Peer CJ, Goey AK, Sissung TM, Erlich S, Lee MJ, Tomita Y, et al. UGT1A1 genotype-dependent dose adjustment of belinostat in patients with advanced cancers using population pharmacokinetic modeling and simulation. *J Clin Pharmacol*. 2016;56(4):450–60.

126. FDA. NDA 215383 Belzutifan Label 2021 [Available from: https://www.accessdata.fda.gov/drugsatfda_docs/label/2021/215383s000lbl.pdf].

127. George B, Lumen A, Nguyen C, Wesley B, Wang J, Beitz J, et al. Application of physiologically based pharmacokinetic modeling for sertraline dosing recommendations in pregnancy. *NPJ Syst Biol Appl.* 2020;6(1):36.

128. Coppola P, Kerwash E, Cole S. Physiologically based pharmacokinetics model in pregnancy: A regulatory perspective on model evaluation. *Front Pediatr.* 2021;9:524.

129. Szeto KX, Le Merdy M, Dupont B, Bolger MB, Lukacova V. PBPK modeling approach to predict the behavior of drugs cleared by kidney in pregnant subjects and fetus. *AAPS J.* 2021;23(4):89.

130. Badhan RKS, Gittins R. Precision dosing of methadone during pregnancy: A pharmacokinetics virtual clinical trials study. *J Subst Abuse Treat.* 2021;130:108521.

131. Ke AB, Nallani SC, Zhao P, Rostami-Hodjegan A, Unadkat JD. Expansion of a PBPK model to predict disposition in pregnant women of drugs cleared via multiple CYP enzymes, including CYP2B6, CYP2C9 and CYP2C19. *Br J Clin Pharmacol.* 2014;77(3):554–70.

132. Abduljalil K, Badhan RKS. Drug dosing during pregnancy-opportunities for physiologically based pharmacokinetic models. *J Pharmacokinet Pharmacodyn.* 2020;47(4):319–40.

133. Abduljalil K, Ning J, Pansari A, Pan X, Jamei M. Prediction of maternal and fetoplacental concentrations of cefazolin, cefuroxime, and amoxicillin during pregnancy using bottom-up physiologically based pharmacokinetic models. *Drug Metab Dispos.* 2022;50(4):386–400.

134. Abduljalil K, Pansari A, Jamei M. Prediction of maternal pharmacokinetics using physiologically based pharmacokinetic models: Assessing the impact of the longitudinal changes in the activity of CYP1A2, CYP2D6 and CYP3A4 enzymes during pregnancy. *J Pharmacokinet Pharmacodyn.* 2020;47(4):361–83.

135. Abduljalil K, Pansari A, Ning J, Jamei M. Prediction of maternal and fetal acyclovir, emtricitabine, lamivudine, and metformin concentrations during pregnancy using a physiologically based pharmacokinetic modeling approach. *Clin Pharmacokinet.* 2022;61(5):725–48.

136. Pasquiers B, Benamara S, Felices M, Nguyen L, Decleves X. Review of the existing translational pharmacokinetics modeling approaches specific to monoclonal antibodies (mAbs) to support the first-in-human (FIH) dose selection. *Int J Mol Sci.* 2022;23(21):12754.

137. Jones HM, Chen Y, Gibson C, Heimbach T, Parrott N, Peters SA, et al. Physiologically based pharmacokinetic modeling in drug discovery and development: A pharmaceutical industry perspective. *Clin Pharmacol Ther.* 2015;97(3):247–62.

138. Huth F, Gardin A, Umehara K, He HD. Prediction of the impact of cytochrome P450 2C9 genotypes on the drug-drug interaction potential of siponimod with physiologically-based pharmacokinetic modeling: A comprehensive approach for drug label recommendations. *Clin Pharmacol Therapeut.* 2019;106(5):1113–24.

139. FDA. NDA 213535 Risdiplam Label 2020 [Available from: https://www.accessdata.fda.gov/drugsatfda_docs/label/2020/213535s000lbl.pdf].

140. Cleary Y, Gertz M, Grimsey P, Gunther A, Heinig K, Ogungbenro K, et al. Model-based drug-drug interaction extrapolation strategy from adults to children: Risdiplam in pediatric patients with spinal muscular atrophy. *Clin Pharmacol Ther.* 2021;110(6):1547–57.

141. FDA. NDA 213535 Risdiplam Clinical Pharmacology and Biopharmaceutics Review(s) 2020 [Available from: https://www.accessdata.fda.gov/drugsatfda_docs/nda/2020/213535Orig1s000ClinPharmR.pdf].

142. FDA. NDA 209092 Ribociclib Label 2017 [Available from: https://www.accessdata.fda.gov/drugsatfda_docs/label/2017/209092s000lbl.pdf].

143. FDA. NDA 209092 Ribociclib Review 2017 [Available from: https://www.accessdata.fda.gov/drugsatfda_docs/nda/2017/209092Orig1s000MultidisciplineR.pdf].

144. FDA. NDA 210861 Larotrectinib Approval Letter 2018 [Available from: https://www.accessdata.fda.gov/drugsatfda_docs/appletter/2018/210861Orig1s000ltr.pdf].

145. FDA. NDA 210656 Glasdegib Maleate Approval Letter 2018 [Available from: https://www.accessdata.fda.gov/drugsatfda_docs/appletter/2018/210656Orig1s000ltr.pdf].

146. FDA. NDA 211810 Pexidartinib Approval Letter 2019 [Available from: https://www.accessdata.fda.gov/drugsatfda_docs/appletter/2019/211810Orig1s000ltr.pdf].

147. FDA. NDA 212327 Fedratinib Approval Letter 2019 [Available from: https://www.accessdata.fda.gov/drugsatfda_docs/appletter/2019/212327Orig1s000ltr.pdf].

12 Physiologically-Based Biopharmaceutics Modeling in Support of Drug Product Specifications and Biowaiver

Xavier Pepin, Fang Wu, Tycho Heimbach, Filippos Kesisoglou, Haritha Mandula, Rodrigo Cristofoletti, and Sandra Suarez

12.1 INTRODUCTION

12.1.1 Regulatory Landscape

The development of pharmaceutical drug products is, in general a long, complex process. In particular, the traditional drug product development process necessitates a great deal of time and resources before a molecule is launched into the market. And despite all these huge efforts, the chances of a lead molecule to enter the market are low. In fact, only about 10%–20% of novel candidate molecules gain market approval, and their journey remains unpredictable throughout their lifecycle [1]. Once a new drug product (innovator) is approved and marketed, changes to the manufacturing process, formulation, addition of new strengths, etc., may occur. Moreover, as the innovator drug product is going off patent, development and manufacturing of a generic equivalent is anticipated, and the pharmaceutical industry may file, e.g., in the US, an abbreviated new drug application (ANDA) for generic drug approval [2,3].

Any manufacturing changes implemented post-approval to the innovator product, including the generic equivalents should have the same safety and effectiveness as the original approved new drug product (innovator). The innovator serves as a reference or standard for comparison for the post-changed drug product and generic equivalents (i.e., multi-source drug products). To ensure safety and effectiveness of the post-changed drug product and/or generic versions, bioequivalence (BE) must be established versus the reference listed drug (RLD). Per the Code of Federal Regulations (Title 21), two drug products will be considered bioequivalent if they are pharmaceutical equivalents or pharmaceutical alternatives whose rate and extent of absorption do not show a significant difference when administered at the same molar dose of active moiety under similar experimental conditions, either single dose or multiple doses [4].

Many aspects of the drug development process and market approval focus on satisfying the regulatory requirements of drug licensing to ensure quality, efficacy, and safety of drug products. To support the pharmaceutical industry in complying with all these requirements, regulatory agencies have published several guidance documents that facilitate the process throughout the lifecycle, especially when it comes to addressing chemistry, manufacturing, and control (CMC) changes. Some regulatory guidance documents (e.g., IVIVC guidance documents) [5,6] reflect the agencies' position to aid in decreasing the regulatory and manufacturing burden (e.g., via biowaiver requests) by embracing the use of modeling and simulation to support major CMC changes. Most recently, the Food and Drug Administration (FDA) published the draft guidance for the industry on the use of physiologically-based pharmacokinetic analyses-biopharmaceutics applications for oral drug product development, manufacturing changes and controls [7].

In response to this guidance, biopharmaceutics computational modeling applications are gaining prominence not only during early drug development but also through the life cycle of the product [8–10]. Quality target product profile (QTPP) is a prospective summary of the quality characteristics of a drug product that ideally will be achieved to ensure the desired quality, taking into account safety and efficacy of the drug product [11]. Biopharmaceutics modeling techniques may help identify formulations with desired QTPP. These strategies assist in determining optimal drug product dosage forms and routes of delivery. In vitro tests in many cases can serve as a surrogate for the recommended bioequivalence studies following major CMC changes and can help determine in vivo outcomes of drug product variants. To this end, in vitro dissolution is the in vitro test that could help assess the impact of CMC changes on the systemic exposure, provided a quantitative relationship between in vitro dissolution, in vivo dissolution, and the PK profiles has been established. The lack of this essential in vitro in vivo link would render the in vitro dissolution mainly serving for quality control.

Models with biopharmaceutics input data are key elements in model informed drug development and are known as Physiologically-Based Biopharmaceutics Models (PBBM). PBBM is a

DOI: 10.1201/9781003031802-12

fit-for-purpose modeling approach [8,12–14], which is to emphasize the role of biopharmaceutics modeling combined with PBPK analysis to facilitate the establishment of the in vitro (i.e., dissolution) in vivo link which is essential to ensure patient-centric drug product quality and gain manufacturing flexibility. It should be noted that the concept of physiologically-based models to address CMC changes has evolved in the past decade. Although there is a trend for utilizing the term PBBM to address drug product quality applications, some scientists still utilize general terms such as PBPK models or PBPK absorption modeling (PBAM) for such applications.

PBBM shares some common steps with PBPK (baseline) model building such as the calibration of disposition and absorption models and their validation using appropriate data. However, PBBM's main purpose is to provide a mechanistic understanding of in vivo drug release with emphasis on the effect of formulation and manufacturing changes. Another key difference is that, to evaluate the in vivo impact of CMC changes, a safe space, which are boundaries defined by in vitro specifications, such as dissolution or other relevant drug product quality attributes, within which drug product variants are anticipated to be bioequivalent to one another [7], can be built using PBBM via the construction of an in vitro in vivo relationship (IVIVR) or IVIVC, which means that one needs to include in vitro dissolution data as an input [15]. It should be noted that during early phases of drug product development, the need for extrapolation (absence of safe space due to the lack of relevant clinical data) is expected and constitutes a plausible and proven path for successful formulation selection, e.g., between a capsule and tablet formulations [16].

Once a PBBM is established and validated, the impact of formulation variants and any other CMC changes on in vivo performance throughout the drug product's lifecycle can be predicted and enlightened based on the model's predictive capability. The traditional approach to IVIVC has resulted in poor success rate due to lack of physiological relevance [17]. With early modeling approaches including PBBM, not only can the success rate of these IVIVC models be improved, but this path offers a greater likelihood of building IVIVRs resulting in a feasible alternate path to biowaivers, especially for IR products for which the success rate of building and validating an IVIVC is rather low. Akin to IVIVC, PBBM-IVIVR can then reduce the regulatory burden since it can be used in lieu of in vivo studies for life cycle management of drug products, including enabling the incorporation of clinical relevance into real time releasing testing (RTRT) manufacturing approaches.

In addition, PBBM is a tool being used to promote patient-centric quality standards (PCQS) based on risk assessment and setting clinically relevant specifications [18]. PCQS which is a set of criteria and acceptance ranges to which drug products should conform to deliver the therapeutic benefits indicated in the label allowing to balance of risk/benefit, and patient needs/regulatory challenges. PBBM aids in promoting PCQS through the development of predictive in vitro dissolution models based on risk assessment. To aid in this process, framework and decision trees have been developed portraying initial biopharmaceutics risk assessment in the Knowledge Aided Structured Assessment (KASA) process defining when PBBM has the highest regulatory utility [19]. Other applications are sporadically seen, such as drug absorption prediction in pediatrics for formulation selection, the evaluation of the effect of gastric pH or food on drug absorption and predicting bioavailability following formulation changes (Figure 12.1) [9]. In generic drug development, the regulatory questions that PBPK absorption modeling/PBBM can help answer include setting dissolution safe space, evaluating the impact of changes in critical quality attributes and assessing the risk of release mechanism change, pH-dependent drug–drug interaction (DDI) potential (following formulation changes), predicting gastrointestinal (GI) local concentration, supporting bioequivalence (BE) assessment in specific populations, and waiving of in vivo studies [8]. To facilitate the regulatory decision-making process related to pH-related DDIs, the FDA has also issued the guidance on evaluation of gastric pH-dependent drug interactions [20], where PBPK absorption model applications are very promising to reduce the regulatory burden.

In this chapter, we describe several case studies that offer the opportunity to further reflect on the application of PBBM and PBPK absorption modeling in support of regulatory decision-making. These case studies demonstrate the successful integration of in vitro dissolution data via the development of mechanistic dissolution models informed by drug and product attributes and parameters to predict in vivo dissolution and systemic exposure and bioequivalence.

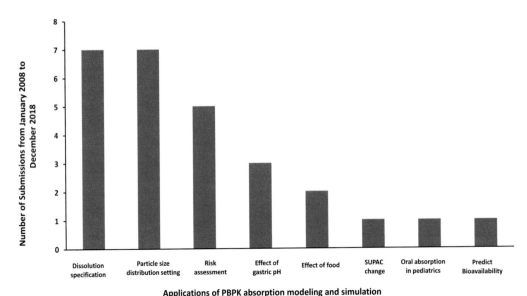

Figure 12.1 Applications of PBPK absorption modeling and simulations in the new drug applications submissions. *Note that in some cases, the same model was used for multiple purposes, e.g., setting of both particle size specification and dissolution acceptance criteria.

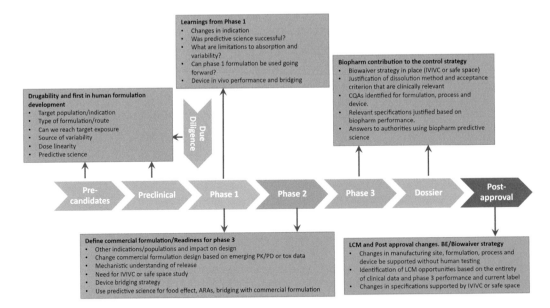

Figure 12.2 Utility of PBBM throughout drug product development and post-approval.

12.2 UTILITY OF PBBM IN SUPPORT OF THE DEVELOPMENT OF NEW DRUGS APPLICATIONS. FOCUS ON QUALITY DECISIONS

12.2.1 Setting Clinically Relevant Product Specifications

PBBM can be used throughout drug product development to explore product performance and how product quality attributes and manufacturing process parameters are linked to in vivo exposure (Figure 12.2). During the clinical phases of drug product development, information on human PK

PBBM (Subset of PBPK) Examples in Oral Formulation Development

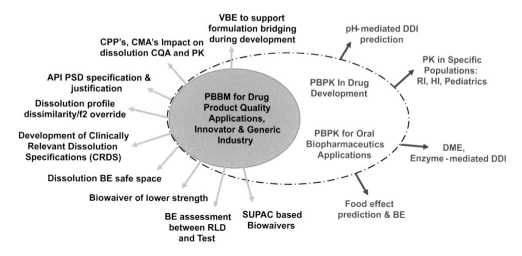

Figure 12.3 PBBM for drug product quality applications.

and drug product performance is verified, and more precision is gained to refine the models in terms of input. The models can be informed and verified with commercial representative drug substance and drug product properties, and this allows prediction of Phase 3 and commercial product exposure. The clinical PK data may originate from multiple independent studies as well as bioequivalence studies. In addition, as PK/PD models emerge from Phase 2 and Phase 3 data, the definition of the drug product safe space can also rely on the combination of PBBM and PK/PD models.

In the field of drug substance and drug product quality, the specifications that can be supported by PBBM are quite numerous, and these are illustrated in Figure 12.3. To be implemented in the model, the variations in product quality whether linked to the formulation, quality of drug substance, excipient performance or process parameters, need to show an impact in vitro on the drug product quality. This drug product quality is mainly assessed through the product dissolution in a discriminatory and biopredictive method.

12.2.1.1 Dissolution: A Tool Not for the Fool!

Dissolution methods can be of many kinds and serve specific purposes during the drug product development. They cannot all be used for the purpose of modeling batch performance in a PBBM. There are several types of dissolution methods based on the apparatus and media used, and their ability to discern for aberrant batches and to mimic the systemic exposure.

Quality Control Dissolution Methods: Historically, quality control dissolution methods (also called new drug application [NDA] methods) were primarily used to release clinical and commercial batches of drug products in the R&D and commercial production sites. These methods use typically USP2 or USP1 apparatuses with media, the composition of which relies on synthetic buffers and sometimes surfactants, the level of which has been justified in view of the drug substance solubility vs pH profile, type and strength of dosage form. The assays are conducted in media volumes typically ranging from 500 to 1,000 mL at 37°C. The agitation rate is typically 50 rpm for USP2 or 100 rpm in USP1 and has been justified to avoid bias due to drug and excipient sedimentation for example. The medium should be stable and as much as possible inert toward the drug substance and the excipients. The regulatory agencies' approved dissolution method may be deemed discriminatory, biorelevant, clinically relevant, or biopredictive.

Biorelevant Dissolution Methods: Biorelevant dissolution methods will attempt to mimic the physiological reality of the administration route. The media in these methods can be more or less complex in terms of composition and presence of micellar phases and may also change with time. These methods can capture more than drug dissolution and connect different compartments. The drug precipitation can be recreated in vitro, and the drug absorption can be present as well in the form of sink compartment of absorptive membranes. Drugs and fluids may also be transferred

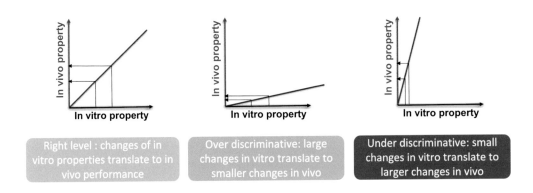

Figure 12.4   Illustration of the discriminatory level for dissolution methods.

from compartments in a dynamic fashion to reproduce fluid composition changes or emptying of gastro-intestinal (GI) compartments [21,22]. The devices used to conduct dissolution with biorelevant methods can also be USP apparatuses with choices of USP1-4. In more sophisticated models such as TIM-1 for example [23], the effect of peristalsis or inter-digestive myoelectric complex in the fasted and fed states can also be reproduced with the addition of mechanical forces on the luminal contents.

Biorelevant methods from simple to more complex are typically used to assess formulation and manufacturing process changes, the effect of food or the effect of pH-related DDI in vitro to guide the need for human evaluation.

Discriminatory Dissolution Methods: Ideally, all dissolution methods should show a certain level of discrimination, i.e., the drug product should dissolve differently in these methods when the quality attributes of the drug substance or the drug product are varied in typical ranges used during formulation and process development. The right level of discrimination is achieved when changes of in vitro properties lead to changes in in vivo properties of the same magnitude. A dissolution method can also be over-discriminative when large changes in dissolution lead to smaller changes in vivo and finally methods can be under-discriminative when small changes in vitro lead to large changes in vivo. The right level of discrimination is always desirable and if slightly over-discriminative methods can be accepted as QC methods, under-discriminatory methods are never acceptable since they will not anticipate changes in vivo (Figure 12.4). Depending on the type of formulation and mechanism of release the variations of quality attributes that are classically explored in the context of QbD to understand the drug product failure modes could comprise (but are not limited to):

- **Immediate Release Formulations**: drug substance particle size, polymorphic form, drug product granule size or density, binder amount, and compression force.

- **Modified Release Matrix Formulations**: different grades/amounts of matrix forming agents, molecular weight or viscosity of the polymers.

- **Modified Release Pellet Formulations**: Coating level/thickness, molecular weight or viscosity of the polymer, mature and content of pore-forming agent.

- **Eroding Tablet Formulations**: surface to volume ratio, compression force.

- **Formulations Containing Amorphous Drug Substance**: Surface to volume ratio, crystalline drug substance (spiking of formulations with crystalline material).

Clinically Relevant Dissolution Method: This attribute means that once the pharmacokinetics of formulation variants has been determined, the observed dissolution rate of these variants in the method of interest will rank order with for example in vivo C_{max} or calculated in vivo absorption rate. Note that some deviation to the in vitro in vivo rank ordering could be expected inside of the safe space (i.e., where dissolution rate is not expected to limit in vivo exposure) or when other phenomena such as regional drug absorption, chemical instability or first pass gut degradation, may lead to lower dissolving formulations reaching a higher exposure than fast dissolving formulations for another reason than drug dissolution.

Biopredictive Dissolution Methods: A method is termed biopredictive, when the dissolution data resulting from such a method can be integrated in the PBBM to provide for a quantitative prediction of human PK profiles. The integration of the dissolution data will depend on the type of formulation, mechanism of release as explained later.

12.2.1.1.1 Methods for Modeling in vitro Dissolution

In silico twins for biorelevant methods are being developed with the ambition to understand the differences in hydrodynamics for example between USP-type apparatuses and these more complex devices [24], to extract key drug and formulation-related parameters such as the drug precipitation at different super-saturation levels in the presence or absence of selected excipients using transfer methods. As mentioned above, the main purpose of a discriminatory dissolution method is to quantify the impact of critical material attributes (CMAs) and critical process parameter (CPPs) changes on the performance of the drug product in vivo. Dissolution data in multiple media and agitation conditions generated for pivotal clinical batches or batches which were used in clinical pharmacology PK studies (e.g., impact of dose, formulation changes, manufacturing process changes, and prandial state) are therefore of immense value to build the PBBM and allow to demonstrate the biopredictive nature of a dissolution method. Depending on the drug product mechanism of release and drug substance properties, the way to integrate dissolution in the PBBM should be carefully chosen and analyzed.

There are several methods to integrate drug product dissolution in a PBBM and the assumptions made when choosing a particular method over another are illustrated in Figure 12.5.

Direct Input: This method is by far the simplest. Measured percent dissolved vs time is entered in the PBBM and the software is let to interpolate percent dissolved between two measured points. If the drug dissolution is not conducted until 100% dissolved, the software will extrapolate to 100 % dissolved using the last two measured points. The caveat to using a direct input of dissolution in a PBBM is the issue related to inter- or extrapolation which may lead to inadequate prediction of in vitro and in vivo percent dissolved. To avoid this issue, it is recommended to use this method only if the frequency of sampling is high during dissolution rate measurement.

Weibull Function: A Weibull function is in the form of:

$$F(t) = P_{max}\left(1 - \exp\left(-\frac{(t - t_{lag})^b}{A}\right)\right)$$

(12.1)

where A is the time scaling factor, t_{lag} the lag time to dissolution, and b is the shape factor. Multiple phase Weibull functions (which ascribe fraction of the drug load to different Weibull functions) are also available in most PBBM software platforms to be able to model multiphasic in vitro release. Weibull function combinations are very flexible and allow to work with sparse sampling in dissolution since the interpolation between points of measured percent dissolved is not linear.

When integrating dissolution with the direct input method or Weibull fit of dissolution data, the assumptions made are that neither the drug dose, solubility or medium volume are limiting the

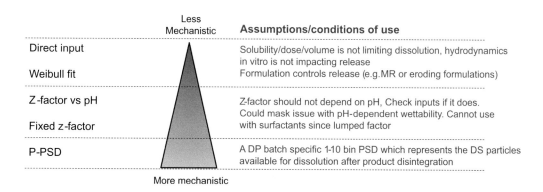

Figure 12.5 Methods for integrating and modeling dissolution profile data in PBBM.

in vitro and in vivo dissolution and that the hydrodynamics in the in vitro test are representative of the in vivo hydrodynamics. This may be the case for Biopharmaceutics Classification System (BCS) class 1 or 3 drugs when the formulation excipients control the drug release and there is little impact of solubility on controlling in vitro dissolution. Typically, this is the case for modified release formulations. Both direct integration and Weibull fit of the dissolution data are therefore not mechanistic models for dissolution since the in vivo release will be matching the entered in vitro profile and will only depend on time but not on the local GI conditions of e.g., pH, volume, or concentration of bile salts.

z-factor: the z-factor was proposed by Takano et al. [25]. It is an aggregated factor which is in the form of

$$z = \frac{3D}{\rho h r_0} \tag{12.2}$$

where D is the drug diffusion coefficient, ρ is the drug crystal density, h is the thickness of the unstirred water layer, and r_0 is the initial particle size radius. The z-factor is an aggregated factor and its utilization as a single batch representative of impact of formulation on dissolution is subject to these parameters being constant across different in vitro or in vivo conditions. Since drug may partition between aqueous phases and micellar phases in vitro and in vivo, the effective drug diffusion coefficient will be dependent on the micelle concentration, since micelle bound drug typically diffuse much slower compared to free drug due to the size difference between micelles and free drug. This parameter should be carefully evaluated when applying the z-factor to fit observed in vitro dissolution data or predict in vitro and in vivo dissolution. In addition, since the z-factor comprises the initial particle size distribution, the fit of dissolution data may sometimes be more adequate for initial time points than later timepoints. Finally, since there is only one z-factor fitted to a batch dissolution data, complex dissolution profiles that deviate from first-order release are hard to fit adequately. Hofsäss et al. [26] have proposed refined ways of fitting z-factor to immediate release formulations in the presence of coning or slow disintegration. The z-factor should not theoretically depend on pH unless the excipients in the formulation show a sensitivity to pH which can be fitted with the z-factor, the z-factor versus pH could not be used as an input to PBBMs.

P-PSD: The product particle size distribution (P-PSD) was introduced by Pepin et al. [27–29] where the reduction of solid drug mass vs time is expressed as:

$$\frac{dm_{\text{solid}}}{dt} = -A(t) \times \left(f_u \times \frac{D_u}{h_u(t)} + \frac{1 - f_u}{f_u} \times \frac{D_b}{h_b(t)} \right) \times \left(C_{S,u} - C_u(t) \right) \tag{12.3}$$

where $f_u = \dfrac{C_u(t)}{C(t)}$ is the drug fraction unbound, D_u the unbound drug diffusion coefficient, D_b is the micelle bound diffusion coefficient, $A(t)$ is the available drug substance area at time t, $h_u(t)$ the unbound unstirred water layer thickness, $h_b(t)$ the micelle bound unstirred water layer thickness, $C_{S,u}$ the unbound drug solubility at the surface of the crystal and $C_u(t)$ the unbound drug bulk concentration at time t. $A(0)$ is the initial drug substance surface area which can be represented as a 1–10 bin spherical particle size distribution, the P-PSD. This approach was proposed as a development of the Gamsiz et al. approach [30] assuming immediate partitioning of drugs to micelles at the surface of the drug, and different thicknesses for unstirred water layer for free and micelle bound drug. These thicknesses are related by the following equation, which was proposed by Pohl et al. [31]:

$$\frac{h_b}{h_u} = \sqrt[3]{\frac{D_b}{D_u}} \tag{12.4}$$

P-PSD particles incorporate the effect of wetting, formulation excipients and process parameters in the drug substance area made available to the dissolution vessel. Like for the z-factor the particles are assumed to be immediately available. In silico, these released particles will travel along the GI tract, dissolve preferentially according to their size. The dissolution of these particles would be sensitive to local volume, pH, and bile salt concentration, which will determine the fraction drug unbound and the total solubility. Recently, two additional models for P-PSD were proposed which integrate the fluid velocity in USP2 dissolution apparatus, one ignoring the effect of drug and formulation sedimentation (P-PSD HD) and one comprising a simulation of the drug and excipient sedimentation and potential formation of a cone at the bottom of the USP2 vessel (P-PSD HDC) [32]. These latter models are important to remove the potential bias coming from formulation coning during dissolution or to account for the fluid velocity in USP2, which is particularly important for large particles or large dosage forms such as eroding tablets or pellets [33,34]. Since the P-PSD can comprise from 1 to 10 bins, there is enough granularity to fit complex dissolution profiles including those presenting multiple phases.

Combination of Methods: An interesting feature of some PBBM software platforms is the ability to combine non-mechanistic and mechanistic models to predict in vivo dissolution, which provides for more flexibility to integrate diverse mechanisms that could be observed on product dissolution. For example, in GastroPlus™, a Weibull function can be combined to a "controlled release undissolved" formulation to handle a potential lag time observed due to product disintegration. The dissolution of undissolved drugs resulting from Weibull predictions of drug release can then be modeled mechanistically using either z-factor or P-PSD approaches. This would allow the in vivo dissolution to occur after a predefined transit time in a section of the GI tract where the drug solubility and available volume for dissolution would uniquely control in vivo dissolution.

Discussion on the Methods: Overall, when reviewing PBBM literature and ways of integrating dissolution, all the methods detailed above for integrating dissolution of immediate release products have been utilized. Anand et al. [35] have shown that out of 27 case studies where dissolution was integrated into a PBBM, the methods detailed above were each used in 4–7 case studies. These authors also showed that for drug products containing low solubility drugs, the use of mechanistic models for integrating dissolution was more frequent than for high solubility drugs.

The advantage of mechanistic dissolution models, such as the z-factor or P-PSD, is that they will account for the specific in vitro conditions of dose, volume, solubility, and sometimes agitation, to derive a batch-specific input to the PBBM. The in vivo drug dissolution predicted from these models will then be dependent on the volume, pH, bile salt concentration, precipitation rate, permeability, efflux, and transit time in the GI tract at any given time during the simulation, since all these parameters will play a role on the drug lumen solubility and concentration. The in vivo dissolution time profile may therefore be significantly different from the in vitro dissolution time profile for a drug product comprising a BCS class 2 drug. However, the dissolution method may still be biopredictive if modeled mechanistically. In addition, because of their mechanistic nature, these models are also applicable to predicting in vivo dissolution in other healthy physiologies such as pediatric patients, or in altered physiologies due to the co-administration of an excipient or a drug, which will change the local conditions in the lumen of the GI tract or the transit of the dosage form. The effect of food or pH-related DDI can be better predicted with these mechanistic models since physiological changes in transit and lumen composition will directly impact the in vivo dissolution rate and extent. Finally, mechanistic models are also recommended to verify or predict the outcome of regional absorption studies where a telemetric capsule delivers the drug load in vivo in a specific GI compartment after radio activation outside the body during the monitoring of capsule transit along the GI tract.

12.2.1.1.2 Steps for Mechanistic in vitro Dissolution Modeling

Prior to introduction in the PBBM, it is recommended to verify that mechanistic models can predict the dissolution of specific batches in different conditions. Typically, dissolution in multiple media can be used to verify if the z-factor and P-PSD can predict in vitro dissolution to an acceptable level of accuracy. The model validation is achieved if predefined acceptance criteria for model prediction performance are met when the batch-specific z-factor or P-PSD predicts the dissolution of the batch in other media just by varying the drug solubility in the appropriate media or the amount of surfactant and size of micelles where relevant. The acceptance criteria can be similar to those used for PK prediction fitting such as the average fold error (AFE) and absolute average fold error (AAFE). The choice of the best performing model can be made by comparing prediction performance. Figure 12.6 shows that for acalabrutinib maleate tablets the prediction performance of the P-PSD model was two times more accurate than for the z-factor on three product batches comprising drug substances of increasing particle size [36].

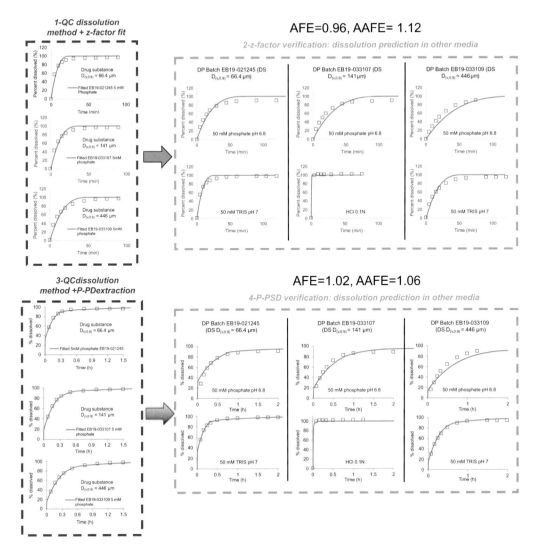

Figure 12.6 Illustration of the two-step method for fitting and verification of mechanistic dissolution models prior to introduction in PBBM. (From Ref. [36].)

12.2.1.2 Type of Drug Product Quality Changes that Can Be Supported by PBBM

12.2.1.2.1 Drug Substance

Synthetic Impurities: Impurities present in a crystalline form will change the drug substance solubility and it is therefore recommended to remeasure drug solubility pH profile and drug solubility in biorelevant media along the development in order to quantify the magnitude of these changes and propose models, which are specific to each development phases including commercial and post-approval phases [37,38].

Polymorphic Impurity: The drug may present more or less expected changes during stability, some of which may impact the exposure. Polymorphic changes during storage whether related to salt disproportionation or transition from an amorphous drug to a crystalline drug will likely impact the drug exposure if the solubility of the polymorphic impurity is limiting drug dissolution and the level of polymorphic impurity is high enough. The example summarized in Table 12.1 shows that PBBM was successfully utilized to support the evaluation of a polymorphic transition for a crystalline drug (JnJ-X).

Table 12.1: Summary Example of JnJ-X PBBM to Evaluate Risk of Polymorphic Transition

Drug Name	JnJ-X
Literature references	[14,39]
Purpose of the model	Establish the safe space for drug substance particle size using DP dissolution. Establish risk of polymorphic transition
BCS class reported	4
Compound nature	crystalline
pKa values (A or B)	Neutral
Log P or log D at pH	~3
Clinical reference	IR Tablets with registered polymorph
Variants	Different doses, variants comprising different particle sizes and new polymorph
Dose or dose range (mg)	50–300 mg
Change to default absorption model	NR
Dissolution method (s) used	2 stage Biorelevant (SGF+FaSSIF)
Integration of dissolution in PBBM	1-Direct input	
	2-Data fitted with Weibull	Weibull used to deconvolute PK
	3-Constant z-factor	
	4-z-factor vs pH	
	5-DS PSD+DLM (Simcyp)	
	6-P-PSD (Simcyp or GastroPlus)	
Batches for model validation are tested in the clinic?	Yes
A-Multiple dissolution conditions for single batch	NR
B-If A-YES, Model able to reproduce all in vitro data?	NA
Comments on dissolution	Large effect of bile salts on solubilization leading to rapid dissolution in FaSSIF medium
Model validation	Model validated on 9 clinical scenarios in the fasted and fed states
Model outcome	Safe space for dissolution established based on PSA on z-factor. Polymorphs are anticipated to be BE (confirmed in clinic)
CRS: How was the edge of safe space defined PSA or VBE?	PSA on z factor
Bridging: How was the BE established?	PSA on z factor for both polymorphs at higher strength

Stereoisomers: Although pure enantiomers of a chiral molecule have the same physical properties (but may have different pharmacokinetics and pharmacodynamics), the racemic mixture of enantiomers will show different thermodynamic properties due to different crystal lattice conformations [40]. In addition, the crystallization of enantiopure drugs in the presence of the opposite enantiomer may lead to inclusion of defects in the crystal lattice and changes in drug solubility [41]. This situation can be treated by PBBM applying different biological properties to the enantiomers and different solubilities of the racemic or impure enantiomer compared to pure enantiomer [42].

Particle Size and Shape: During the drug substance development process and as required by the properties of the drug, exposure required to reach efficacy in the clinic and the type of drug product developed, a reduction of the drug substance particle size can be envisaged. When particles are highly wettable or when surfactants are added to the formulation, a size reduction will lead to more surface generated and therefore a higher dissolution rate. However, for poorly wettable drug substances, and in the absence of enough surfactant in the formulation, small drug particles will not wet compared to large ones, and the drug product dissolution rate could be slower as a result of the drug substance size reduction. This is illustrated by the graph of Figure 12.7 showing the area of spontaneous wetting for a sphere of drug substance as a function of its particle radius. These simulations were conducted by varying the liquid-to-solid Young contact angle for a particle density of

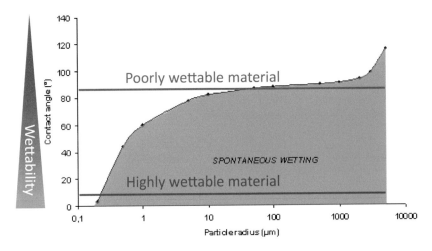

Figure 12.7 Spontaneous wetting of a solid sphere on a liquid-air interface.

1.2 g/mL, liquid density of 1 g/mL, liquid kinematic viscosity of 1 mPa.s, and predicting whether the acceleration due to gravity would be sufficient to allow the particle to cross the liquid-air interface by integration of the free energy variation on the system. Figure 12.7 illustrates that a direct input of measured drug substance particle size distribution may not be a good representation of the drug substance surface area available for dissolution in the tablet formulation. Additional caveats such as the lack of spherical morphology for most pharmaceutical drug substances, the potential formation of drug substance aggregates of smaller primary particles [28], or the preferential wetting of crystal surfaces when placed in water [43], make it very difficult to use sizing methods of drug substances (typically particle size distribution by laser diffraction) as a direct input method to predict drug product performance. In addition, when drug substances are formulated in a tablet for example, compression forces during the manufacturing process may lead, when applied to brittle drug substances, to a reduction in the size of primary drug substance particles, which creates more surface area available for dissolution [44].

The link of drug substance particle size which is a quality attribute of drug substance batches to in vivo human exposure has to be achieved through product performance. In other words, a link between drug substance particle size and drug product dissolution must be proven, and the justification of drug substance particle size can be made indirectly through specifications on the drug product.

12.2.1.2.2 Drug Product

Excipients Type: Some immediate release formulations comprise a large amount of insoluble excipients, utilized as fillers, disintegrants, glidants, or lubricants. The size, density, and swelling properties of these excipients will define, in given hydrodynamic conditions, the amount of formulation that may sediment in the dissolution vessel, forming a cone which may entrap drug substance particles, leading to a slower dissolution compared to conditions where no sedimentation occurs [32,45]. Although this coning or sedimentation in vitro is considered as a bias of the in vitro technique, it may impair the biopredictive nature of the method and lead to artificial incomplete dissolution profiles in conditions where the drug is fully soluble. Beyond the stomach where phases of very low agitation are found in the fasted state, there is no reason why formulation induced drug sedimentation may delay in vivo drug absorption since particles are dispersed along the GI tract due to peristalsis. Preclinical evidence shows that lighter or denser than water particles display delayed gastric emptying in the dog compared to particles with water equivalent density at equivalent sizes [46]. In addition, many immediate release formulations of drugs which can be considered markers of gastric emptying (such as weak acids with high solubility and permeability beyond the stomach) show multiple concentration-time profile peaks during the absorption phase which is related to partial gastric emptying of the formulation [27,28,47–49]. There is not enough evidence to link multiple peaking phenomena due to the presence of dense excipients and more research is needed to fully understand and model the various phases of gastric emptying in silico. In vitro, the bias due to sedimentation can be eliminated, for example, by recovering a batch-specific product particle size which can be integrated in PBBMs [32].

Level or Type of Acidifier or Surfactant: Acidifiers are commonly used in formulations comprising weak bases to manipulate the micro-environmental pH and provide for an improved drug dissolution. Badawy and Hussain [50] reported that a level of 16.7% intra-granular or extra-granular tartaric acid in BMS-561389 tablets allowed to reach full release in acetate buffer, pH 5.5, where the drug products without tartaric acid would only dissolve to a 40% plateau. By changing the micro-environmental pH around the dissolving drug, the acidifier puts the drug in solution and if the super-saturation is not too high compared to the drug thermodynamic equilibrium solubility at the pH of the medium, it can be maintained long enough for the drug to be absorbed. This spring effect can also be mediated by surfactants comprised in the formulation, which will locally aid the wettability of the drug or its solubility in the dissolution medium. Qualitative and quantitative changes made to these excipients may impact drug product dissolution in discriminatory conditions, which could be qualified via PBBM.

Excipients Which Are Absorbed: Some excipients can be absorbed from the GI tract alongside the drug and may change the pharmacokinetics or toxicokinetics of a drug product. A famous example is that of propylene glycol, which can be absorbed from the GI tract and protects against liver injury related to acetaminophen reduction since propylene glycol is a competitive inhibitor of CYP2E1 [51]. PBBM could be used to account for the joint effect of formulation and excipient drug–drug interaction on the parent and downstream metabolite pharmacokinetics.

Poorly Absorbable Osmotic Agents: fructose, mannitol [52], sorbitol [53], and high molecular weight PEG [54] can increase the osmotic pressure in the lumen of the GI tract and since they are poorly absorbed, they can lead to transit acceleration and an increase in luminal volume in the intestine [55]. This can have an effect on the absorption of drugs such as cimetidine for example [56]. PBBM was successfully utilized on a variety of drugs to determine a provisional no effect threshold for mannitol [57]. In addition, these excipients are also shown in the rat to be able to open the tight junction of the enterocytes, which may affect the paracellular absorption of small molecules [58].

Performance of the Disintegrants: The disintegrants present in tablet formulations may show impaired performance after storage due to the combined action of humidity and high temperature [59]. If the delay in tablet disintegration has been demonstrated but quality attributes of the drug substance(s) are not altered in the formulation, i.e., there is only a delay to capsule or tablet disintegration but the rate and extent of dissolution are the same, the impact of this product change can be evaluated with PBBM by applying a delay to the tablet disintegration with a Weibull function combined with the rapid dissolution of undissolved drug, which can dissolve according to a mechanistic dissolution model, for example.

Variability in Capsule Opening: Capsule opening times in vitro can show variations related to temperature, pH, and the type of capsule shell utilized in the formulation. HPMC capsules are less prone to crosslinking and show less dependence on temperature compared to Gelatin capsules, but at pH 6.8, the dissolution of HPMC capsules is more variable and longer on the average than gelatin capsules [60]. Crosslinking of gelatin capsule upon storage when the shell reacts with certain excipients in the formulations has shown little impact in vivo [61], and the in vivo significance of this change in product quality attributes is anticipated by running in vitro dissolution with and without pepsin or pancreatin. In addition, the prandial state of an individual can also influence the capsule opening time, and lag times are frequently observed with capsules administered in the fed state compared to tablets [62]. The delay in drug release from formulation can typically be modeled with a PBBM [63].

Magnesium Stearate: Magnesium stearate is a common lubricant used in tablet manufacturing. This flake-like excipient typically exhibits a large surface area and poor mechanical resistance [64]. This excipient-specific surface can vary significantly from different suppliers and different batches and may impact beyond the manufacturing process or tablet appearance. Magnesium stearate is very hydrophobic, and depending on the blending process, amount utilized in the formulation, and specific surface area, it may lead to variation in apparent drug substance surface energy [65], which will lead to wettability issues during dissolution or changes in apparent drug solubility [66].

In addition, during drug product stability, magnesium stearate present in formulations comprising HCl salts of weak bases was shown to promote salt disproportionation in certain storage conditions [67]. This would be anticipated to impact the drug solubility, drug product dissolution, and ultimately the exposure to the drug. Variations in the dissolution profiles of formulations comprising magnesium stearate are frequent, and they can be covered with a PBBM approach as was shown for Priadel® [10].

Excipients that Are PgP Inhibitors. PEG stearates, PEG glyceryl fatty acid compounds, PEG fatty acid esters, polysorbates, and poloxamers have been reported to inhibit PgP [68]. If drug products are formulated with excipients that are PgP inhibitors, any change in the PgP inhibitor level in a formulation should be carefully justified, with in vitro data and potentially preclinical data. In addition, PBBM can support some of these changes provided the effect of PgP inhibition is appropriately modeled based on clinical data such as PK DDI with cyclosporin A or Rifampicin, for example [69]. In this case, the definition of a dissolution safe space will not be possible since the formulation composition may impact the influx and similarly dissolving drug products could lead to different exposure.

12.2.2 Supporting Manufacturing and Process Changes
12.2.2.1 Introduction

There are many manufacturing process parameters that may influence the drug product quality attributes. During commercial drug product (DP) manufacturing process development, robustness studies are typically conducted following the QbD approach to define the knowledge space of the product and process performance, by varying the manufacturing process parameters and material attributes in order to define their criticality with regard to product in vitro and in vivo performance.

Dissolution data generated on formulation variants resulting from these studies using discriminatory methods will reveal the outcome of these variations on the in vitro dissolution of drug products. Pharmaceutical companies rely more on virtual twins of pharmaceutical processes to evaluate the complex synergies and antagonisms of the combined manufacturing process parameters and formulation attributes on end product performance [70]. Using these simulation tools, the knowledge space is explored and validated against actual experiments to be able to define edges of failure in a more systematic way. This in silico evaluation is coupled with PBBM predictions to evaluate the consequences of these changes on human exposure. The combination of in silico modeling and in vitro or in vivo verification and model validation represents a powerful tool that forms an integral part of quality by design.

12.2.2.2 Case Study: 300 mg Diltiazem MR: PBBM to Support Manufacturing Site Change [71]

Diltiazem HCl modified release capsules, 300 mg comprising populations of immediate release (IR) and extended release (ER) pellets were manufactured in a reference site A [71]. Some work was undertaken to move the manufacture to plant B to improve the supply chain flexibility. The modified coating technology for prolonged release pellets was an over-coat with Eudragit RS/RL polymer. Batches manufactured in plant A and proposed plant B in the QC medium (0.1N HCl) showed some minor differences at release and after 3-month storage, but this did not prevent the relative BA from being conducted. The relative BA study between the two batches failed. The plant B/A C_{max} ratio was of 0.84 [0.79–0.9] while the area under the concentration-time curve (AUC) ratio was of 0.94 [0.88–0.99] (Figure 12.8). A GastroPlus model was set up to deconvolute human observed PK profiles during the relative BA study using a biphasic Weibull function combined with a compartmental model previously developed with appropriate separate clinical data. Comparison of in vivo dissolution with in vitro dissolution revealed a 6 hour more rapid in vivo dissolution compared to in vitro dissolution for the ER part of the drug load but with a similar profile (Figure 12.9). A root cause analysis was conducted, and it was concluded that the chloride ion present in the QC medium (HCl) prevents the prolonged release coat on the ER pellet to hydrate. The percent weight increase of dry films of Eudragit RS/RL placed in different aqueous solutions of various buffers composition and in water, was measured at room temperature and both HCl or NaCl reduced film hydration compared to water or phosphate (Figure 12.10). Eudragit RS/RL is indeed a resin that comprises chloride ions in its scaffold. The presence of additional chloride in the medium was able to retard the hydration and drug release from coated pellets. The 0.1N HCl used as a medium for the QC dissolution method was neither discriminant nor biopredictive for this product. A new dissolution medium made of pH6.8 phosphate was recommended to improve the QC method and dissolve the test batches manufactured on both plants. The correlation between in vitro and in vivo dissolution was greatly improved illustrating the difference of behavior between these two batches while providing excellent in vitro in vivo correlation.

An additional learning from this PBBM is that it allowed to explain the higher relative exposure of females compared to males during the relative BA study. Indeed, even considering body weight correction, females in the study were systematically showing a higher exposure to diltiazem. Due to the prolonged drug release of these MR formulations (over 25 hours), the drug was predominantly absorbed from the caecum (16%) and ascending colon (40%) the overall absorption counting

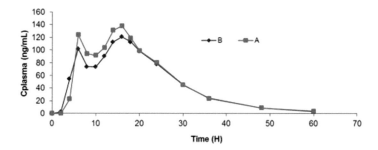

Figure 12.8 Average PK profiles following 300 mg Diltiazem, HCl MR capsule administration from different manufacturing site A and B.

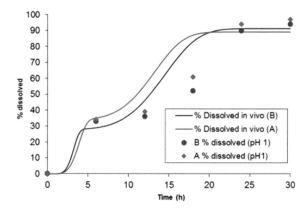

Figure 12.9 Deconvoluted in vivo dissolution (solid line) for products from plant A and B compared to measured in vitro dissolution of products (symbols) with the QC dissolution method.

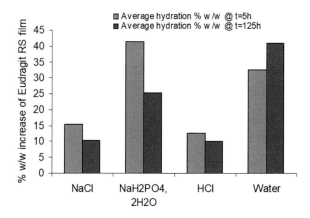

Figure 12.10 Swelling of Eudragit RS/RL films in various aqueous media at room temperature.

the upper segments of the GI tract amounted to 73% and was therefore incomplete due to lack of release prior to the end of physiological transit. The reason for the higher exposure of females to the drug was mechanistically explained by considering that they typically show a slower transit in the large intestine which can amount to 4-hour more residence per segment of the large intestine [72]. Using these adjustments in the physiology, the increase in ascending colon residence time to 20 hours for females compared to 12 hours for males allowed to reproduce the observed exposure ratios between females and males.

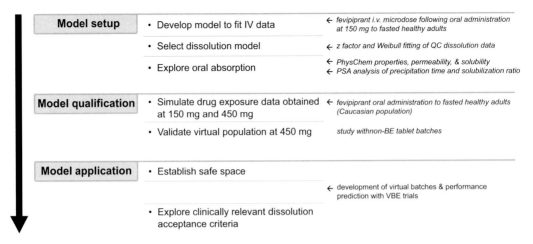

Model setup	• Develop model to fit IV data	← *fevipiprant i.v. microdose following oral administration at 150 mg to fasted healthy adults*
	• Select dissolution model	← *z factor and Weibull fitting of QC dissolution data*
	• Explore oral absorption	← *PhysChem properties, permeability, & solubility* ← *PSA analysis of precipitation time and solubilization ratio*
Model qualification	• Simulate drug exposure data obtained at 150 mg and 450 mg	← *fevipiprant oral administration to fasted healthy adults (Caucasian population)*
	• Validate virtual population at 450 mg	*study withnon-BE tablet batches*
Model application	• Establish safe space	
		← *development of virtual batches & performance prediction with VBE trials*
	• Explore clinically relevant dissolution acceptance criteria	

Figure 12.11 PBBM workflow strategy to define fevipiprant knowledge space and safe space to define CRDS (Modified from Ref. [73].)

12.2.2.3 Case Study – PBBM to Support Drug Product Quality and CRDS for Fevipiprant IR Formulations

12.2.2.3.1 Background and PBBM Purpose

Fevipiprant is a zwitterionic, low molecular weight, BCS class IV drug substance. PBBM was used to aid in clinically relevant dissolution specification setting for fevipiprant [73]. This case study includes clinical pharmacokinetic data for two doses with BE and clinically observed non-BE data. Moreover, IV micro-dosing data were used to describe disposition parameters. The objective was to define the fevipiprant critically relevant dissolution specifications (CRDS) and the bioequivalence safe space for the QC dissolution method. The general workflow is shown in Figure 12.11.

12.2.2.3.2 Software and Model Set-Up

The interested reader is referred to the PBBM publication by Kourentas et.al. [73] including the supplemental files [73] for model parameters, simulation settings, and parameter sensitivity analyses. All simulations were conducted in GastroPlus v 9.7 (Simulations Plus, Lancaster, CA) using the advanced compartmental absorption and transit (ACAT) model. In the ACAT model, the default values for compartment volume percent occupation by water in the small intestine and colon (40% and 10%) were used for fasted state simulations. Human pharmacokinetic (PK) parameters were determined via a population pharmacokinetic (pop-PK) analysis of the pooled individual ($n=16$) concentration-time profiles from Weiss et al. [74], as described in the supplementary material (Part A) [73]. Input PK parameters to the biopharmaceutics model, such as plasma clearance and volume of distribution of fevipiprant were determined by fitting individual concentration- time profiles after a single intravenous dose of 0.1 mg by a 2-compartment PK model with a linear clearance. Table 12.2 lists PK and physicochemical input parameters for the PBBM.

Percent drug absorption for the BE and non-BE batches was simulated using effective permeability (P_{eff}) and determination of physicochemical characteristics including drug solubility in bio-relevant media (Table 12.2) and aqueous buffers; see supplemental section [73]. As C_{max} is sensitive to dissolution profiles and relevant to demonstrate bioequivalence, parameter sensitivity analysis (PSA) was conducted with varying permeability and the Weibull time scaling factor.

12.2.2.3.3 API Physicochemical Properties

The physicochemical properties used as input for simulations are shown in Table 12.2.

12.2.2.3.4 Systemic Disposition Parameters

Systemic disposition parameters were obtained from a 100 µg intravenous data along with a 150 mg oral dose, thus avoiding non-linearities with clearance [74]. A one-compartment model was used. The V_c and CL values as well as the FPE are shown in Table 12.2.

Table 12.2: Fevipiprant (QAW039) Physicochemical, Pharmacokinetic Parameters and Dissolution Model

Parameter	Value	Source/Comment
Compound	Fevipiprant	
Mol wt	426.4 g/mol	Measured
Log P	2.36	Calculated with ADMET Predictor
pKa	pKa_1: 2.9 (acidic), pKa_2: 4.1 (basic)	Determined after fitting pH-solubility profile. Estimated data were in line with experimental values
Sol_factors	193.2 for pKa_1 & 772.9 for pKa_2	Determined after fitting pH-solubility profile
Biorelevant solubilities at 37°C	0.08 mg/mL in SGF (final pH 1.6[a]) 1.1155 mg/mL in FaSSIF-v2[b] (final pH 6.3[a])	Determined when using the salt form
Dissolution model	Weibull Function	Kourentas et al. [73]
Dissolution data	Quality Control method, pH 6.8	Kourentas et al. [73]
Solubilization ratio	17,600	Calculated in GastroPlus™ based on solubility in biorelevant media
Nanoparticle effect	Deactivated	No nanosized formulation investigated
Reference solubility	7.0E-3 mg/mL at pH 4	Determined when using the salt form
Precipitation time *vs.* pH	NA[c]	Use of fixed (constant) value
Diffusion coefficient	0.66×10^{-5} cm²/s	Calculated from the molecular weight in GastroPlus™
Drug particle density	1.2 g/mL	GastroPlus™ default value
Chemical degradation	Not taken into account as it is negligible	-
Human P_{eff}	0.43×10^{-4} cm/s	Calculated by an in-house formula using Caco-2 data (internal data)
Blood/plasma conc. ratio	0.56	Internal data
Adj plasma Fup [%]	11.8	
CL [L/h]	18.7	PK disposition parameters were derived from a 100 µg *i.v.* micro dose in combination with a 150 mg oral dose [74] and supplementary material, part A [73]
V_c [16]	6.99	
V_p [16]	102	
Q [L/h]	8.37	
$T_{1/2}$ [h]	12.31	
FPE [%]	37.1[d]	GastroPlus™ estimated value based on the derived CL value via population PK analysis

[a] Reported pH indicates the values in the equilibrium.
[b] The bile salts concentration was 3 mM for the FaSSIF-v2.
[c] NA: Not applicable.
[d] Calculated using a body weight of 70 kg, CL of 33.4 L/h with blood to plasma ratio of 0.56, and the default GastroPlus™ liver blood flow rate.

12.2.2.3.5 Dissolution Data

Key dissolution data that were evaluated in clinical studies included three batches, which were *Clinical_batch_150 mg, Clinical_batch_450 mg_Fast* and a non-bioequivalent *Clinical_batch_450 mg_Slow*. A final drug product batch (*FDP_450_mg*) was included in the PBBM-generated safe space, but this batch was not tested in the clinic.

For all batches, the in vivo dissolution was investigated by utilizing in vitro dissolution, which was monitored using the QC method, supplemental section E [73]. The in vitro testing conditions were determined at 900 mL (USP) phosphate buffer pH 6.8 (37°C) in a USP II apparatus with a rotation speed at 75 rpm. In all dissolution tests, the percent coefficient of variation (%CV) calculated at all-time points was not more than 5%.

Virtual dissolution profiles were generated in GastroPlus™ to investigate the edge of BE failure. A batch, *virtual_batch_450 mg_75%*, which exhibited 75% amount dissolved at 45 minutes and amount dissolved calculated at 100%; this batch defined the edge of failure.

12.2.2.3.6 Dissolution Model

Two models for dissolution were used. The mean dissolution profiles (i.e., % mean dissolved amount vs. time) were fitted by following two approaches:

a. Use of dissolution Takano model where dose, volume, and equilibrium solubility were considered for the z-factor calculations.

b. Use of single Weibull function where the dosage form switched to CR: Gastric Release and the Weibull parameters of %total released, time scale factor, and shape were calculated. For PSA, the Weibull time scale factor was varied. To generate virtual release profiles with varied release characteristics, the Weibull model was used.

12.2.2.3.7 Results and BE Safe Space Generation

For fevipiprant 450 mg formulations, slower dissolution leads to lower percent dissolved in vivo and lower percent absorbed (Figure 12.12a and b) [73]. The lower boundary of the safe space was defined by the dissolution profiles of two virtual batches identified by parameter sensitivity analyses of the Weibull time scale factor. These batches were *"virtual batch_450_mg_80%"* and the *"virtual batch_450_mg_75%"*, whichever was lower (Figure 12.13). The batch *"clinical batch_450 mg_slow"* with known bio-nonequivalence in the clinic fell below the virtual batches

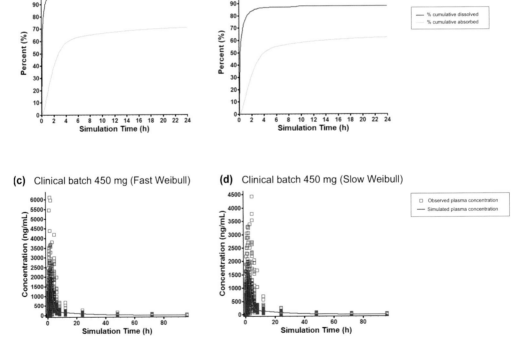

Figure 12.12 Simulated %cumulative dissolved (red line) or absorbed (light blue line) amounts vs. time profiles (a and b) and the simulated vs. plasma concentration -time profiles (blue lines; c and d) for *Clinical batch_450 mg_Fast* (a and c) and *Clinical batch_450 mg_Slow*, non-BE, (b and d). Open squares are the observed individual C_p time profiles. (Modified from Ref. [73].)

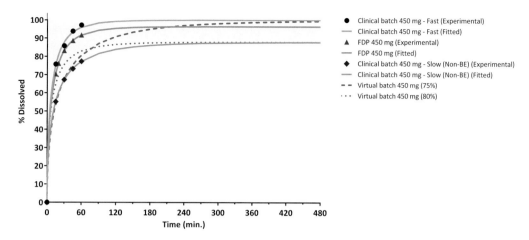

Figure 12.13 Bioequivalence safe space plot (green area) including the clinically tested dissolution knowledge space, the non-BE batch and chosen virtual profiles. Calculated dissolution profiles *virtual_batch_450_mg_80%* (dotted green line), *virtual_batch_450_mg_75%* (dashed green line), and clinical batch *FDP_450* mg using the single Weibull equation (solid purple line). For comparative purposes, % mean experimental ($n=6$; symbols) and fitted dissolved amount (solid lines) vs. time with *clinical batch_450 mg_fast* (black circles; solid brown line), *clinical batch_450 mg_slow* with known bio-nonequivalence (purple diamonds; solid pink line), and *FDP_450* mg (blue triangles) are also presented. The brown and pink solid lines define the IR knowledge space. The green area represents the safe space for fevipiprant at the dose level of 450 mg. A % dissolved value of 80% at 60 minutes was chosen to support QC criteria and is above the edge of failure determined by the *virtual_batch_450_mg_75%* batch. (Modified from Ref. [73].)

in % release at all timepoints (Figure 12.13). The safe space is shown in Figure 12.13. A $Q=80\%$ dissolved after 60 minutes for an IR oral solid dosage form reflected the boundaries of the fevipiprant BE safe space.

12.2.3 Impact of Formulation Changes on Food Effect

12.2.3.1 Introduction

The impact of food on drug absorption has been long recognized and extensively reviewed in the literature. [75,76] Studying the interaction of drug compounds with food is a critical component of preclinical and clinical development and informs product labeling recommendations. [77] While the BCS and the Biopharmaceutics Drug Disposition Classification System (BDDCS) have been extensively used as early predictors of food effect [78], in recent years there's been increasing interest in the application of PBPK absorption models as a means to more quantitatively predict food effect [79,80]. In a recent review article, Vinarov et al. cited 22 published manuscripts that have reported PBPK food effects predictions for more than 30 compounds. [77] Note that the focuses are different when using PBPK/PBBM to predict food effect or to predict the food impact on bioequivalence, which is more associated with formulation-food interaction. This section is more focused on using PBPK to predict the food effect.

Application of PBPK absorption models for food effects lies at the intersect of clinical and CMC activities. While, as suggested by BCS and BDDCS, food effect is often seen as a compound property that is taken into consideration to inform dosing instructions during clinical development, it is also well recognized that food effect can be formulation-dependent. Regulatory guidance documents specifically highlight this consideration and recommend the conduct of clinical food effect studies after significant formulation changes for new drugs or the conduct of bioequivalence studies in the fed state for generic drug products [81,82].

Successful application of PBPK absorption models for formulation-dependent food effects relies on the same principles around the incorporation of formulation/drug product-related measurements that apply to PBBM in the drug product quality space and have been described in earlier sections of this book chapter. Incorporation of biorelevant solubility and dissolution data in media simulating fed and fasted state, typically fed state simulated intestinal fluid (FeSSIF) and fasted state simulated intestinal fluid (FaSSIF), is a key component of the model. Researchers have proposed high-level workflows for the development of such models that generally rely on the development and validation of the model against fasted state data before proceeding with food effect prediction, and ideally with confirmation of the food effect prediction against clinical data for application of the model for late-stage development and regulatory applications [83].

The role of formulation on food effect for aprepitant, a BCS IV compound, is well documented in the literature [84,85]. An early-development formulation based on micronized API showed a significant food effect with approximately 3-fold and 4.5-fold increase in AUC at 100 and 300 mg, respectively. To address the food effect, a nanocrystalline formulation of aprepitant was developed as the final market formulation. Capsules with nanosized API show no significant food effect at the doses of 80 and 125 mg used in the final commercial product. PBPK absorption models to simulate the aprepitant food effect have been reported in the literature by several authors. Parrott et al. first reported a PBPK model with biorelevant solubility as input using the GastroPlus software [86]. Shono et al. subsequently reported a model using a custom PBPK model developed in the STELLA software, incorporating dissolution kinetics in biorelevant media [87]. More recently Pepin et al. reported models developed as part of the IQ Consortium PBPK Food Effect WG to develop a standardized workflow for food effect predictions [88]. The case study described below attempts to capture the best practices from these publications and presents a somewhat standardized approach to food effect prediction for different formulations.

12.2.3.2 Case Study – Prediction of Formulation-Dependent food Effect for Aprepitant
12.2.3.2.1 Software
For the purposes of this example, all simulations were conducted in GastroPlus™ v 9.8.3 (Simulations Plus, Lancaster, CA) using the ACAT model. The readers can refer to the published literature [87,88] for simulation settings for alternative software. The same principles described below are applicable across other software/absorption models.

12.2.3.2.2 API Physicochemical Properties
Physicochemical properties used as input for simulations are shown in Table 12.3.

As with other PBPK absorption modeling and PBBM applications, the incorporation of biorelevant solubility data is key to the model success for food effect prediction. At minimum, solubilities in biorelevant media simulating the intestine need to be incorporated. As shown in Table 12.3, solubility in v2 of FaSSIF and FeSSIF was used for the simulation in this example. It should be noted that the presence of food could also alter solubility in the stomach. In practice, the primary absorption driving force in the model is intestinal solubility. Shono et al. demonstrated that the incorporation of biorelevant solubilities for the stomach compartment did not significantly impact the simulation of food effect [87].

12.2.3.2.3 Systemic Disposition Parameters
Systemic disposition parameters were obtained from intravenous data. A one-compartment model was used. The V_c and CL values are shown in Table 12.3.

12.2.3.2.4 Accounting for Formulation Differences
The micronized and nanosized formulations have an average particle size of 7 and 0.12 μm, respectively [89]. Simply adjusting for particle size in the software is not enough to simulate the absorption difference [89]. Shono et al. [87] reported differential solubility measurements for the two formulations. As seen in Table 12.3, the apparent solubility of the nanosized formulation was ~2–2.5-fold higher in FaSSIF v2 (13.6 vs 5.4 μg/mL) or simple media (e.g. 16.6 vs 6.6 μg/mL in FaSSGF) but comparable in FeSSIF v2 (102 vs 92.4 μg/mL). Incorporating this solubility difference is critical to capture directionally the improvement of bioavailability of the nanosized material.

12.2.3.2.5 Dissolution Input
Two models for dissolution were attempted. As reported by Pepin et al. [88] the micronized dissolution in FaSSIF was modeled by the z-factor model. Alternatively, the Johnson model based on

Table 12.3: Physicochemical and Pharmacokinetic Input Parameters for Aprepitant PBPK Absorption Model

Parameter	Value	Reference/Rationale
Molecular weight	534.4	From structure
pKa	2.8	Optimized to fit the pH-solubility profile, final value is close to the reported pKa. The acidic pKa outside physiologically pH range was not included.
Log$P$	4.8	[84]
fu plasma	0.05	[88]
B/P ratio	0.86	[88]
Fu enterocyte (%)	100	Default value
Human P_{eff} (10^{-4} cm/s)	2.416	[88]
Formulation	IR	
Dose	100 mg (micronized) 125 mg (nanosized)	
Precipitation	T_p=9,000 seconds	Precipitation removed
Intrinsic solubility (μg/mL)	0.7 μg/mL for micronized, 1.3 μg/mL for nanosized	Based on SIFsp data [87]
FaSSIF Solubility (μg/mL)	5.4 (micro), 13.6 (nano)	v2 for either media [87]
FeSSIF Solubility (μg/mL)	92.4 (micro), 102 (nano)	
FaSSGF Solubility (μg/mL)	6.6 μg/mL (micro), 16.6 μg/mL (nano)	[87]
Solubilization ratio	6.24E+8, N=2.4669 (micro) 1.33E+7, N=1.7546 (nano)	Fitted to FaSSIF and FeSSIF (v2) solubility data in the software
Model for dissolution	z-factor	[88]
Particle diameter (μm)	7 (micro), 0.12 (nano)	[84, 87]
z factor (mL/mg/s)	0.00704 (micro)	Fitted to FaSSIF dissolution data
PK Model	1 compartment model	
V_c (L/kg)	0.944	Based on IV data [88]
IV Clearance (L/h/kg)	0.07234	Based on IV data [88]

the particle size radius was used. The dissolution of the nanosized material is immediate to the solubility plateau and thus only the Johnson model was used.

12.2.3.2.6 Absorption Model (ACAT) Physiology Settings

The default OptLogD v 6.1 absorption scale factor (ASF) model was used, but absorption in the large intestine (caecum and colon) was removed by setting the ASF values to 0. As reported by Wu et al., even nanosized formulations showed very low exposure after direct colonic administration in dogs [84]. The default caecum/colonic ASFs would significantly overestimate colonic absorption.

12.2.3.2.7 Results, Model Optimization, and Model Adjustments

First, the model for the micronized formulation was attempted. The model using particle size as input resulted in a higher bioavailability prediction in the fasted state compared to the model using z-factor as input. Absorption in the fasted state is predominantly dictated in the simulation by solubilization in the stomach due to the higher solubility in the more acidic environment. The simulation results are shown in Figure 12.14. The prediction using the Johnson model is within the range of exposures seen for the micronized formulation in clinical studies. The prediction of fasted exposure for nanosized formulation is shown in Figure 12.15. The model directionally predicts an approximately 2-fold increase in bioavailability for the nanosized formulation which is in line with the bioavailability increase observed clinically, once corrected for the dose difference. However, the absolute prediction of the profile is significantly lower than the observed clinical data, with the caveat that study variability could account for some of the difference. Contrary to

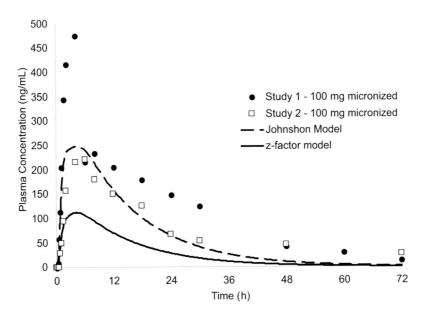

Figure 12.14   Fasted state exposure prediction for micronized formulation.

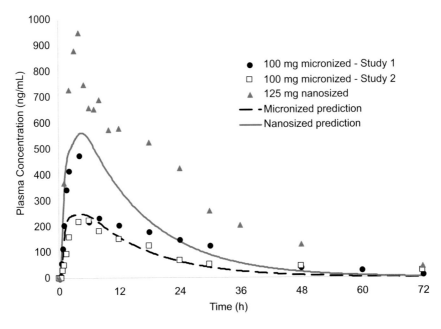

Figure 12.15   Prediction of fasted state exposure for nanosized vs micronized formulation.

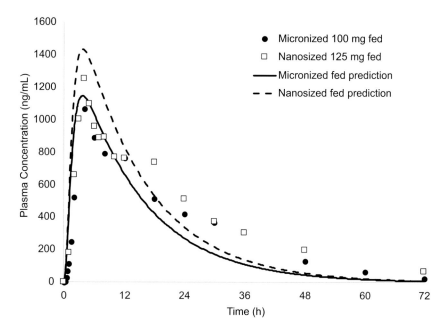

Figure 12.16 Prediction of fed state exposure for nanosized vs micronized formulation.

the fasted state prediction, prediction for fed state is not sensitive to dissolution input. Keeping the same dissolution model, the prediction for the micronized and nanosized formulations is shown in Figure 12.16. Fed state exposure is accurately predicted for either formulation. Considering the results from Figures 12.15 and 12.16, the model accurately predicts the magnitude of the food effect for the micronized formulation but doesn't fully predict the elimination of the food effect for the nanosized formulation. The underprediction of fasted state exposure for the nanosized formulation is perhaps not surprising as the mechanism for increased bioavailability of nanosuspensions is still being debated in the literature and may require model modifications beyond what is currently attempted. However, the example provides the reader with a general workflow for applying the model to such formulation-dependent food effect questions.

Emami Riedmaier et al. [80] have evaluated the food effects of 30 drugs using a controlled, pre-defined in vitro, and bottom-up modeling methodology. High confidence (exposure ratios predicted within 0.8–1.2) predictions were obtained in half of the cases and moderate confidence (exposure ratios predicted within 0.5–2) in 27% of the cases. Some food effect mechanisms leading to current prediction issues by PBPK models were also identified such as the presence of a salt form for the drug, the impact of drug precipitation, the impact of chyme viscosity on the dissolution of IR formulations or the impact of physiological buffers on the dissolution of drugs. The prediction for moderate- and low-confidence drugs was found to be improved using a middle out approach where fasted state data is utilized to inform the model [88], or additional in vitro data is generated to better characterize the impact of physiological buffers on the drug dissolution especially for acidic or basic compounds when there is an acid-base reaction during dissolution [90]. In conclusion, with current PBPK tools, food effect prediction is accurate in a majority of cases.

12.2.4 Impact of Formulation Changes on pH Effects

12.2.4.1 Introduction

Acid-reducing agents (ARAs) are frequently utilized as co-medications, especially in the treatment of cancer of all types. Smelick et al. reported that the prevalence of ARA administration in cancer patients ranged from 20% to 65% with a median value of about 30% [91]. If the pharmacokinetics of a cancer drug is significantly affected by ARA, the label may exclude the use of this drug with certain types of ARAs or recommend staging of the drugs administration to avoid the interaction. PBBM which are developed with mechanistic dissolution models are able to evaluate the impact of acid-reducing agents. There are three main types of acid-reducing agents: Antacids, H2-receptor antagonist (H2RA) and proton pumps inhibitors (PPIs). Antacids are typically salts that have a

273

direct buffering action on the protons in the stomach, while H2RA and PPI inhibit the secretion of HCl. H2RA competitively binds to the histamine receptors on gastric parietal cells, inhibiting histamine-induced acid secretion, while PPI inhibits the hydrogen pumps of parietal cells [92]. PPIs are the most prescribed ARAs [91]. The effect of PPI can be predicted using PBBM when the model uses a mechanistic model since a change of pH in the stomach will enable a different in vivo dissolution rate to be predicted (Table 12.4). For weak bases, an increase in stomach pH due to the co-administration of ARAs, typically can slow the in vivo dissolution rate and lead to a reduction in C_{max} or AUC. For weak bases that have been formulated as salts or co-crystals, the reduction in exposure can be greatly attenuated or even reversed [93]. For example for HCl salts of weak bases, the action of PPI or H2RA reduces the stomach concentration in chlorides compared to fasted state stomach conditions [94]. For HCl salts where the common ion effect is important and with low intrinsic salt solubility, a reduction in chloride concentration in a stomach resulting from a treatment with H2RA or PPI will lead to a higher solubility of the salt in the stomach compared to the absence of treatment. Upon stomach emptying, the precipitation of weak bases should be considered and in vivo data are still needed to inform the model regarding the precipitation parameters to use, since most in vitro transfer assays are not biopredictive and tend to overestimate the extent of precipitation [95]. If the weak base does not precipitate at the target clinical dose following a rapid pH shift experiment [22], the likelihood of in vivo precipitation is low. This in vitro observation needs to be controlled with in vivo or preclinical data [28]. If precipitation is observed in vitro, it is important to use human data to verify the conditions where precipitation happens and which precipitation parameter to apply. Typically, this can be achieved with variants of the target commercial formulations or leveraging the information coming from all the clinical phases including the effects of food or ascending dose studies [33]. Table 12.4 gives a few summary examples of PBBM which were used to assess the impact of ARAs on human exposure. Successful predictions of the ARAs effect on four weak bases (tapentadol, darunavir, erlotinib, and saxagliptin) were also reported by Dong et al. [96].

12.2.4.2 Case Study: Acalabrutinib Maleate Tablets: Use of PBBM to Support Dissolution Specifications When the Drug Is Administered with PPI

Acalabrutinib as a 100 mg free base capsule is subject to label restrictions when it needs to be administered with ARAs. PPIs are contra-indicated and acalabrutinib should be administered 2 hours apart from the administration of antacids or H2RAs. A new formulation of acalabrutinib which comprises a maleate salt to 100 mg free base equivalent was developed and tested in the clinic for the effect of food, and effect of PPI. This formulation was also demonstrated to be bioequivalent to 100 mg acalabrutinib free base capsules in the fasted state [99]. The purpose of the PBBM was to propose and justify dissolution specifications for acalabrutinib maleate tablets, which would guarantee product efficacy and safety for all patients with and without PPI co-administration. The PBBM relied on clinical data generated with formulation variants comprising drug substances of increasing particle size and also an oral solution extemporaneously prepared with the clinical reference acalabrutinib maleate tablet [99].

12.2.4.3 Software

All simulations were conducted in GastroPlus v 9.8.2 (Simulations Plus, Lancaster, CA. For more details, the readers can refer to the published literature [28,29,36].

12.2.4.4 Drug Substance and Drug Product Physicochemical Properties

Acalabrutinib maleate has a specific pH solubility profile, which is dependent on the pKa values of maleic acid, acalabrutinib and the solubility product of the salt (Table 12.5). In addition, the salt is able to reduce the micro-environmental pH around the surface of the crystals and therefore increase the drug surface solubility compared to acalabrutinib [36]. As a result, the surface solubility of acalabrutinib maleate is higher than the surface solubility of acalabrutinib at all physiological pH, Drug product dissolution is more complete and faster for acalabrutinib maleate tablets compared to acalabrutinib capsules in all the dissolution conditions tested.

12.2.4.5 Systemic Disposition Parameters

Systemic disposition parameters were obtained from intravenous data on acalabrutinib. A two-compartment model was used and fitted to individual subjects. A representative population was therefore created based on real subjects and kept constant to predict average exposure with different formulations. Distribution parameters fitted to individual IV data can be found in

Table 12.4: Summary Examples Drugs for Which the Effect of Acid-Reducing Agents Were Anticipated with PBBM

Drug Name		Ribociclib Succinate	Entrectinib	Acalabrutinib
Literature references		[10,16,97]	[98]	[28,29]
Purpose of the model		Bridging hard gelatin Capsule and film coated Tablet, prediction of PPI and food effect	Establish a design space to understand impact of commercial formulation changes	Choice of clinically relevant dissolution method, safe space for Drug substance (DS)-Particle Size Distribution (PSD)
BCS class reported		4	4	2
Compound nature		Crystalline	Crystalline	Crystalline
pKa values (A or B)		5.5(B), 8.6(B)	2.54 (B), 7.54 (B)	3.54 (B), 5.77 (B), 12.1(A)
Log P or log D at pH		1.954	3.96 at pH 7.4	2
Clinical reference		200 mg IR Capsule	200 mg hard gelatin IR formulation with tartaric acid (F06)	Roller compacted, Capsule
Variants		200 mg IR Tablet with slower dissolution (BE ref batch) and 200 mg IR Tablet (commercial batch BE test batch)	200 mg hard gelatin IR formulation without acidulant (F01)	4 other Capsule batches (RC Capsule and binary blend Capsules), doses from 2.5 to 400 mg
Dose or dose range (mg)		600 mg	600 mg	100 mg
Change to default absorption model		NR	Large precipitation time (based on in vitro data)	SI and colon % volume occupation reduced to 7.5% and 2%. Individual gastric emptying profiles added
Dissolution method (s) used		900 mL pH 1, 2, 4.5 and 6.8 USP2 5 rpm and USP1 100 rpm.	USP2, 75rpm HCL pH 1 or pH 4	QC + exploratory. QC was demonstrated clinically relevant
Integration of dissolution in PBBM	1-Direct input	Yes		
	2-Data fitted with Weibull			
	3-Constant z-factor	Yes		
	4-z-factor vs pH	Yes		
	5-DS PSD+DLM (Simcyp)			
	6-P-PSD (Simcyp or GastroPlus)	Yes	Yes	Yes

(Continued)

275

Table 12.4: (Continued) Summary Examples Drugs for Which the Effect of Acid-Reducing Agents Were Anticipated with PBBM

Drug Name	Ribociclib Succinate	Entrectinib	Acalabrutinib
Batches for model validation are tested in the clinic?	Yes	Yes	Yes
A-Multiple dissolution conditions for single batch	Yes	Yes	Yes (pH, agitation, bile salt or SLS concentration)
B- If A-YES, Model able to reproduce all in vitro data?	NR	Yes provided surface pH was used in the model	Yes
Comments on dissolution	All data was used to fit pH-dependent z-factor, product particle size (P-PSD) with DDDPlus. pH2 was also integrated with a Weibull function. pH-dependent z-factor was preferred	DDDPlus® used to fit in vitro data for both formulations	QC method was clinically with pH 6.8 method. Since P-PSD is predictive of other dissolution conditions
Model validation	Prediction of Tablets and Capsule oral PK data in fasted and fed states	Model validated against 4 clinical studies on F01 and F06 variants in fasted and fed states, with and without PPI	Model able to reproduce the BE and non-BE study results across all the clinical experience with change in formulation, dissolution rate, stomach pH or DDI with grapefruit juice
Model outcome	Safe space around the reference Tablet and commercial Tablet batch established. Dissolution integration methods were equivalent. Large safe space for poorly permeable drugs Absorption was not altered as a function of gastrointestinal pH [97]	Sensitivity analysis allowed to evaluate the impact of micronization on the exposure for various scenarios	Safe space for DS PSD illustrated. Advantage of P-PSD as a method for integrating dissolution in PBBM.
CRS: How was the edge of safe space defined PSA or VBE?	10 VBE trials with real to virtual batches	PSA	PSA on PSD for in vivo dissolution
Bridging: How was the BE established?	VBE	NA	NA

Table 12.5: Drug Related Parameters for the PBBM for Acalabrutinib and Acalabrutinib Maleate

Parameter (Unit)	Selected Value	Justification
Molecular weight (g/mol)	465.5 (acalabrutinib), 599.59 (acalabrutinib maleate)	From structure
pKa values in physiological range	Acalabrutinib: 3.54 (B) and 5.77 (B) Maleic acid: 2.27 (A) and 5.99 (A)	Acalabrutinib: Measured [28] Maleic acid from Schwarz et al. [100]
Log P	2.0	Measured [28]
Diffusion coefficient (10^{-5} cm^2/s)	0.6069	Calculated by model based on density and molecular weight
True density (g/mL)	Acalabrutinib: 1.34 Acalabrutinib maleate: 1.36	Measured (see [28] for free base)
Intrinsic solubility @ pH 8 (µg/mL)	Acalabrutinib: 48 Acalabrutinib maleate: 2,190	Measured (see [28] for free base)
Aqueous solubility vs pH	Calculated from intrinsic solubility data and pKa of relevant moieties	See section on solubility vs pH profile
FaSSIF-v2 solubility (mg/mL)	0.12 (free base)	Measured [28]
FeSSIF solubility (mg/mL)	0.67 (free base)	Measured [28]
Precipitation time (seconds)	100,000	Precipitation not present based on in vitro and preclinical in vivo data [28]
Fraction unbound in plasma (%)	2.6	Measured *in vitro* in human plasma [28]
Blood to plasma ratio	0.787	Measured *in vivo* in human blood [28]
Effective permeability 10^{-4} cm/s	5.4	Constant from MDCK-MDR1 data [28]
Bile salt effect for dissolution	ON	NA
Solubilization ratio (no unit)	1.2E4	Calculated by model based on FaSSIF-v2 & FeSSIF solubility data
The diffusion coefficient is adjusted for bile salt effect	ON	Default model option
Dissolution model	Johnson model with a maximum diffusion layer thickness of 30 microns	Default model mechanistic dissolution model
P-PSD	P-PSD extracted from *in vitro* product dissolution data	Batch-specific input parameter to the PBBM [29], see main text
Gut V_{max} CYP3A4 (mg/s)	Variable	Fitted to individual oral profiles from clinical study ACE-HV-009 [28]
Gut K_m CYP3A4 (mg/L)	20	Constant fitted to oral profiles from clinical study ACE-HV-009 [28]
Drug substance particle size	P-PSD extracted from *in vitro* product dissolution data	See section on drug product dissolution
Gut V_{max} P-gp (mg/s)	4.22E-03	Constant and extracted from *in vitro* data from MDCK-MDR1 cells [28]
Gut K_m P-gp (mg/L)	2.78	Constant and extracted from *in vitro* data from MDCK-MDR1 cells [28]

the literature. The first pass gut extraction and first pass liver extraction were made mechanistic by the addition of CYP3A4 enzyme in the gut and liver and utilization of Michaelis-Menten parameters to match individual differences observed in the study used to set up the model.

12.2.4.6 Dissolution Input

The apparent drug solubility in the dissolution medium without pH adjustment, i.e. letting the pH drift in an excess of powder was measured and used as an input to predict in vitro dissolution at multiple pH. The dissolution of various clinical and technical drug products was fitted with a P-PSD model, similar to that used for acalabrutinib free base capsules [29]. To predict in vivo dissolution, the surface solubility versus bulk pH is utilized as an input to the PBBM, and the pH in the various compartments of the ACAT model is left at the default values. The P-PSD model verification is shown in Figure 12.6.

12.2.4.7 Absorption Model (ACAT) Physiology Settings

Default fasted and fed state physiologies were utilized. For simulations of the action of PPI on the stomach pH, the value of stomach pH was raised to 6. The volumes in the GI tract, small intestine, and colon were reduced to 7.5% and 2%, respectively as was done for the acalabrutinib free base model. These values are closer to measurements of free water in the lumen of the GI tract by MRI [101]. In addition, for fasted state and PPI stomach conditions, a gastric retention was accounted for: The drug product is dosed at time 0, but remains in the stomach for a predetermined time and is then released. The use of the "mixed multiple dose" feature of GastroPlus allowed to reproduce this gastric retention. The gastric emptying profiles were not changed compared to the previous acalabrutinib free base model [28,36]. Acalabrutinib has displayed alongside other drugs multiple peaks in the PK which were related to gastric retention and partial emptying. This phenomenon is observed in other drugs, which are markers of gastric emptying [27,47,49,102].

12.2.4.8 Results and Discussion

The PBBM was validated using drug product batch P-PSD to handle in vivo dissolution. The model was able to evaluate the effect of PPI on drug dissolution and the effect of food on the pharmacokinetics for the acalabrutinib maleate tablet. C_{max} and AUC predictions were aligned with the predictions observed with the free base model (Figure 12.17) and were of good quality: AFE=1.01 and average absolute prediction error (AAPE)=6.7% for C_{max} predictions. AFE=1.05 and AAPE=8.5% for AUC_{0-t} prediction. After model validation, the model was used to define the edge of failure for drug product dissolution. Two virtual batches A and B, which dissolved slower than clinical batches, were utilized in the model to predict their relative exposure to the clinical reference dosed in the fasted state. If the stomach pH is acidic, all the clinical batches including

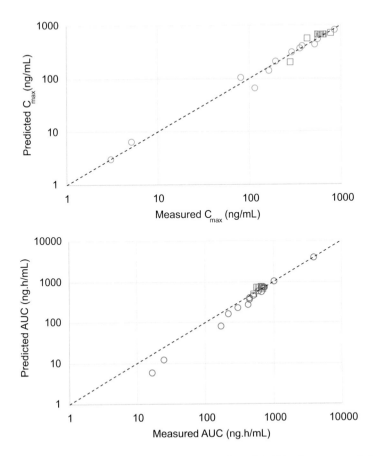

Figure 12.17 Measured vs predicted C_{max} (upper panel) and AUC_{0-t} (lower panel) for acalabrutinib capsules (blue) and acalabrutinib maleate tablets (orange).

VBA and VBB are anticipated to be bioequivalent to one another. If the subject is pre-treated with PPI and the stomach pH equals 6, there is an observable reduction in exposure for product which dissolves slower. In this case, both the C_{max} ratio of VBA and VBB fall below the 80% bioequivalence threshold compared to the clinical reference in acidic conditions. Similarly, the AUC ratio for VBB falls below the 80% bioequivalence threshold, while the AUC ratio of VBA in neutral stomach conditions is just above this threshold. In all likelihood, if a bioequivalence study was conducted in these scenarios, both VBA and VBB would fail the study acceptance criteria.

In parallel to the PBBM, a PKPD relationship was built between acalabrutinib steady state C_{max} and AUC and the target receptor occupancy: Bruton Tyrosine Kinase (BTK). The engagement to this receptor triggers the pharmacological action of acalabrutinib and it constitutes therefore a good marker of clinical efficacy. The absolute exposure achieved by VBA and VBB in terms of C_{max} and AUC when co-administered with PPI was used to predict the BTK occupancy which would result. These values of BTK occupancy were comparable to the levels achieved during pivotal clinical phases where the drug was demonstrated active. It was concluded that despite a lower exposure when dosed with PPI compared to dosed in the fasted state, the variants tested in the PBBM were anticipated to be safe and effective. The combination of the PBBM and PKPD allowed for a wider safe space to be defined for acalabrutinib maleate tablet dissolution in the QC medium and ultimately to justify the proposed dissolution specification.

12.3 UTILITY OF PBPK/PBBM IN SUPPORT OF THE DEVELOPMENT OF ABBREVIATED NEW DRUG APPLICATION-EXAMPLES

12.3.1 Biowaiver

One of the applications of PBPK/PBBM is to support waiving of in vivo studies. Generally, waiver of in vivo PK studies for lower strength can be dependent on several CFR requirements such as formulation composition proportionality, dissolution similarity, and bioequivalence on other strength. However, for the cases where dissolution profiles between strengths are different or formulations are different, PBPK absorption modeling/PBBM can be used to predict the impact of deviation of critical quality attributes (e.g., dissolution) on drug exposure and reduce the burden of conducting in vivo studies for lower strengths of products. As a case study example, a drug product (IR formulation) has dissimilar dissolution profiles for lower strength of the Test product. For this case, PBPK/PBBM modeling was used for predicting the impact of faster release of lower strength on the bioequivalence under fasting and fed conditions. Several limitations were identified in the submitted model and recommendations were provided by U.S. Food and Drug administration, including but not limited to (i) validating the model for the intended purpose using different strengths or using data from formulations with different release rates; (ii) demonstrate prediction performance for pharmacokinetic data of bio-strength under both fasted and fed conditions. Thus, assessing model performance in the proposed context of use and establishing confidence in the developed model would be important before using the PBPK/PBBM model in assessing the impact of dissolution differences on in vivo performance/BE [19].

Another evolving area is using PBPK absorption modeling to evaluate the food impact on drug exposure and BE and support waiving of fed BE studies for generic drugs. Food can increase liver and portal vein blood flow, increase the release of bile salt from the gall bladder, increase gastric pH, delay gastric emptying, and increase GI tract motility, volume and viscosity of the stomach and intestine fluid, etc. In generic drug area, researchers have developed a PBPK model for acyclovir oral IR tablet with the aim of assessing the impact of food on BE studies using virtual population simulation, commonly known as virtual bioequivalence (VBE). Data collection related to the physicochemical properties and PK studies of the drug was the first step of this PBPK modeling followed by the development and validation of an acyclovir PBPK model for intravenous (i.v.) infusion to get the disposition parameters, such as apparent volume of distribution and clearance. Later, an oral PBPK model for acyclovir 200 mg IR tablet was developed with the inclusion of in vitro permeability data into the PBPK modeling platform. Model validation is an inevitable part of the PBPK model development process, and different doses of acyclovir i.v. infusion and oral IR tablets along with independent clinical studies from published literature and ANDA reports were used to validate the i.v. and oral acyclovir PBPK model in this case. Next, the validated acyclovir PBPK model was used to predict the acyclovir plasma profile under the fed condition by replacing the fasting physiology of a PBPK model with a high fat fed physiology. In vitro dissolution data were used as the PBPK model input and showed good prediction of the acyclovir plasma profile for 800-mg IR tablet under both fasted and fed conditions. Finally, the VBE simulations were conducted in healthy virtual subjects and showed that the test and reference acyclovir 800 mg IR tablets were bioequivalent to each other under both fasted and fed conditions, similar to the outcomes observed in the ANDA results [103].

When using PBPK models for supporting risk assessment and biowaiver, there are some challenges. The challenges include but are not limited to the modeling of in vitro dissolution profiles, the combination of drug- and formulation-specific properties with GI variability, and the impact of the formulation/excipients on permeation, especially for BCS Class III drugs. The models should be informed with appropriate estimates of subject variability, which can be obtained from a previously conducted in vivo pharmacokinetic study or included in the system parameters. Research has been conducted to support addressing these challenges and move this area ahead [19,104].

12.3.2 Support of PBBM in Settting Clinically Relevant Drug Product Specifications

According to the US Code of Federal Regulations [105], drug product applications must include the specifications necessary to ensure the identity, strength, quality, purity, potency, and bioavailability of the drug product, including acceptance criteria relating to, dissolution rate. As such, setting drug substance and drug product specifications is an intrinsic step in the drug product development process and constitutes a regulatory requirement to ensure consistent product quality throughout the drug product's lifecycle. The traditional approach for specification setting (e.g., based on process capability) lacks understanding in the relationship between CMAs, CPPs, dissolution and clinical outcome for the identification of the critical biopharmaceutics attributes (CBA). This gap may lead to drug substance and drug product specifications (e.g., acceptance criterion) limits that are overly wide, unnecessarily tight or might result in the in vitro performance not being reflective of the expected drug product's systemic exposure, efficacy, and safety profile.

The identification of the CBAs is a multidisciplinary effort and in many cases requires introducing deliberate but meaningful variations to the CMAs and CPPs identified based on risk assessment to establish the in vitro in vivo link which is essential for setting specifications that are clinically relevant. Due to the critical role that dissolution plays in defining the bioavailability (BA) of the drug, in vitro dissolution, if identified as a CQA, can serve as a relevant predictor of the in vivo performance of the drug product. To this end, CRDS (and thus, clinically relevant drug product specifications (CRDPS) ensure consistent in vivo performance as proven by their ability to pass only batches with adequate in vivo performance, thus ensuring consistent efficacy and safety profiles [106].

There are several general approaches for establishing CRDPS ranging from conventional to mechanistic approaches [107]. These approaches enable dissolution testing to define the boundaries of a safe space. Under the safe space paradigm, all lots that have dissolution profiles within the upper and lower limits of the specifications are bioequivalent [7]. Expansion of the safe space limits (defined by comparing upper to lower bounds) may be possible based on exposure-response data (for the innovator drug) and by identifying lots exhibiting dissolution profiles at the upper and lower dissolution limits that are bioequivalent to the clinical/BA lots or to an appropriate reference standard which in the case of ANDAs should include the RLD [5].

The mechanistic approach to setting CRDPS (i.e., via PBBM) facilitates the establishment of the essential in vitro in vivo link, and thus the construction of in vitro in vivo relationships (IVIVRs) offering a simpler and feasible path to biowaivers, for IR drug products) for which the rate of success of IVIVCs is rather low [17]. In addition, PBBM tools streamline the drug product development process for generic drug products by relying on the totality of data available in the literature or internal to the company thus decreasing the burden of conducting PK studies which are essential for establishing a safe space and thus CRDPS. Furthermore, the implementation of PBBM tools has the potential to expand the safe space limits, resulting in wider manufacturing and regulatory flexibility than one based on conventional approaches.

In vitro dissolution data is one of the key inputs into PBBM. Thus, before PBBM implementation, one should determine whether dissolution has been identified as CQA and the rate-limiting step toward drug absorption. To aid in this process, framework and decision trees have been developed portraying initial biopharmaceutics risk assessment in the KASA process defining when PBBM has the highest regulatory utility [19]. However, a validated PBBM has the potential to also expand the manufacturing and regulatory flexibility delineated under several regulatory frameworks such as BCS, IVIVC, and similarity testing by facilitating the establishment of CRDPS as exemplified by case studies below.

Bisoprolol fumarate, formulated as IR oral tablet (case study 1) is considered to be a BCS class I compound with more than 85% dissolved within 15 minutes. Over the years, slight differences in dissolution of bisoprolol batches were observed not meeting the criterion of rapidly dissolving [108]. A PBBM for bisoprolol was then built and validated using GastroPlus® software (Figure 12.18) to evaluate the clinical relevance (i.e., impact on PK exposure) of variability in dissolution (e.g., wider dissolution profiles) of bisoprolol fumarate IR tablets. Based on virtual BE trials (Figure 12.19), safe space expansion was explored using hypothetical dissolution data. A formulation with in vitro dissolution reaching 70% dissolved in 15 minutes and 79.5% in 30 minutes was shown to be BE to classical fast dissolution of bisoprolol (>85% within 15 minutes), as point estimates and 90% confidence intervals of the maximum plasma concentration and area under the concentration-time

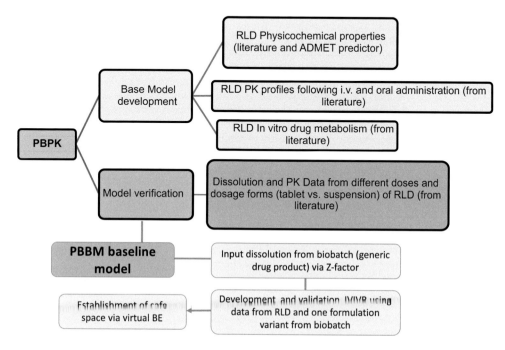

Figure 12.18 Workflow for PBBM building, validation and establishing of safe space (adapted from original workflow). (Adapted from Ref. [108].)

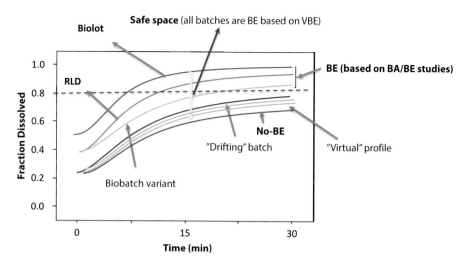

Figure 12.19 Safe space established based on VBE for bisoprolol fumarate IR tablets. (Adapted from Ref. [108].)

curve were within the BE limits. The authors concluded that in vitro dissolution was not critical for the systemic exposure of bisoprolol over a wide range of tested values. It should be noted that the safe space boundaries were defined based on extrapolation outside the knowledge space. However, based on biopharmaceutics risk assessment (e.g., formulation has not been modified and the process has not changed considerably), the risk is considered very low and thus, extrapolation may be possible for BCS class 1/3 IR products.

12.3.2.1 Generic Drug Case study: PBBM to Support Lower Strength Biowaiver in Case of f2 Mismatch (f2 Fails/Virtual BE Passes)

12.3.2.1.1 Background and PBBM Purpose

The generic compound PBBM is described by Wu et al. [109]. Generic compound is a weakly acidic molecule formulated as an IR tablet with five strengths: 40, 80, 120, 160, and 320 mg. The compound can be classified as a BCS III drug with Log D of −1.17 (pH 7) with acidic pKa of 5.6 and 3.7. The solubility is low in acidic condition (0.045 mg/mL at pH 1.2) and as pH increases, the solubility increases (0.333 mg/mL at pH 4.5 and 3.029 mg/mL at pH 6.8). After oral administration, the absorption was rapid with a t_{max} of 2–4 hours with linear pharmacokinetics. Dr. Reddy's developed generic IR test formulation for all strengths, and as per regulatory guidance, a crossover bioequivalence study in the fasting study was conducted at higher strength of 320 mg in healthy human subjects, and bioequivalence was achieved between reference and generic formulations.

Based on the successful bioequivalence study on higher strength 320 mg, the waiver for 40, 80, 120, 160 mg was requested. To obtain biowaiver for all lower strengths, dissolution tests in multimedia (pH 1.2, pH 4.5, and pH 6.8, 1,000 mL, 50 rpm, USP II (Paddle) at $37 \pm 0.5°C$) were performed for all strengths as per the current EMA regulatory guidance [110]. The estimated similarity factor (f2) values were found >50 for all the batches, except for the lowest strength of test formulations, 40 mg, for which f2 was found to be 43 and less than 50 in pH 4.5 acetate buffer. Based on this f2 value, the regulatory agency denied the waiver for lower strength 40 mg, and hence the possibility of conducting a separate bioequivalence study for 40 mg study was anticipated. However, to obtain a waiver for the 40 mg bioequivalence study, PBBM was conducted to assess the impact of this lower f2 value on in vivo pharmacokinetics (PK) of the molecule.

12.3.2.1.2 Simulation Methodology

The PBBM modeling and simulation were used to justify the impact of failing f2 on the bioequivalence. A workflow is shown in Figure 12.20. The modeling strategy included utilizing the pH-solubility profile generated in-house along with Log P and pKa values (Table 12.6). Particle size (D_{10}, D_{50}, and D_{90}) tested for in-house formulations of 40 and 320 mg was used for test product and reference standard. The human effective permeability value was optimized to capture in vivo behavior and the default precipitation time was used. Plasma protein binding and blood to plasma ratio were obtained from the literature and used in simulations. Elimination parameters were obtained by fitting literature-based intravenous pharmacokinetic profiles into the PKPlus module.

To simulate PK profiles, the rate of dissolution described by z-factor as a function of pH was estimated by fitting multimedia in vitro dissolution profiles to built-in z-factor model in GastroPlus®. Overall, the PBBM model was developed using i.v. disposition parameters, physicochemical properties, and dissolution rate (z-factor) vs pH data, and the model was validated against C_p-time profiles of pivotal test and reference formulations from clinical BE study, which was conducted by Dr. Reddy's Laboratories in healthy volunteers in the fasting condition. The model validation was conducted with virtual population as well. Once the model was validated, the dissolution profiles of 40 mg strength were fitted with a z-factor vs pH model and used as input for 320 mg strength. This represented the worst-case simulation scenario wherein 40 mg dissolution data were used as input for simulating the highest strength 320 mg PK. These simulated concentration-time profiles following oral administration using in vitro data of the test batch of 40 mg (given as input for 320 mg) were compared with clinical data of pivotal 320 mg test and reference formulations.

12.3.2.1.3 Results and Discussion

The PBBM model integrated generic compound physicochemical properties with the use of the z-factor dissolution model (multi pH vs z-factor) method (Figure 12.21) and a single compartmental model (top-down approach). The simulated plasma concentration-time profiles with virtual bioequivalence simulations of 68 subjects predicted the observed concentrations well (Figure 12.22)

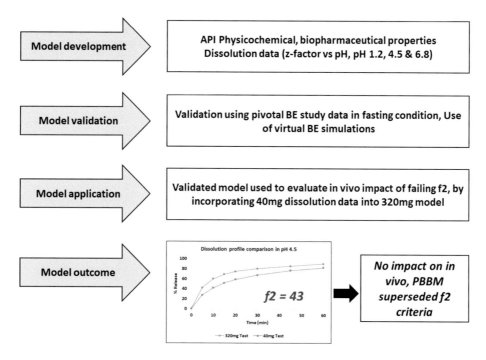

Figure 12.20 Case study Generic Drug PBBM modeling workflow.

Table 12.6: Key Input Parameters for Simulations for PBBM Generics Drug

Property	Value
Model application	Demonstration that f2 is non-biopredictive, widening of dissolution safe space
Molecular weight (g/mol)	435.53
Log P	Log D -1.17 at pH 7
pKa	5.6, 3.7 (acid)
pH – solubility profile (mg/mL)	pH 1.2: 0.045 pH 4.5: 0.333 pH 6.8: 3.029
Effective human permeability (cm/s)	0.2×10^{-4} (optimized value)
Precipitation time (s)	900
Dissolution model	z-factor vs pH
Dissolution method	Multimedia (pH 1.2, pH 4.5 and pH 6.8)
Surface pH correction[a]	No
Interpolation	PBBM to supersede f2 criteria
Disposition data	Intravenous bolus data at 20 mg dose
Disposition model parameters	V_c=0.069 L/kg CL=0.026 L/h/kg k_{10}=0.384 L/h k_{12}=0.245 L/h k_{21}=0.134 L/h $t_{1/2}$=9.26 hours FPE =3.21%
Chosen model acceptance criteria	%PE<10%

Source: Partially reprinted from Wu et.al. [109].

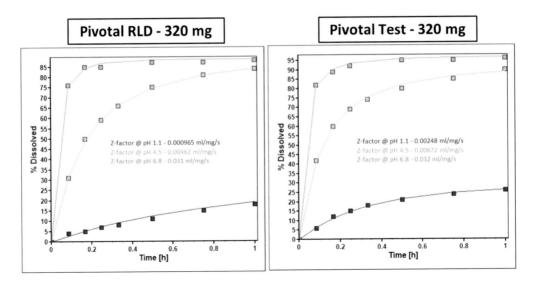

Figure 12.21 Case study for Generic drug, Dissolution profiles of pivotal RLD and Test 320 mg products along with z-factor fitting at various pH conditions. The dissolution rate is highest at pH 6.8, moderate at pH 4.5 and slowest at pH 1.1 for both formulations. At pH 4.5 (middle profile), a dissolution mismatch with f2 < 50, was observed.

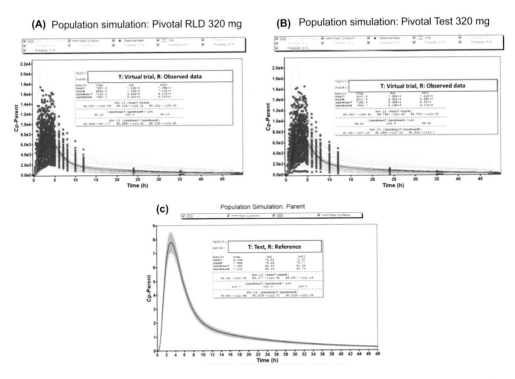

Figure 12.22 Case study for Generic drug, Virtual BE simulations with 68 subjects (a) population simulation of pivotal RLD 320 mg (b) population simulation of pivotal test 320 mg. In Figure (a) and (b), individual PK profiles (pink dots) was compared with simulated mean exposure profiles (solid blue line), where simulations with a different level of confidence interval were presented as light blue line. (c) Virtual BE of pivotal RLD (pink: reference) vs test 320 mg (green: test). The probability contours are shown in thin blue lines in (a) and (b). Highlighted green box in the middle of each Figure represents a bioequivalence comparison of two batches at 90% confidence interval.

Table 12.7: Generics Case Study, DRL Compound (a Given Drug Name), Predicted and Observed T/R Ratio's for Fasting Clinical Study of 320 mg

	Predicted		Observed		
Parameter	T/R Ratio	90% Confidence Interval	T/R Ratio	90% Confidence Interval	%Prediction Error (PE)[a]
C_{max}	100.7	90.83–111.66	92.6	83.74–102.39	8.7
AUC_{0-inf}	100.4	90.03–112.07	94.9	86.98–103.64	5.8
AUC_{0-t}	100.5	90.12–112.04	94.8	86.75–103.55	6.0

[a] %PE = ((predicted − observed)/observed)*100

Table 12.8: Generics Case Study, Population Simulation Results for 40 mg Test Compared Against 320 mg Test and Reference Batches

Dissolution Input	C_{max}		AUC_{0-t}		AUC_{0-inf}	
	Geomean T/R	Geomean 90% CI	Geomean T/R	Geomean 90% CI	Geomean T/R	Geomean 90% CI
T/R against pivotal test 320 mg	99.36	89.65–110.12	99.44	89.13–110.95	99.40	89.14–110.83
T/R against pivotal RLD 320 mg	100.1	90.27–110.91	99.88	89.53–111.44	99.88	89.58–111.37

with prediction errors lower than 10% and were considered acceptable from a model validation perspective (Table 12.7).

The predicted *T/R* ratios correlated well with predicted *T/R* ratios of the pivotal study, and confidence intervals were within 80%–125%, indicating the robustness of the PBBM model (Table 12.8).

The validated model was subsequently applied to 40 mg batch where dissolution mismatch was observed in pH 4.5 media. Virtual BE trial was then performed with the previously validated population using *z*-factor vs pH data of lower strength test formulation batch of 40 mg as dissolution input. This represents worst-case simulations wherein 40 mg dissolution data were used as input for simulating the highest strength 320 mg PK. These simulated concentration-time profiles following oral administration using in vitro data of the test batch of 40 mg were within BE limits (C_{max}, AUC_{0-t}, and AUC_{0-inf} well within 0.80%–1.25% range) of clinically observed mean PK data for the test batch of 320 mg.

Hence PBBM simulations were utilized to justify the f2 mismatch of the lower strength of 40 mg. However, for this case, it would be good to conduct virtual BE for 40 mg in addition to 320 mg strength to confirm the BE results. In addition, the modeling and simulation work implemented shows the relevance of PBBM to evaluate the biopredictive ability and establish the clinical relevance of the dissolution methods. In this case, if the 40 mg is shown to be bioequivalent despite f2 mismatch, one could conclude that the dissolution method is over-discriminating. It should be noted that having a method that is over-discriminating does not pose a risk to the patient. On the contrary, if any, it will ensure that no product batches will be released with performance outside the approved specifications. On the other hand, establishing a safe space renders the dissolution method clinically relevant as this exercise informs the sampling time and *Q* value within which the dissolution method will no longer reject batches that are expected to be bioequivalent to the biolot /RLD.

12.4 CHALLENGES AND FUTURE PERSPECTIVES

Challenges in the broad utilization of PBBM by the pharmaceutical industry during development and post-approval are mainly related to the lack of training of scientists and also the limited number of regulatory submissions where PBBM is applied to setting quality specifications for drug substances and drug products.

In addition, the lack of harmonized guidelines on the acceptability and application of PBBM worldwide does not encourage the industry to develop and submit these models to regulatory agencies. Overall, based on a survey conducted among the participants of the workshop: "Current

State and Future Expectations of Translational Modeling Strategies to Support Drug Product Development, Manufacturing Changes and Controls" that took place on September 23–25, 2019 at the University of Maryland in College Park, Maryland [13], the acceptance rate of submitted PBBM models was of around 40%, and the three main reasons why models were rejected by the agencies were that (i) models were not fit for purpose (35%), (ii) Model was not fitting the clinical data adequately (22%), and (iii) the model was not predicting variation in exposure, i.e. the knowledge space was not large enough (14%) [18]. More work is therefore needed to define the scope for model and what variants should be tested in the clinic to support model validation and ensure that they are fit for purpose. In addition, the definition of clear acceptance criteria for model validation is needed so that the two main reasons for model rejection are addressed. To this effect, the scientific community is working to generate enough published examples and provide training to all involved parties so that more standardization be brought to the content of PBBM submissions and so that the acceptance rate of model informed biowaivers or definition of safe spaces be improved. In particular, the initiative brought by the IQ group together with M-CERSI and regulators from the USA, Canada, Brazil, Great Britain, Europe, and Japan is of great importance. In this proposed work, the regulatory agencies have agreed to review mock submission of PBBM and provide their feedback during a 3-day workshop where the merits and drawbacks of each approach will be discussed, and paths toward standardization will be proposed.[1]

As was illustrated in this book chapter, the benefits of using PBBM during drug product development and after registration are important and can be summarized below:

1. **Mechanistic Understanding of Product Performance**: PBBM are mechanistic models and link product quality attributes to in vivo dissolution and therefore exposure to a drug product. They can be applied to all human body compartments and therefore predict systemic as well as local tissue or gut lumen concentration of a drug. The understanding of what limits drug absorption or dissolution in relevant matrixes can guide formulation scientists to improve drug substance or drug product robustness to the inherent variation of the human physiology within and between subjects. By combining PBBM and PKPD models, the design of the right molecule for the target indication can also be attempted. For example, for a prolonged release intra-articular drug, which is locally acting, a low solubility compound may be desirable, whereas for a systematically active drug where broad tissue distribution is required and oral administration is envisaged, minimum thresholds of solubility and permeability can be defined to reach a target plasma exposure using PBBM. It is well known that the use of PBBM can guide scientists to develop and select the desired commercial formulation, avoid clinical (bridging) studies between phase 1 and phase 3 formulations and therefore accelerate drug product development.

2. **Manufacturing and Regulatory Flexibility for the Commercial Drug Product**: Once the commercial formulation has been defined and the design space for the material attributes and process parameters has been studied, it is recommended to test in the clinic relevant commercial formulation variants and verify if the PBBM is able to predict observed variation in exposure resulting from these clinical studies. If such is the case, the use of PBBM within the knowledge space can help define a safe space resulting in manufacturing flexibility for post-approval changes within this space. This allows for seamless manufacturing site changes and can help manufacturers adjust their release specifications to ensure manufacturing ability while maintaining the expected product quality.

3. **Biowaivers**: PBBM can be used in lieu of clinical trials to bridge formulations when they are different from what was tested in the clinic. Such biowaivers can reduce the cost of the clinical trial and also development time from the manufacture of clinical batches to the reporting of the clinical trial results. In addition to time and money saving, using modeling and simulation to replace human evaluation also has ethical aspects, since healthy volunteers would not be subjected to a drug from which they receive no benefit, or patients would not be subjected to trial medicines which they would not necessarily benefit to the fullest for their treatment. In addition, virtual trials allow the testing of multiple scenarios or more subjects than real clinical trials which limits the chance of false positive or false negative results. Finally, the nature of variation in exposure can be interrogated mechanistically and assigned to formulation behavior or to physiological variables.

---

[1] Physiologically-Based Biopharmaceutics Modeling (PBBM) Best Scientific Practices to Drive Drug Product Quality: Latest Regulatory and Industry Perspectives. http://www.pharmacy.umaryland.edu/pbbm2023.

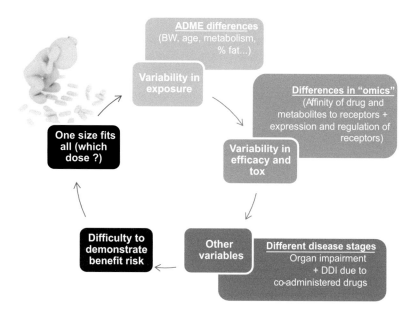

Figure 12.23 Limitations to finding the right 'one size fits all' dose.

Beyond the applications illustrated above, PBBM and in general PBPK absorption models hold an even greater promise for patient centricity, which is to allow the calculation of dose, release rate, and scheduling requirements for each patient [111]. This concept is often referred to as precision dosing [112] or model-informed precision dosing (MIPD) [113,114].

There are limitations to the current paradigm of 'one size fits all' to find the 'right dose' (Figure 12.23). As a consequence, the pharmaceutical industry worldwide spends considerable energy and resources in drug development with a low (14%) probability of drug success from phase 1 to market [115]. It is estimated that late-stage clinical failures lead to the loss of tens of billions of USD in pivotal clinical trials only each year.[2] More specifically, the lack of individual approach to dosing leads to variable exposure (PK) and variable efficacy or toxicity, without an obvious link between these two when the pharmacological or toxicological target engagement or expression is variable between subjects. This variability in clinical endpoints and lack of clear exposure response relationship forces the industry to generate larger data volume to which statistical methods are applied to be able to demonstrate equivalency or superiority of a treatment over another one. In addition, when no safe and effective dose can be found for example when there is a drug–drug interaction or when patients show organ disfunction, patients are excluded from the treatment, or the drug is abandoned altogether (Figure 12.23). The concept of precision dosing is not novel and has been applied without resorting to modeling tools to handle warfarin dosing for example based on the drug concentration (pharmacokinetic marker) or the clinical effect of the drug (clinical endpoint or phenotype). Genotyping can help stratify populations and is linked to variable expression of enzymes or pharmacological targets throughout the human body but cannot be used quantitatively to inform precision dosing calculations. Clinicians rely currently on the phenotypes for personal dosing, which requires a theragnostic drug administration [116–118]. As human proteome constantly changes during life, following aging, environmental stress, and disease, the use of messenger RNA (mRNA), allows to quantify the expression of enzymes and pharmacological receptors in given organs in the body through minimally invasive sampling techniques such as liquid biopsies. This field has been utilized for example to reach a diagnostic on the presence of cancer [119–121], but was also applied to quantify the expression of metabolizing enzymes in the liver [122].

The idea behind the use of PBBM to support MIPD is to create a virtual twin for each patient, and utilize this model to calculate the dose, release rate or scheduling requirement [113,123–126].

---

[2] https://www.genengnews.com/a-lists/unlucky-13-top-clinical-trial-failures-of-2018.

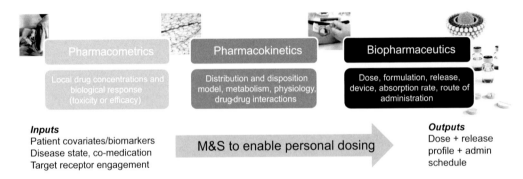

Figure 12.24 Input and output parameters required for MIPD.

This information would then be used to manufacture a patient-specific formulation for example through 3D printing [114,127–129] or to determine the dose which should be delivered by a drug delivery device for example [111]. The current modeling tools could be directly applied to MIPD with new definitions of input and output parameters (Figure 12.24).

The input parameters for a virtual twin PBBM would be the patient's covariates, disease state, and co-medications, and the outputs would be the required dose, drug release profile, and scheduling requirements. There are many benefits for patients, global health, global environment, countries health systems, or private health cover payors to start applying MIPD. These benefits are outlined below

- **Patient Centricity**: every patient will receive an adapted treatment (dose, schedule and/or release rate), and could stay on treatment despite drug–drug interactions.

- **Increased Medical Value for Drug Therapies**: higher efficacy, lower side effects, reduced healthcare costs, easier differentiation.

- **Reduced Drug Development Costs and Environmental Impact:** smaller model-informed clinical trials, reduced late phase project attrition, better translational tools, smaller batch manufacture or local compounding.

- **Higher Regulatory and Payers' Acceptability**: lower risks for patients in the commercial phase since individualized treatment, smart pharmacovigilance → model verification during the product life.

Overall, the use of PBBM as virtual twins to enable model informed precision dosing will represent a big step for the patients.

12.5 CONCLUSION

One of the central components of patient-centric drug product development is drug product quality. PBBM has emerged strongly into this space by enabling the establishment of a link between vitro product performance and in vivo exposure, a key element for enabling enhanced drug product understanding and building clinical relevance into drug product design and control. Many gaps remain to gain the full potential of PBBM tools in terms of knowledge, science, and global harmonization, and this chapter can help bring insight into current examples of PBBM applications. Looking into the future, PBBM could be utilized to help understand excipient effects and also set acceptable limits or define acceptable specifications for them. This would be particularly interesting for BCS class 3 drugs, where permeability or transit could be key elements to determine exposure. Finally, PBBM may also be used in the spirit of patient-centric design as a virtual twin for each patient and enable the individual dose, release rate, and scheduling requirements adapted to the disease state of the patient and potentially their co-medications.

DISCLAIMER

The views expressed in this book chapter are those of the authors and should not be construed to represent the US Food and Drug Administration's views or policies. The mention of commercial products, their sources, or their use in connection with material reported herein is not to be construed as either an actual or implied endorsement of such products by the US Food and Drug Administration.

REFERENCES

1. Yamaguchi, S., M. Kaneko, and M. Narukawa, Approval Success Rates of Drug Candidates Based on Target, Action, Modality, Application, and Their Combinations. *Clinical and Translational Science*, 2021. **14**(3): pp. 1113–1122.

2. CRS, *How FDA Approves Drugs and Regulates Their Safety and Effectiveness*, C. R. Service, Editor. 2018.

3. FDA. *Generic Drug Development*. 2021; Available from: https://www.fda.gov/drugs/abbreviated-new-drug-application-anda/generic-drug-development.

4. USA_Federal_Government, *Code of Federal Regulations. Part 320-Bioavailability and Bioequivalence Requirements*. 2023.

5. FDA, *Extended Release Oral Dosage Forms: Development, Evaluation, and Application of In Vitro/In Vivo Correlations*, CDER, Editor. 1997, CDER.

6. EMA, Guideline on the pharmacokinetic and clinical evaluation of modified release dosage forms (EMA/CPMP/EWP/280/96 Corr1). 2014.

7. FDA, *The Use of Physiologically Based Pharmacokinetic Analyses - Biopharmaceutics Applications for Oral Drug Product Development, Manufacturing Changes, and Controls*, CDER, Editor. 2020.

8. Wu, D. and M. Li, Current State and Challenges of Physiologically Based Biopharmaceutics Modeling (PBBM) in Oral Drug Product Development. *Pharmaceutical Research*, 2023. **40**(2): pp. 321–336.

9. Wu, F., et al., Biopharmaceutics Applications of Physiologically Based Pharmacokinetic Absorption Modeling and Simulation in Regulatory Submissions to the U.S. Food and Drug Administration for New Drugs. *AAPS Journal*, 2021. **23**(2): p. 31.

10. Heimbach, T., et al., Dissolution and Translational Modeling Strategies toward Establishing an In Vitro-In Vivo Link-a Workshop Summary Report. *The AAPS Journal*, 2019. **21**(2): 15 pp.

11. ICH, International Conference on Harmonisation of Technical Requirements for Registration of Pharmaceuticals for Human Use Considerations (ICH) Guideline Q8 (R2) on Pharmaceutical Development. (Accessed on June 5, 2023), ICH, Editor. 2009.

12. Abend, A., et al., Dissolution and Translational Modeling Strategies Enabling Patient-Centric Drug Product Development: the M-CERSI Workshop Summary Report. *The AAPS Journal*, 2018. **20**(3): 8 pp.

13. Pepin, X.J.H., et al., Current State and Future Expectations of Translational Modeling Strategies to Support Drug Product Development, Manufacturing Changes and Controls: A Workshop Summary Report. *Journal of Pharmaceutical Sciences*, 2021. **110**: pp. 555–566.

14. Heimbach, T., et al., Establishing the Bioequivalence Safe Space for Immediate-Release Oral Dosage Forms using Physiologically Based Biopharmaceutics Modeling (PBBM): Case Studies. *Journal of Pharmaceutical Sciences*, 2021. **110**(12): pp. 3896–3906.

15. Bhattiprolu, A.K., et al., Utility of Physiologically Based Biopharmaceutics Modeling (PBBM) in Regulatory Perspective: Application to Supersede f2, Enabling Biowaivers & Creation of Dissolution Safe Space. *Journal of Pharmaceutical Science*, 2022. **111**(12): pp. 3397–3410.

16. Laisney, M., et al., Physiologically Based Biopharmaceutics Modeling to Demonstrate Virtual Bioequivalence and Bioequivalence Safe-Space for Ribociclib Which Has Permeation Rate-Controlled Absorption. *Journal of Pharmaceutical Sciences*, 2021. **111**(1): pp. 274–284.

17. Suarez-Sharp, S., et al., Regulatory Experience with In Vivo In Vitro Correlations (IVIVC) in New Drug Applications. *The AAPS Journal*, 2016. **18**(6): pp. 1379–1390.

18. Mitra, A., et al., Applications of Physiologically Based Biopharmaceutics Modeling (PBBM) to Support Drug Product Quality: A Workshop Summary Report. *Journal of Pharmaceutical Sciences*, 2021. **110**: pp. 594–609.

19. Wu, F., et al., Regulatory Utility of Physiologically-Based Pharmacokinetic Modeling to Support Alternative Bioequivalence Approaches and Risk Assessment: A Workshop Summary Report. *CPT Pharmacometrics & System Pharmacology*, 2023. **12**: pp. 585–597.

20. FDA, *Evaluation of Gastric pH-Dependent Drug Interactions with Acid-Reducing Agents: Study Design, Data Analysis, and Clinical Implications Guidance for Industry*, CDER, Editor. 2023.

21. Mann, J., et al., Validation of Dissolution Testing with Biorelevant Media: An OrBiTo Study. *Molecular Pharmaceutics*, 2017. **14**(12): pp. 4192–4201.

22. Berben, P., et al., Biorelevant Dissolution Testing of a Weak Base: Interlaboratory Reproducibility and Investigation of Parameters Controlling In Vitro Precipitation. *European Journal of Pharmaceutics and Biopharmaceutics*, 2019. **140**: pp. 141–148.

23. Barker, R., B. Abrahamsson, and M. Kruusmägi, Application and Validation of an Advanced Gastrointestinal In Vitro Model for the Evaluation of Drug Product Performance in Pharmaceutical Development. *Journal of Pharmaceutical Sciences*, 2014. **103**(11): pp. 3704–3712.

24. Hopgood, M., G. Reynolds, and R. Barker, Using Computational Fluid Dynamics to Compare Shear Rate and Turbulence in the TIM-Automated Gastric Compartment with USP Apparatus II. *Journal of Pharmaceutical Sciences*, 2018. **107**(7): pp. 1911–1919.

25. Takano, R., et al., Oral Absorption of Poorly Water-Soluble Drugs: Computer Simulation of Fraction Absorbed in Humans from a Miniscale Dissolution Test. *Pharmaceutical Research*, 2006. **23**(6): pp. 1144–1156.

26. Hofsäss, M.A. and J. Dressman, Suitability of the z-Factor for Dissolution Simulation of Solid Oral Dosage Forms: Potential Pitfalls and Refinements. *Journal of Pharmaceutical Sciences*, 2020. **109**(9): pp. 2735–2745.

27. Pepin, X.J., et al., Justification of Drug Product Dissolution Rate and Drug Substance Particle Size Specifications Based on Absorption PBPK Modeling for Lesinurad Immediate Release Tablets. *Molecular Pharmaceutics*, 2016. **13**(9): pp. 3256–3269.

28. Pepin, X.J.H., et al., Bridging In Vitro Dissolution and In Vivo Exposure for Acalabrutinib. Part II. A Mechanistic PBPK Model for IR Formulation Comparison, Proton Pump Inhibitor Drug Interactions, and Administration with Acidic Juices. *European Journal of Pharmaceutics and Biopharmaceutics*, 2019. **142**: pp. 435–448.

29. Pepin, X.J.H., et al., Bridging In Vitro Dissolution and In Vivo Exposure for Acalabrutinib. Part I. Mechanistic Modelling of Drug Product Dissolution to Derive a P-PSD for PBPK Model Input. *European Journal of Pharmaceutics and Biopharmaceutics*, 2019. **142**: pp. 421–434.

30. Gamsiz, E.D., et al., Predicting the Effect of Fed-State Intestinal Contents on Drug Dissolution. *Pharmaceutical Research*, 2010. **27**(12): pp. 2646–2656.

31. Pohl, P., S.M. Saparov, and Y.N. Antonenko, The Size of the Unstirred Layer as a Function of the Solute Diffusion Coefficient. *Biophysical Journal*, 1998. **75**(3): pp. 1403–1409.

32. Pepin, X., M. Goetschy, and S. Abrahmsén-Alami, Mechanistic Models for USP2 Dissolution Apparatus, Including Fluid Hydrodynamics and Sedimentation. *Journal of Pharmaceutical Sciences*, 2021. **111**(1): pp. 185–196.

33. Pepin, X.J.H., et al., Physiologically Based Biopharmaceutics Model for Selumetinib Food Effect Investigation and Capsule Dissolution Safe Space - Part I: Adults. *Pharmaceutical Research*, 2022. **40**(2): pp. 387–403.

34. Scholz, A., et al., Can the USP Paddle Method Be Used to Represent In-Vivo Hydrodynamics? *Journal of Pharmacy and Pharmacology*, 2003. **55**(4): pp. 443–451.

35. Anand, O., et al., The Use of Physiologically Based Pharmacokinetic Analyses-in Biopharmaceutics Applications -Regulatory and Industry Perspectives. *Pharmaceutical Research*, 2022. **39**(8): pp. 1681–1700

36. Pepin, X., et al., Acalabrutinib Maleate Tablets: The Physiologically Based Biopharmaceutics Model behind the Drug Product Dissolution Specification. *Molecular Pharmaceutics*, 2023. **20**(4): pp. 2181–2193.

37. Keshavarz, L., et al., Influence of Impurities on the Solubility, Nucleation, Crystallization, and Compressibility of Paracetamol. *Crystal Growth & Design*, 2019. **19**(7): pp. 4193–4201.

38. Capellades, G., H. Wiemeyer, and A.S. Myerson, Mixed-Suspension, Mixed-Product Removal Studies of Ciprofloxacin from Pure and Crude Active Pharmaceutical Ingredients: The Role of Impurities on Solubility and Kinetics. *Crystal Growth & Design*, 2019. **19**(7): pp. 4008–4018.

39. McAllister, M., et al., Developing Clinically Relevant Dissolution Specifications for Oral Drug Products-Industrial and Regulatory Perspectives. *Pharmaceutics*, 2020. **12**(1): p. 19.

40. Buchholz, H.K., et al., Thermochemistry of Racemic and Enantiopure Organic Crystals for Predicting Enantiomer Separation. *Crystal Growth & Design*, 2017. **17**(9): pp. 4676–4686.

41. Duddu, S.P., F.K.Y. Fung, and D.J.W. Grant, Effects of Crystallization in the Presence of the Opposite Enantiomer on the Crystal Properties of (SS)-(+)-Pseudoephedrinium Salicylate. *International Journal of Pharmaceutics*, 1996. **127**(1): pp. 53–63.

42. Hanke, N., et al., A Mechanistic, Enantioselective, Physiologically Based Pharmacokinetic Model of Verapamil and Norverapamil, Built and Evaluated for Drug-Drug Interaction Studies. *Pharmaceutics*, 2020. **12**(6). p. 556.

43. Heng, J.Y., et al., Anisotropic Surface Chemistry of Aspirin Crystals. *Journal of Pharmaceutical Sciences*, 2007. **96**(8): pp. 2134–2144.

44. Skelbæk-Pedersen, A.L., et al., Investigation of the Effects of Particle Size on Fragmentation during Tableting. *International Journal of Pharmaceutics*, 2020. **576**: p. 118985.

45. Mann, J., et al., Stimuli to the Revision Process: The Case for Apex Vessels Stimuli articles do not necessarily reflect the policies of the USPC or the USP Council of Experts. *Dissolution Technologies*, 2021. **28**: p. 6.

46. Meyer, J.H., et al., Effect of Size and Density on Canine Gastric Emptying of Nondigestible Solids. *Gastroenterology*, 1985. **89**(4): pp. 805–813.

47. Andreas, C.J., et al., Mechanistic Investigation of the Negative Food Effect of Modified Release Zolpidem. *European Journal of Pharmaceutical Sciences*, 2017. **102**: pp. 284–298.

48. Bermejo, M., et al., A Mechanistic Physiologically-Based Biopharmaceutics Modeling (PBBM) Approach to Assess the In Vivo Performance of an Orally Administered Drug Product: From IVIVC to IVIVP. *Pharmaceutics*, 2020. **12**(1): p. 74.

49. Li, M., et al., Understanding In Vivo Dissolution of Immediate Release (IR) Solid Oral Drug Products Containing Weak Acid BCS Class 2 (BCS Class 2a) Drugs. *The AAPS Journal*, 2021. **23**(6): p. 113.

50. Badawy, S.I.F. and M.A. Hussain, Microenvironmental pH Modulation in Solid Dosage Forms. *Journal of Pharmaceutical Sciences*, 2007. **96**(5): pp. 948–959.

51. Ganetsky, M., et al., Effect of Excipients on Acetaminophen Metabolism and Its Implications for Prevention of Liver Injury. *Journal of Clinical Pharmacology*, 2013. **53**(4): pp. 413–420.

52. Adkin, D., et al., The Effect of Different Concentrations of Mannitol in Solution on Small Intestinal Transit: Implications for Drug Absorption. *Pharmaceutical Research*, 1995. **12**(3): pp. 393–396.

53. Madsen, J.L., J. Linnet, and J.J. Rumessen, Effect of Nonabsorbed Amounts of a Fructose-Sorbitol Mixture on Small Intestinal Transit in Healthy Volunteers. *Digestive Diseases and Sciences*, 2006. **51**(1): pp. 147–153.

54. Basit, A.W., et al., The Effect of Polyethylene Glycol 400 on Gastrointestinal Transit: Implications for the Formulation of Poorly-Water Soluble Drugs. *Pharmaceutical Research*, 2001. **18**(8): pp. 1146–1150.

55. Grimm, M., et al., Gastric Emptying and Small Bowel Water Content after Administration of Grapefruit Juice Compared to Water and Isocaloric Solutions of Glucose and Fructose: A Four-Way Crossover MRI Pilot Study in Healthy Subjects. *Molecular Pharmaceutics*, 2018. **15**(2): pp. 548–559.

56. Adkin, D.A., et al., The Effect of Mannitol on the Oral Bioavailability of Cimetidine. *Journal of Pharmaceutical Sciences*, 1995. **84**(12): pp. 1405–1409.

57. Yamane, M., et al., The Provisional No-Effect Threshold of Sugar Alcohols on Oral Drug Absorption Estimated by Physiologically Based Biopharmaceutics Model. *Journal of Pharmaceutical Sciences*, 2021. **110**(1): pp. 467–477.

58. Mineo, H., et al., Indigestible Disaccharides Open Tight Junctions and Enhance Net Calcium, Magnesium, and Zinc Absorption in Isolated Rat Small and Large Intestinal Epithelium. *Digestive Diseases and Sciences*, 2004. **49**(1): pp. 122–132.

59. Maclean, N., et al., Investigating the Role of Excipients on the Physical Stability of Directly Compressed Tablets. *International Journal of Pharmaceutics: X*, 2022. **4**: p. 100106.

60. Chiwele, I., B.E. Jones, and F. Podczeck, The Shell Dissolution of Various Empty Hard Capsules. *Chemical and Pharmaceutical Bulletin (Tokyo)*, 2000. **48**(7): pp. 951–956.

61. Digenis, G.A., T.B. Gold, and V.P. Shah, Cross-Linking of Gelatin Capsules and Its Relevance to Their In Vitro-In Vivo Performance. *Journal of Pharmaceutical Sciences*, 1994. **83**(7): pp. 915–921.

62. Johnson, M., et al., Relative Bioavailability and Food Effect of GSK3640254 Tablet and Capsule Formulations in Healthy Participants. *Clinical Pharmacology in Drug Development*, 2022. **11**(5): pp. 632–639.

63. Lin, H.P., et al., Physiologically Based Pharmacokinetic Modeling for Substitutability Analysis of Venlafaxine Hydrochloride Extended-Release Formulations Using Different Release Mechanisms: Osmotic Pump Versus Openable Matrix. *Journal of Pharmaceutical Sciences*, 2016. **105**(10): pp. 3088–3096.

64. Wang, J., H. Wen, and D. Desai, Lubrication in Tablet Formulations. *European Journal of Pharmaceutics and Biopharmaceutics*, 2010. **75**(1): pp. 1–15.

65. Swaminathan, V., J. Cobb, and I. Saracovan, Measurement of the Surface Energy of Lubricated Pharmaceutical Powders by Inverse Gas Chromatography. *International Journal of Pharmaceutics*, 2006. **312**(1–2): pp. 158–165.

66. Zarmpi, P., et al., Impact of Magnesium Stearate Presence and Variability on Drug Apparent Solubility Based on Drug Physicochemical Properties. *The AAPS Journal*, 2020. **22**(4): pp. 1–18.

67. John, C.T., et al., Formulating Weakly Basic HCl Salts: Relative Ability of Common Excipients to Induce Disproportionation and the Unique Deleterious Effects of Magnesium Stearate. *Pharmaceutical Research*, 2013. **30**(6): pp. 1628–1641.

68. Wang, S.W., et al., Determination of P-Glycoprotein Inhibition by Excipients and Their Combinations Using an Integrated High-Throughput Process. *Journal of Pharmaceutical Sciences*, 2004. **93**(11): pp. 2755–2767.

69. Yamazaki, S., et al., Physiologically-Based Pharmacokinetic Modeling Approach to Predict Rifampin-Mediated Intestinal P-Glycoprotein Induction. *CPT: Pharmacometrics* & Systems Pharmacology, 2019. **8**(9): pp. 634–642.

70. Martin, N.L., et al., Process Modeling and Simulation of Tableting-An Agent-Based Simulation Methodology for Direct Compression. *Pharmaceutics*, 2021. **13**(7): p. 996.

71. Pepin, X. Use of IVIVc and IVIVe to support formulation development - Industrial case studies. In *AAPS Meeting - 4th November 2014*. 2014. San Diego, USA.

72. Valentin, J., Basic Anatomical and Physiological Data for Use in Radiological Protection: Reference Values. *Annals of the ICRP*, 2002. **32**(3–4): pp. 1–277.

73. Kourentas, A., et al., Establishing the Safe Space via Physiologically Based Biopharmaceutics Modeling. Case Study: Fevipiprant/QAW039. *AAPS J*, 2023. **25**(1): p. 25.

74. Weiss, H.M., et al., A Study of the Effect of Cyclosporine on Fevipiprant Pharmacokinetics and its Absolute Bioavailability Using an Intravenous Microdose Approach. *Drug Metabolism and Disposition*, 2020. **48**(10): p. 917.

75. Fleisher, D., et al., Drug, Meal and Formulation Interactions Influencing Drug Absorption after Oral Administration. Clinical Implications. *Clinical Pharmacokinetics*, 1999. **36**(3): pp. 233–254.

76. Koziolek, M., et al., The Mechanisms of Pharmacokinetic Food-Drug Interactions - A Perspective from the UNGAP Group. *European Journal of Pharmaceutical Sciences: Official Journal of the European Federation for Pharmaceutical Sciences*, 2019. **134**: pp. 31–59.

77. Vinarov, Z., et al., Assessment of Food Effects during Clinical Development. *International Journal of Pharmaceutics*, 2023. **635**: p. 122758.

78. Custodio, J.M., C.Y. Wu, and L.Z. Benet, Predicting Drug Disposition, Absorption/Elimination/Transporter Interplay and the Role of Food on Drug Absorption. *Advanced Drug Delivery Reviews*, 2008. **60**(6): pp. 717–733.

79. Kesisoglou, F., Can PBPK Modeling Streamline Food Effect Assessments? *The Journal of Clinical Pharmacology*, 2020. **60**(S1): pp. S98–S104.

80. Emami Riedmaier, A., et al., Use of PBPK Modeling for Predicting Drug-Food Interactions: An Industry Perspective. *The AAPS Journal*, 2020. **22**(123): pp. 1–15.

81. CDER, F., *Assessing the Effects of Food on Drugs in INDs and NDAs - Clinical Pharmacology Considerations Guidance for Industry*, CDER, Editor. 2019, CDER.

82. CDER, F., *Bioequivalence Studies with Pharmacokinetic Endpoints for Drugs Submitted under an ANDA, Guidance for Industry*, CDER, Editor. 2021, CDER.

83. Tistaert, C., et al., Food Effect Projections Via Physiologically Based Pharmacokinetic Modeling: Predictive Case Studies. *Journal of Pharmaceutical Sciences*, 2019. **108**(1): pp. 592–602.

84. Wu, Y., et al., The Role of Biopharmaceutics in the Development of a Clinical Nanoparticle Formulation of MK-0869: A Beagle Dog Model Predicts Improved Bioavailability and Diminished Food Effect on Absorption in Human. *International Journal of Pharmaceutics*, 2004. **285**(1–2): pp. 135–146.

85. Kesisoglou, F. and A. Mitra, Crystalline Nanosuspensions as Potential Toxicology and Clinical Oral Formulations for BCS II/IV Compounds. *AAPS Journal*, 2012. **14**(4): pp. 677–687.

86. Parrott, N., et al., Predicting Pharmacokinetics of Drugs Using Physiologically Based Modeling--Application to Food Effects. *AAPS Journal*, 2009. **11**(1): pp. 45–53.

87. Shono, Y., et al., Forecasting In Vivo Oral Absorption and Food Effect of Micronized and Nanosized Aprepitant Formulations in Humans. *European Journal of Pharmaceutics and Biopharmaceutics*, 2010. **76**(1): pp. 95–104.

88. Pepin, X., et al., Understanding Mechanisms of Food Effect and Developing Reliable PBPK Models Using a Middle-Out Approach. *AAPS Journal*, 2021. **23**: pp. 1–14.

89. Kesisoglou, F. and Y. Wu, Understanding the Effect of API Properties on Bioavailability through Absorption Modeling. *AAPS Journal*, 2008. **10**(4): pp. 516–525.

90. Wagner, C., et al., Use of Physiologically Based Pharmacokinetic Modeling for Predicting Drug-Food Interactions: Recommendations for Improving Predictive Performance of Low Confidence Food Effect Models. *The AAPS Journal*, 2021. **23**(4): p. 85.

91. Smelick, G.S., et al., Prevalence of Acid-Reducing Agents (ARA) in Cancer Populations and ARA Drug-Drug Interaction Potential for Molecular Targeted Agents in Clinical Development. *Molecular Pharmaceutics*, 2013. **10**(11): pp. 4055–4062.

92. Segregur, D., et al., Impact of Acid-Reducing Agents on Gastrointestinal Physiology and Design of Biorelevant Dissolution Tests to Reflect These Changes. *Journal of Pharmaceutical Sciences*, 2019. **108**(11): pp. 3461–3477.

93. Kesisoglou, F., M. Vertzoni, and C. Reppas, Physiologically Based Absorption Modeling of Salts of Weak Bases Based on Data in Hypochlorhydric and Achlorhydric Biorelevant Media. *AAPS PharmSciTech*, 2018. **19**(7): pp. 2851–2858.

94. Litou, C., et al., Characteristics of the Human Upper Gastrointestinal Contents in the Fasted State under Hypo-and A-Chlorhydric Gastric Conditions under Conditions of Typical Drug-Drug Interaction Studies. *Pharmaceutical Research*, 2016. **33**(6): pp. 1399–1412.

95. O'Dwyer, P.J., et al., In Vitro Methods to Assess Drug Precipitation in the Fasted Small Intestine - A PEARRL Review. *Journal of Pharmacy and Pharmacology*, 2019. **71**: pp. 536–556.

96. Dong, Z., et al., Application of Physiologically-Based Pharmacokinetic Modeling to Predict Gastric pH-Dependent Drug-Drug Interactions for Weak Base Drugs. *CPT: Pharmacometrics & Systems Pharmacology*, 2020. **9**(8): pp. 456–465.

97. Samant, T.S., et al., Ribociclib Bioavailability Is Not Affected by Gastric pH Changes or Food Intake: In Silico and Clinical Evaluations. *Clinical Pharmacology and Therapeutics*, 2018. **104**(2): pp. 374–383.

98. Parrott, N., et al., Physiologically Based Absorption Modelling to Explore the Impact of Food and Gastric pH Changes on the Pharmacokinetics of Entrectinib. *The AAPS Journal*, 2020. **22**(4): pp. 1–13.

99. Sharma, S., et al., Bioequivalence and Relative Bioavailability Studies to Assess a New Acalabrutinib Formulation that Enables Coadministration with Proton-Pump Inhibitors. *Clinical Pharmacology in Drug Development*, 2022. 11(11): pp. 1294–1307.

100. Schwarz, J.A., et al., Determination of Dissociation Constants of Weak Acids by Deconvolution of Proton Binding Isotherms Derived from Potentiometric Data. *Journal of Solution Chemistry*, 1996. **25**(9): pp. 877–894.

101. Mudie, D.M., et al., Quantification of Gastrointestinal Liquid Volumes and Distribution Following a 240 mL Dose of Water in the Fasted State. *Molecular Pharmaceutics*, 2014. **11**(9): pp. 3039–3047.

102. Hens, B., et al., Dissolution Challenges Associated with the Surface pH of Drug Particles: Integration into Mechanistic Oral Absorption Modeling. *The AAPS Journal*, 2022. **24**(1): p. 17.

103. Al Shoyaib, A., et al., Regulatory Utility of Physiologically Based Pharmacokinetic Modeling for Assessing Food Impact in Bioequivalence Studies: A Workshop Summary Report. *CPT: Pharmacometrics & Systems Pharmacology*, 2023. **12**: pp. 610–618.

104. Wu, F., et al., Scientific Considerations to Move towards Biowaiver for Biopharmaceutical Classification System Class III Drugs: How Modeling and Simulation Can Help. *Biopharmaceutics & Drug Disposition*, 2021. **42**(4): pp. 118–127.

105. USA_Federal_Government, *Code of Federal Regulations. Part 314.50-Content and Format of an NDA.* 1985.

106. Suarez-Sharp, S., et al., Applications of Clinically Relevant Dissolution Testing: Workshop Summary Report. *The AAPS Journal*, 2018. **20**(6): 14 pp.

107. Kakhi M, Delvadia P, Suarez-Sharp S. Biopharmaceutic Considerations in Drug Product Design and In Vitro Drug Product Performance. In: Ducharme MP Shargel L, eds. Shargel and Yu's *Applied Biopharmaceutics and Pharmacokinetics*, McGraw-Hill Education; 2022. Accessed April 18, 2024. https://accesspharmacy.mhmedical.com/content.aspx?bookid=3127&sectionid=264439163.

108. Macwan, J.S., et al., Application of Physiologically Based Biopharmaceutics Modeling to Understand the Impact of Dissolution Differences on In Vivo Performance of Immediate Release Products: The Case of Bisoprolol. *CPT: Pharmacometrics & Systems Pharmacology*, 2021. **10**(6): pp. 622–632.

109. Wu, D., et al., Physiologically Based Pharmacokinetics Modeling in Biopharmaceutics: Case Studies for Establishing the Bioequivalence Safe Space for Innovator and Generic Drugs. *Pharmaceutical Research*, 2022. **40**(2): pp. 337–357.

110. EMA, Guideline on the Investigation of Bioequivalence, 2010.

111. Geraili, A., M. Xing, and K. Mequanint, Design and Fabrication of Drug-Delivery Systems toward Adjustable Release Profiles for Personalized Treatment. *View*, 2021. **2**(5): p. 20200126.

112. Peck, R.W., Precision Dosing: An Industry Perspective. *Clinical Pharmacology & Therapeutics*, 2021. **109**(1): pp. 47–50.

113. Darwich, A.S., et al., Model-Informed Precision Dosing: Background, Requirements, Validation, Implementation, and Forward Trajectory of Individualizing Drug Therapy. *Annual Review of Pharmacology and Toxicology*, 2021. **61**(1): pp. 225–245.

114. Pérez-Blanco, J.S. and J.M. Lanao Model-Informed Precision Dosing (MIPD). *Pharmaceutics*, 2022. **14**. DOI: 10.3390/pharmaceutics14122731.

115. Wong Chi, H., W.E.I. Siah Kien, and W. Lo Andrew, Estimation of Clinical Trial Success Rates and Related Parameters. *Biostatistics*, 2019. **20**(2): pp. 273–286.

116. Linder, M.W., et al., Warfarin Dose Adjustments Based on CYP2C9 Genetic Polymorphisms. *Journal of Thrombosis and Thrombolysis*, 2002. **14**(3): pp. 227–232.

117. Ansell, J., A. Holden, and N. Knapic, Patient Self-Management of Oral Anticoagulation Guided by Capillary (Fingerstick) Whole Blood Prothrombin Times. *Archives of Internal Medicine*, 1989. **149**(11): pp. 2509–2511.

118. Carlquist, J.F. and J.L. Anderson, Using Pharmacogenetics in Real Time to Guide Warfarin Initiation. *Circulation*, 2011. **124**(23): pp. 2554–2559.

119. Hulstaert, E., et al., RNA Biomarkers from Proximal Liquid Biopsy for Diagnosis of Ovarian Cancer. *Neoplasia*, 2022. **24**(2): pp. 155–164.

120. Lone, S.N., et al., Liquid Biopsy: A Step Closer to Transform Diagnosis, Prognosis and Future of Cancer Treatments. *Molecular Cancer*, 2022. **21**(1): p. 79.

121. Trujillo, B., et al., Blood-Based Liquid Biopsies for Prostate Cancer: Clinical Opportunities and Challenges. *British Journal of Cancer*, 2022. **127**(8): pp. 1394–1402.

122. Achour, B., et al., Liquid Biopsy Enables Quantification of the Abundance and Interindividual Variability of Hepatic Enzymes and Transporters. *Clinical Pharmacology and Therapeutics*, 2021. **109**(1): pp. 222–232.

123. Darwich, A.S., et al., Why Has Model-Informed Precision Dosing Not Yet Become Common Clinical Reality? Lessons from the Past and a Roadmap for the Future. *Clinical Pharmacology & Therapeutics*, 2017. **101**(5): pp. 646–656.

124. Keizer, R.J., et al., Model-Informed Precision Dosing at the Bedside: Scientific Challenges and Opportunities. *CPT: Pharmacometrics & Systems Pharmacology*, 2018. **7**(12): pp. 785–787.

125. Polasek, T.M. and A. Rostami-Hodjegan, Virtual Twins: Understanding the Data Required for Model-Informed Precision Dosing. Clinical Pharmacology & Therapeutics, 2020. **107**(4): pp. 742–745.

126. Abdulla, A., et al., Model-Informed Precision Dosing of Antibiotics in Pediatric Patients: A Narrative Review. *Frontiers in Pediatrics*, 2021. **9**. p. 624639.

127. Vaz, V.M. and L. Kumar, 3D Printing as a Promising Tool in Personalized Medicine. *AAPS PharmSciTech*, 2021. **22**(1): p. 49.

128. Tan, Y.J.N., et al., On-Demand Fully Customizable Drug Tablets Via 3D Printing Technology for Personalized Medicine. *Journal of Controlled Release*, 2020. **322**: pp. 42–52.

129. Bhuskute, H., P. Shende, and B. Prabhakar, 3D Printed Personalized Medicine for Cancer: Applications for Betterment of Diagnosis, Prognosis and Treatment. AAPS PharmSciTech, 2021. **23**(1): p. 8.

13 Integrating PBPK Modeling and Organ-on-a-Chip Systems to Inform Drug Development

Nicolò Milani, Neil Parrott, Yumi Yamamoto, Claire Simonneau, Nenad Manevski, Wen Li Kelly Chen, Martina Pigoni, and Stephen Fowler

13.1 OVERVIEW

The International Consortium for Innovation and Quality in Pharmaceutical Development (IQ), defined microphysiological systems as "going beyond traditional 2D culture by including several of the following design aspects: a multicellular environment within biopolymer or tissue-derived matrix; a 3D structure; the inclusion of mechanical cues such as stretch or perfusion for breathing, gut peristalsis, flow; incorporating primary or stem cell-derived cells; and/or inclusion of immune system components" [1]. A recent review described Organ-on-Chips as "systems containing engineered or natural miniature tissues grown inside microfluidic chips" [2]. Microphysiological Systems (MPS) and Organ-on-Chip (OoC) definitions therefore overlap and the terminology is sometimes used interchangeably. Both incorporate cell cultures or co-cultures often supported via some type of microfabricated scaffold and usually have media flow as an important element in the long-term maintenance of cellular morphology and activities. In this chapter, we refer to the described advanced cellular systems as OoC throughout, for consistency.

Physiologically-based pharmacokinetic (PBPK) modeling is a technique for prediction of human pharmacokinetics which integrates *in vitro* measured drug properties in a simulated physiological framework. Applications in drug discovery and development are numerous and include prediction of human doses, prediction of drug–drug interaction potential and prediction of the effects of formulation modification. PBPK combines drug parameters such as solubility, permeability, plasma protein binding and hepatic intrinsic clearance with physiological system parameters such as gastrointestinal pH, transit times, organ weights, blood flows, enzyme expression and transporter expression. Prediction of pharmacokinetics in special populations, for example patients with hepatic impairment or pediatric patients, can be made by modifying the physiological parameters while leaving drug properties unchanged. Alternatively, PK predictions for different formulations or administration routes can be made by changing the drug input properties. The drug-specific parameters such as physicochemical properties and absorption, distribution, metabolism and excretion (ADME) parameters are usually measured independently in individually optimized experiments. Parameters measured under different experimental conditions then need to be combined in the PBPK model. This combination needs to be performed based on free drug parameters which are calculated or measured for each of the different media employed in the individual experiments. While PBPK modeling can be very powerful, it is clear that many input data from separate experiments must be combined and this introduces uncertainty. Furthermore, the division into many separate *in vitro* experiments can hamper the capture of the effects when parameters are mutually dependent. Therefore the opportunity to derive high-quality data from a smaller number of more physiologically relevant experiments is highly attractive. OoC systems have the potential to offer such an opportunity. Examples of three major benefits are:

1. More accurate *in vitro* input parameter estimates. This may be because the tissue phenotype is closer to the *in vivo* phenotype or because measurement limitations can be overcome. For example, incubations in OoC systems can be performed over longer times than current systems.

2. The opportunity to study metabolites generated within the system. These may affect ADME and PD parameters in a manner that is not predictable using the metabolite separately as a test reagent or not possible due to the unavailability or transient nature of the metabolite involved.

3. Generation of self-consistent PK datasets for multiple tissues linked in a realistic configuration by a single common medium containing drug.

At the same time, multi OoC system usage is currently restricted by low capacity and by delivering holistic and complex data, rather than individual parameters. These limitations make OoC less suited to applications requiring multiple drug concentrations to be tested (e.g., enzyme kinetics) and are more suited to time-based assessment of ongoing processes (e.g., drug permeation and intrinsic clearance).

DOI: 10.1201/9781003031802-13

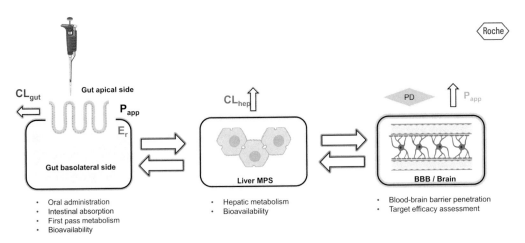

Figure 13.1 Parameter evaluation in a hypothetical PKPD model using a Gut-Liver OoC coupled with the brain tissue as target compartment of the tested drug.

There is a fundamental difference between studying the effect of a drug on the activities of cells (pharmacodynamic experiments and toxicology experiments) compared with studying the effect of the cells on the drug (pharmacokinetic and drug metabolism experiments). *In vitro* pharmacodynamics and toxicology experiments usually apply the drug at chosen fixed concentrations and the effect on the cells is measured at defined incubation time points. The use of large media volumes relative to the mass of tissue enables the maintenance of drug and nutrient concentrations throughout the experiment and permits straightforward assignment of cellular changes to drug exposure. The mass of cellular material employed may be quite small, since sensitive measurement technologies (imaging methodologies, mRNA and protein expression, cell morphology, cell toxicity markers) can be employed. In contrast, for pharmacokinetics and metabolism studies a change in concentration of drug with time must be determined quantitatively, e.g., as the drug permeates through a barrier tissue, accumulates within cells, is depleted due to metabolism or metabolite products are generated. For drug metabolism studies, the combination of intrinsic metabolic activity, tissue mass and media volume must result in drug and metabolite concentrations measurably changing during the experiment. For metabolite formation studies, sufficient metabolite amounts must be generated by the cells to be measurable following dilution into the media. For permeation and distribution studies there needs to be sufficient media to measure changes in drug concentrations on both sides of the barrier tissue.

This chapter does not aim to cover topics such as drug formulation or dissolution that are important for bioavailability but are not measured using OoC experiments. Instead, we will review advances made using OoC for three tissue examples that are essential to PBPK modeling: gut for drug absorption and first pass clearance; liver for first pass and systemic clearance and brain as an example of a barrier-protected target tissue (Figure 13.1). We will also consider in detail the combined gut-liver OoC system that has particular relevance for human pharmacokinetics and bioavailability prediction. We will discuss how current or anticipated advances in OoC could result in improved PK assessment and thereby in better PK/PD predictions. In addition, we will look at how PBPK modeling approaches can assist in the design of OoC experiments to obtain the best quality data outputs when investing in OoC experiments.

13.2 INTESTINAL OOC AND PBPK MODELING

13.2.1 Introduction

Adequate bioavailability (F) is key to the developability of an orally administered drug. Accurate prediction of bioavailability is therefore essential when selecting drug candidates. Oral bioavailability can be broken down into three main components, the fraction of drug entering the gut wall from the lumen (F_a), the fraction of drug escaping gut metabolism in the gut wall (F_g) and the fraction that escapes metabolism during the first pass through the liver (F_h). These components combine to determine F, where $F=F_a*F_g*F_h$. Individual components can be characterized using a range of *in vitro* tools of varying complexity and predictive accuracy depending on compound properties. Although *in vitro* methods for estimating cellular permeability and hepatic clearance are relatively well established for conventional small molecules (e.g., Lipinski's Rule of Five for drug absorption [3]), the emergence of "beyond Rule-of-Five" (bRo5) molecules (e.g., macrocycles, degraders, and peptides) to expand the druggable space is accompanied by challenges such as poor oral absorption and extra-hepatic and/or non-CYP-mediated metabolic pathways, which are difficult to predict with existing tools. Moreover, retrospective analysis of animal versus human oral bioavailability across 184 compounds indicated limited *quantitative* correlations between human and animal data [4,5]. Therefore, new human-centric experimental and *in silico* tools are urgently needed to support compound optimization, mechanistic understanding of ADME processes and translation to the clinic. In the following sections, we focus on the prediction of intestinal availability ($F_a \times F_g$) and highlight opportunities where data generated with advanced *in vitro* systems may improve PBPK prediction. We will also discuss how PBPK modeling can help validate the *in vitro* models by calibrating the predictions with clinical data.

13.2.2 Absorption (F_a)

The absorption of an orally administered drug depends on compound solubility and cellular permeability. For solid dosage forms, understanding of drug dissolution is generally obtained using standard macroscale dissolution studies that are integrated into physiologically-based biopharmaceutics models [6]. Once in solution, the drug must permeate the intestinal membranes. This may involve paracellular transport, passive transcellular diffusion, or active transport across the intestinal epithelium. Permeability measurements across Caco2 monolayers (P_{app}, A → B) have been successfully used to classify the extent of drug absorption in humans for passively transported drugs [7]. Caco2 cells are derived from a human colorectal adenocarcinoma cell line [8] and permeability measured in the apical to basolateral direction (P_{app} A → B) is often used together with compound solubility to predict drug absorption [9]. This data is commonly integrated with PBPK modeling and is an important contribution to human dose prediction. However, compared to the native small intestine, Caco2 monolayers are known to under-predict the absorption of paracellularly transported drugs due to overly tight intercellular junctions, attributable to their colorectal adenocarcinoma origin [10]. Indeed, Caco2 cells show trans-epithelial electrical resistance (TEER) values of 300–2,400 Ohm cm^2 which is much higher than the relevant values in human small and large intestines which range from 35 to 120 Ohm cm^2 [11,12]. Another reported drawback of Caco2 cells is that different subclones and culture conditions used across laboratories may yield variable TEER values, leading to different P_{app} estimation [13,14]. Caco2 co-cultured with HT29-MTX cells has been demonstrated to reduce excessively tight junctions [11] and can achieve a more relevant paracellular permeability which is important for the absorption of small hydrophilic drugs. Other cell models such as Madin-Darby canine kidney (MDCK) and Lewis lung carcinoma-porcine kidney 1 (LLCPK1) cells are alternatives to Caco2 for studying cellular permeability and can be transfected with human transporters for mechanistic studies [15]. Caco2 monolayers do express the common intestinal efflux and uptake transporters (PS_{inf} and PS_{eff}) but their expression levels compared to the *in vivo* regional expression are unclear [12,13]. The role of the P-glycoprotein (Pgp) intestinal transporter has been investigated with Caco2 cells for different compounds [16,17]. For highly soluble compounds, high luminal concentrations are likely to saturate the transporters, resulting in predominantly passive diffusion-driven absorption. However, for compounds with low solubility or very low doses, non-saturable transport processes may dictate the absorption. To this end, intestinal organoid or iPSC-derived monolayer models in transwells or in microfluidic chips with *in vivo* relevant transporter profiles have been developed [18–20]. Comparison of the gene expression profile of Caco2, duodenum organoid-derived monolayer and the native duodenum tissue revealed unusually high OATP2B1 and OCT1 expression in Caco2 cells but more comparable transporter profile in the duodenum organoid-derived monolayers and the native tissue [18]. A different example reported that the nucleoside transporter (CNT3) is markedly absent from Caco2 cells but is expressed in intestinal stem cell-derived monolayers, which correlated with improved permeability of nucleoside transporter substrates *in vitro* and improved prediction of human F_a [10].

13.2.3 Intestinal Metabolism (F_g)

While Caco2 cells can be used for predicting permeability [12,21], they are either deficient or low in the major cytochrome P450 enzymes (CYPs) and uridine 5'-diphospho-glucuronosyltransferases (UGTs) [12,13,22] and overexpress carboxylesterase 1 (CES1) compared to the small intestine [23], and thus unsuited to metabolic studies. Instead, models such as intestinal microsomes, permeabilized enterocytes, and cryopreserved intestinal mucosal epithelium have been used to study intestinal metabolism and F_g prediction [24]. Davies et al. [24], evaluated F_g estimation from these three models across a chemically diverse set of 32 compounds with available observed F_g data. Overall, it was shown that human F_g can be adequately predicted for high-F_g compounds ($F_g > 0.7$), but the prediction accuracy declines for the low and moderate F_g compounds ($F_g < 0.7$), potentially due to contribution from uptake and efflux transporters. However, correct prediction of $F_g > 0.7$ can also be difficult where there is insufficient metabolic activity in the intestinal cell system. In this case, more physiologically relevant cellular models with the full complement of metabolic enzymes and transporters that are functional in long-term cultures would be invaluable to interrogate the interplay between transport and metabolism and improve the overall prediction of human $F_a \times F_g$.

Jones et al., reported several case studies from AstraZeneca where unanticipated or underestimated intestinal metabolism resulted in program termination due to significant underprediction of first pass clearance and over-prediction of bioavailability [25]. A common theme emerging from these examples of preclinical-to-clinical disconnect is that it occurs for compounds outside of the BCS I classification, where poor permeability and/or solubility-limited absorption is accompanied by increased intestinal extraction due to the long residence time in the gut and/or inability to achieve sufficiently high free drug concentrations to saturate metabolism and efflux. This type of problem can be exacerbated in cases where intestine-specific non-CYP metabolism (e.g., UGT1A10 [26]) is involved because it is hard to detect in conventional screening cascades and can be poorly predicted by preclinical animal experiments. Human jejunal and colon tissue explants in the Ussing chamber have proven useful for predicting region-specific drug absorption and metabolism [27], and transporter-metabolism interplay was used to explain the underprediction of clinical PK due to intestinal loss [25]. However, routine access to fresh human tissues is challenging in early drug discovery projects, and stem cell-derived intestinal models are emerging with promise for these investigations.

Recently, intestinal organoids [28–31] have shown promise for ADME studies. Cui et al. reported on the ADME properties of a human stem cell-derived intestinal microtissue grown on a transwell that exhibited superior metabolic function compared to Caco2. *In vitro* intestinal bioavailability, estimated as drug recovery in the basolateral chamber after 24 hours, qualitatively correlated with the observed human $F_a \times F_g$ data [32]. Although organoid- and iPSC-derived intestinal monolayers have shown improved metabolic enzyme expression at the mRNA level [18,19], comprehensive functional characterization using marketed drugs with a range of F_g is currently lacking.

13.2.3.1 How to Predict Intestinal Metabolism with PBPK Models?

When a drug is orally administered it has undergone a combination of process that are considered in a PBPK model. Commonly a mechanistic absorption model considers an additional compartment, usually named as absorption compartment, which takes into account different processes such as solubility, dissolution, partitioning into micelles, particle size, particle growth, and precipitation. In addition, the biological processes such as the membrane permeability with the integration of the physiology in different regions of the gastrointestinal tract (fluid volumes, transit times, areas and luminal pH) are also included [33] within the transit absorption model. They are dynamic compartmental models which are able to predict the intestinal drug absorption in linked compartment that represent the individual intestinal tracts.

PBPK models [34–38], predict intestinal metabolism at a given instantaneous drug concentration using the Michaelis-Menten equation, where the rate of metabolism in enterocytes (v_{ent}) is calculated as (Equation 13.1):

$$v_{ent} = \frac{v_{max}\, C_{ent,total}\, f_{u,ent}}{K_M + C_{ent,total}\, f_{u,ent}}$$

(13.1)

where v_{max} and K_M are the limiting velocity and the Michaelis-Menten constant of the enzymatic reaction, respectively, $C_{ent,total}$ is the predicted total concentration of the compound in the enterocyte, and $f_{u,ent}$ is the unbound fraction of drug in the enterocyte. The v_{ent} is calculated for each relevant drug-metabolizing enzyme in the intestine, meaning that individual v_{max} and K_M values should be known. Further, as protein expression of individual enzymes varies between intestinal compartments, the overall rate of intestinal metabolism (v_{int}) can be calculated as (Equation 13.2):

$$v_{int} = \sum_e \sum_c v_{ent(e)} ESF_{(e,c)}$$

(13.2)

where $v_{ent(e)}$ is the individual rate of metabolism for enzyme e and ESF is the individual enzyme scaling factor for enzyme e and intestinal compartment c. Additionally, to accurately predict the $C_{ent,total}$, one needs information about compounds' oral dose, solid form and formulation, intrinsic and biorelevant media solubility, passive permeability across cellular membranes, and efflux or uptake transporters that may affect disposition in enterocytes. Table 13.1 provides an overview of information needed for a successful PBPK model of intestinal drug metabolism.

As Table 13.1 illustrates, the bottom-up PBPK approach is information-intensive, requiring mechanistic understanding of both (1) compound- and (2) system-specific parameters. While system-specific parameters are sometimes already included within commercially available PBPK software, many compound-specific parameters still need to be measured (or predicted). Many ADME assays are available for this purpose and are also summarized in Table 13.1. In return, once established, PBPK models offer a dynamic simulation with insights into intestinal metabolism across dose levels and formulation scenarios (e.g., immediate vs. sustained release). This allows for predictions of fraction escaping gut metabolism (f_g), as well as modeling of intestinal drug interactions.

Despite best efforts, drug discovery teams will often miss one or more piece of information from Table 13.1. Indeed, many mechanistic ADME assays including enzyme and transporter phenotyping, as well as enzyme kinetic measurements and biorelevant media solubilities, are performed during nonclinical and clinical development, rather than drug discovery. From that perspective, complete bottom-up PBPK models of gut disposition are often used *retrospectively*, to rationalize and mechanistically explain clinical and nonclinical observations. The question arises as to what drug discovery teams can do to predict intestinal metabolism *prospectively*, to guide compound series optimization and candidate selection?

As cellular (e.g., cryopreserved enterocytes) and subcellular (e.g., intestinal microsomes) models of intestinal metabolism are readily available, one pragmatic option is to measure the intrinsic clearance (CL_{int}) of a drug in these models, similar to well-established assays with liver microsomes and hepatocytes. The CL_{int} is usually measured at the low concentration of drug (e.g., 0.5–1 µM), under (implicit) assumptions that this concentration is (1) therapeutically relevant and (2) below the K_M value(s) of responsible drug-metabolizing enzymes. Indeed, if the enterocyte concentration is lower than K_M (i.e., $C_{ent,total} \ll K_M$), Equation 13.2 for the rate of intestinal metabolism can be simplified as (Equation 13.3):

$$v_{ent} = \frac{v_{max}\ C_{ent,total}\ f_{u,ent}}{K_M + C_{ent,total}\ f_{u,ent}} \simeq \frac{v_{max}}{K_M}\ C_{ent,total}\ f_{u,ent} = CL_{int}\ C_{ent,total} f_{u,ent} \tag{13.3}$$

This simplification allows for measured v_{max} and K_M values to be replaced with their simple ratio, namely CL_{int} measured in available *in vitro* intestinal models such as subcellular fractions, enterocytes or organoids. The CL_{int} measurements are often performed by following the disappearance of the test compound over incubation time, to determine the elimination rate constant (k_{el}; 1/min) via nonlinear regression with the monoexponential decay equation ($C_t = C_0 e^{-k_{el}t}$). The CL_{int} is then calculated as (Equation 13.4):

$$CL_{int} = \frac{v_{inc}}{m(\text{enzyme source})} \tag{13.4}$$

where v_{inc} is the volume of the incubation and m(enzyme source) is either the total amount of protein (e.g., microsomal incubations) or the total number of cells (enterocyte incubations) used in the assay.

In fact, to use bottom-up PBPK models, teams may face the challenge of estimating v_{max} and K_M values (required by PBPK software) from available CL_{int} values (measured *in vitro* from substrate disappearance). If CL_{int} values are measured across the concentration range (e.g., 0.1–10 µM), this will be possible by fitting substrate depletion data with the Michaelis-Menten equation using multiple nonlinear regression.

As $C_t = C_0 e^{-k_{el}t}$ and $v_{ent} = \dfrac{v_{max}\ C_{ent,total}\ f_{u,ent}}{K_M + C_{ent,total}\ f_{u,ent}}$, then $v_{ent} = \dfrac{v_{max,app}\ C_{ent,total}\ f_{u,ent}}{K_{M,app} + C_{ent,total}\ f_{u,ent}}\ e^{-k_{el}t}$ where $v_{max,app}$

and $K_{M,app}$ are apparent v_{max} and K_M values estimated by simultaneous fitting of the equations to all concentration-time profiles using nonlinear regression. If only a single CL_{int} value is available (as is likely when using OoC systems with limited capacity and therefore testing only a single

Table 13.1: Overview of PBPK Input Parameters/Information, Gut System-Related Parameters with the Respective Experimental Origins of the Data and Opportunities for MPS

Drug-Specific Parameters

Measured Parameter	Cell Type	Application	Limitations	Scaling Method	Emergent OoC (Technology)
Intestinal Permeability (P_{app})	Caco2	Passive drug transport		P_{app}-P_{eff} conversion based on calibration against human P_{eff} values of a range of marketed drugs	• Stem cell-derived organoids in monolayer format • Region-specific models possible • Cross-species comparisons possible
Intestinal metabolism ($CL_{int,gut}$)	• Subcellular fractions • Enterocytes • Mucosa	Predictive for high-F_g compounds ($F_g > 0.7$),	Poor prediction accuracy for low to moderate F_g compounds ($F_g < 0.7$)	Enzyme-specific inputs and scaling factors (mg of protein/g of tissue) not readily available due to region-specific differences in cell and enzyme abundance	• Region-specific models • Cross-species comparisons
Hepatic metabolism ($CL_{int,hep}$)	• Subcellular fractions • Suspension hepatocytes • Long-term hepatocyte co-cultures	Predictive for CYP, UGT, and FMO-mediated pathways	Low sensitivity for low Clint due to limited incubation times	Tissue scaling factors available assuming homogeneous distribution of cells and enzymes	3D perfused primary hepatocyte models
Intestinal transport (Er)	Transfected cell lines overexpressing specific animal or human transporters	• Endogenous expression level is not accurately captured • Region-specific expression not captured		Transporter-specific inputs (v_{max} and K_M)	• Stem cell-derived organoids in monolayer format • Region-specific models • Cross-species comparisons

(Continued)

Table 13.1: (Continued) Overview of PBPK Input Parameters/Information, Gut System-Related Parameters with the Respective Experimental Origins of the Data and Opportunities for MPS

Drug-Specific Parameters

Additional Information	Comment	Available Assay(s)
Drug-Specific Information		
Knowledge of individual enzymes involved in intestinal drug metabolism	One should understand which enzymes are responsible for the metabolism of the compound in intestinal tissues (e.g., CYP3A4, UGT1A10, or CES2).	Phenotyping with recombinant enzymes and/or with enzyme selective chemical inhibitors. Assays in organoids with single enzyme knock-outs
K_M for each enzyme (and metabolite)	The Michaelis-Menten constant of the enzyme-specific metabolic reaction	Metabolite formation kinetic studies. Substrate depletion across several concentrations
v_{max} for each enzyme (and metabolite)	Maximum rate of the specific metabolic reaction	Metabolite formation kinetic studies. Substrate depletion across several concentrations
Physicochemical properties (e.g., $\log D/\log P$ and pKa)	Lipophilicity and acid-base ionization constants are needed for modeling of absorption and tissue partitioning in PBPK models	Shake-flask (or similar) method for $\log D$. Potentiometric or colorimetric titration for pKa
Passive cellular permeability (P_{app})	The rate of passive permeation across the enterocytes	Permeability across cellular monolayers with tight junctions in the presence of transporter inhibitors
$f_{u,ent}$	Fraction unbound in enterocytes	Measured with equilibrium dialysis or estimated from physicochemical properties of the compound
Gut System-Specific Parameters		
Physiological parameters of the gastrointestinal tract	Length, volume, radius, transit time, blood flow, pH, and other information about individual gut compartments	
Expression and regional distribution of intestinal enzymes	As PBPK models typically divide the gastrointestinal tract into physiological sections (e.g., duodenum, jejunum, and ileum), one should provide enzyme expression data for each individual section. Commercial software often incorporates expression data for several enzymes	
Expression and regional distribution of efflux and uptake transporters	Similar to drug-metabolizing enzymes	

303

drug concentration e.g., 1 μM), however, correct assignment of v_{max} and K_M are infeasible. In this case, under the assumption of $C_{ent,total} \ll K_M$, one can propose empirical values of v_{max} and K_M whose ratio will correspond to observed CL_{int} (e.g., if observed CL_{int} at 1 μM of substrate is 5 μL/min/mg, empirical approximations of v_{max} and K_M could be 50 and 10, providing a correct v_{max}/K_M ratio of 5) while still enabling some estimation of metabolism saturation to be included in the modeling.

The use of CL_{int} instead of v_{max} and K_M resolves some of the complexities but others will remain untackled, especially the question of which drug-metabolizing enzymes are involved. While this question is difficult to answer without dedicated enzyme phenotyping studies, measurements of CL_{int} in the presence and absence of specific enzyme inhibitors may provide an initial insight (e.g., erythromycin [39], itraconazole [40], or azamulin [41] for CYP3A4). Other input parameters for PBPK models can sometimes be approximated with computational predictions, for example via machine learning models developed based on historical data or quantitative structure-activity models.

If available *in vitro* data is insufficient to support PBPK modeling, a simple alternative may be to use a static model of intestinal metabolism [24,42]. While static models tend to ignore many relevant compound and system parameters (e.g., oral dose, solubility, gut motility, etc.), they provide an approximation that can be used for compound ranking and initial assessment of metabolic liability. The Q_{gut} model is one example, inspired by the well-stirred liver model often used to predict liver metabolism [43]. In addition to experimental CL_{int} values, the Q_{gut} model requires measurements of passive intestinal cellular permeability (P_{app}), intestinal surface area (A_{int}), and enterocytic blood flow (Q_{ent}). First, the permeability clearance (CL_{perm}), is calculated as a product of P_{app} and A_{int} ($CL_{perm} = P_{app} \cdot A_{int}$). Next, the CL_{perm} and Q_{ent} are combined to calculate the Q_{gut}, a hybrid parameter of permeability through the enterocyte membrane and Q_{ent} (Equation 13.5).

$$Q_{gut} = \frac{CL_{perm} \; Q_{ent}}{CL_{perm} + Q_{ent}} \qquad (13.5)$$

Finally, the fraction escaping gut metabolism (f_g) can be approximated as (Equation 13.6):

$$f_g = \frac{Q_{gut}}{Q_{gut} + CL_{int} \dfrac{f_{u,gut}}{f_{u,inc}}} \qquad (13.6)$$

where $f_{u,gut}$ and $f_{u,inc}$ represent the fraction unbound in the intestine and *in vitro* incubations, respectively.

As exemplified in this section, for a well-characterized compound with understood biotransformation pathways, intestinal metabolism can be simulated with PBPK models. If some of the parameters are missing, teams can resort to approximations (e.g., CL_{int} instead of v_{max} and K_M) and computational predictions. Given the number of model parameters and their experimental uncertainty, it is likely that validation (and calibration) of PBPK models with nonclinical data is needed prior to predictions of human outcomes. Static models such as Q_{gut} can lead to further simplifications, albeit at the significant loss of mechanistic insight. Readers may also notice an increasing divergence between bottom-up requirements of PBPK models (each mechanistic parameter is required separately) and recent research in human *in vitro* models showing a tendency toward holistic models with multiple cell types and complex readouts. Indeed, if the physiologically relevant human intestinal organoids offer an integrated assessment of intestinal metabolism and permeability, the question arises how can these results be used in PBPK models? One possible answer is that existing PBPK approaches will require a modification, to allow for scaling of results from single organ organotypic models. An alternative could be that organotypic models are assayed in the mechanistic mode, allowing for deconvolution of parameters needed for bottom-up PBPK models. Both approaches will require a close collaboration between experimental and modeling scientists, to leverage the strengths of both approaches and fill the existing gaps.

13.3 LIVER OOCS AND PBPK MODELING

The liver is a crucial organ in the metabolism of most drugs and contributes significantly to first pass and systemic drug clearance via metabolism and biliary elimination and the prediction of hepatic clearance is a vital element for a basic PBPK model for a new drug. A short introduction about the Liver OoCs in DMPK is provided here, as is propaedeutic for the next paragraph about the Gut-Liver OoC. Different *in vitro* assays for determining hepatic intrinsic clearance, such as human liver microsomes or suspension cultures of human hepatocytes, have been used for the prediction of hepatic clearance for many years. These systems have the advantage of simplicity and high throughput but may be limited by the length of incubation before drug-metabolizing enzyme activity is lost. This may preclude the detection of drug depletion for highly metabolically stable compounds [44]. The use of suspended cultures of cryopreserved primary hepatocytes allows members of multiple metabolic enzyme families to act simultaneously on the drug in the presence of physiologically relevant cofactor concentrations. In recent years, long-term hepatocyte co-cultures have been validated and adopted for intrinsic clearance assessment as they provide the long-term incubations necessary to measure the turnover of highly metabolically stable drugs. (For further information on this approach, see recent case study for risdiplam [45]). A liver OoC could incorporate 3D cell cultures such as hepatocyte-derived spheroids, stem cell-derived liver organoids or hepatocyte co-cultures. Also microfluidic devices using cell lines such as immortalized human hepatocellular carcinoma (HepG2) and human bi-potent progenitor (HepaRG) have been reported in several studies [46,47]. An advantage of HepG2 and HepaRG is their relative stability, availability, and reproducible culture characteristics [48,49]. However, they may suffer from poor metabolic activity compared with primary hepatocytes [50]. Indeed, it was recently demonstrated that LoCs with plated cryopreserved primary hepatocytes can be successfully applied for long-term incubation. The cells grown under 3D conditions in the presence of microphysiological flow were viable in incubations lasting up to 4 days without change of media [51,52]. Furthermore, in the shear stress conditions available in OoC devices, seeded human hepatocytes were demonstrated to have some predictivity for *in vivo* hepatic clearance. Although liver OoCs with primary hepatocytes are promising tools, they still need further improvement and development for full DMPK applications. One current disadvantage is the lack of multi-donor pooled hepatocyte cultures exhibiting good activity. Since *in vitro* predictions should be representative of a relevant population, the use of a pool of cell donors is a requirement in order to avoid bias due to an individual donor expression pattern. This has previously been achieved through the generation of commercially available pooled HLM, suspension hepatocytes, and micropatterned hepatocyte co-cultures which were suitable for *in vivo* clearance prediction [53,54]. However, the low culture viability of cells from many donors in OoC systems makes the establishment of a good pool of donors challenging. In the future, the development of scaffolds that promote the growth of hepatocytes from a wider number of donors will help to alleviate both the pooled donor problem and the limitation in supply of cells from viable donors. Additional challenges include the small tissue mass vs media volume, the lack of enzymatic activity retention for more than 3–4 days, and the impossibility to assess transporter-mediated uptake and efflux.

13.4 GUT-LIVER OOCS AND PBPK MODELING

13.4.1 Introduction

As reported in the previous section, the drug crossing the gut wall may also represent an opportunity for first pass metabolism ($CL_{int,gut}$). Drug is then transferred via the portal vein to the liver where further transport and metabolism ($CL_{int,hep}$) can occur. Rather than requiring independent experiments for these steps, the Gut-Liver OoC integrates all processes into one experiment and thus permits observation of how drugs, metabolites, and different tissues may interact with each other (Figure 13.2).

The metabolism data generated via single organ systems cannot capture more complex interactions where the activity of one organ is influenced by processes occurring in another organ. For example, valacyclovir is a prodrug that is actively taken up by intestinal transporters and then activated by a combination of gut and liver esterases to generate the active antiviral agent acyclovir [55,56]. Another example could be when metabolites inhibit the metabolism of a parent drug. The integration of data generated in OoC systems into PBPK models is required since while the Gut-Liver OoC can in principle capture the interplay of processes within a single *in vitro* device the mismatch between tissue mass, activity and medium volume/composition *in vitro* and *in vivo* means that there is still a need to scale up to the *in vivo* setting using physiological scaling techniques for both gut and liver. This involves the extraction of fundamental intrinsic parameters (e.g., P_{app}, PS_{inf}, PS_{eff}, $CL_{int,gut}$, and $CL_{int,hep}$) via modeling of the *in vitro* system and scaling to *in vivo* using *in vitro* system and *in vivo* physiological factors.

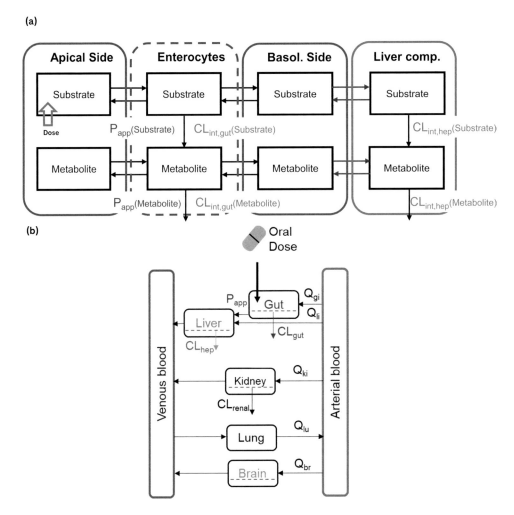

Figure 13.2 (a) General model of a hypothetical compound which is administered in the apical side of a Gut-Liver OoC device. The compound is metabolized in the gut compartment and in the liver compartment after crossing the *in vitro* intestinal cell barrier. Analogous to the parent compound, the metabolite is also metabolized in the liver or can recirculate back to the basolateral side and cross the intestinal barrier or be further metabolized in the gut cells. (b) Use of the DMPK drug parameters from the *in vitro* investigation in the PBPK modeling.

Table 13.2 summarizes prior publications reporting the use of Gut-Liver OoC in DMPK and shows information on the studied drugs and the specific cell systems used for the intestinal and hepatic compartments. Also detailed in Table 13.2 is the *in silico* model used for DMPK parameter estimation and translation to *in vivo*.

13.4.2 Cell Cultures Used in Current Gut-Liver OoC
13.4.2.1 Design of the Gut-Liver OoC

Gut-Liver OoC devices include both intestinal and hepatic tissues physically located in different compartments. The intestinal compartment is separated into apical and basolateral sides which represent the lumen and the blood circulation of the intestinal tract, respectively. The apical and basolateral sides are typically supplied in the form of a transwell® with the cells seeded on the apical side. The basolateral side of the transwell sits within the basolateral compartment of the OoC which is linked to the liver compartment either thorough a microflow system or by forming a single compartment with the liver cells. The continuous flow in the basolateral compartment may promote measurement of net drug absorption since the media flow removes the drug arriving in the basolateral

Table 13.2: Current Available Gut-Liver OoCs Applied in the DMPK Field

Ref.	Compartment		Test Compound	In silico Application
	Intestine	Liver		
Maschmeyer et al. [60]	Small intestine epithelial cells from the ileum section of small intestine tissue	HepaRG	Troglitazone	• No in silico activity was reported
Lee et al. [59]	Caco2	HepG2	Paracetamol	• Flow velocity and shear stress inside a gut-liver chip • Compartmental model with three compartments • IVIVE
Choe et al. [61]	Caco2	HepG2	Apigenin	• Simulation of compound transport inside the chip • Semi-quantitative comparison with the in vivo rat data
Tsamandouras et al. [57]	Caco2-BBe epithelial cells and mucin-producing goblet cells (HT29-MTX) at a 9:1 ratio, plus monocyte-derived dendritic cells	Human hepatocytes and Kupffer cells	Diclofenac and hydrocortisone	• Compartmental model • MCMC for the evaluation the difference among the three independent experimental conditions due to organ cross-talk
Arakawa et al. [62]	Caco2	HepaRG	Triazolam	• Fitting by compartmental analysis of in vitro data to predict DMPK parameters • IVIVE using empirical scaling factor
Milani et al. [58]	Caco2-HT29 cells	Human hepatocytes	Mycophenolate Mofetil	• Fitting by compartmental analysis of in vitro data to predict DMPK parameters • Statistical analysis to evaluate gut-liver, gut-only, and liver-only experiment

compartment in a similar way as blood flow *in vivo*. Certain devices may also contain a compartment named the mixing chamber which denotes the systemic circulation [57]. The microflow is separated into intra and inter-compartment flows and is usually generated by a system of peristaltic micro-pumps. This flow is able to mix the media and guarantees well-stirred conditions in the basolateral compartment. (The intra-compartmental flow that links the gut basolateral compartment with the liver compartment does not come into contact with the cells if they are seeded on the apical side.) The intra-compartment microflow is available in the liver compartment and is reported to contribute a physiological cell shear stress helps to maintain hepatocyte differentiation and increases cell longevity favoring prolonged cell viability and expression of drug-metabolizing enzymes [51,54].

13.4.2.2 PK Processes in the Gut-Liver OoC

In the Gut-Liver OoC, the drug is usually introduced into the apical side medium, and after permeation through the intestinal cells, it is released in the basolateral side and then moved to the liver compartment by media flow. After absorption into the intestinal cells, the drug can also be metabolically transformed into metabolite(s) which are released back to the apical or the basolateral side. In the liver compartment, the drug and metabolites can be further metabolized or recirculate back to the basolateral compartment (see Figure 13.2). The drug and metabolite(s) are commonly detected and quantified by sampling from the apical side, the basolateral side, and the liver compartment. *In silico* modeling of this multi-compartmental Gut-Liver OoC requires detailed mathematical models to estimate the *in vitro* parameters from multiple readouts for both the drug and the metabolite(s). The most common models use a compartmental framework captured as a system of ordinary differential equations (ODEs). The ODE system is used for fitting to the observed data in each compartment and for all the detected compounds in order to predict the *in vitro* DMPK parameters required for scale up in a PBPK framework.

As shown in Table 13.2, the majority of systems reported in the literature exploited Caco2 cells as a monoculture or as a co-culture with HT-29 cells in the intestinal compartment with the limitation reported in the previous paragraph. Cells in the hepatic compartment are commonly cryopreserved primary hepatocytes or immortalized hepatic cells such as HepaRG and HepG2 [57–62].

Another important point is the quantification of the number of viable cells over the incubation time since this is essential for proper quantitative scaling of *in vitro* parameters to *in vivo*. The measured intestinal and hepatic clearance values are scaled based on the number of viable cells [52,58]. In addition, the use of biomarkers such as urea production for hepatocytes can provide further information on the stability of the cell viability [52]. The number of the gut cells for scaling the intestinal clearance can also be evaluated by confocal laser scanning microscopy (CLSM) as reported by Milani et al. [58] since the transwell is transparent and the cells form a monolayer which permits optical quantification.

13.4.3 Mechanistic Modeling Applied to the Gut-Liver OoC

As described above, the combination of intestinal and hepatic cells in one device allows the simultaneous evaluation of multiple DMPK processes. However, quantitative translation requires mathematical modeling of the *in vitro* experiments to estimate *in vitro* DMPK parameters from the concentration vs time profiles of the drug and metabolite(s) in all sampled compartments. Commonly, compartmental models are used although the simultaneous evaluation of multiple processes in one device makes the parameter estimation much more complex than is the case for standard *in vitro* devices. Indeed, in addition to the intrinsic complexity given by the multiple DMPK processes, the Gut-Liver OoC also has several additional variables that can greatly influence the experimental outcome and the parameter estimation.

13.4.3.1 Typical Parameters in the Gut-Liver OoC

In the multi-OoC *in vitro* systems, all the parameters connected to the design of the device need to be included in the mechanistic model in addition to the DMPK processes of the test compound and the impact of their values and uncertainties carefully evaluated in the parameter estimation phase [63]. In a Gut-Liver OoC, we can consider three different types of parameters (Table 13.3): the drug parameters and system parameters related to OoC design and system parameters related to OoC tissue biology such as the cell donors, the time for which the biological activity is retained, and the volume of the cells. The drug parameters are represented by the intestinal and hepatic clearance, the intestinal permeability, and in case of active uptake the efflux ratio and they are the parameters that are estimated from the experiment. The drug parameters are also influenced by the cells used since the activity of certain metabolic enzymes or membrane transporters is highly

Table 13.3: Major Design, Biological, and Drug Parameters Available in a Gut-Liver OoC Experiment

Parameter in Gut-Liver OoC	Parameter Type
System Design	
Inter-compartmental media flow rates	Design
Intra-compartmental media flow rates	
Surface area and apical volume of the intestinal transwell	
Number of intestinal and hepatic cells	
Media volume reduction for sampling and potential evaporation	
Biological	
Volume of cells	Biological
Time for which biological activity is retained	
Cells donor and associated enzyme expression	
Drug-Specific Properties	
Intestinal permeability	Drug
(population average) Intestinal Intrinsic Clearance	
(population average) Hepatic Intrinsic Clearance	
(population average) Efflux ratio	
Unbound fraction in the media	

variable among different subjects. In addition, another compound-parameter is the unbound fraction of the compounds in the apical and basolateral media, which needs to be measured independently or predicted. Regarding the system-parameter, it was reported that the experimental uncertainty of the media flow rate that connects the basolateral and liver compartments might play an important role in certain experimental conditions [58]. In addition, the impact of the volume of all compartments in the DMPK prediction needs to be carefully evaluated. The relatively small volume of some system compartments might also require consideration of volume changes over the incubation time. Indeed, the reduction of volume due to the sampling volume and the media evaporation entails a volume reduction [52,58]. The volume reduction for sampling is dependent on the sampling volume and the sampling frequency. The media evaporation is highly influenced by the design of the device and in particular it depends on many features, such as the position and heat output of the micro-pumps that may increase the local temperature of the plate. An experimental estimation of the evaporation rate can be easily performed and included in the model as zero order kinetic process [58]. The different impact of the media reduction due to sampling and media evaporation on the concentration vs time profile is not only related to the Gut-Liver OoC, but also in mono OoC devices such as the liver-OoC [52]. In certain conditions, even biological parameters such as the average volume of the cells can have a very high influence on parameter estimation. It was reported that the cell volume of the intestinal cells was able to impact the P_{app}(MPAG) of mycophenolic acid by around 40% just varying the volume of the Caco2 and the enterocytes as input parameter in the model [58,64–66].

A proper application of the *in silico* modeling can help in the investigation of an additional positive effect in the multi-OoCs: the organ-cross talking in the *in vitro* experiments which was extensively debated in recent time [67–69]. Regarding the Gut-Liver OoC, different papers reported that having the gut and the hepatic cells in the same device allowed to improve the metabolic activity of both compartments [57,62,70]. The authors supposed that the effect of a higher metabolic activity was due to the effect of physiological signal of the hepatic and intestinal cells. The effect was evaluated from the absolute value of the predicted parameters in monoculture (e.g., gut-only and liver-only) and in the multi-organ condition [57,58,62]. The authors compared the data in mono and multi-tissue systems and they reported a higher DMPK activity in the multi-OoC conditions. However, to properly evaluate the difference in the parameter values, the predicted parameters need to be associated with an accurate estimation of their uncertainty. Commonly, the parameter uncertainty is reported as ±SD but it assumes that the uncertainty is normal distributed around the predicted value. However, as reported in the Gut-Liver OoC, the normality of the uncertainty has to be evaluated and the range of the values within a certain confidence level needs to be used when the distribution of the uncertainty is not normal [58]. In this way, a more robust and unbiased comparison from quantitative data might better highlight the actual organ-cross talking. Organ cross-talk would optimally be demonstrated in future studies by removing the comparing the activities of co-cultured and not co-cultured tissues in single organ experiments.

13.4.3.2 *Application of Gut-Liver OoC in the IVIVE*

Although the main ADME application of the Gut-Liver OoC is the generation of accurate ADME parameters and subsequent IVIVE performance, there are only two articles currently available that describe this. Arakawa et al. used the Gut-Liver OoC PK model to predict the *in vivo* profile of the triazolam and two major metabolites. With a bottom-up approach, the authors were able to predict relatively well the *in vivo* plasma profiles of triazolam and the two metabolites when appropriate empirical scaling factors (SFs) were also included with the *in vitro* predicted DMPK parameters [62]. Similarly, Lee et al. compared the scaled *in vitro* peak time, peak concentration, and half-life time parameters of paracetamol from the Gut-Liver OoC with those available *in vivo* [59]. Therefore, it was demonstrated the benefit of having a multi-OoC device such as the Gut-Liver system to predict the *in vivo* profile of a test compound.

13.5 BLOOD-BRAIN BARRIER (BBB) MODELS AND PBPK MODELING

13.5.1 Introduction

The development of drugs for neurological disorders, where the drug target is located in the brain, remains challenging although there is a huge unmet medical need [71]. One of the factors for the high attrition rate of drug development is the lack of understanding about drug concentrations at the target site in the central nervous system (CNS) [72].

The measurement of target site concentrations in human CNS is highly limited due to ethical and practical constraints. While cerebrospinal fluid (CSF) collected from the lumbar region is often used as a surrogate of brain exposure in clinical settings [73], it may not always reflect the drug concentration in the target site of the brain, particularly in cases involving low passive permeability, active transporters, or diseased conditions [74–77]. *In vivo* intracerebral microdialysis for small molecules [78–80] and large pore microdialysis for large molecules [81–83] are the techniques which are often used to provide drug time-concentration profiles in the brain extracellular fluid (brainECF) of different brain regions. However, the use of microdialysis in humans is highly restricted despite being minimally invasive.

A translational physiologically-based pharmacokinetic (PBPK) model framework for the CNS is of great interest, as it enables the prediction of drug concentrations at therapeutic target sites in humans based on preclinical data [84–86]. PBPK models explicitly distinguish between system physiology and drug characteristics, which interact to govern the drug distribution in different compartments. Performance of the PBPK model predictions relies on the quality and availability of data which is required for the model development.

The *in vitro* modeling of the BBB is a relatively new approach to investigate drug transport across the BBB. This technology has been developed to mimic the complex structure and function of the BBB *in vitro*, allowing for the study of drug transport across the barrier in a more realistic and physiologically relevant manner. Although the BBB *in vitro* models are still in the early stages of development, some of them have already been used to investigate drug transport at the BBB, and their ability to predict *in vivo* brain uptake seems particularly promising. Additionally, given the limitations mentioned earlier, the use of *in vitro* models to parameterize PBPK models is becoming increasingly relevant.

In this section, we will introduce the main *in vitro* BBB models currently available, discussing the advantages and disadvantages of the different cell types, and platforms used. We will also describe the different *in vitro* model systems and present their applications in the context of brain drug delivery. Finally, PBPK models focusing on predicting drug concentration in action sites in the CNS for small and large molecules will be summarized along with the current challenges. The potential of brain OoC to refine and improve the current CNS PBPK model will also be discussed.

13.5.2 BBB Models for Drug Delivery to the Brain

13.5.2.1 *Main Cell Types Used in BBB Models*

The BBB is a very complex and highly selective barrier that strictly controls permeation and transport to the brain parenchyma [87,88]. Highly specialized cells and very specific structural organization are key elements for the correct functionality of the BBB. In the BBB, brain endothelial cells are surrounded by pericytes and the astrocyte endfeet. Both pericytes and astrocytes are important for regulating the integrity and functionality of the endothelium, through mechanisms involving direct contact interactions but also communication via soluble factors. Here we briefly summarize the different sources of cells most commonly used for BBB *in vitro* modeling, focusing in particular on cells derived from hiPSC.

13.5.2.2 Human Brain Endothelial Cells

Endothelial cells from animal origin have been extensively used to model the BBB *in vitro*. Their tight endothelial monolayers with a high transendothelial resistance made them a good model to study small molecule transport through the BBB (see for example the model based on porcine brain endothelial cells established by Patabendige and colleagues) [89,90]. Nevertheless, a big limitation of these cells are the intrinsic species-specific features that might limit their translatability, especially in terms of differences in protein binding affinity and transport rate [91,92]. In addition to this, primary mouse and rat cells also have very low yields, which makes high throughput use of the cells extremely difficult. Primary sources of human brain endothelial cells have been considered for *in vitro* modeling of BBB [93,94] and more commercial vendors are now offering this cell type. This cell type overcomes the problem related to interspecies differences and shows high similarity of gene expression with *in vivo* models, but it introduces other limitations such as batch to batch variability, still limited cell supply and cell identity changes with diminish similarity with the *in vivo* counterpart when cells are kept in culture [95,96]. Immortalized endothelial cells can potentially overcome some of these limitations since they can be expanded *in vitro* and their identity monitored during time. Several immortalized lines have been generated (TY10, BB19, hBMEC, [97–99]) from brain tissue and, among those, hCMEC/D3 [100] are extensively used and characterized [101,102]. Even if multiple studies have confirmed the presence of endothelial specific markers in hCMEC/D3 cells [103,104], their level of expression and the relatively low junctional tightness of the formed monolayer represents still a limitation [102,105,106].

iPSC-derived endothelial cells represent a renewable and scalable source of cells, potentially also bringing to the system a higher degree of robustness and reproducibility. Additionally, considering the well-established editing methods and the possibility of deriving iPSC cells from patients, an *in vitro* BBB model derived from iPSC represents an unprecedented opportunity for modeling BBB dysfunctions and studying disease mechanisms. The first and the most used protocols to derive brain endothelial cells (iBMEC) was established by Lippmann and colleagues in 2012 and it is based on a differentiation strategy that promotes neural and endothelial co-differentiation [107–110]. Alternative methods based on mesodermal induction and Wnt pathway activation have also been published and optimized by several groups [111–115]. While the use of the first differentiation model leads to cell monolayers with high TEER and low permeability values [106], the identity of the iBMEC obtained was recently challenged and shown to be partially epithelial rather than recapitulating a full endothelial identity [116]. In the coming years, the field will have to face the challenge of validating these new iPSC-derived brain endothelial models, not only from the identity and functional point of view but also in terms of *in vivo* translatability.

13.5.2.3 Human Brain Pericytes and Astrocytes

Similar to brain endothelial cells, primary and immortalized pericytes and astrocytes have been used *in vitro* to model BBB and improve its functionality [117,118]. Nowadays, primary human brain pericytes and astrocytes can be purchased from different companies (e.g., ScienCell Research Laboratories, Cell systems, iXCells Biotechnologies, and Lonza), and several immortalized cell lines have been generated [119–121]; nevertheless, the same problems related to primary sources and immortalization described for brain endothelial cells can be extended also to pericytes and astrocytes.

Protocols for the generation of iPSC-derived pericytes have been recently established by several groups [122–125]. In particular, Stebbin and colleagues proposed a pericyte differentiation protocol based on neural crest stem cells-derivation [125]. Additionally, Faal and colleagues established two protocols that rely on either mesoderm or neural crest induction to generate brain-specific pericytes [123]. Even if the authors show that these pericyte populations express pericyte markers and improve BBB features when in culture with primary endothelial cells, a deep characterization of their identity and comparison with *in vivo* counterparts are still missing [123,125].

Several protocols for the generations of iPSC-derived astrocytes were developed based on neural induction followed by specific astrocyte differentiation mediated by extrinsic soluble factors [126–129]. In addition to this approach, iPSC-induced astrocytes can also be obtained with alternative methods for example by isolating them from cerebral organoids derived from human pluripotent stem cells [130,131] or by intrinsic activation of transcription factors critical for astrocyte differentiation [132].

13.5.2.4 Different Types of BBB in vitro Models

The purpose of *in vitro* modeling is to reproduce experimentally a microphysiological environment that could help better assess physiological or pathological processes to eventually bridge the gap between *in vivo* and *in vitro* findings.

In the context of the BBB, a large variety of *in vitro* models has been established to facilitate CNS drug discovery. Most of the models are used to assess the permeation of drug candidates, mainly small molecules. These models are often simplistic *in vitro* models that can be easily scaled up and compatible with high throughput screenings. New models have recently emerged, usually more complex ones that can better reproduce the physiological features of the BBB. These innovative models have been essentially developed to evaluate the potential of CNS therapeutics to bypass the resistance feature of the BBB, a strategy that is often seen in the development of biologics.

In this section, we focus on describing some of the BBB models that are currently used to better predict the distribution of drugs (small and large molecules) against neurological disorders (Table 13.4).

13.5.2.4.1 2D Models

Conventional 2D models are still a gold standard in drug discovery since they are relatively simple, affordable, reproducible, and compatible with high throughput.

13.5.2.4.1.1 Monolayer of Cells The first *in vitro* BBB models developed were monocultures of cells cultivated on plastic dishes, usually brain endothelial cells (BECs) [101,133,134]. This type of assay rapidly showed limitations in transport studies. Indeed the stiffness of the plastic surface, combined with the absence of matrix and the absence of two distinct compartments were key missing elements.

To overcome these limitations, monolayers of cells are now seeded in a transwell model [135–140] a microporous membrane suspended in a well that can separate the vascular side from the brain parenchymal side. The main application of such a model is for the assessment of brain penetration of drugs, typically small molecules. In this system, permeability is measured by the transfer rate between the two compartments that are separated by the monolayer of cells, usually epithelial cells overexpressing human transporters or BECs. Thanks to its ease of use and scalability, the transwell assay represents today the most established assay in the BBB field and remains extensively used during the first stages of the drug discovery process (e.g., drug permeability screening) [141]. The standardized dimensions of the transwell and their physical transferability confer the capability for QC prior to inclusion in a larger experiment and flexibility to use in multiple types of OoC systems. Despite this practicability, the system has also shown some limitations in terms of barrier properties, mainly due to the lack of cell–cell and cell–matrix interactions but also shear stress that could better mimic blood flow.

13.5.2.4.1.2 Co-culture models To overcome the absence of cell communication in such a system, scientists have introduced co-cultures models. Indeed, Hartmann et al. have shown the importance of co-cultivating BECs with astrocytes or pericytes to increase barrier function by improving the tightness of cell monolayers [142,143]. Usually, BECs are seeded in the transwell insert and supporting cells like astrocytes and/or pericytes are grown on the other side of the insert [144–147]. In this setup, even though BECs are not in direct contact with the other cell types, the system allows cellular communication via the secretion of soluble factors. This indirect interaction is sufficient to increase TEER (transendothelial electrical resistance), barrier tightness and leads to better predictability of transport studies. Interestingly, these findings showed that mimicking the neurovascular unit environment in an *in vitro* system is key for the production of more efficacious transport studies [148].

In the late 2010s, 2D OoC models were developed to incorporate shear stress in existing BBB models [149–154]. These chips are very similar to the transwell system since they are made of two different channels separated by a porous membrane. Usually, BECs are seeded in one channel and astrocytes and/or pericytes are seeded in the other channel. In this device, flow is connected to the endothelial channel and allows the application of fluid shear stress. These devices are relatively easy to use and easily accessible since a lot of companies are now commercializing such systems.

Table 13.4: Applications, Advantages and Limitations of Current BBB *in vitro* Models

Model Type	Model Subtype	Cell Types	Application	Advantages	Limitations
Monolayer of cells	2D	BECs, Epithelial cells overexpressing specific transporters/ receptors	Drug transport[a], Permeability	Cost, HTP, TEER, Reproducibility	Barrier properties, Cellular interactions, Microvascular geometry, Shear stress
Co-culture	2D	BECs, +Astrocytes, +Pericytes	Drug transport[a], Permeability	HTP, TEER, Reproducibility	Barrier properties, Cellular interactions, Microvascular geometry, Shear stress
Organs-on-chip	2D	BECs, + Astrocytes, + Pericytes, + Immune cells	Drug transport[a], Permeability, Barrier integrity	TEER, Shear stress	LTP, Cellular interactions, Microvascular geometry, Expensive
Tubular channels	3D	BECs, + Astrocytes, + Pericytes, + Immune cells	Drug transport[a], Permeability, Barrier integrity, Disease modeling	MTP, TEER, Shear stress, Reproducibility	Cellular interactions, Microvascular geometry, Expensive
Organoids	3D	BECs, + Astrocytes, + Pericytes	Drug transport[a], Permeability, Disease modeling	MTP, Reproducibility	Microvascular geometry, Shear stress, TEER, Expensive
Microvascular networks	3D	BECs, + Astrocytes, + Pericytes, + Immune cells	Drug transport[a], Permeability, Barrier integrity, Disease modeling	Cellular self-organization	LTP, Technically complex, Shear stress, Reproducibility, TEER, Expensive

BECs, Brain Endothelial Cells; LTP, Low Throughput; HTP, High Throughput; MTP, Moderate Throughput; TEER, high transepithelial electrical resistance indicating tight junction barrier formation.

a Drug transport for both small and large molecule in vitro studies.

Thanks to the addition of shear stress, these models have demonstrated improved transport functions and are usually used to perform drug transport studies in combination with barrier integrity assessments (e.g., reduction of mitoxantrone flux, increase of rhodamine 123 accumulation with vinblastine, increase of angiopep-2 and anti-transferrin antibody transcytosis) [153–156]. Although these models have shown better barrier functions, they are technically more complex and less reproducible than the transwell model, which limits their scalability and use as a standard screening assay. While for early screening, direct cell interactions and shear stress are not necessary, the need of models that can better mimic BBB functions are needed for mechanistic studies and disease modeling. Many groups have shown now the relevance of introducing 3D models to reproduce the 3D cellular organization of the BBB *in vitro*.

13.5.2.4.2 3D Models

One of the big advantages of 3D BBB models is their ability to assess drug effects in physiological and pathological conditions. Moreover, like all BBB *in vitro* models, 3D models can predict the permeability of drugs but they are also compatible with imaging methods which give them an advantage compared to the more simplistic 2D models to answer mechanistic questions.

13.5.2.4.2.1 Tubular Channels Recently, new microfluidic models consisting of 3D tubular channels have been introduced [152,157–160]. These 3D tubular systems are made of a minimum of two rectangular cross-sectioned channels. Usually, BECs are seeded into one channel and are connected to the second channel filled with a collagen gel matrix supplemented or not with supporting cells. This model has shown improved barrier properties which are mainly due to the presence of cell-matrix interactions and the addition of flow. Microfluidic models with cylindrical channels have also emerged in order to ensure a more consistent shear stress along the luminal endothelial wall [161–163] but their characterization in terms of barrier tightness assessment remains difficult due to the cylindrical geometry of the channel. Currently, the advantage of such models is their compatibility with a moderate throughput plate-based format that can be used for drug screening [118]. In this setup, shuttling of drugs (e.g., P-gp substrates) or large molecules (e.g., anti-transferrin receptor antibodies) can relatively easily be measured by media sampling or fluorescence detection. Although these models demonstrate better BBB properties, the morphology of the vasculature as well as the permeability values still remain larger than those observed *in vivo*.

13.5.2.4.2.2 BBB Organoids A new 3D model of the BBB formed by the self-organization of human BECs, pericytes, and astrocytes has recently been developed [164,165]. BBB organoids allow direct cell–cell interactions in the absence of artificial membranes and can recapitulate functional and morphological features of the BBB *in vivo*. Several methods have been implemented to generate the organoids, from ultra-low attachment plates to micropatterned hydrogel platforms. These models have been used mainly to study BBB penetration of small molecules or peptides but also to assess the transport of large molecules via receptor-mediated transcytosis [164–170]. Despite their ease of manipulation, the bioanalytical methods required to assess absolute drug concentrations in these models usually limit their scalability.

13.5.2.4.2.3 Microvascular Networks 3D co-culture microvascular networks represent the most recent models established in the field of BBB biology. These models are based on the self-assembly of hydrogel-embedded BBB cells into a microvascular network [150,171–175]. Several groups showed that these models acquire permeability values comparable to those found *in vivo* [176]. This is not surprising because in this setup cells are well connected to each other, leading to the creation of a microenvironment that allows spontaneous vasculogenesis. To enhance barrier function, perfusion has also been tested in this model [174,176] but the majority of 3D vasculogenesis models have been implemented without these flow conditions. Currently, because of their complexity, low reproducibility, and difficult scalability, microvascular network models are only used to assess permeability changes in the context of CNS disorder.

To summarize, a lot of *in vitro* BBB models have been established and are extensively used today to support CNS drug discovery. Nevertheless, the variety of data outputs extracted from each of these models remains limited. It is now well admitted that a combination of *in vitro* models would be the method of choice and would provide the most relevant information regarding the potential of a drug to penetrate the BBB and thereby increase its chance of reaching its target site in the CNS.

13.5.3 PBPK Models to Predict Drug Target Site Concentrations in Brain
13.5.3.1 Small Molecules

The CNS physiology and physicochemical properties of small molecules which interplay and determine the distribution of small molecules in the CNS are well investigated [177]. The CNS physiological compartments consist of the brain microvasculature, brain intracellular fluid (brainICF), brainECF, lysosomes, and several CSF compartments including compartment-specific pH [77,177]. In addition, physiological flows such as the cerebral blood flow, brainECF bulk flow and CSF flow take an important role in drug distribution together with different drug transport modes including paracellular, transcellular, and active transport across the BBB and the blood-CSF barrier (BCSFB).

Several animal PBPK models to predict drug target site concentrations in the brain have been developed using *in vivo* data on the compounds ranging from simple to more comprehensive [85,86,178–184]. A comprehensive brain PBPK model was developed based on rat brain microdialysis data for several compounds with different physicochemical properties. This model was successfully translated to humans, describing the drug concentration profiles for acetaminophen, methotrexate, and morphine in various compartments in the human CNS [85,86,183]. This approach required measurements of drug concentrations in multiple locations in the CNS using microdialysis which is not routinely performed in industrial settings. Therefore, approaches to predict drug concentration-time profiles at target site without *in vivo* animal data were of great interest.

A 4-compartmental permeability-limited brain (4Brain) model was developed under an IVIVE-PBPK framework, demonstrating its ability to predict drug concentrations for paracetamol and phenytoin in the human CNS [185]. This 4Brain model is nested within the human whole body PBPK model of the Simcyp Simulator. One limitation of this model may be a lack of complexity in the brain compartment, which is critical for predicting receptor-binding kinetics for drugs that act on membrane-bound receptors.

More recently, a comprehensive rat CNS PBPK model which consists of brainECF, brainICF, and four CSF compartments was proposed [186]. This model can predict the concentration-time profiles of small molecules at the drug action site based solely on plasma pharmacokinetics (PK), drug physicochemical properties including active transporters involved, CNS physiology, and *in vitro* information. The rat CNS PBPK model was scaled for use in humans mainly by substituting the values of rat-specific parameters with their corresponding human values, and by converting the contribution of active transport at the BBB and the BCSFB from rat to human based on reported differences in the expression of active transporters (Figure 13.3). The human CNS PBPK model has demonstrated its ability to accurately predict concentration-time profiles in multiple human CNS compartments for acetaminophen, oxycodone, morphine, and phenytoin [186,187]. This model can be applied to any compounds for which their physicochemical properties and information on the active transporters involved are available. The model has been further improved by accounting for brain non-specific binding, incorporating pH effect on drug ionization and refining passive transports [77]. The model showed the potential to predict PK profiles of small molecules in multiple CNS compartments under different physiological conditions [188,189].

Current CNS PBPK models for small molecules face multiple challenges. Firstly, there is a lack of information on the expression levels and activity of active transporters at the BBB and BCSFB, with the exception of major transporters like P-gp and MRP that have been well investigated for interspecies differences in expression and activity [103,190]. Secondly, there is limited quantitative information available on pathophysiological changes in brain and CSF physiology, BBB functionality and intra-brain distribution in CNS disease [191–196] as well as in aging conditions [197–201]. These pathophysiological changes can lead to a distinct CNS pharmacokinetic profile compared to healthy conditions, and the lack of knowledge on pathophysiological parameters prevents accurate prediction of drug concentrations in the brain under specific disease conditions and populations. *In vitro* BBB models may offer a solution to the challenges mentioned above (Table 13.4). For example, several BBB OoC recapitulating the complex brain physiology have been used to understand the changes that occur under CNS disease states [156,202–204]. Incorporating the quantitative information of these pathophysiological changes from BBB models may be able to inform the system-specific parameters in the PBPK models and consequently improve the prediction of drug concentrations in the human brain under disease conditions. Recently, Ito et al. have designed a BBB transwell model which is capable of providing BBB permeability parameters for drugs and predicting the brain drug concentration profile in humans when combined with a CNS PBPK model [205]. This is one of the first reports demonstrating the potential use of *in vitro* BBB models in conjunction with CNS PBPK modeling to predict brain drug concentration profiles for small molecules. Although further optimization is necessary (such as integrating *in vitro-in vivo* correlation data of multiple drugs and conducting whole proteome analysis of transporter expression) to validate the feasibility, the integration of information from *in vitro* BBB models into CNS PBPK modeling is expected to become an increasingly promising approach for predicting drug concentration profiles in human brain.

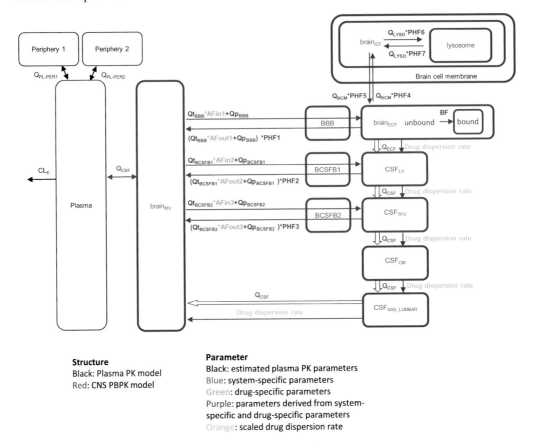

Figure 13.3 The human CNS PBPK model structure [186].

The model consists of a plasma PK model and a CNS PBPK model with estimated plasma PK parameters, and system-specific and drug-specific parameters (colors) for CNS. Brain$_{MV}$: brain microvascular, BBB: blood-brain barrier, BCSFB: blood-CSF barrier, brain$_{ECF}$: brain extra cellular fluid, brain$_{ICF}$: brain intra-cellular fluid, CSF$_{LV}$: CSF in the lateral ventricle, CSF$_{TFV}$: CSF in the third and fourth ventricle, CSF$_{CM}$: CSF in the cisterna magna, CSF$_{SAS\_LUMBAR}$: CSF in the subarachnoid space and lumbar region, Q_{CBF}: cerebral blood flow, Qt$_{BBB}$: transcellular diffusion clearance at the BBB, Qp$_{BBB}$: paracellular diffusion clearance at the BBB, Qt$_{BCSFB1}$: transcellular diffusion clearance at the BCSFB1, Qp$_{BCSFB1}$: paracellular diffusion clearance at the BCSFB1, Qt$_{BCSFB2}$: transcellular diffusion clearance at the BCSFB2, Qp$_{BCSFB2}$: paracellular diffusion clearance at the BCSFB2, Q_{BCM}: passive diffusion clearance at the brain cell membrane, Q_{LYSO}: passive diffusion clearance at the lysosomal membrane, Q_{ECF}: brainECF flow, Q_{CSF}: CSF flow, AFin1–3: asymmetry factor into the CNS compartments 1–3, AFout1–3: asymmetry factor out of the CNS compartments 1–3, PHF1–7: pH-dependent factor 1–7, BF: binding factor.

13.5.3.2 *Monoclonal Antibodies (mAbs)*

There are distinct differences between PBPK models for small molecules and large molecules due to the differences in size and drug disposition characteristics [206,207]. Typical PBPK models for monoclonal antibodies (mAbs) consisting of organ compartments interconnected by both blood and lymph flows were proposed [207–209]. Since PBPK models for mAbs have been developed extensively to characterize plasma and tissue disposition, the brain is often excluded or treated similarly to other peripheral tissues. Recently a brain PBPK model for mAbs was proposed that characterizes brain disposition of mAbs in different regions of the brain across several species [210]. The model accounts for the CNS physiology, as in the PBPK models for small molecules, and also incorporates the differential entry of mAbs across BBB and BCSFB via paracellular transport, pinocytosis and Fc receptor (FcRn)-mediated transcytosis. The model also includes the CSF circulation and intra-brain distribution via the perivascular pathway to describe the kinetics of mAbs in brainECF and CSF. The PBPK model was simplified or refined to enhance its applicability or further validated using mAb concentrations in brainECF and CSF measured with microdialysis for multiple compounds and animals [211–213]. The studies showed that the PBPK model not only quantifies mAb concentrations in different regions of the brain but also provides a quantitative platform of clinical translation of mAbs targeting the CNS.

The limitation of the current mAb brain PBPK model is a lack of understanding of BBB transport and intra-brain distribution of large molecules although a lot of effort has been made [214–217]. In addition, the accuracy of the model predictions relies on the extent and quality of available literature, and some parameters are currently missing or inaccurate. Further experiments providing physiological parameters, understanding and quantifying the mechanism of the BBB transport and intra-brain distribution will be a key to improve the mAbs brain PBPK model.

In vitro BBB models may be able to provide quantitative information on how mAbs are transported across the BBB and how they distribute within the brain. Some recent studies demonstrated the potential of BBB OoC to be used to measure *in vitro* the distribution of mAbs (e.g., anti-transferrin receptor antibodies) [119,153]. Since transferrin receptor-mediated transcytosis is currently the preferred pathway for mAb delivery to the brain, a BBB model that could address *in vitro* para- and transcellular dispositions of anti-transferrin antibodies could potentially be one promising first approach to be used as input for mAbs CNS PBPK modeling [218].

13.6 CHALLENGES AND FUTURE PERSPECTIVES

PBPK modeling is an established discipline making use of *in vitro* ADME parameters to predict human pharmacokinetics, therapeutic doses, and drug–drug interactions. OoC can add value where they can contribute better data or provide data that could not previously be measured. Because PBPK is a quantitative science and the parameter data that are used need to be reliably scaled to *in vivo* drug properties, the requirements for OoC performance are very high. Over the past decade, OoC has progressed substantially and this can be observed in the measures of success reported. For instance, the culture of hepatocytes on new scaffolds that maintain morphology and continue to secrete albumin and urea for multiple days was an important initial achievement. Subsequently, the culture of hepatocytes that were sensitive to some level of CYP3A induction by prototypical inducers demonstrated potential application. More recent reports of OoC that are competent in the generation of metabolites involving multiple classes of drug-metabolizing enzymes and produce intrinsic clearance data that can be scaled to some extent, represent another step forward. In the future, OoC that can reliably provide permeability values, intestinal and hepatic intrinsic clearance data, tissue-specific uptake rates, and fraction metabolized estimations for the different enzyme pathways involved in drug metabolism will be developed. The improved *in vitro* data will enhance predictions of bioavailability, clearance, target tissue drug concentrations, and drug–drug interaction potential. Most of these assessments will still need to be made via an integrative computational framework such as PBPK modeling.

The preceding sections have described recent advances in cellular systems for the gut, liver, and brain through the application of new technologies, including microphysiological systems and the advances in cell culture methodologies. We set out three areas where OoC can potentially enhance PBPK predictions:

1. Generation of more accurate ADME / PD parameters.

2. Potential to better account for metabolites.

3. The generation of consistent, multi-tissue, datasets.

The greatest current opportunity for OoC to rapidly improve human pharmacokinetics and dose prediction is by providing models for the different tissues that are more representative of the *in vivo* phenotype. Drug-metabolizing enzyme and drug transporter phenotypes have been improved by the addition of media flow, optimizing the microenvironment of the cells, making combinations of different cell types within a system, or the ability to culture the cells for a longer period of time. Further improvements are anticipated and will be needed for these *in vitro* tissues to reproduce representative *in vivo* activities.

When considering the implementation of new tools it is important to be objective about where gains can be made and prioritize the development of those with greatest impact. For instance, PK predictions for BCS1 high permeability/high solubility drugs cleared via hepatic metabolism will only improve to a small extent from the application of advanced gut models. In contrast, more physiologically relevant permeability and first pass drug metabolism measurements will benefit PK prediction for low permeability 'beyond rule of 5' drugs, such as macrocyclic peptides and protacs/degraders [219,220]. In addition, drugs targeting gastrointestinal disease, where systemic exposure should be restricted, need better ADME models for both healthy and diseased gut. Prediction of prodrug activation in the gut will be improved when gut models express the correct balance of human carboxylesterase enzymes (i.e., high CES2 and low CES1 expression). Prediction of high first pass gut extraction that limits bioavailability will be enhanced with higher expression of CYP and UGT enzymes closer matching mean *in vivo* activities. Drugs with high gut extraction include HIV protease inhibitors such as saquinavir, calcium channel blockers such as nifedipine and immunosuppressants such as tacrolimus [37].

Advanced *in vitro* liver models that enable long-term hepatocyte incubations to be performed have already shown benefits, improving PK prediction for low-clearance drugs [53,54]. Current challenges include the establishment of hepatocyte cultures or co-cultures that possess and maintain population-average drug-metabolizing enzyme and drug transporter activities and increasing the tissue mass/media volume ratio to address drug turnover/incubation time limitations. Brain OoC exemplifies the needs when trying to understand drug penetration of target tissues protected by specialized barrier tissues. At the same time as developing the required physiology, consideration needs to be made of the drug measurement requirements for generation of the quantitative data outputs required for extrapolation to the *in vivo* situation. This could be in terms of the ability to sample on either side of the barrier tissue or the need for quantitation of imaging readouts to enable drug flux rate calculations. The well-established transwell system has the advantages of standardization and transferability, enabling different barrier tissue cultures to easily be introduced into OoC systems of different designs. In this chapter, the BBB has been used as an example. The same principles can be applied to other tissues such as the testis and kidney when suitable cell cultures become available. A greater level of challenge may exist to combine alternative barrier tissue model designs (e.g., tubular tissue models) in a modular way with other OoC components, but these may offer more promise for establishing *in vivo*-like phenotypes. Media sampling and tissue imaging protocols will also need to be standardized to enable applications to proceed from assessment of cytotoxicity (e.g., barrier function breakdown) into more useful drug permeation rates and active uptake/efflux measurements.

Superficially, multi OoC systems may appear to eliminate the need for PBPK with its requirement to combine data from many individual experiments: They allow multiple tissues to be combined in a single system with the different tissues linked by media flow and present drug concentration-time profiles that may resemble *in vivo* pharmacokinetics. At present, it is important not to forget that although OoC may be more physiological than standard *in vitro* experimental systems, the fluid flows, binding of drug to media proteins and ratio of media volume to tissue mass are very different from those in the body. For instance, incubation media typically includes maximally 10% fetal calf serum in comparison to undiluted human plasma and the cells/media flow rates are quite different *in vitro* and *in vivo*. A liverchip system explored recently by Docci et al reported a media flow rate of 0.3 mL/min transiting through ~0.3 million hepatocytes (~1 mL/min/million hepatocytes) [52]. In contrast, a human liver has a >100-fold higher drug extraction capacity, based upon simple comparison of hepatic blood flow and organ mass [221]. Until microphysiological systems evolve to truly mimic human physiology it will remain necessary to extract the ADME parameters from OoC experiments and use these, via PBPK modeling, to simulate the *in vivo* situation (Figure 13.2).

In the meantime, clarity about what parameters from organ OoC and multi-organ OoC will be transferred to a PBPK model for human PK prediction can be helpful when designing or modifying the OoC. In addition, modeling approaches can be applied to OoC experimental design to give the best chance for unambiguous and accurate ADME parameter estimates to be derived, within the constraints of the drug tested and system used.

OoC development can be expected to proceed hand in hand with PBPK modeling: OoC can offer additional and more accurate parameter estimates to include in PBPK models and may in the future bring parameters needed for PBPK modeling that are not currently available from *in vitro* experiments, such as renal and biliary secretion rates and accurate tissue compartment concentration measurements. In the GI tract simulations, PBPK can make use of OoC measurements for a single gut element and extrapolate to other regions of the gut. In addition, modeling approaches can be used to enhance the probability of successful OoC experiment performance and enable experimental designs to focus on optimal parameter estimation.

REFERENCES

1. Fabre K, Berridge B, Proctor WR, Ralston S, Will Y, Baran SW, et al. Introduction to a manuscript series on the characterization and use of microphysiological systems (MPS) in pharmaceutical safety and ADME applications. *Lab on a Chip*. 2020;20(6):1049–57.

2. Leung CM, De Haan P, Ronaldson-Bouchard K, Kim G-A, Ko J, Rho HS, et al. A guide to the organ-on-a-chip. *Nature Reviews Methods Primers*. 2022;2(1):33.

3. Lipinski CA, Lombardo F, Dominy BW, Feeney PJ. Experimental and computational approaches to estimate solubility and permeability in drug discovery and development settings. *Advanced Drug Delivery Reviews*. 2012;64:4–17.

4. Musther H, Olivares-Morales A, Hatley OJ, Liu B, Hodjegan AR. Animal versus human oral drug bioavailability: do they correlate? *European Journal of Pharmaceutical Sciences*. 2014;57:280–91.

5. Hatley OJ, Jones CR, Galetin A, Rostami-Hodjegan A. Quantifying gut wall metabolism: methodology matters. *Biopharmaceutics & Drug Disposition*. 2017;38(2):155.

6. Jamei M, Abrahamsson B, Brown J, Bevernage J, Bolger MB, Heimbach T, et al. Current status and future opportunities for incorporation of dissolution data in PBPK modeling for pharmaceutical development and regulatory applications: OrBiTo consortium commentary. *European Journal of Pharmaceutics and Biopharmaceutics*. 2020;155:55–68.

7. Artursson P, Karlsson J. Correlation between oral drug absorption in humans and apparent drug permeability coefficients in human intestinal epithelial (Caco-2) cells. *Biochemical and Biophysical Research Communications*. 1991;175(3):880–5.

8. Bohets H, Annaert P, Mannens G, Anciaux K, Verboven P, Meuldermans W, et al. Strategies for absorption screening in drug discovery and development. *Current Topics in Medicinal Chemistry*. 2001;1(5):367–83.

9. Thomas S, Brightman F, Gill H, Lee S, Pufong B. Simulation modelling of human intestinal absorption using Caco-2 permeability and kinetic solubility data for early drug discovery. *Journal of Pharmaceutical Sciences*. 2008;97(10):4557–74.

10. Takenaka T, Harada N, Kuze J, Chiba M, Iwao T, Matsunaga T. Human small intestinal epithelial cells differentiated from adult intestinal stem cells as a novel system for predicting oral drug absorption in humans. *Drug Metabolism and Disposition*. 2014;42(11):1947–54.

11. Hilgendorf C, Spahn-Langguth H, Regårdh CG, Lipka E, Amidon GL, Langguth P. Caco-2 versus caco-2/HT29-MTX co-cultured cell lines: permeabilities via diffusion, inside-and outside-directed carrier-mediated transport. *Journal of Pharmaceutical Sciences*. 2000;89(1):63–75.

12. van Breemen RB, Li Y. Caco-2 cell permeability assays to measure drug absorption. *Expert Opinion on Drug Metabolism & Toxicology*. 2005;1(2):175–85.

13. Hayeshi R, Hilgendorf C, Artursson P, Augustijns P, Brodin B, Dehertogh P, et al. Comparison of drug transporter gene expression and functionality in Caco-2 cells from 10 different laboratories. *European Journal of Pharmaceutical Sciences*. 2008;35(5):383–96.

14. Walter E, Kissel T. Heterogeneity in the human intestinal cell line Caco-2 leads to differences in transepithelial transport. *European Journal of Pharmaceutical Sciences*. 1995;3(4):215–30.

15. Billat P-A, Roger E, Faure S, Lagarce F. Models for drug absorption from the small intestine: where are we and where are we going? *Drug Discovery Today*. 2017;22(5):761–75.

16. Hochman JH, Chiba M, Nishime J, Yamazaki M, Lin JH. Influence of P-glycoprotein on the transport and metabolism of indinavir in Caco-2 cells expressing cytochrome P-450 3A4. *Journal of Pharmacology and Experimental Therapeutics*. 2000;292(1):310–8.

17. Chiu Y-Y, Higaki K, Neudeck BL, Barnett JL, Welage LS, Amidon GL. Human jejunal permeability of cyclosporin A: influence of surfactants on P-glycoprotein efflux in Caco-2 cells. *Pharmaceutical Research*. 2003;20:749–56.

18. Kasendra M, Luc R, Yin J, Manatakis DV, Kulkarni G, Lucchesi C, et al. Duodenum intestine-chip for preclinical drug assessment in a human relevant model. *Elife*. 2020;9:e50135.

19. Yoshida S, Honjo T, Iino K, Ishibe R, Leo S, Shimada T, et al. Generation of human-induced pluripotent stem cell-derived functional enterocyte-like cells for pharmacokinetic studies. *Stem Cell Reports*. 2021;16(2):295–308.

20. Kulkarni G, Apostolou A, Ewart L, Lucchesi C, Kasendra M. Combining human organoids and organ-on-a-chip technology to model intestinal region-specific functionality. *Journal of Visualized Experiments: Jove*. 2022;183:e63724.

21. Chow E, Liu S, Du Y, Pang K. The Caco-2 cell monolayer: usefulness and limitations AU-Sun, Huadong. *Expert Opinion on Drug Metabolism & Toxicology*. 2008;4:395–411.

22. Zhang H, Tolonen A, Rousu T, Hirvonen J, Finel M. Effects of cell differentiation and assay conditions on the UDP-glucuronosyltransferase activity in Caco-2 cells. *Drug Metabolism and Disposition*. 2011;39(3):456–64.

23. Ishiguro N, Kishimoto W, Volz A, Ludwig-Schwellinger E, Ebner T, Schaefer O. Impact of endogenous esterase activity on *in vitro* p-glycoprotein profiling of dabigatran etexilate in Caco-2 monolayers. *Drug Metabolism and Disposition*. 2014;42(2):250–6.

24. Davies M, Peramuhendige P, King L, Golding M, Kotian A, Penney M, et al. Evaluation of *in vitro* models for assessment of human intestinal metabolism in drug discovery. *Drug Metabolism and Disposition*. 2020;48(11):1169–82.

25. Jones CR, Hatley OJ, Ungell A-L, Hilgendorf C, Peters SA, Rostami-Hodjegan A. Gut wall metabolism. Application of pre-clinical models for the prediction of human drug absorption and first-pass elimination. *The AAPS Journal*. 2016;18:589–604.

26. Neradugomma N, Basit A, Takahashi R, Fan P, Smith B, Murray B, et al. A10-Characterization of differential tissue abundance of major non-cyp enzymes in human. *Drug Metabolism and Pharmacokinetics*. 2020;35(1):S21.

27. Sjöberg Å, Lutz M, Tannergren C, Wingolf C, Borde A, Ungell A-L. Comprehensive study on regional human intestinal permeability and prediction of fraction absorbed of drugs using the Ussing chamber technique. *European Journal of Pharmaceutical Sciences*. 2013;48(1–2):166–80.

28. Ozawa T, Takayama K, Okamoto R, Negoro R, Sakurai F, Tachibana M, et al. Generation of enterocyte-like cells from human induced pluripotent stem cells for drug absorption and metabolism studies in human small intestine. *Scientific Reports*. 2015;5(1):1–11.

29. Takenaka T, Harada N, Kuze J, Chiba M, Iwao T, Matsunaga T. Application of a human intestinal epithelial cell monolayer to the prediction of oral drug absorption in humans as a superior alternative to the Caco-2 cell monolayer. *Journal of Pharmaceutical Sciences*. 2016;105(2):915–24.

30. Yoshida S, Miwa H, Kawachi T, Kume S, Takahashi K. Generation of intestinal organoids derived from human pluripotent stem cells for drug testing. *Scientific Reports*. 2020;10(1):1–11.

31. Zietek T, Giesbertz P, Ewers M, Reichart F, Weinmüller M, Urbauer E, et al. Organoids to study intestinal nutrient transport, drug uptake and metabolism-update to the human model and expansion of applications. *Frontiers in Bioengineering and Biotechnology*. 2020;8:577656.

32. Cui Y, Claus S, Schnell D, Runge F, MacLean C. In-depth characterization of EpiIntestinal microtissue as a model for intestinal drug absorption and metabolism in human. *Pharmaceutics*. 2020;12(5):405.

33. Sjögren E, Westergren J, Grant I, Hanisch G, Lindfors L, Lennernäs H, et al. *In silico* predictions of gastrointestinal drug absorption in pharmaceutical product development: application of the mechanistic absorption model GI-Sim. *European Journal of Pharmaceutical Sciences*. 2013;49(4):679–98.

34. Reddy MB, Bolger MB, Fraczkiewicz G, Del Frari L, Luo L, Lukacova V, et al. PBPK modeling as a tool for predicting and understanding intestinal metabolism of uridine 5′-diphospho-glucuronosyltransferase substrates. *Pharmaceutics*. 2021;13(9):1325.

35. Yau E, Petersson C, Dolgos H, Peters SA. A comparative evaluation of models to predict human intestinal metabolism from nonclinical data. *Biopharmaceutics & Drug Disposition*. 2017;38(3):163–86.

36. Heikkinen AT, Baneyx G, Caruso A, Parrott N. Application of PBPK modeling to predict human intestinal metabolism of CYP3A substrates - an evaluation and case study using GastroPlus. *European Journal of Pharmaceutical Sciences*. 2012;47(2):375–86.

37. Gertz M, Houston JB, Galetin A. Physiologically based pharmacokinetic modeling of intestinal first-pass metabolism of CYP3A substrates with high intestinal extraction. *Drug Metabolism and Disposition*. 2011;39(9):1633–42.

38. S Darwich A, Neuhoff S, Jamei M, Rostami-Hodjegan A. Interplay of metabolism and transport in determining oral drug absorption and gut wall metabolism: a simulation assessment using the "Advanced Dissolution, Absorption, Metabolism (ADAM)" model. *Current Drug Metabolism*. 2010;11(9):716–29.

39. Chan TS, Scaringella Y-S, Raymond K, Taub ME. Evaluation of erythromycin as a tool to assess CYP3A contribution of low clearance compounds in a long-term hepatocyte culture. *Drug Metabolism and Disposition*. 2020;48(8):690–7.

40. Klammers F, Goetschi A, Ekiciler A, Walter I, Parrott N, Fowler S, et al. Estimation of fraction metabolized by cytochrome P450 enzymes using long-term cocultured human hepatocytes. *Drug Metabolism and Disposition*. 2022;50(5):566–75.

41. Chanteux H, Rosa M, Delatour C, Nicolaï J, Gillent E, Dell'Aiera S, et al. Application of aza-mulin to determine the contribution of CYP3A4/5 to drug metabolic clearance using human hepatocytes. *Drug Metabolism and Disposition*. 2020;48(9):778–87.

42. Peters SA, Jones CR, Ungell A-L, Hatley OJ. Predicting drug extraction in the human gut wall: assessing contributions from drug metabolizing enzymes and transporter proteins using preclinical models. *Clinical Pharmacokinetics*. 2016;55:673–96.

43. Yang J, Jamei M, Yeo KR, Tucker GT, Rostami-Hodjegan A. Prediction of intestinal first-pass drug metabolism. *Current Drug Metabolism*. 2007;8(7):676–84.

44. Hutzler JM, Ring BJ, Anderson SR. Low-turnover drug molecules: a current challenge for drug metabolism scientists. *Drug Metabolism and Disposition*. 2015;43(12):1917–28.

45. Fowler S, Brink A, Cleary Y, Günther A, Heinig K, Husser C, et al. Addressing today's Absorption, Distribution, Metabolism, and Excretion (ADME) challenges in the translation of *in vitro* ADME characteristics to humans: a case study of the SMN2 mRNA splicing modifier risdiplam. *Drug Metabolism and Disposition*. 2022;50(1):65–75.

46. Lee SY, Kim D, Lee SH, Sung JH. Microtechnology-based *in vitro* models: mimicking liver function and pathophysiology. *APL Bioengineering*. 2021;5(4):041505.

47. Zanelli U, Caradonna NP, Hallifax D, Turlizzi E, Houston JB. Comparison of cryopreserved HepaRG cells with cryopreserved human hepatocytes for prediction of clearance for 26 drugs. *Drug Metabolism and Disposition*. 2012;40(1):104–10.

48. Donato MT, Tolosa L, Gómez-Lechón MJ. Culture and functional characterization of human hepatoma HepG2 cells. *Protocols in* in vitro *Hepatocyte Research*. 2015:77–93.

49. Arzumanian VA, Kiseleva OI, Poverennaya EV. The curious case of the HepG2 cell line: 40 years of expertise. *International Journal of Molecular Sciences*. 2021;22(23):13135.

50. Kratochwil NA, Meille C, Fowler S, Klammers F, Ekiciler A, Molitor B, et al. Metabolic profiling of human long-term liver models and hepatic clearance predictions from *In vitro* data using nonlinear mixed-effects modeling. *The AAPS Journal*. 2017;19(2):534–50.

51. Rubiano A, Indapurkar A, Yokosawa R, Miedzik A, Rosenzweig B, Arefin A, et al. Characterizing the reproducibility in using a liver microphysiological system for assaying drug toxicity, metabolism and accumulation. *Clinical and Translational Science*. 2020;14(3):1049–61.

52. Docci L, Milani N, Ramp T, Romeo AA, Godoy P, Franyuti DO, et al. Exploration and application of a liver-on-a-chip device in combination with modelling and simulation for quantitative drug metabolism studies. *Lab on a Chip*. 2022;22(6):1187–205.

53. Umehara K, Cantrill C, Wittwer MB, Di Lenarda E, Klammers F, Ekiciler A, et al. Application of the Extended Clearance Classification System (ECCS) in drug discovery and development: selection of appropriate in vitro tools and clearance prediction. *Drug Metabolism and Disposition*. 2020;48(10):849–60.

54. Docci L, Klammers F, Ekiciler A, Molitor B, Umehara K, Walter I, et al. *In vitro* to *in vivo* extrapolation of metabolic clearance for UGT substrates using short-term suspension and long-term co-cultured human hepatocytes. *The AAPS Journal*. 2020;22(6):1–12.

55. Balimane PV, Sinko PJ. Effect of ionization on the variable uptake of valacyclovir via the human intestinal peptide transporter (hPepT1) in CHO cells. *Biopharmaceutics & Drug Disposition*. 2000;21(5):165–74.

56. MacDougall C, Guglielmo BJ. Pharmacokinetics of valaciclovir. *Journal of Antimicrobial Chemotherapy*. 2004;53(6):899–901.

57. Tsamandouras N, Chen WLK, Edington CD, Stokes CL, Griffith LG, Cirit M. Integrated gut and liver microphysiological systems for quantitative *in vitro* pharmacokinetic studies. *The AAPS Journal*. 2017;19(5):1499–512.

58. Milani N, Parrott N, Franyuti DO, Godoy P, Galetin A, Gertz M, et al. Application of a gut-liver-on-a-chip device and mechanistic modelling to the quantitative *in vitro* pharmacokinetic study of mycophenolate mofetil. *Lab on a Chip*. 2022;22(15):2853–68.

59. Lee DW, Ha SK, Choi I, Sung JH. 3D gut-liver chip with a PK model for prediction of first-pass metabolism. *Biomedical Microdevices*. 2017;19(4):1–13.

60. Maschmeyer I, Hasenberg T, Jaenicke A, Lindner M, Lorenz AK, Zech J, et al. Chip-based human liver-intestine and liver-skin co-cultures-A first step toward systemic repeated dose substance testing *in vitro*. *European Journal of Pharmaceutics and Biopharmaceutics*. 2015;95:77–87.

61. Choe A, Ha SK, Choi I, Choi N, Sung JH. Microfluidic Gut-liver chip for reproducing the first pass metabolism. *Biomedical Microdevices*. 2017;19(1):1–11.

62. Arakawa H, Sugiura S, Kawanishi T, Shin K, Toyoda H, Satoh T, et al. Kinetic analysis of sequential metabolism of triazolam and its extrapolation to humans using an entero-hepatic two-organ microphysiological system. *Lab on a Chip*. 2020;20(3):537–47.

63. Milani N, Parrott N, Galetin A, Fowler S, Gertz M. In silico modeling and simulation of organ-on-a-chip systems to support data analysis and a priori experimental design. *CPT: Pharmacometrics & Systems Pharmacology*. 2024;13(4):524–43. https://ascpt.onlinelibrary.wiley.com/doi/10.1002/psp4.13110.

64. Ho M-CD, Ring N, Amaral K, Doshi U, Li AP. Human enterocytes as an *in vitro* model for the evaluation of intestinal drug metabolism: characterization of drug-metabolizing enzyme activities of cryopreserved human enterocytes from twenty-four donors. *Drug Metabolism and Disposition*. 2017;45(6):686–91.

65. Tahara M, Inoue T, Miyakura Y, Horie H, Yasuda Y, Fujii H, et al. Cell diameter measurements obtained with a handheld cell counter could be used as a surrogate marker of G2/M arrest and apoptosis in colon cancer cell lines exposed to SN-38. *Biochemical and Biophysical Research Communications*. 2013;434(4):753–9.

66. Tan CW, Gardiner BS, Hirokawa Y, Layton MJ, Smith DW, Burgess AW. Wnt signalling pathway parameters for mammalian cells. *PLoS One*. 2012;7(2):e31882.

67. Fernández-Costa JM, Ortega MA, Rodríguez-Comas J, Lopez-Muñoz G, Yeste J, Mangas-Florencio L, et al. Training-on-a-chip: a multi-organ device to study the effect of muscle exercise on insulin secretion *in vitro*. *Advanced Materials Technologies*. 2022;8(7):2200873.

68. Schimek K, Frentzel S, Luettich K, Bovard D, Rütschle I, Boden L, et al. Human multi-organ chip co-culture of bronchial lung culture and liver spheroids for substance exposure studies. *Scientific Reports*. 2020;10(1):7865.

69. Bauer S, Wennberg Huldt C, Kanebratt KP, Durieux I, Gunne D, Andersson S, et al. Functional coupling of human pancreatic islets and liver spheroids on-a-chip: towards a novel human ex vivo type 2 diabetes model. *Scientific Reports*. 2017;7(1):14620.

70. Chen WL, Edington C, Suter E, Yu J, Velazquez JJ, Velazquez JG, et al. Integrated gut/liver microphysiological systems elucidates inflammatory inter-tissue crosstalk. *Biotechnology and Bioengineering*. 2017;114(11):2648–59.

71. Gribkoff VK, Kaczmarek LK. The need for new approaches in CNS drug discovery: why drugs have failed, and what can be done to improve outcomes. *Neuropharmacology*. 2017;120:11–9.

72. Danhof M, de Jongh J, De Lange EC, Della Pasqua O, Ploeger BA, Voskuyl RA. Mechanism-based pharmacokinetic-pharmacodynamic modeling: biophase distribution, receptor theory, and dynamical systems analysis. *Annual Review of Pharmacology and Toxicology*. 2007;47:357–400.

73. Liu X, Smith BJ, Chen C, Callegari E, Becker SL, Chen X, et al. Evaluation of cerebrospinal fluid concentration and plasma free concentration as a surrogate measurement for brain free concentration. *Drug Metabolism and Disposition*. 2006;34(9):1443–7.

74. Lin JH. CSF as a surrogate for assessing CNS exposure: an industrial perspective. *Current Drug Metabolism*. 2008;9(1):46–59.

75. de Lange EC. Utility of CSF in translational neuroscience. *Journal of Pharmacokinetics and Phar macodynamics*. 2013;40(3):315–26.

76. Shen DD, Artru AA, Adkison KK. Principles and applicability of CSF sampling for the assessment of CNS drug delivery and pharmacodynamics. *Advanced Drug Delivery Reviews*. 2004;56(12):1825–57.

77. Saleh MAA, Loo CF, Elassaiss-Schaap J, De Lange ECM. Lumbar cerebrospinal fluid-to-brain extracellular fluid surrogacy is context-specific: insights from LeiCNS-PK3.0 simulations. *Journal of Pharmacokinetics and Pharmacodynamics*. 2021;48(5):725–41.

78. de Lange EC, Danhof M, de Boer AG, Breimer DD. Critical factors of intracerebral microdialysis as a technique to determined the pharmacokinetics of drugs in rat brain. *Brain Research*. 1994;666(1):1–8.

79. Hammarlund-Udenaes M. The use of microdialysis in CNS drug delivery studies: pharmacokinetic perspectives and results with analgesics and antiepileptics. *Advanced Drug Delivery Reviews*. 2000;45(2–3):283–94.

80. Hammarlund-Udenaes M, Paalzow LK, de Lange EC. Drug equilibration across the blood-brain barrier-pharmacokinetic considerations based on the microdialysis method. *Pharmaceutical Research*. 1997;14:128–34.

81. Chang HY, Morrow K, Bonacquisti E, Zhang W, Shah DK. Antibody pharmacokinetics in rat brain determined using microdialysis. *MAbs*. 2018;10(6):843–53.

82. Chang HY, Wu S, Li Y, Zhang W, Burrell M, Webster CI, et al. Brain pharmacokinetics of anti-transferrin receptor antibody affinity variants in rats determined using microdialysis. *MAbs*. 2021;13(1):1874121.

83. Janson J, Andersson G, Bergquist L, Eriksson M, Folgering JHA. Impact of chemical modification of sulfamidase on distribution to brain interstitial fluid and to CSF after an intravenous administration in awake, freely-moving rats. *Molecular Genetics and Metabolism Reports*. 2020;22:100554.

84. Yamamoto Y, Danhof M, de Lange ECM. Microdialysis: the key to physiologically based model prediction of human CNS target site concentrations. *AAPS Journal*. 2017;19(4):891–909.

85. Westerhout J, Ploeger B, Smeets J, Danhof M, de Lange EC. Physiologically based pharmacokinetic modeling to investigate regional brain distribution kinetics in rats. *AAPS Journal*. 2012;14(3):543–53.

86. Westerhout J, Van den Berg D-J, Hartman R, Danhof M, de Lange EC. Prediction of methotrexate CNS distribution in different species-Influence of disease conditions. *European Journal of Pharmaceutical Sciences*. 2014;57:11–24.

87. Abbott NJ, Rönnbäck L, Hansson E. Astrocyte-endothelial interactions at the blood-brain barrier. *Nature Reviews Neuroscience*. 2006;7(1):41–53.

88. Stern L, Gautier R. II.-Les Rapports Entre Le Liquide Céphalo-Rachidien Et Les éléments Nerveux De L'axe Cerebrospinal. *Archives Internationales de Physiologie*. 1922;17(4):391–448.

89. Patabendige A, Skinner RA, Abbott NJ. Establishment of a simplified *in vitro* porcine blood-brain barrier model with high transendothelial electrical resistance. *Brain Research*. 2013;1521:1–15.

90. Patabendige A, Skinner RA, Morgan L, Abbott NJ. A detailed method for preparation of a functional and flexible blood-brain barrier model using porcine brain endothelial cells. *Brain Research*. 2013;1521:16–30.

91. Warren MS, Zerangue N, Woodford K, Roberts LM, Tate EH, Feng B, et al. Comparative gene expression profiles of ABC transporters in brain microvessel endothelial cells and brain in five species including human. *Pharmacological Research*. 2009;59(6):404–13.

92. Uchida Y, Ohtsuki S, Katsukura Y, Ikeda C, Suzuki T, Kamiie J, et al. Quantitative targeted absolute proteomics of human blood-brain barrier transporters and receptors. *Journal of Neurochemistry*. 2011;117(2):333–45.

93. Cucullo L, Couraud PO, Weksler B, Romero IA, Hossain M, Rapp E, et al. Immortalized human brain endothelial cells and flow-based vascular modeling: a marriage of convenience for rational neurovascular studies. *Journal of Cerebral Blood Flow and Metabolism: Official Journal of the International Society of Cerebral Blood Flow and Metabolism*. 2008;28(2):312–28.

94. Urich E, Lazic SE, Molnos J, Wells I, Freskgård PO. Transcriptional profiling of human brain endothelial cells reveals key properties crucial for predictive *in vitro* blood-brain barrier models. *PLoS One*. 2012;7(5):e38149.

95. Bouïs D, Hospers GA, Meijer C, Molema G, Mulder NH. Endothelium *in vitro*: a review of human vascular endothelial cell lines for blood vessel-related research. *Angiogenesis*. 2001;4(2):91–102.

96. Sabbagh MF, Nathans J. A genome-wide view of the de-differentiation of central nervous system endothelial cells in culture. *eLife*. 2020;9:e51276.

97. Prudhomme JG, Sherman IW, Land KM, Moses AV, Stenglein S, Nelson JA. Studies of Plasmodium falciparum cytoadherence using immortalized human brain capillary endothelial cells. *International Journal for Parasitology*. 1996;26(6):647–55.

98. Stins MF, Badger J, Sik Kim K. Bacterial invasion and transcytosis in transfected human brain microvascular endothelial cells. *Microbial Pathogenesis*. 2001;30(1):19–28.

99. Maeda T, Sano Y, Abe M, Shimizu F, Kashiwamura Y, Ohtsuki S, et al. Establishment and characterization of spinal cord microvascular endothelial cell lines. *Clinical and Experimental Neuroimmunology*. 2013;4(3):326–38.

100. Weksler BB, Subileau EA, Perrière N, Charneau P, Holloway K, Leveque M, et al. Blood-brain barrier-specific properties of a human adult brain endothelial cell line. *FASEB Journal: Official Publication of the Federation of American Societies for Experimental Biology*. 2005;19(13):1872–4.

101. Helms HC, Abbott NJ, Burek M, Cecchelli R, Couraud PO, Deli MA, et al. *In vitro* models of the blood-brain barrier: an overview of commonly used brain endothelial cell culture models and guidelines for their use. *Journal of Cerebral Blood Flow and Metabolism: Official Journal of the International Society of Cerebral Blood Flow and Metabolism*. 2016;36(5):862–90.

102. Rahman NA, Rasil ANa HM, Meyding-Lamade U, Craemer EM, Diah S, Tuah AA, et al. Immortalized endothelial cell lines for *in vitro* blood-brain barrier models: a systematic review. *Brain Research*. 2016;1642:532–45.

103. Ohtsuki S, Ikeda C, Uchida Y, Sakamoto Y, Miller F, Glacial F, et al. Quantitative targeted absolute proteomic analysis of transporters, receptors and junction proteins for validation of human cerebral microvascular endothelial cell line hCMEC/D3 as a human blood-brain barrier model. *Molecular Pharmaceutics*. 2013;10(1):289–96.

104. Weksler B, Romero IA, Couraud PO. The hCMEC/D3 cell line as a model of the human blood brain barrier. *Fluids and Barriers of the CNS*. 2013;10(1):16.

105. Eigenmann DE, Xue G, Kim KS, Moses AV, Hamburger M, Oufir M. Comparative study of four immortalized human brain capillary endothelial cell lines, hCMEC/D3, hBMEC, TY10, and BB19, and optimization of culture conditions, for an *in vitro* blood-brain barrier model for drug permeability studies. *Fluids and Barriers of the CNS*. 2013;10(1):33.

106. Kim BJ, Shusta EV, Doran KS. Past and current perspectives in modeling bacteria and blood-brain barrier interactions. *Frontiers in Microbiology*. 2019;10:1336.

107. Hollmann EK, Bailey AK, Potharazu AV, Neely MD, Bowman AB, Lippmann ES. Accelerated differentiation of human induced pluripotent stem cells to blood-brain barrier endothelial cells. *Fluids and Barriers of the CNS*. 2017;14(1):9.

108. Lippmann ES, Al-Ahmad A, Azarin SM, Palecek SP, Shusta EV. A retinoic acid-enhanced, multicellular human blood-brain barrier model derived from stem cell sources. *Scientific Reports*. 2014;4(1):4160.

109. Lippmann ES, Azarin SM, Kay JE, Nessler RA, Wilson HK, Al-Ahmad A, et al. Derivation of blood-brain barrier endothelial cells from human pluripotent stem cells. *Nature Biotechnology*. 2012;30(8):783–91.

110. Neal EH, Marinelli NA, Shi Y, McClatchey PM, Balotin KM, Gullett DR, et al. A simplified, fully defined differentiation scheme for producing blood-brain barrier endothelial cells from human iPSCs. *Stem cell Reports*. 2019;12(6):1380–8.

111. Lian X, Bao X, Al-Ahmad A, Liu J, Wu Y, Dong W, et al. Efficient differentiation of human pluripotent stem cells to endothelial progenitors via small-molecule activation of WNT signaling. *Stem Cell Reports*. 2014;3(5):804–16.

112. Patsch C, Challet-Meylan L, Thoma EC, Urich E, Heckel T, O'Sullivan JF, et al. Generation of vascular endothelial and smooth muscle cells from human pluripotent stem cells. *Nature Cell Biology*. 2015;17(8):994–1003.

113. Qian T, Maguire SE, Canfield SG, Bao X, Olson WR, Shusta EV, et al. Directed differentiation of human pluripotent stem cells to blood-brain barrier endothelial cells. *Science Advances*. 2017;3(11):e1701679.

114. Nishihara H, Gastfriend BD, Soldati S, Perriot S, Mathias A, Sano Y, et al. Advancing human induced pluripotent stem cell-derived blood-brain barrier models for studying immune cell interactions. *FASEB Journal: Official Publication of the Federation of American Societies for Experimental Biology*. 2020;34(12):16693–715.

115. Gastfriend BD, Nishihara H, Canfield SG, Foreman KL, Engelhardt B, Palecek SP, et al. Wnt signaling mediates acquisition of blood-brain barrier properties in naïve endothelium derived from human pluripotent stem cells. *eLife*. 2021;10:e70992.

116. Lu TM, Houghton S, Magdeldin T, Durán JGB, Minotti AP, Snead A, et al. Pluripotent stem cell-derived epithelium misidentified as brain microvascular endothelium requires ETS factors to acquire vascular fate. *Proceedings of the National Academy of Sciences of the United States of America*. 2021;118(8):e2016950118.

117. Gastfriend BD, Palecek SP, Shusta EV. Modeling the blood-brain barrier: beyond the endothelial cells. *Current Opinion in Biomedical Engineering*. 2018;5:6–12.

118. Schreiner TG, Creangă-Murariu I, Tamba BI, Lucanu N, Popescu BO. *In vitro* modeling of the blood-brain barrier for the study of physiological conditions and Alzheimer's disease. *Biomolecules*. 2022;12(8):1136.

119. Wevers NR, Kasi DG, Gray T, Wilschut KJ, Smith B, van Vught R, et al. A perfused human blood-brain barrier on-a-chip for high-throughput assessment of barrier function and antibody transport. *Fluids and Barriers of the CNS*. 2018;15(1):1–12.

120. Furihata T, Ito R, Kamiichi A, Saito K, Chiba K. Establishment and characterization of a new conditionally immortalized human astrocyte cell line. *Journal of Neurochemistry*. 2016;136(1):92–105.

121. Umehara K, Sun Y, Hiura S, Hamada K, Itoh M, Kitamura K, et al. A new conditionally immortalized human fetal brain pericyte cell line: establishment and functional characterization as a promising tool for human brain pericyte studies. *Molecular Neurobiology*. 2018;55(7):5993–6006.

122. Kusuma S, Shen YI, Hanjaya-Putra D, Mali P, Cheng L, Gerecht S. Self-organized vascular networks from human pluripotent stem cells in a synthetic matrix. *Proceedings of the National Academy of Sciences of the United States of America*. 2013;110(31):12601–6.

123. Faal T, Phan DTT, Davtyan H, Scarfone VM, Varady E, Blurton-Jones M, et al. Induction of mesoderm and neural crest-derived pericytes from human pluripotent stem cells to study blood-brain barrier interactions. *Stem Cell Reports*. 2019;12(3):451–60.

124. Jamieson JJ, Linville RM, Ding YY, Gerecht S, Searson PC. Role of iPSC-derived pericytes on barrier function of iPSC-derived brain microvascular endothelial cells in 2D and 3D. *Fluids and Barriers of the CNS*. 2019;16(1):15.

125. Stebbins MJ, Gastfriend BD, Canfield SG, Lee M-S, Richards D, Faubion MG, et al. Human pluripotent stem cell-derived brain pericyte-like cells induce blood-brain barrier properties. *Science Advances*. 2019;5(3):eaau7375.

126. Shaltouki A, Peng J, Liu Q, Rao MS, Zeng X. Efficient generation of astrocytes from human pluripotent stem cells in defined conditions. *Stem Cells (Dayton, Ohio)*. 2013;31(5):941–52.

127. Hedegaard A, Monzón-Sandoval J, Newey SE, Whiteley ES, Webber C, Akerman CJ. Promaturational effects of human iPSC-derived cortical astrocytes upon iPSC-derived cortical neurons. *Stem Cell Reports*. 2020;15(1):38–51.

128. Leventoux N, Morimoto S, Imaizumi K, Sato Y, Takahashi S, Mashima K, et al. Human astrocytes model derived from induced pluripotent stem cells. *Cells*. 2020;9(12):2680.

129. Voulgaris D, Nikolakopoulou P, Herland A. Generation of human iPSC-derived astrocytes with a mature star-shaped phenotype for CNS modeling. *Stem Cell Reviews and Reports*. 2022;18(7):2494–512.

130. Dezonne RS, Sartore RC, Nascimento JM, Saia-Cereda VM, Romão LF, Alves-Leon SV, et al. Derivation of functional human astrocytes from cerebral organoids. *Scientific Reports*. 2017;7(1):45091.

131. Sloan SA, Darmanis S, Huber N, Khan TA, Birey F, Caneda C, et al. Human astrocyte maturation captured in 3D cerebral cortical spheroids derived from pluripotent stem cells. *Neuron*. 2017;95(4):779–90.e6.

132. Leng K, Rose IVL, Kim H, Xia W, Romero-Fernandez W, Rooney B, et al. CRISPRi screens in human iPSC-derived astrocytes elucidate regulators of distinct inflammatory reactive states. *Nature Neuroscience*. 2022;25(11):1528–42.

133. Borges N, Shi F, Azevedo I, Audus KL. Changes in brain microvessel endothelial cell monolayer permeability induced by adrenergic drugs. *European Journal of Pharmacology*. 1994;269(2):243–8.

134. Hartz AM, Miller DS, Bauer B. Restoring blood-brain barrier P-glycoprotein reduces brain amyloid-beta in a mouse model of Alzheimer's disease. *Molecular Pharmacology*. 2010;77(5):715–23.

135. Shayan G, Choi YS, Shusta EV, Shuler ML, Lee KH. Murine *in vitro* model of the blood-brain barrier for evaluating drug transport. *European Journal of Pharmaceutical Sciences*. 2011;42(1–2):148–55.

136. Silwedel C, Forster C. Differential susceptibility of cerebral and cerebellar murine brain microvascular endothelial cells to loss of barrier properties in response to inflammatory stimuli. *Journal of Neuroimmunology*. 2006;179(1–2):37–45.

137. Dehouck MP, Meresse S, Delorme P, Fruchart JC, Cecchelli R. An easier, reproducible, and mass-production method to study the blood-brain barrier *in vitro*. *Journal of Neurochemistry*. 1990;54(5):1798–801.

138. Pardridge WM, Triguero D, Yang J, Cancilla PA. Comparison of *in vitro* and *in vivo* models of drug transcytosis through the blood-brain barrier. *Journal of Pharmacology and Experimental Therapeutics*. 1990;253(2):884–91.

139. Abbott NJ, Hughes CC, Revest PA, Greenwood J. Development and characterisation of a rat brain capillary endothelial culture: towards an *in vitro* blood-brain barrier. *Journal of Cell Science*. 1992;103 (Pt 1):23–37.

140. Stone NL, England TJ, O'Sullivan SE. A novel transwell blood brain barrier model using primary human cells. *Frontiers in Cellular Neuroscience*. 2019;13:230.

141. Passeleu-Le Bourdonnec C, Carrupt PA, Scherrmann JM, Martel S. Methodologies to assess drug permeation through the blood-brain barrier for pharmaceutical research. *Pharmaceutical Research*. 2013;30(11):2729–56.

142. Gaillard PJ, Voorwinden LH, Nielsen JL, Ivanov A, Atsumi R, Engman H, et al. Establishment and functional characterization of an *in vitro* model of the blood-brain barrier, comprising a co-culture of brain capillary endothelial cells and astrocytes. *European Journal of Pharmaceutical Sciences*. 2001;12(3):215–22.

143. Hartmann C, Zozulya A, Wegener J, Galla HJ. The impact of glia-derived extracellular matrices on the barrier function of cerebral endothelial cells: an *in vitro* study. *Experimental Cell Research*. 2007;313(7):1318–25.

144. Abbott NJ, Dolman DE, Drndarski S, Fredriksson SM. An improved *in vitro* blood-brain barrier model: rat brain endothelial cells co-cultured with astrocytes. *Methods in Molecular Biology*. 2012;814:415–30.

145. Hind WH, Tufarelli C, Neophytou M, Anderson SI, England TJ, O'Sullivan SE. Endocannabinoids modulate human blood-brain barrier permeability *in vitro*. *British Journal of Pharmacology*. 2015;172(12):3015–27.

146. Wang Y, Wang N, Cai B, Wang GY, Li J, Piao XX. *In vitro* model of the blood-brain barrier established by co-culture of primary cerebral microvascular endothelial and astrocyte cells. *Neural Regeneration Research*. 2015;10(12):2011–7.

147. Appelt-Menzel A, Cubukova A, Gunther K, Edenhofer F, Piontek J, Krause G, et al. Establishment of a human blood-brain barrier co-culture model mimicking the neurovascular unit using induced pluri- and multipotent stem cells. *Stem Cell Reports*. 2017;8(4):894–906.

148. Sivandzade F, Cucullo L. In-vitro blood-brain barrier modeling: a review of modern and fast-advancing technologies. *Journal of Cerebral Blood Flow & Metabolism*. 2018;38(10):1667–81.

149. Booth R, Kim H. Characterization of a microfluidic *in vitro* model of the blood-brain barrier (muBBB). *Lab on a Chip*. 2012;12(10):1784–92.

150. Griep LM, Wolbers F, de Wagenaar B, ter Braak PM, Weksler BB, Romero IA, et al. BBB on chip: microfluidic platform to mechanically and biochemically modulate blood-brain barrier function. *Biomedical Microdevices*. 2013;15(1):145–50.

151. Wang YI, Abaci HE, Shuler ML. Microfluidic blood-brain barrier model provides *in vivo*-like barrier properties for drug permeability screening. *Biotechnology and Bioengineering*. 2017;114(1):184–94.

152. Brown JA, Pensabene V, Markov DA, Allwardt V, Neely MD, Shi M, et al. Recreating blood-brain barrier physiology and structure on chip: a novel neurovascular microfluidic bioreactor. *Biomicrofluidics*. 2015;9(5):054124.

153. Park TE, Mustafaoglu N, Herland A, Hasselkus R, Mannix R, FitzGerald EA, et al. Hypoxia-enhanced Blood-Brain Barrier Chip recapitulates human barrier function and shuttling of drugs and antibodies. *Nature Communications*. 2019;10(1):2621.

154. Vatine GD, Barrile R, Workman MJ, Sances S, Barriga BK, Rahnama M, et al. Human iPSC-derived blood-brain barrier chips enable disease modeling and personalized medicine applications. *Cell Stem Cell*. 2019;24(6):995–1005 e6.

155. Elbakary B, Badhan RK. A dynamic perfusion based blood-brain barrier model for cytotoxicity testing and drug permeation. *Scientific Reports*. 2020;10(1):3788.

156. Wang JD, Khafagy el S, Khanafer K, Takayama S, ElSayed ME. Organization of endothelial cells, pericytes, and astrocytes into a 3D microfluidic *in vitro* model of the blood-brain barrier. *Molecular Pharmaceutics*. 2016;13(3):895–906.

157. Adriani G, Ma D, Pavesi A, Kamm RD, Goh EL. A 3D neurovascular microfluidic model consisting of neurons, astrocytes and cerebral endothelial cells as a blood-brain barrier. *Lab on a Chip*. 2017;17(3):448–59.

158. Linville RM, DeStefano JG, Sklar MB, Xu Z, Farrell AM, Bogorad MI, et al. Human iPSC-derived blood-brain barrier microvessels: validation of barrier function and endothelial cell behavior. *Biomaterials*. 2019;190:24–37.

159. Herland A, van der Meer AD, FitzGerald EA, Park T-E, Sleeboom JJ, Ingber DE. Distinct contributions of astrocytes and pericytes to neuroinflammation identified in a 3D human blood-brain barrier on a chip. *PLoS One*. 2016;11(3):e0150360.

160. Shin Y, Choi SH, Kim E, Bylykbashi E, Kim JA, Chung S, et al. Blood-brain barrier dysfunction in a 3D *in vitro* model of Alzheimer's disease. *Advanced Science (Weinheim)*. 2019;6(20):1900962.

161. Chrobak KM, Potter DR, Tien J. Formation of perfused, functional microvascular tubes *in vitro*. *Microvascular Research*. 2006;71(3):185–96.

162. van Der Helm MW, Van Der Meer AD, Eijkel JC, van den Berg A, Segerink LI. Microfluidic organ-on-chip technology for blood-brain barrier research. *Tissue Barriers*. 2016;4(1):e1142493.

163. Kim JA, Kim HN, Im SK, Chung S, Kang JY, Choi N. Collagen-based brain microvasculature model *in vitro* using three-dimensional printed template. *Biomicrofluidics*. 2015;9(2):024115.

164. Urich E, Patsch C, Aigner S, Graf M, Iacone R, Freskgard PO. Multicellular self-assembled spheroidal model of the blood brain barrier. *Scientific Reports*. 2013;3:1500.

165. Cho CF, Wolfe JM, Fadzen CM, Calligaris D, Hornburg K, Chiocca EA, et al. Blood-brain-barrier spheroids as an *in vitro* screening platform for brain-penetrating agents. *Nature Communications*. 2017;8:15623.

166. Bergmann S, Lawler SE, Qu Y, Fadzen CM, Wolfe JM, Regan MS, et al. Blood-brain-barrier organoids for investigating the permeability of CNS therapeutics. *Nature Protocols*. 2018;13(12):2827–43.

167. Nzou G, Wicks R, Wicks E, Seale S, Sane C, Chen A, et al. Human cortex spheroid with a functional blood brain barrier for high-throughput neurotoxicity screening and disease modeling. *Scientific Reports*. 2018;8(1):1–10.

168. Nzou G, Wicks RT, VanOstrand NR, Mekky GA, Seale SA, El-Taibany A, et al. Multicellular 3D neurovascular unit model for assessing hypoxia and neuroinflammation induced blood-brain barrier dysfunction. *Scientific Reports*. 2020;10(1):9766.

169. Sokolova V, Mekky G, van der Meer SB, Seeds MC, Atala AJ, Epple M. Transport of ultrasmall gold nanoparticles (2 nm) across the blood-brain barrier in a six-cell brain spheroid model. *Scientific Reports*. 2020;10(1):18033.

170. Simonneau C, Duschmalé M, Gavrilov A, Brandenberg N, Hoehnel S, Ceroni C, et al. Investigating receptor-mediated antibody transcytosis using blood-brain barrier organoid arrays. *Fluids and Barriers of the CNS*. 2021;18(1):1–17.

171. Campisi M, Shin Y, Osaki T, Hajal C, Chiono V, Kamm RD. 3D self-organized microvascular model of the human blood-brain barrier with endothelial cells, pericytes and astrocytes. *Biomaterials*. 2018;180:117–29.

172. Hajal C, Offeddu GS, Shin Y, Zhang S, Morozova O, Hickman D, et al. Engineered human blood-brain barrier microfluidic model for vascular permeability analyses. *Nature Protocols*. 2022;17(1):95–128.

173. Xu H, Li Z, Yu Y, Sizdahkhani S, Ho WS, Yin F, et al. A dynamic *in vivo*-like organotypic blood-brain barrier model to probe metastatic brain tumors. *Scientific Reports*. 2016;6:36670.

174. Bang S, Lee SR, Ko J, Son K, Tahk D, Ahn J, et al. A low permeability microfluidic blood-brain barrier platform with direct contact between perfusable vascular network and astrocytes. *Scientific Reports*. 2017;7(1):8083.

175. Lee S, Chung M, Lee SR, Jeon NL. 3D brain angiogenesis model to reconstitute functional human blood-brain barrier *in vitro*. *Biotechnology and Bioengineering*. 2020;117(3):748–62.

176. Offeddu GS, Haase K, Gillrie MR, Li R, Morozova O, Hickman D, et al. An on-chip model of protein paracellular and transcellular permeability in the microcirculation. *Biomaterials*. 2019;212:115–25.

177. de Lange EC. The mastermind approach to CNS drug therapy: translational prediction of human brain distribution, target site kinetics, and therapeutic effects. *Fluids and Barriers of the CNS*. 2013;10:1–16.

178. Hansen D, Scott D, Otis K, Lunte S. Comparison of *in vitro* BBMEC permeability and *in vivo* CNS uptake by microdialysis sampling. *Journal of Pharmaceutical and Biomedical Analysis*. 2002;27(6):945–58.

179. Bourasset F, Scherrmann JM. Carrier-mediated processes at several rat brain interfaces determine the neuropharmacokinetics of morphine and morphine-6-beta-D-glucuronide. *Life Sciences*. 2006;78(20):2302–14.

180. Kielbasa W, Stratford RE, Jr. Exploratory translational modeling approach in drug development to predict human brain pharmacokinetics and pharmacologically relevant clinical doses. *Drug Metabolism and Disposition*. 2012;40(5):877–83.

181. Trapa PE, Belova E, Liras JL, Scott DO, Steyn SJ. Insights from an integrated physiologically based pharmacokinetic model for brain penetration. *Journal of Pharmaceutical Sciences*. 2016;105(2):965–71.

182. Westerhout J, Smeets J, Danhof M, de Lange EC. The impact of P-gp functionality on non-steady state relationships between CSF and brain extracellular fluid. *Journal of Pharmacokinetics and Pharmacodynamics*. 2013;40(3):327–42.

183. Yamamoto Y, Valitalo PA, van den Berg DJ, Hartman R, van den Brink W, Wong YC, et al. A generic multi-compartmental CNS distribution model structure for 9 drugs allows prediction of human brain target site concentrations. *Pharmaceutical Research*. 2017;34(2):333–51.

184. Ball K, Bouzom F, Scherrmann JM, Walther B, Decleves X. Physiologically based pharmacokinetic modelling of drug penetration across the blood-brain barrier--towards a mechanistic IVIVE based approach. *AAPS Journal*. 2013;15(4):913–32.

185. Gaohua L, Neuhoff S, Johnson TN, Rostami-Hodjegan A, Jamei M. Development of a permeability-limited model of the human brain and cerebrospinal fluid (CSF) to integrate known physiological and biological knowledge: estimating time varying CSF drug concentrations and their variability using *in vitro* data. *Drug Metabolism and Pharmacokinetics*. 2016;31(3):224–33.

186. Yamamoto Y, Valitalo PA, Huntjens DR, Proost JH, Vermeulen A, Krauwinkel W, et al. Predicting drug concentration-time profiles in multiple CNS compartments using a comprehensive physiologically-based pharmacokinetic model. *CPT: Pharmacometrics & Systems Pharmacology*. 2017;6(11):765–77.

187. Yamamoto Y, Valitalo PA, Wong YC, Huntjens DR, Proost JH, Vermeulen A, et al. Prediction of human CNS pharmacokinetics using a physiologically-based pharmacokinetic modeling approach. *European Journal of Pharmaceutical Sciences*. 2018;112:168–79.

188. Saleh MAA, Bloemberg JS, Elassaiss-Schaap J, de Lange ECM. Drug distribution in brain and cerebrospinal fluids in relation to IC(50) values in aging and Alzheimer's disease, using the physiologically based LeiCNS-PK3.0 model. *Pharmaceutical Research*. 2022;39(7):1303–19.

189. Saleh MAA, Hirasawa M, Sun M, Gulave B, Elassaiss-Schaap J, de Lange ECM. The PBPK LeiCNS-PK3.0 framework predicts Nirmatrelvir (but not Remdesivir or Molnupiravir) to achieve effective concentrations against SARS-CoV-2 in human brain cells. *European Journal of Pharmaceutical Sciences*. 2023;181:106345.

190. Aday S, Cecchelli R, Hallier-Vanuxeem D, Dehouck MP, Ferreira L. Stem cell-based human blood-brain barrier models for drug discovery and delivery. *Trends in Biotechnology.* 2016;34(5):382–93.

191. Gustafsson S, Lindstrom V, Ingelsson M, Hammarlund-Udenaes M, Syvanen S. Intact blood-brain barrier transport of small molecular drugs in animal models of amyloid beta and alpha-synuclein pathology. *Neuropharmacology.* 2018;128:482–91.

192. Ravenstijn PG, Drenth HJ, O'Neill MJ, Danhof M, de Lange EC. Evaluation of blood-brain barrier transport and CNS drug metabolism in diseased and control brain after intravenous L-DOPA in a unilateral rat model of Parkinson's disease. *Fluids Barriers CNS.* 2012;9:4.

193. Ederoth P, Tunblad K, Bouw R, Lundberg CJ, Ungerstedt U, Nordstrom CH, et al. Blood-brain barrier transport of morphine in patients with severe brain trauma. *British Journal of Clinical Pharmacology.* 2004;57(4):427–35.

194. Tunblad K, Ederoth P, Gardenfors A, Hammarlund-Udenaes M, Nordstrom CH. Altered brain exposure of morphine in experimental meningitis studied with microdialysis. *Acta Anaesthesiologica Scandinavica.* 2004;48(3):294–301.

195. Gynther M, Puris E, Peltokangas S, Auriola S, Kanninen KM, Koistinaho J, et al. Alzheimer's disease phenotype or inflammatory insult does not alter function of L-type amino acid transporter 1 in mouse blood-brain barrier and primary astrocytes. *Pharmaceutical Research.* 2018;36(1):17.

196. De Lange ECM, Vd Berg DJ, Bellanti F, Voskuyl RA, Syvanen S. P-glycoprotein protein expression versus functionality at the blood-brain barrier using immunohistochemistry, microdialysis and mathematical modeling. *European Journal of Pharmaceutical Sciences.* 2018;124:61–70.

197. Resnick SM, Pham DL, Kraut MA, Zonderman AB, Davatzikos C. Longitudinal magnetic resonance imaging studies of older adults: a shrinking brain. *Journal of Neuroscience.* 2003;23(8):3295–301.

198. Sigurdsson S, Aspelund T, Forsberg L, Fredriksson J, Kjartansson O, Oskarsdottir B, et al. Brain tissue volumes in the general population of the elderly: the AGES-Reykjavik study. *Neuroimage.* 2012;59(4):3862–70.

199. May C, Kaye J, Atack JR, Schapiro M, Friedland R, Rapoport S. Cerebrospinal fluid production is reduced in healthy aging. *Neurology.* 1990;40(3 Part 1):500.

200. Oner Z, Sagsmall i UKA, Kose E, Oner S, Kavaklsmall i UA, Cay M, et al. Quantitative evaluation of normal aqueductal cerebrospinal fluid flow using phase-contrast cine MRI according to age and sex. *Anatomical Record (Hoboken).* 2017;300(3):549–55.

201. Nagra G, Johnston MG. Impact of ageing on lymphatic cerebrospinal fluid absorption in the rat. *Neuropathology and Applied Neurobiology.* 2007;33(6):684–91.

202. Kim J, Lee KT, Lee JS, Shin J, Cui B, Yang K, et al. Fungal brain infection modelled in a human-neurovascular-unit-on-a-chip with a functional blood-brain barrier. *Nature Biomedical Engineering.* 2021;5(8):830–46.

203. Lyu Z, Park J, Kim KM, Jin HJ, Wu H, Rajadas J, et al. A neurovascular-unit-on-a-chip for the evaluation of the restorative potential of stem cell therapies for ischaemic stroke. *Nature Biomedical Engineering.* 2021;5(8):847–63.

204. Seo S, Nah SY, Lee K, Choi N, Kim HN. Triculture model of *in vitro* BBB and its application to study BBB-associated chemosensitivity and drug delivery in glioblastoma. *Advanced Functional Materials*. 2021;32(10):2106860.

205. Ito R, Morio H, Baba T, Sakaguchi Y, Wakayama N, Isogai R, et al. *In vitro-In vivo* correlation of blood-brain barrier permeability of drugs: a feasibility study towards development of prediction methods for brain drug concentration in humans. *Pharmaceutical Research*. 2022;39(7):1575–86.

206. Ferl GZ, Theil FP, Wong H. Physiologically based pharmacokinetic models of small molecules and therapeutic antibodies: a mini-review on fundamental concepts and applications. *Biopharmaceutics & Drug Disposition*. 2016;37(2):75–92.

207. Wong H, Chow TW. Physiologically based pharmacokinetic modeling of therapeutic proteins. *Journal of Pharmaceutical Sciences*. 2017;106(9):2270–5.

208. Shah DK, Betts AM. Towards a platform PBPK model to characterize the plasma and tissue disposition of monoclonal antibodies in preclinical species and human. *Journal of Pharmacokinetics and Pharmacodynamics*. 2012;39(1):67–86.

209. Glassman PM, Balthasar JP. Physiologically-based modeling to predict the clinical behavior of monoclonal antibodies directed against lymphocyte antigens. *MAbs*. 2017;9(2):297–306.

210. Chang HY, Wu S, Meno-Tetang G, Shah DK. A translational platform PBPK model for antibody disposition in the brain. *Journal of Pharmacokinetics and Pharmacodynamics*. 2019;46(4):319–38.

211. Bloomingdale P, Bakshi S, Maass C, van Maanen E, Pichardo-Almarza C, Yadav DB, et al. Minimal brain PBPK model to support the preclinical and clinical development of antibody therapeutics for CNS diseases. *Journal of Pharmacokinetics and Pharmacodynamics*. 2021;48(6):861–71.

212. Van De Vyver AJ, Walz AC, Heins MS, Abdolzade-Bavil A, Kraft TE, Waldhauer I, et al. Investigating brain uptake of a non-targeting monoclonal antibody after intravenous and intracerebroventricular administration. *Frontiers in Pharmacology*. 2022;13:958543.

213. Wu S, Le Prieult F, Phipps CJ, Mezler M, Shah DK. PBPK model for antibody disposition in mouse brain: validation using large-pore microdialysis data. *Journal of Pharmacokinetics and Pharmacodynamics*. 2022;49(6):579–92.

214. Pardridge WM. Delivery of biologics across the blood-brain barrier with molecular Trojan horse technology. *BioDrugs*. 2017;31(6):503–19.

215. Yu YJ, Watts RJ. Developing therapeutic antibodies for neurodegenerative disease. *Neurotherapeutics*. 2013;10(3):459–72.

216. Haqqani AS, Delaney CE, Brunette E, Baumann E, Farrington GK, Sisk W, et al. Endosomal trafficking regulates receptor-mediated transcytosis of antibodies across the blood brain barrier. *Journal of Cerebral Blood Flow & Metabolism*. 2018;38(4):727–40.

217. Pizzo ME, Wolak DJ, Kumar NN, Brunette E, Brunnquell CL, Hannocks MJ, et al. Intrathecal antibody distribution in the rat brain: surface diffusion, perivascular transport and osmotic enhancement of delivery. *Journal of Physiology*. 2018;596(3):445–75.

218. Sato S, Liu S, Goto A, Yoneyama T, Okita K, Yamamoto S, et al. Advanced translational PBPK model for transferrin receptor-mediated drug delivery to the brain. *Journal of Controlled Release.* 2023;357:379–93.

219. Pike A, Williamson B, Harlfinger S, Martin S, McGinnity DF. Optimising proteolysis-targeting chimeras (PROTACs) for oral drug delivery: a drug metabolism and pharmacokinetics perspective. *Drug Discovery Today.* 2020;25(10):1793–800.

220. Cantrill C, Chaturvedi P, Rynn C, Schaffland JP, Walter I, Wittwer MB. Fundamental aspects of DMPK optimization of targeted protein degraders. *Drug Discovery Today.* 2020;25(6):969–82.

221. Molina DK, DiMaio VJ. Normal organ weights in men: part II-the brain, lungs, liver, spleen, and kidneys. *American Journal of Forensic Medicine and Pathology.* 2012;33(4):368–72.

Index

Note: **Bold** page numbers refer to tables and *italic* page numbers refer to figures.